HANDBOOK OF PSYCHIATRY IN PALLIATIVE MEDICINE

HANDBOOK OF

PSYCHIATRY IN PALLIATIVE MEDICINE

EDITED BY

Harvey Max Chochinov, M.D., PH.D.

William Breitbart, M.D.

OXFORD
UNIVERSITY PRESS

OXFORD

UNIVERSITY PRESS

Oxford   New York
Athens   Auckland   Bangkok   Bogotá   Buenos Aires   Calcutta
Cape Town   Chennai   Dar es Salaam   Delhi   Florence   Hong Kong   Istanbul
Karachi   Kuala Lumpur   Madrid   Melbourne   Mexico City   Mumbai
Nairobi   Paris   São Paulo   Singapore   Taipei   Tokyo   Toronto   Warsaw

and associated companies in
Berlin   Ibadan

Library of Congress Cataloging-in-Publication Data
Handbook of psychiatry in palliative medicine /
edited by Harvey M. Chochinov, William Breitbart.
p.   cm.
Includes bibliographical references and index.
ISBN 0-19-509299-6
1. Palliative treatment—Psychological aspects.   2. Terminal care—Psychological aspects.
3. Critically ill—Medical care—Psychological aspects.   I. Chochinov, Harvey M.   II.
Breitbart, William, 1951—   .
[DNLM: 1. Palliative Care.   2. Terminally Ill.   3. Neoplasms—Psychology.
4. Psychotherapy.   5. Family—psychology.   6. Ethics.   WB 310 P9735 2000]
R726.8.P778   2000
362.1'75—dc21   99-011188

9 8 7 6 5 4 3 2 1

Printed in the United States of America
on acid-free paper

For my parents, Dave and Shirley Chochinov; my dear wife, Michelle; and our beloved daughters, Lauren and Rachel. In memory of my grandparents, Max and Pessa Chochinov and Joseph and Florence Wolodarsky; my Aunt Marilyn Levitt, and my brother-in-law, Shep Nerman.

For my wife, Rachel Breitbart, and my son, Samuel Benjamin Breitbart.

Who can find a good woman?
    She is precious beyond all things.
Her husband's heart trusts her completely
    She is his best reward

Who can hope for a good son?
    He too is precious beyond all things.
His parents love him completely
    He is their blessing for eternity.

Adapted from Proverbs 31:10–11

Foreword

Neil MacDonald, C.M., M.D., FRCP(C), FRCP(Edin)
Director, Cancer Ethics Program
Center for Bioethics
Clinical Research Institute of Montreal
Professor, Oncology, McGill University

When confronted by patients with incurable cancer, traditional oncology research and practice prioritized efforts to reduce tumor size in anticipation that these approaches would prolong life. Relatively less attention was devoted to symptoms induced by the biological activity of the tumor or to the neuropsychiatric manifestations of cancer. Tumor mass, *primus inter pares*, was regarded as "the enemy," while the impact of cancer on human suffering and the effects of unbridled suffering on patient quality of life and survival were assigned second-echelon status.

For some years, Dr. Jimmie Holland and her associates at Memorial Sloan-Kettering Cancer Center have endeavored to bridge these "two solitudes" and to teach us to regard cancer control as a three-dimensional exercise embracing biological and psychosocial issues in a seamless fashion. A continuing line of bright, innovative clinician-scientists has emerged from Dr. Holland's program. Two of these protégés, Dr. Harvey Chochinov and Dr. William Breitbart, have recruited an excellent team of contributors to provide us with a seminal account of the role of psychiatry in the care of palliative-care patients. The title *Handbook of Psychiatry in Palliative Medicine* is not fully illustrative of the book's contents.

The editors have wisely complemented traditional psychiatric topics with a broad analysis of critical social and ethical issues that come to the fore at the end of life. Examples include a discussion by Nathan Cherny on the nature of suffering in the dying cancer patient, a chapter on spiritual issues, and a number of chapters that consider ethical topics.

My perspective on palliative care is that of the medical oncologist. The editors and authors wisely recognize the benefits of palliative care for all patients with life-threatening illnesses. This is not a textbook on "palliative care in cancer." Rather, the value of applying the principles of palliative care to the care of AIDS patients, children (commonly dying from illnesses other than cancer), and other disorders is clearly emphasized.

Handbook of Psychiatry in Palliative Medicine should be read by palliative-care health professionals. Because of the breadth of its approach to the problems of dying patients, this book will also grace the libraries of a wider range of thoughtful individuals who are concerned about modern approaches and attitudes toward end of life care. Recently, deficiencies in our care of patients with life-threatening illnesses have been clearly brought to our attention. (See M.J. Field and C.K.

Cassel (eds), *Approaching Death: Improving Care at the End of Life* [Washington, DC: National Academy Press: 1997].) The communities we serve expect us to change the mosaic of educational programmes, care policies, and financial regulations that have often combined to create a pattern of neglect.

Drs. Chochinov, Breitbart, and their collaborators present us with a panoramic view that reaches beyond the title of the textbook and will inform the reflections and the work of all who labor to redress the factors that limit fair patient access to superb palliative care. I offer my congratulations on a job well done, and my encouragement to others to profit from this initiative.

Foreword

Jimmie Holland, M.D.
Chair, Department of Psychiatry
and Behavioral Sciences
Memorial Sloan-Kettering Cancer Center
New York, New York

The emerging interest in the care of patients with advanced and terminal illness has been a gratifying global change in health care. As research interest has flourished in this area, studies have increasingly shown the centrality of psychiatric and psychosocial issues in the delivery of optimal palliative care. It is a particular pleasure for me to see this book being published, since both authors were trained in our program and I have had the opportunity to see their careers develop and to see them become important contributors to the research base in this area of palliative care. They have, through the book, brought together the best thinking of the best people in this new field, providing a reference text from which those new to the field can readily apprise themselves of the basic principles of the psychiatric dimensions of palliative medicine. Beginning with the psychiatric complications, which are so common and which cause so much of the suffering in terminal illness, the chapters put the issues of anxiety, depression, and delirium and their management in the proper clinical perspective. Moving on to symptom management, psychotherapeutic interventions, issues particular to children and families, and the ethical and spiritual domains, both the topics and the choice of outstanding authors ensure that the reader is provided with the latest synthesis of the available information in that particular area.

The editors are to be commended for integrating, for the first time, the available clinical and research information on psychiatric complications of palliative medicine and placing them in one book. This volume should rapidly join the general textbooks of palliative medicine as a reference text from which one can access both theoretical and clinical information. This book makes me feel more secure that the psychiatric and psychosocial domains of palliative care will receive the attention that they deserve to ensure that patients receive optimal care in these domains, which are so central to their well-being.

Preface

We offer this new textbook as our contribution to modern palliative care and the development of a new area of palliative medicine one might term Psychiatric Palliative Care. We were obviously inspired by two recent textbooks published by Oxford University Press that we were both privileged to contribute to: *The Oxford Textbook of Palliative Medicine*, edited by Derek Doyle, Geoffrey W. C. Hanks, and Neil Mac-Donald; and *Psycho-oncology*, edited by Jimmie C. Holland. This new textbook represents, in some ways, the result of a fusion or marriage of these two texts. The "offspring" has features reminiscent of both intellectual parents, but has unique characteristics of its own. We are indeed proud parents of this project, and we owe a great debt of gratitude to our teachers, who taught us and nurtured us, and to the stellar group of contributors to this text, who have given it the strength and vitality to stand on its own as an important text that broadens the perspective of modern palliative medicine.

To a large degree, this book grew out of our contributions to *The Oxford Textbook of Palliative Medicine*, in particular the chapter entitled "Psychiatric Aspects of Palliative Care" by Breitbart, Chochinov, and Passik. We realized that the subject matter covered in this chapter could easily be expanded into a text that would stand on its own and become an important addition to the palliative medicine literature. We were guided by one critically important belief derived from our clinical work and research as psychiatrists working with patients with life-threatening illness. This belief is that concepts of adequate palliative care must be expanded in their focus beyond pain and physical symptom control to include psychiatric, psychosocial, existential, and spiritual domains of care. We felt we had the ability and opportunity to expand the scope of what constituted optimal palliative care to include psychiatric dimensions of palliative medicine by bringing together the most renowned experts in the field of psychiatry and palliative care to produce what we believe is a landmark publication.

Along with John L. Shuster, Jr., M.D., we had the great privilege to serve on the Ad Hoc Committee on End-of-Life Care of the Academy of Psychosomatic Medicine. This committee produced a position statement on psychiatric aspects of care provided to patients nearing the end of life entitled "Psychiatric Aspects of Excellent End-of-Life Care" that was endorsed by the academy in 1997. The full text is available on the academy's Web site: www.apm.org. The opening paragraph of the position statement best expresses the need for this textbook on psychiatry in palliative medicine:

Psychiatric morbidity at the end of life is significant and causes substantial, potentially remediable pain and suffering to dying patients and their families. Despite the fact that quality care for the psychiatric complications of terminal illness is and should be an integral component of excellent, comprehensive End-of-Life care, few hospices and palliative care services have access to personnel with the experience or expertise to address psychiatric morbidity in the terminally ill patient. Mental pain and emotional suffering, especially that stemming from depression, appear to play a major role in patient requests for assisted dying. For these reasons, psychiatric aspects of excellent end-of-life care deserve the attention of consultation-liaison psychiatrists and palliative care practitioners alike.

This book is a comprehensive and practical resource to palliative care practitioners, psychiatrists, psychologists, mental health professionals, and all others involved in the care of the terminally ill for the assessment and management of psychiatric, psychosocial, and existential concerns of patients with life-threatening illness. The contributors to this text have been chosen for their unique ability to bring a combination of clinical and research experience to the review of these issues. We are proud that the contributors to this text are indeed the internationally recognized experts in their respective fields, and we are extremely grateful for their participation in this project. The text has 28 chapters and is divided into 7 parts: I, Psychiatric Complications of Terminal Illness; II, Symptom Management; III, Psychotherapeutic Intervention and Palliative Care; IV, Pediatric Palliative Care; V, Family and Staff Issues; VI, Ethical and Spiritual Issues; VII, Research Issues.

Part I consists of 7 chapters, including chapters on a psychiatric perspective on hospice by Colin Murray Parkes; care and management of the patient at the end of life by Ned Cassem; diagnosis and management of depression by Keith Wilson, Harvey Chochinov, William Breitbart, et al; suicide, assisted suicide, and euthanasia by Barry Rosenfeld, William Breitbart, Harvey Chochinov, et al.; anxiety in palliative care by David Payne and Mary Jane Massie; delirium in the terminally ill by William Breitbart and Kenneth Cohen; and palliative care in the chronically mentally ill by Jimmie Holland, Sherry Schachter, and David Goldenberg. Part II contains 4 chapters on pain, fatigue, eating disor-

ders, and an overview of physical symptom management in the terminally ill for mental health professionals by Russell Portenoy, William Breitbart, David Payne, Lynna Lesko and Susan Abbey. Part III is a unique and extremely valuable collection of chapters focusing on psychotherapy issues and the terminally ill. Chapters in this section include contributions from Gary Rodin, James Spira, Milton Viederman, Dennis Turk, and David Spiegel. They cover the gamut of psychotherapy interventions from individual therapies, existential psychotherapy, and cognitive-behavioral interventions to group psychotherapies. Part IV focuses on pediatric palliative care and includes two chapters by Margaret Stuber and Barbara Sourkes that are invaluable contributions to the literature on psychiatric and psychological care of the dying child. Part V focuses on the family and staff, with contributions by David Wellisch on family issues and palliative care; communication with terminally ill patients and their relatives by Peter Maguire; burnout and staff stress by Mary Vachon; and bereavement by Sidney Zisook. Part VI includes important contributions on ethics by Edmund D. Pellegrino and on spiritual care of the dying by Balfour Mount and Michael Kearney. Additional chapters include one on the treatment of suffering by Nathan Cherny, and addressing the needs of patients who request euthanasia by Margaret McDonald, Steven Passik, and Nessa Coyle. Part VII completes the text with chapters by Irene Higginson and Eduardo Bruera on the current state and future needs of research in psychiatric and psychosocial aspects of palliative care.

We are sincerely grateful, and wish to thank all the individuals who contributed to helping us succeed in this endeavor. To our contributors we offer our profound thanks and respect. To the editorial staff at Oxford University Press, especially Joan Bossert and Cynthia Garver, thank you for your guidance and especially your kind patience. We are deeply indebted to our colleagues, fellows, trainees, and support staff at Memorial Sloan-Kettering Cancer Center in the Department of Psychiatry and Behavioral Sciences, the Department of Neurology, Pain and Palliative Care Service, and the Pain Service, Department of Anesthesiology, and at the University of Manitoba Department of Psychiatry and CancerCare Manitoba. We have been extremely proud of our association with the Project on Death in America (PDIA) as PDIA Faculty Scholars and are extremely grateful to Kathleen Foley, M.D., Susan Block, M.D., Mary Callaway, the PDIA board and our fellow PDIA scholars for their constant support, encouragement, and inspiration. We owe a special debt of gratitude and respect to our esteemed teachers and mentors; in particular, we wish to express our deepest thanks to Jimmie Holland, Ned Cassem, Neil MacDonald, Balfour Mount, Eduardo Bruera, Keith Wilson, Linda Kristjanson, Leslie Degner, John Farber, Russell Portenoy, Richard Payne, Nessa Coyle, Sherry Schachter, and Subash Jain. We would also like to thank our friends in the Brazilian Palliative Care Association, particularly Ana Georgia de Melo, and Victoria and Mario Herzberg, for their inspiration and their gifts of love and support. This book could not have been possible without the dedicated work of our assistants David Strout, Betty Fleck, Holly Callaghan, and Brenda Doerksen. We thank them for putting up with our

anxious moments. We are also, of course, indebted to our patients who taught us so much.

Finally, we cannot end the preface of this book, our first such collaboration, without acknowledging the profound importance of what has now grown to be a close personal friendship and academic collaboration of almost 15 years. It all began in 1986 when a young Canadian psychiatrist from the prairies of Winnipeg and a spanking new attending psychiatrist at Memorial Sloan-Kettering Cancer Center in New York met as supervisee and supervisor, only to become fast friends and valued colleagues. Editing this book together had its moments of both joy and hardship, but we are so proud that we have created something that will live on as a testament not only to the truth we struggle to reveal, but to a friendship we hope will endure two lifetimes.

New York, N.Y.   W.B.
Winnipeg, Manitoba   H.M.C.
August 1999

Contents

Contributors

Susan Abbey, M.D., FRCPC
Director, Program in Medical Psychiatry
The Toronto Hospital
and Assistant Professor, Department of Psychiatry
University of Toronto
Toronto, Ontario

William Breitbart, M.D.
Attending Psychiatrist/Chief, Psychiatry Service
Department of Psychiatry and Behavioral Sciences
Memorial Sloan-Kettering Cancer Center
and Attending Psychiatrist, Pain and Palliative Care
   Service
Department of Neurology, Memorial Sloan-Kettering
   Cancer Center
and Professor of Clinical Psychiatry, Department of
   Psychiatry
The Weill Medical College of Cornell University
and Soros Faculty Scholar, Project on Death in
   America
New York, NY

Eduardo Bruera, M.D.
Professor and Chair
Department of Palliative Care
University of Texas
M. D. Anderson Cancer Center
Houston, TX

Brenda Bursch, Ph.D.
Assistant Clinical Professor
UCLA Neuropsychiatric Institute
Los Angeles, CA

Edwin H. Cassem, M.D.
Professor, Department of Psychiatry
Harvard Medical School
and Chief of Psychiatry
Massachusetts General Hospital
Boston, MA

Nathan I. Cherny, MBBS., FRACP
Chief and Director of Cancer Pain and Palliative
   Care Unit
Department of Medical Oncology
Shaare Zedek Medical Center
Jerusalem, Israel

Harvey Max Chochinov, M.D., Ph.D., FRCPC
Professor, Departments of Psychiatry and Family
   Medicine
(Division of Palliative Care), University of Manitoba
and Soros Faculty Scholar, Project on Death in America
and Medical Research Council of Canada Scientist
Department of Psychosocial Oncology, CancerCare
   Manitoba
Winnipeg, Manitoba

Kenneth Cohen, M.D.
Department of Psychiatry
The Weill Medical College of Cornell University
New York, NY

Nessa Coyle, R.N., M.S.
Director, Supportive Care Program
Pain and Palliative Care Service, Department of
  Neurology
Memorial Sloan-Kettering Cancer Center
New York, NY

Barbara J. de Faye, M.A.
School of Psychology, University of Ottawa
Ottawa, Ontario

Susan Diamond, L.C.S.W.
Department of Psychiatry and Behavioral Sciences
Stanford University School of Medicine
Stanford, CA

Tamara Z. Earhart, B.A.
Department of Psychiatry and Behavioral Sciences
Stanford University School of Medicine
Stanford, CA

Caryn S. Feldman, Ph.D.
Department of Anesthesiology
University of Washington
Seattle, WA

Laurie A. Gillies, Ph.D. Cpsych
Head, Interpersonal Therapy Clinic
The Clarke Division of the Centre for Addiction
  and Mental Health
and Assistant Professor, University of Toronto
  Department of Psychiatry
Toronto, Ontario

Irene J. Higginson, B. Med. Sci., BMBS, MFPHM,
  Ph.D.
Senior Lecturer and Consultant
Palliative Care Research Group
Health Services Research Unit
London School of Hygiene and Tropical Medicine
London, England

Jimmie C. Holland, M.D.
Chair, Department of Psychiatry and
  Behavorial Sciences
Memorial Sloan-Kettering Cancer Center
and Professor, Department of Psychiatry
The Weill College of Medicine of Cornell
  University
New York, NY

Michael Kearney, M.D.
Medical Director
Our Lady's Hospice
Harold's Cross
Dublin, Ireland

Suzanne Krivo, M.D.
Psychiatric Resident
University of California, San Diego
Department of Psychiatry
San Diego, CA

Lynna M. Lesko, M.D., Ph.D.
Consultant, Department of Psychiatry and
  Behavioral Sciences
Memorial Sloan Kettering Cancer Center
and Adjunct Attending, Department of Psychiatry
The Weill Medical College of Cornell University
New York, NY
and Associate Director, General Medicine
Clinical Research
Boehringer Ingelheim Pharmaceutical, Inc.
Ridgefield, Connecticut

Neil MacDonald, CM, M.D., FRCP(C), FRCP(Edin)
Director, Cancer Ethics Program
Centre for Bioethics
Clinical Research Institute of Montreal
and Professor, Department of Oncology, McGill
  University
Montreal, Quebec

Peter Maguire, M.D.
Honorary Consultant Psychiatrist
Director, CRC Psychological Medicine Group
Stanley House
Christie Hospital
Manchester, England

Mary Jane Massie, M.D.
Attending Psychiatrist and Director, Barbara White
    Fishman Center for Psychological Counseling
Department of Psychiatry and Behavioral Sciences
Memorial Sloan-Kettering Cancer Center
and Professor of Clinical Psychiatry, Department of
    Psychiatry
The Weill Medical College of Cornell University
New York, NY

Margaret V. McDonald, M.S.W.
Research Associate
Visiting Nurse Service
New York, NY

Balfour Mount, CM OQ M.D., FRCPC
Eric M. Flanders Professor of Palliative Medicine
McGill University
and Director, Palliative Care Services, Royal Victoria
    Hospital
Montreal, Quebec

Colin Murray Parkes, M.D.
Senior Lecturer in Psychiatry, The London Hospital
    Medical College
and Consultant Psychiatrist to the Royal London
    Hospital
and St. Christopher's Hospice
London, England

Steven D. Passik, Ph.D.
Director, Oncology Symptom Control Research
Community Cancer Care, Inc.
Indianapolis, IN

David K. Payne, Ph.D.
Clinical Assistant Psychologist, Department of
    Psychiatry and Behavioral Sciences
Memorial Sloan-Kettering Cancer Center
New York, NY

Edmund D. Pellegrino, M.D.
Clinical Director, Centre for Bioethics
Georgetown University Medical Center
and John Carroll Professor of Medicine and Medical
    Ethics
Washington, DC

Russell K. Portenoy, M.D.
Chairman, Department of Pain Medicine and
    Palliative Care
Beth Israel Medical Center
New York, NY

Gary Rodin, M.D., FRCPC
Professor, Department of Psychiatry, University of
    Toronto
and Head, Mental Health Program, The Toronto
    Hospital
and Head, Psychosocial Oncology Program, The
    Toronto Hospital
Princess Margaret Hospital

Barry Rosenfeld, Ph.D.
Assistant Professor, Department of Psychology
Long Island University
Brooklyn, NY

Sherry Schachter, Ph.D., R.N.
Pain and Palliative Care Service, Department of
    Neurology
Memorial Sloan-Kettering Cancer Center
New York, NY

Barbara M. Sourkes, Ph.D.
Intensive Ambulatory Care Service
The Montreal Children's Hospital
McGill University
Montreal, Quebec

David Spiegel, M.D.
Professor, Department of Psychiatry and Behavioral
    Sciences
Stanford University School of Medicine
Stanford, CA

James L. Spira, Ph.D.
MPH, Director
Assistant Clinical Professor, Department of
    Psychiatry
and Assistant Research Professor, Department of
    Medicine
Duke University School of Medicine
Program in Health Psychology
Durham, NC
and Visiting Associate Professor
UNC-CH School of Medicine
University of North Carolina
Chapel Hill, NC

Sara L. Stein, M.D.
Postdoctoral Research Fellow
Department of Psychiatry and Behavioral Sciences
Stanford University School of Medicine
Stanford, CA

Margaret L. Stuber, M.D.
Associate Professor, Department of Psychiatry and
  Behavioral Sciences
UCLA Neuropsychiatric Institute
and Director, Pediatric C-L Psychiatry
UCLA Children's Hospital
Los Angeles, CA

Dennis C. Turk, Ph.D.
John and Emma Bonica Professor
  of Anesthesiology and Pain Research
Department of Anesthesiology
University of Washington
Seattle, WA

Mary L. S. Vachon, R.N., Ph.D.
Consultant in Psychosocial Oncology and Palliative
  Care
Toronto-Sunnybrook Regional Cancer Centre
Toronto, Ontario

Milton Viederman, M.D.
Professor of Clinical Psychiatry
The Weill Medical College of Cornell University
and Director, Consultation-Liaison Service
New York Presbyterian Hospital
and Training and Supervising Analyst
Center for Psychoanalytic Training and Research
Columbia University
New York, NY

David K. Wellisch, Ph.D.
Professor in Residence, Department of Psychiatry
  and Behavioral Sciences
UCLA, Neuropsychiatric Institute
Los Angeles, CA

Keith G. Wilson, Ph.D.
Institute for Rehabilitation Research and
  Development
The Rehabilitation Centre
and Department of Medicine, University of Ottawa
School of Psychology, University of Ottawa
Ottawa, Canada

Sidney Zisook, M.D.
UCSD, Department of Psychiatry OPD Services
and Professor of Psychiatry, UCSD School
  of Medicine
San Diego, CA

PART I
Psychiatric Complications of Terminal Illness

Hospice: A Psychiatric Perspective

Colin Murray Parkes, M.D.

Hospice, as we know it today, is a concept originated by Cicely Saunders and her colleagues at St. Christopher's Hospice, Sydenham, and developed across the world. From the start it contained two elements: (1) prompt and effective control of the pain and other symptoms of patients with terminal illnesses and (2) psychological, social, and spiritual care for patients and their families. The former was achieved largely through the sophisticated use of morphine, the latter through a network of professional staff and volunteers who supported patients and family members throughout the terminal illness (defined as the period from the end of active or curative treatment to death) and supported the family in bereavement.

Saunders became aware of the need for improving the care of the dying while working as a nurse at St. Thomas' Hospital. She subsequently began to realize how this could be achieved at St. Luke's Hospital in Bayswater, where she worked for 7 years as a volunteer. Here she learned to use morphine for pain and was impressed by the personal care given by Dr. Howard Barrett and described in his annual reports. She entered medicine with the express purpose of caring for this group of patients and took a post in clinical research at a small hospital run by the Sisters of Charity, St. Joseph's Hospice, Hackney. She

worked there from 1958 to 1965. Here she refined her methods of using regular morphine for pain and developed the style of personal care that was to become her hallmark. St. Joseph's Hospice emphasized the importance of humane spiritual care, but the psychological care provided there was unsophisticated, was focused on the patient, and ended with the patient's death. It was Saunders who drew attention to the need for reform and whose total commitment to this field brought into being St. Christopher's Hospice, which was the test bed for the development of the sophisticated care that we now associate with the better hospices. This, in turn, eventually helped bring about the new field of palliative medicine.

I first met Saunders while she was still working at St. Joseph's Hospice. I was conducting research into the psychological consequences of bereavement, and I remember her telling me how dissatisfied she felt with the care that she was able to offer to the families of her patients. She recognized that she often got very close to family members while caring for the patient but had to break off that contact with them at a time when they needed her most—when the patient died.

In this chapter I describe how this work developed and the contribution that psychiatrists have made and continue to make in this field. My own work did not, of course, take place in a vacuum, and it is notable that several other psychiatrists made important contributions to our thinking during the early days of the development of hospice. A colleague at the Maudsley Hospital in the early 1960s was John Hinton. While I was studying bereavement, he was studying psychological aspects of cancer. Hinton[1] convincingly demonstrated the frequency with which patients with terminal illnesses were aware of their diagnosis and prognosis at a time when most medical and nursing staff thought it better to conceal this information. In later years he was to carry out one of the first scientific comparisons of the impact of three types of palliative care on the psychological state of patients, work that demonstrated that patients under the care of a hospice suffered less emotional distress than those in the other two settings.[2]

While Hinton was carrying out his initial studies, Glaser and Strauss[3] and Weisman and Hacket[4] were studying the ways in which cancer patients, their families, and their medical attendants dealt with their anxiety in the face of death by denying, avoiding, or postponing full realization. Their work helped to point up the need for better communication with the dying and set the scene for death education in the US, which originated as an attempt to bring the whole subject of death out of the closet.

Another early contribution was by Knight Aldrich,[5] who was then professor of psychiatry at Billings Hospital in Chicago. His paper "The Dying Patient's Grief" drew attention to the losses faced by terminally ill patients and helped to spur one of his trainee psychiatrists, Elisabeth Kübler-Ross, to undertake her own studies. She it was who adapted the "phases of grief," which had been developed by James Robertson and John Bowlby in the course of their studies of children separated from their mothers,[6] to designate "phases of dying."[7] While the concept of "phases" has proved inadequate to describe the complexity of responses to terminal illness, the phenomena that she described undoubtedly occur and provided us, for the first time, with a psychological frame of reference for helping the "hopeless case" (as such patients were then seen).

My own earliest studies, at the Maudsley, were of psychiatric patients whose illness had come on following a bereavement. They enabled me to build on Lindemann's earlier work[8] and to formulate a classification of pathological grief that

is still widely used today.[9,10] Little was known, at that time, about the normal pattern of grief, and I subsequently joined John Bowlby's research unit at the Tavistock Institute of Human Relations, where I was able to study an unselected group of young and middle-aged widows, to describe their reaction to bereavement, and to link my own studies of grief in adult life with Bowlby's studies of grief in childhood.[11,12]

Another area in which psychiatrists were making important contributions was that of the "therapeutic community." This term was originated by Maxwell Jones[13,14] to describe an innovative way of caring for psychiatric patients in mental hospitals. Coming, as it did, at a time when psychiatry was under attack for the damaging effects of "institutionalism," the attempts of Jones and others to make use of the psychodynamic forces at work in institutions and to break down the barriers between psychiatric patients and the multidisciplinary team who cared for them came as a breath of fresh air, which was taken up with enthusiasm across the United Kingdom and which subsequently spread to the United States in the era of community mental health. Under its influence, most psychiatric wards were unlocked, physical methods of restraint were minimized, and padded cells were made obsolete. The discovery of the phenothiazine drugs had made "chemical restraint" an alternative option, but Jones's work at Dingleton Hospital, which had opened its doors before the discovery of chlorpromazine, proved that the therapeutic community was capable of reducing the need for coercion and, indeed, for inpatient treatment of the mentally disturbed. The significance of this work extended beyond psychiatry and was to be recognized in institutions of all kinds, including hospitals, prisons, and orphanages.

Also contributing, at this time, to the management of acute psychiatric disorder was the concept of crisis intervention, which was a major part of the community mental health program advocated by Gerald Caplan[15] at his influential Laboratory of Community Psychiatry at Harvard University. Caplan regarded bereavement as a prime example of a life event that carries a risk to mental health, and he encouraged the development of services for the bereaved that can be seen as models for preventive psychiatry. I spent a year at Caplan's Laboratory in 1966, directing the Harvard Bereavement Project, and while I was there Cicely Saunders came to stay, bringing with her her plans for her new hospice. We spent some days discussing these, and I realized this was an opportunity to put into practice some ideas I had been developing about how to prepare people for loss and how to prevent psychiatric problems after bereavement. She subsequently invited me to act as consultant psychiatrist to St. Christopher's Hospice, a post I have occupied ever since the facility opened in 1967.

These various studies reflect the ideas that were around in psychiatry when Saunders opened the doors on her own "therapeutic community." They not only indicate the influences these ideas had on the development of hospice but also explain why hospice made sense to many people who were familiar with these fields. As Saunders herself said, the psychiatrists who supported her helped make hospice "respectable."

THE CHANGING ROLES OF THE PSYCHIATRIST AT ST. CHRISTOPHER'S HOSPICE

My own experience as consultant psychiatrist to St. Christopher's caused me to revise my views on liaison psychiatry. It was clear that the traditional ways of treating emotionally disturbed patients by means of drugs or individual psychotherapy were unlikely to help more than a small proportion of the people who were referred to me. Few had clearcut psychiatric illnesses, and most of those who did would be unlikely to live long enough to benefit from weekly psychotherapy or drugs that might take several weeks to become effective. Clearly, if I was to be of any use to these people, I had to take a different approach. I needed to work with and through their families and the multidisciplinary team of fellow staff members and volunteers at the hospice. This network of people constitute the "community" around the sick person; they are present throughout the day, and it is they who must become psychiatrists to the patient and to the patient's family.

The slogan "No service without research, no research without service," which was often quoted in the Tavistock at that time, also applies well to the early days at St. Christopher's Hospice. Each case was a challenge to be discussed with the staff team. Innovative ideas were welcomed, and the institution was still small enough for the entire staff to meet regularly to discuss the policies and principles that were being established. I found myself moving between patient-focused consultation, family-focused consultation, staff-focused consultation, and institution-focused consultation, any or all of which might be needed in any of the individual and group encounters with which I became involved. Caplan had helped me to understand the difference among these types of consultation and to move among them without getting lost too often.

In the early years the majority of our patients were referred because of pain, and it was the success of the pain control that was the most obvious benefit to arise. Our success in this field helped to maintain staff morale and to get us through the first few years when we were still struggling with the more complex and difficult problems of psychosocial care. A study of the views of relatives of patients who had died of cancer in the hospice and in other hospitals in the vicinity in 1972–73 confirmed this impression.[16] By this time the work of the hospice was becoming known, and the hospice's methods of symptom control were soon adopted elsewhere. When this study was replicated 10 years later,[17] other hospitals were achieving comparable pain control, but several indices showed that the psychosocial care that patients and their families received was still better at the hospice than at other hospitals.

Few people would argue that it is necessary to have hospices in order to achieve adequate control of symptoms in most patients with terminal illness. Where hospices still provide and are likely to continue to provide superior care is in the psychological, social, and spiritual dimensions. Of course, the very nature of hospice has changed from its original model. At its inception, St. Christopher's Hospice provided inpatient care and outpatient consultation, but this was only part of Saunders's plan. Within a few years, the home care program had started, and before long "the tail had begun to wag the dog." At the present time more care is given in the patient's home than in the hospice itself, thanks to the work of the home care team. In the United States, which lacks the British tradition of family medicine by general practitioners who visit the home, the whole idea of home care for the dying was an innovation, and hospice is widely associated with home care as opposed to inpatient care in a hospital.

My own studies have shown that, while the addition of home care to our hospice program undoubtedly increased the length of time that patients spend at home, the strain on the family was also increased, sometimes considerably.[18] It is hard for visiting nursing staff to provide the same support at home that can be given to patients and family on a hospice ward. This said, the combination of a well-integrated inpatient and home-care hospice program does constitute a better model than either on its own.

The addition of a bereavement service and, much later, a day hospice, both of which were and continue to be largely staffed by volunteers, reduces strain on the family and ensures that they have the best possible chance of continuing to cope while the patient is alive and to emerge unharmed by bereavement.

Although we had informed bereaved people of our wish to help from the time the hospice opened, the bereavement care service proper was not launched until 1970 because of opposition from members of staff who disliked the idea of a proactive approach to bereaved people at risk. They held to the view that those who needed help would ask for it and that any attempt to approach people at risk would be intrusive and possibly harmful. Matters came to a head when the widow of one of our patients committed suicide a few weeks after her husband's death. She had not asked for our help, and her death forced the skeptics to allow a trial to be made of an alternative model of service.

In order to test the efficacy of the service, bereaved people who were thought to be at risk (using a formal risk assessment) were assigned at random to two groups. Members of one group were approached by a bereavement counselor with an offer of help, and members of the other group were not approached (although anyone who asked for help would get it). During the first few months of operation of the service, no differences were found between the groups, but thereafter the counseled group reported significantly fewer indicators of anxiety and tension, and the consumption of drugs, alcohol, and tobacco was lower than that of the comparison group, none of whom had asked for help.[19]

Confirmation of the value of short-term support to the bereaved came from a similar study that had been carried out by another psychiatrist, Beverly Raphael, in Australia.[20] She, too, found a significant difference between counseled and uncounseled groups. In her study the counseling was given by a highly qualified psychiatrist, herself; in mine, it was given by carefully selected and trained hospice volunteers. This model of service has been widely copied across the world, but it is sad that it is largely limited to the relatives of patients who have died in a hospice, a group who are likely to be in less need of help than people bereaved by more sudden and traumatic types of death. In Britain the organization Cruse—Bereavement Care uses very similar means of selecting, training, and supporting volunteers to provide counseling to people who have suffered bereavements of all kinds.[21]

Another important aspect of my work at the hospice for many years was support to staff. Much of this was carried out in groups, which were held regularly with ward staff, with the home-care team, with the senior staff members. These groups were forums in which discussion of psychological issues regarding the care of particular patients and family members could take place, and they were also opportunities for staff members to share their own thoughts and feelings about their work and to support each other. Not all staff chose to seek support at these meetings, particularly when the level of trust within a team was not high, and it was important that other sources of support were also available. I saw many staff members on an individual basis, and there were others who sought support from colleagues, senior staff, or the chaplin. Thus, the entire staff of the hospice became part of a network of care that justified the term "community." In addition, a visiting American psychiatrist, Sam Klagsbrun, has made an annual visit for many years in order to provide an opportunity for staff members to review their work with an independent person from outside the community.

It is a reasonable question to ask how much of this work was properly the work of a psychiatrist. If we see the psychiatrist's role as being to diagnose and treat mental illness, we must recognize that most of the psychological problems of patients who are dying and of family members before and after bereavement are not mental illnesses, nor are the day-to-day psychological difficulties of staff and volunteers. If, on the other hand, the psychiatrist's roles include the development of programs to prevent mental illness and research to evaluate and facilitate these programs, then this is precisely what I was doing. The implication of this is that, as with most forms of preventive medicine, once the program had become established, it was appropriate to hand over much of it to nonpsychiatrists. It was, in a sense, part of the object of the exercise to make myself redundant, and, to a large extent, I have succeeded in this. Most of the activities I initiated have now been taken over by a team of social workers who have the skills that are needed to provide support to patients and families, support staff, and run the bereavement service. In other hospices, some of these tasks have been undertaken by psychologists, who have, as a profession, begun to take an interest in the field. All of these developments are to be encouraged.

What remains for the psychiatrist to do? Activities that seem to be appropriate when all of these other gaps have been filled include consultation with patients and family members who are referred by hospice staff (i.e., the orthodox role of the consultant psychiatrist), acting as backup consultants to the front line of social workers and other staff who are carrying out the day-to-day work of psychosocial support, contributing to training programs, chairing case conferences at which staff can meet to discuss problem families, and undertaking innovative research and developments. All of these make the psychiatrist a valuable member of any hospice team, and it is sad that so many hospices lack this kind of help.

THE DISTINCTIVE FEATURES
OF HOSPICE

What distinguished hospices from other types of palliative care? Most hospice staff would use the word "holistic" to describe the distinctive feature of their work. By this they mean that they pay attention to all aspects of the patients and their families, a claim that is self-evidently impossible to fulfill, since nobody can pay attention to all of anything or anybody; we *have* to be selective. Perhaps a better analogy is to microscopy, in which we may choose to use a low-powered or a high-powered magnification. Much of medicine is high powered, focused in great detail on one or a few aspects of a person. Thus, the good radiotherapist knows precisely where to focus radiation and in what dosage in order to kill as many cancer cells as possible without killing the patient. Psycho-

logical skills, while desirable, are not essential to this job, and, given the choice, most people would rather go to a technically skilled radiotherapist than to one who is better with people than machines.

Hospice staff, on the other hand, are often low powered. They are less concerned with the technical aspects of care, and they attempt to take the family (which includes the patient) as the unit of care. Physical, psychological, social, and spiritual needs are all covered, although none of them are likely to be explored in great detail, and a wide range of orthodox and unorthodox approaches is adopted in the mistaken belief that holism means you have to say yes to everything. This sometimes gives an impression of benevolent amateurism to hospice care. Some hospice staff seem to care a great deal in a fuzzy and unfocused way, but they lack the sophistication to focus when focus is needed. This, I hasten to add, is not the case in the better hospices.

To develop the analogy with microscopy further: Good microscopists know that, to get the best results, they need to rack back and forth between high and low powers. The same applies to the good hospices. Hospices have always recognized the need for employing sufficient numbers of staff and volunteers to enable all to have time to develop relationships and to communicate effectively and in depth with patients and their families. This implies that they should train their staff to take a highly sophisticated view of each of the dimensions of care—physical, psychological, social, and spiritual. They should know when and how to pay minute attention to a particular problem in one of these dimensions and when to pull back to take a broader perspective. One example has to suffice to illustrate this issue. Two patients were discussing the nurses on the ward. One of them expressed a preference for nurse A, "who always makes me laugh." Another disagreed: "I prefer nurse B," she said. "You can be serious with her." She then reported a conversation with nurse B in which it was clear that the nurse had helped her come to terms with her cancer by a sensitive and sophisticated interaction in which she had helped the patient clarify the difficulties she faced. When subsequently I reported this conversation to a senior nurse, she observed that both nurses had their strengths and their weaknesses. Nurse A was the pet of the ward; everybody loved her, and she loved everybody. A bright, attractive, cheerful girl, she had a pollyan-nish ability to look on the bright side, yet her contributions to ward discussions in which prob-lems were discussed in depth were abysmal; she never seemed to understand what was going on under the surface. Nurse B, on the other hand, was rather intense. She would spend hours talk-ing in depth to one patient and ignore the needs of others. She was similarly blind to the needs of her colleagues, who often found themselves hav-ing to do her duties because she was too intensely involved with a patient to drag herself away. Ide-ally, we all need to be able to move back and forth between narrow and broad focus and to plan our work in such a way that we can alternate the two to the best advantage of the families we serve.

Most medical and nursing staff are "patient fo-cused." We have been trained to put patients first, and, while most of us pay attention to the fam-ily when necessary, we tend to think of them as an optional extra that we will take on if we have the time. Sometimes family members become a nuisance, demanding our time and interfering with our attempts to treat "our" patients. We eas-ily forget that their knowledge of and rights to be with the patient are greater than ours. As long as the patient is alive, families, too, often minimize or deny their own needs, yet the patient's trou-bles will soon be over, while those of the family may just be beginning.

FAMILY PSYCHOLOGY IN A HOSPICE

It is part of the psychiatrist's responsibility to off-set staff's bias toward patient care over family care by flying a flag for the families (a role that social workers are also well qualified to perform). One of the most important tools of low-powered mi-croscopy in hospice is the genogram. The genogram is the shorthand key to the whole fam-ily. It needs to be clearly displayed whenever a family is being discussed in the team and referred to in many of our interactions with patients and their families. A turning point in the history of St. Christopher's Hospice was reached when staff agreed to place the genogram on the front page of the case notes. Every nurse, doctor, and coun-selor could then become familiar with the family tree of every family in his or her care. The very act of drawing the genogram indicates to the pa-tient that our interest is broader than that of most

other medical and nursing staff whom they have met. Having established the broad picture of the family, it is possible to begin to examine in more detail particular problems in one or other person in the genogram. Most hospices now devote an entire section of the case notes to the family, in-cluding a continuing assessment of family needs, which enables us to identify family members in special need of our help both before and after the patient's death. There is now a sizable body of re-search into bereavement outcome that enables us to identify risk factors before the patient's death that predict who will do well and who badly af-ter that event.[22] Some hospices use formal meth-ods of assessing family need, such as scoreable questionnaires. These are valuable for research purposes, but they lack flexibility. At St. Christo-pher's, a semiformal method is used to flag issues that need to be considered, but the global assess-ment of bereavement need and the decision whether to offer proactive counseling after be-reavement is now made by a social worker rather than by a "risk score."

The psychiatrist brings sophistication on psy-chosocial issues, and we need to be able to focus and to train other members of the team to focus on these issues when the need arises. The best way to do this is to hold case conferences at which we can discuss psychological problems in the fam-ily with other members of the team. To ensure that the necessary time is devoted to exploring the ramifications of the problems under discus-sion, it is seldom a good idea to discuss more than one or two families in a conference of one hours duration. The psychiatrist chairs these and takes an active part in leading the discussion. By ask-ing the right questions and suggesting possible ar-eas for further exploration, we are demonstrating how we think about families and enabling staff to do the same. In time, staff will become so-phisticated in this area, and visiting psychiatrists who have participated in such groups have been surprised at the high level of discussion of family dynamics.

Consultations with patients and family mem-bers who have been referred to the liaison psy-chiatrist constitute another opportunity to teach staff, and it is important to leave sufficient time to provide feedback to the staff on our formula-tion of the problem. Most hospices now adopt a style of care that assigns one or a small number of nurses to each family, and it is important for psychiatrists to meet with a member of that group to find out how the members see the problem and to share our views. This also helps us to become a part of the team.

EDUCATIONAL ROLES

An important function of hospices in Great Britain is to educate members of the caring professions in the skills of palliative and bereavement care. Their staffs develop high levels of expertise in these areas, and many hospices are recognized as centers of excellence with appropriate facilities for study. Both external courses and in-service training are offered, and many staff members come for a limited period to work in the hospice before moving to other settings.

Psychiatrists have useful roles to play in these training programs. If alternative expertise is not available, it may be necessary to teach basic-level programs in the assessment and management of anxiety, fear, psychological trauma, bereavement, confusion, attachment problems, and family dysfunction. Over the years at St. Christopher's Hospice, I have been able to hand over most of this basic training to other professional staff, many of whom were originally trained by me. I now tend to limit my training to advanced-level courses, case conferences, research meetings, and other special meetings.

Hospices can offer useful placements to trainee psychiatrists at the senior level who have an interest in liaison psychiatry. It is, of course, essential for them to receive proper supervision in this work from the hospice's consultant psychiatrist, since the skills they have learned elsewhere are of only limited value in this setting.

THE STAFF "FAMILY" IN A HOSPICE

Most hospices are small units in which all members of the team get to know each other well, and it is this community that the visiting psychiatrist will get to know. Hospices tend to attract caring people who look after one another as well as looking after the families they serve. In many ways they resemble large families, and, while it is often a privilege and a pleasure to become part of such a family, we should also expect to find the same problems that can beset large families. Hos-

pice teams, however caring, are not immune to the problems of rivalry, power struggles, and change that can undermine security and trust and render any family dysfunctional. The loss of established staff members who leave and are replaced by new people often upsets the security of a well-functioning team, as do sickness or end-of-tether behavior among staff, who may have problems outside the hospice that affect their work. Circumstances of this kind, which occur in all caring communities, may have a particular impact in small teams that are working at full stretch. In such circumstances, staff members often neglect their own and one another's needs.

In supporting staff, it is important for us to understand the difference between grief, which is common, and burnout, which is probably rarer in hospice than in other health-care settings. Grief is, of course, the reaction to losses of all kinds, and every nurse or doctor who cares about as well as for people who are facing loss must be prepared to share it. The staff of hospices, because they have to cope with a death rate that is higher than that in any other setting, must learn to live with grief. At times, particularly when a death was not expected, when we have become more than usually involved, or when we have failed to achieve the goals that we have set ourselves, our grief, as well as that of the families we serve, may become hard to bear. At such times, it is important for staff to know that they can share their own grief with colleagues without being labeled "weak" or creating undue anxiety. As one nurse at St. Christopher's Hospice said, "I have learned to cry here." She meant that she had discovered that it was not only patients and their relatives who need and are permitted to express grief in this setting. She had discovered that, when sad things happened, she could withdraw briefly and cry on the shoulder of a friend; she then felt better and could return to the fray.

These problems are not fundamentally different from those that occur in all settings for palliative care, and they are discussed in more detail elsewhere in this volume (see chapters 21 and 22). They are emphasized in this chapter on hospice because of the special prominence that they receive in that setting and the special opportunity that exists in such caring communities to tackle the problems at both individual and institutional level. At the institutional level, the organization of a well-functioning staff support network, which usually includes the psychiatrist, is explicit and important. Everyone acknowledges the importance of spending time communicating with patients and their families, but staff may need to be reminded of the importance of spending time communicating with one another.

THE HOSPICE IDEAL AND ITS PROBLEMS

Many of those who choose to work in hospices have very high ideals. They expect a great deal of themselves and of each other. Hospices are regularly portrayed as "wonderful" places in which the "atmosphere" is always peaceful. To some extent this is a sales pitch by fund-raisers, but it also reflects everyone's need to believe that hospices have some magical means of calming the fears of the dying and assuaging the pains of grief. In the early days of hospice, many of our patients had suffered greatly before they came to us, and their gratitude and relief when their pain was relieved helped to create the myth that everybody dies happy in a hospice. Today this is less likely to be the case, and we may have to work hard to relieve the complex social and emotional problems that we meet. We shall not always succeed. These things considered, it is not surprising that some staff are disillusioned and blame the hospice that does not live up to their exalted expectations; others blame themselves. As one who has worked in hospices for nearly 30 years, I have to say that hospice care can be a rewarding field of work—on balance, the gains outweigh the losses—but we must be prepared for failure as well as for success, and we must take the rough with the smooth.

Within the hospice there is a danger that people will collude with the myth of hospice by keeping their problems to themselves and pretending that all is well. Psychiatrists are, or should be, better than some at reading unspoken messages and recognizing the true situation. We can then give people permission to be human.

Another feature of most hospices is the value that they place on spiritual and religious aspects of care. This, too, is a mixed blessing. If, by spiritual care, we mean an attempt to help people to find meaning in their lives at a time when many feel that life has lost its meaning, then spiritual care is as much a part of the role of the psychia-

trist as it is of the chaplain. We should all be seeking to learn to speak the spiritual language of our clients (which may or may not be a religious language) and to help them to make sense of their lives. On the whole, hospice staff are against proselytizing, although many of them have a strong faith of their own. Problems arise if they assume that any expression of irritation, anger, or grief by themselves or others is evidence of selfishness or of lack of faith. This causes them to adopt a perpetual smile and a polite manner that can be most annoying to people who are spoiling for a fight or who may not feel like smiling back. As one patient put it, "They're all too bloody nice here!" If such staff members should be human enough to lose their temper or "break down," they may need a lot of reassurance that we do not think any the less of them. Humanity is better than niceness.

Contrary to popular belief, psychiatrists and priests are not rivals. Each brings certain skills and viewpoints that may complement those of the other. Each is perceived in different ways by clients, and this too colors the opportunities for and types of communication that they have with patients and their families. Thus, the psychiatrist can prescribe drugs but not rituals; the priest can say a prayer with a patient but will be regarded with suspicion if he or she asks questions about intimate matters. Priests are well trained in theology, but their knowledge of psychology may be poor, whereas the opposite is true of the psychiatrist. Some people eagerly seek the help of a priest but want nothing to do with a psychiatrist; others distrust all priests but respect psychiatrists. It follows that the hospice chaplain and the priest need to work together, to learn each other's roles and to respect each other if they are to be of the best value to their clients. It helps if psychiatrist and chaplain can meet regularly at case conferences or other settings in which they can help each other.

Psychiatrists can make or mar their reputation in the close-knit community of a hospice when things go badly wrong. Perhaps a patient has committed suicide, morale in a team has collapsed, several nurses have resigned, and/or a much-loved member of the senior staff has been found to have cancer. Events of this kind threaten the functioning of the entire group. It is important for us to keep our ear to the ground and take action, if possible, before people start to burn out.

The action is, of course, no different from the action that is needed when families are at the end of their tether. We need to meet with all of those affected by the situation and show them that we care. A group meeting can be a good place to reassure people of our concern for them and our confidence in them. This done, they may feel secure enough to share their thoughts and feelings and to support one another. The psychiatrist acts as a facilitator, a shoulder to cry on, a surrogate parent, and a punching bag.

It will be clear from what has been said that hospices are not fundamentally different from most other settings for palliative care. Their staffs are often more cohesive than most, staffs should be more highly trained in psychosocial skills, and they often have the advantage of a higher staff/patient ratio than other settings. Their high reputation may attract funds that are not available to others who are just as deserving, but it also places on the staff expectations that may be hard to meet. Hospices excite envy, suspicion, adulation, and magical expectations, none of which are justified. Even so, they achieve a great deal and are rewarding places to work.

References

1. Hinton JM. The physical and mental distress of the dying. *Quarterly Journal of Medicine*, 1963; 32:1–21.

2. Hinton JM. Comparison of places and policies for terminal care. *Lancet*, 1979; 6:29–32.

3. Glaser BG, Strauss AL. *Awareness of Dying*. Chicago: Aldine, 1965.

4. Weisman AD, Hacket T. Denial as a social act. In: Levin S, Kahana RJ, eds, *Psychodynamic Studies on Aging: Creativity, Reminiscing, and Dying*. New York: International University Press, 1967.

5. Aldrich CK. 1962. The dying patient's grief. *Journal of the American Medical Association*, 1963; 184:329–331.

6. Robertson J, Bowlby J. Responses of young children to separation from their mothers. *Courier of the International Children's Centre* (Paris), 1952; 2:131–140.

7. Ross EK. *On Death and Dying*. London: Tavistock, 1970.

8. Lindemann E. The symptomatology and management of acute grief. *American Journal of Psychiatry*, 1944; 101:141.

9. Parkes CM. Bereavement and mental illness. Part I. A clinical study of the grief of bereaved psychiatric patients. Part II. A classification of bereavement reactions. *British Journal of Medical Psychology*, 1965; 38:1–26.

10. Jacob S. *Pathologic Grief: Maladaptation to Loss*. Washington, DC: American Psychiatric Proceedings, 1993.

11. Bowlby J, Parkes CM. Separation and loss. In: Anthony EJ, Koupernik C, eds, *The Child in His Family*, Vol. 1: *International Yearbook of Child Psychiatry and Allied Professions*. New York: John Wiley, 1970:180–198.

12. Parkes CM. *Bereavement: Studies of Grief in Adult Life*. New York: International University Press, 1972; 3rd ed, 1995.

13. Jones M et al. *Social Psychiatry*. London: Tavistock, 1952. Subsequently published in the USA as The Therapeutic Community. New York: Basic Books, 1953.

14. Jones M. *Social Psychiatry in Practice*. Harmondsworth: Penguin Books, 1968.

15. Caplan G. *Principles of Preventive Psychiatry*. New York: Basic Books, 1964.

16. Parkes CM. Terminal care: Evaluation of inpatient service at St. Christopher's Hospice. Part I. Views of surviving spouse on effects of service on the patient. Part II. Self-assessment of effects of the service on surviving spouses. *Postgraduate Medical Journal*, 1979; 55:517–527.

17. Parkes CM, Parkes JLN. "Hospice" versus "hospital" care—reevaluation after 10 years as seen by surviving spouses. *Postgraduate Medical Journal*, 1984; 60:120.

18. Parkes CM. Terminal care: Evaluation of an Advisory Domiciliary Service at St. Christopher's Hospice. *Postgraduate Medical Journal*, 1980; 56:685–689.

19. Parkes CM. Evaluation of a bereavement service. *Journal of Preventive Psychiatry*, 1981;1:179–88.

20. Raphael B. Preventive intervention with the recently bereaved. *Archives of General Psychiatry*, 1977; 34:1450–1454.

21. Parkes CM. Bereavement care in Britain: a critical review. In: Chigier E, ed, *First International Symposium on Grief and Bereavement*. Vol. 3: *Community and Support Systems*. London: Freund, 1988.

2

Care and Management of the Patient at the End of Life

Edwin H. Cassem, M.D.

At the end of life, suffering comes in many forms. Palliative care may require an intensity that rivals that of curative care. Keeping the patient clean despite nearly continuous incontinence or diarrhea, neutralizing unpleasant odors, frequently suctioning copious bronchial secretions, controlling peripheral and pulmonary edema, preventing bedsores, containing agitated delirium, and fighting the psychosocial forces that can lead to family fragmentation can tax the ingenuity and equanimity of the most skilled health professionals.[1-5] To the list of symptoms requiring palliation at the end of life must be added those of psychiatric illness and the psychosocial and spiritual suffering these patients face. For patients in this predicament, the request for psychiatric consultation comes most commonly with major depression, delirium and organic brain syndromes, substance abuse, difficulty grieving the pending loss that death will bring, treatment-resistant continuous pain syndromes, and personality disorders, where the patient's splitting, hostility, treatment rejection, litigation threats, or outrage at having the illness disrupt the relationships with family and treatment team. There may also be denial and an inability to accept diagnosis or treatment, unrealistic hopes for miracles, persistent questions such as why there is no improvement, anxiety, often extreme, with near panic and unspecifiable fears about dying, ambivalence and guilt, for example, the ambivalence felt by a daughter with vaginal cancer on learning that the diethylstilbestrol her mother took during pregnancy is implicated, and the guilt felt by her mother; and concerns over how to handle unrelated bad news, for example, whether a dying person should be told of a relative's death when ability to tolerate another trauma is seriously questioned.[3,5,7-4] Religion and spirituality are often extremely important for patients and family at the end of life, and support in this realm is an essential feature of palliative care.[9,10]

When a patient is dying, the entire family is the appropriate focus for medical treatment. A family member may be the first to notice a difficulty (such as a personality change) and therefore serves as an indispensable historian. Or a family member may have more difficulty coping with the illness than the patient and because of his own needs irritate caregivers, distract them from the patient, claim the patient, not he, is anxious, cause isolation of physicians from the family (physicians may time their visits to the patient to avoid the family), and seriously jeopardize treatment and the chance to make death meaningful and dignified.

CARE OF THE PERSON AT THE END OF LIFE

Preliminary Considerations

Breaking Bad News

Because so many reactions to the news of diagnosis are possible, it is helpful to have some plan of action in mind ahead of time that will permit the greatest variation and freedom of response. When the diagnosis is made and it is time to inform the patient, the physician should sit down together with the patient in a private place. The spouse (and sometimes family) should be included in the discussion unless there is a good reason not to do so. If at all possible, the patient should be informed well ahead of time that when all the tests are completed, the physician will sit down with him to go over the information and treatment plans in detail. If the patient is an inpatient, the physician should sit down to deliver bad news. Standing while conveying bad news is regarded by patients as unkind and expressive of wanting to leave as quickly as possible. If the patient is tested as an outpatient and returns home before test results are known, she should be told that diagnostic information is far too important to convey by phone and a meeting to discuss the results arranged. Patients who learn bad news by phone commonly label that approach as thoughtless, even though they may have asked for information. As the appointed day of discussion approaches, the patient should be warned again. This permits those patients who wish no or minimal information to say so.

When the findings are threatening (e.g., when a biopsy is positive for malignancy), how can the news best be conveyed? A good opening statement is one that is (1) rehearsed so that it can be delivered calmly, (2) brief (three sentences or less), (3) designed to encourage further dialogue, and (4) reassuring of continued attention and care. A typical delivery might go as follows: "The tests confirmed that your tumor is malignant [the bad news]. I have therefore asked the surgeon [radiotherapist, oncologist] to come by to speak with you, examine you, and make recommendations for treatment [we will do something about it]. As things proceed, I will discuss them with you and how we should proceed [I will stand by you]." Silence and quiet observation at this point will yield more valuable information about the patient than any other part of the exchange. What are the emotional reactions? What sort of coping is seen at the very start? While observing, one can decide how best to continue with the discussion, but sitting with the patient for a period of time is the most valuable part of this initial encounter with a grim reality that both patient and physician will continue to confront together, possibly for a very long time.

Telling the Truth

Without honesty, human relationships are destined for shipwreck. If truthfulness and trust are so obviously interdependent, how can there be so much conspiracy to avoid truth with the dying? The paradoxical fact is that for terminally ill patients the need for both honesty and the avoidance of the truth can be intense. Sir William Osler is reputed to have said, "A patient has no more right to all the facts in my head than he does to all the medications in my bag." A routine blood smear has just revealed that a 25-year-old man has acute myelogenous leukemia. If he is married and the father of two small children, should he be told the diagnosis? Is the answer obvious? What if he has had two prior psychotic breaks with less serious illness? What if his wife says he once said he never wanted to know if he had a malignancy?

Most empirical studies in which patients were asked whether or not they wanted to be told the truth about malignancy overwhelmingly indicated a desire for truth. When 740 patients in a cancer detection clinic were asked prior to diagnosis if they wanted to be told their diagnosis, 99% said they did.[15] Another group in this same clinic was asked after the diagnosis was established, and 89% of them replied affirmatively, as did 82% of another group who had been examined and found to be free of malignancy. Gilbertsen and Wangensteen[16] asked the same questions of 298 survivors of surgery for gastric, colonic, and rectal cancers and found 82% wanted to be told the truth. The same investigators questioned 92 patients who had advanced cancer and were judged by their physicians to be preterminal and found that 73 (79%) of the patients thought they should be informed of their diagnosis.

How many patients do not want to know the truth or regard it as harmful? The effects of blunt truth telling have been studied empirically in both England and the United States. Aitken-Swan and Easson[17] were told by 7% of 231 patients who were explicitly informed of their diagnosis that the frankness of the consultant was resented. Gilbertsen and Wangensteen[16] observed that 4% of a sample of surgical patients became emotionally upset at the time they were told and appeared to remain so throughout the course of their illness. Gerlé et al.[18] studied 101 patients that were divided into two groups. Members of one group were told, along with their families, the frank truth of their diagnoses. In the other group, an effort was made to maintain a conspiracy of silence with family and physician that excluded the patient from discussion of the diagnosis. At first, greater emotional upset appeared in the group where patient and family were informed together, but the investigators observed in follow-up that the emotional difficulties of the families of those patients shielded from the truth far outweighed those of the patients and families that were told the diagnosis simultaneously. In general, empirical studies support the idea that truth is desired by terminally ill patients and does not harm those to whom it is given. Honesty sustains the relationship with a dying person rather than retarding it.

> Dr. Hackett saw in consultation a 57-year-old housewife with metastatic breast cancer, now far advanced. She reported a persistent headache, which she attributed to nervous tension and asked why she should be nervous. Turning the question back to her, he was told, "I am nervous because I have lost 60 pounds in a year. The priest comes to see me twice a week, which he never did before, and my mother-in-law is nicer to me even though I am meaner to her. Wouldn't this make you nervous?" . . . [He] said to her, "You mean you think you're dying." "That's right, I do," she replied. He paused and said quickly, "You are." She smiled and said, "Well, I've finally broken the sound barrier; someone's finally told me the truth."[19]

Not all patients can be dealt with so directly. A nuclear physicist greeted his surgeon on the day following exploratory laparotomy with the words, "Lie to me, Steve." Individual variations in willingness to hear the initial diagnosis are extreme, and diagnosis is entirely different from prognosis. Many patients have said they were grateful to their physician for telling them they

had a malignancy. Very few, however, reacted positively to being told they are dying. In my experience, "Do I have cancer?" is a common question, whereas "Am I dying?" is a rare one. The question about dying is more commonly heard from patients who are dying rapidly, such as those in cardiogenic shock.

Physicians today generally prefer to tell cancer patients their diagnoses. Oken's study of 1961 documented that 90% of responding physicians preferred not to tell patients the diagnosis.[20] When Novack et al.[21] repeated this questionnaire in 1979, 97% of responding physicians indicated a preference for telling the cancer patient the diagnosis. One hundred percent of the physicians said that patients had a right to know.

Honest communication of the diagnosis (or of any truth) by no means precludes later avoidance or even denial of the truth. In two studies, patients who had been explicitly told their diagnosis (using the word "cancer" or "malignancy") were asked 3 weeks later what they had been told. Nineteen percent of one sample[17] and 20% of the other[16] denied that their condition was cancerous or malignant. Likewise, Croog et al.[22] interviewed 345 men 3 weeks after myocardial infarction and were told by 20% of them that they had not had a heart attack. All had been explicitly told their diagnosis. For a person to function effectively, truth's piercing voice must occasionally be muted or even excluded from awareness. On four consecutive days I spoke with a man who had a widely spread bone cancer. On the first day he said he didn't know what he had and didn't like to ask questions. The second day he said he was "riddled with cancer." On the third day he didn't really know what ailed him. The fourth day he said that even though nobody likes to die that was now his lot.[23]

Truth telling is no panacea. Communicating a diagnosis honestly, though difficult, is easier than the labors that lie ahead. Telling the truth is merely a way to begin, but since it is an open and honest way, it provides a firm basis on which to build a relationship of trust.

Goals of Treatment at the End of Life

Saunders[24] had stated that the aim is to keep patients feeling like themselves as long as possible. For her, dying is also a "coming together time" when patient, family, and staff help one another share the burden of saying appropriate good-byes.

For Kübler-Ross[25] the "unfinished business" of the dying is reconciling and resolving conflicts with loved ones and pursuit of specific remaining hopes. The LeShans[26,27] have deliberately chosen not to focus on dying ("Death is a minor problem") but to search aggressively with patients for what they wish to accomplish in living ("What you do until then is a major problem, and we can work on that."). Weisman and Hackett[28] have coined the term "appropriate death." To achieve this patients should be relatively pain-free, operate on as effective a level as possible within the limits of their disability, recognize and resolve residual conflicts, satisfy those remaining wishes that are consistent with their conditions and ego ideals, and be able to yield control to others in whom they have confidence.

The final phase of a person's life deserves a positive emphasis. Cassell[29] has said that an individual life lived is a work of art. The end of life is part of this artistic product, an opportunity to affirm and celebrate the value of the life and what this individual has accomplished, stood for, and meant to others. While not many may be able to say, as Cardinal Bernardine[30] did a month before he died, that "death is my friend," one might be able to set positive goals, take as much control of life as possible, and so live that the end of life becomes them as much as any other part of it. The mother who faces premature death must decide what and how she will tell her children about her illness and approaching death and how to understand their reactions, support them, and prepare them for their futures without her. What does she want them to know and remember about her? If they are older and in conflict, how can she use her authority to encourage reconciliation? How can she in general use the pulpit of the dying woman? Caring and planning for children, spouse, friends, and work can preoccupy her constructively, giving her concrete goals to attain and a way to sustain for self esteem.

Likewise, the core task for those who love the dying person is to make the patient's remaining time more comfortable and meaningful, and they must examine their relationships to the dying person. How can they help their loved one achieve a dying time she can be proud of and participate so that they themselves can be proud of their own conduct during this time and begin preparing for themselves a memorial of her with which they can live comfortably for the rest of their lives?

Loss of a loved one is what frightens people most when death appears on the horizon. Many other relationships may also be threatened. Help that rallies all to strengthen and improve their relationships addresses this most frightening aspect of death, loss that feels like abandonment.

Perhaps more important than any other principle is that the treatment be individualized. This can be accomplished only by getting to know the patient, responding to his needs and interests, proceeding at this pace, and allowing him to shape the manner in which those in attendance behave. There is no one "best" way to die.

Hospice Care of the Terminally Ill: Psychiatric Component

The World Health Organization (WHO) defines palliative (or hospice) care as "the active total care of patients whose disease is not responsive to curative treatments."[31] This definition does not mention death, an acknowledgment that doing so upsets some patients so much that they will not accept hospice care even when it is desperately needed. This is a common impasse to care. One may have to implore the patient to accept hospice care for the benefit of their family, and occasionally the physician and family may request hospice care despite the patient's opposition. The goals of palliative care can be simply expressed as aggressive minimization of the patient's burdens and maximization of quality of life. The latter generally is an effort to maximize independence and the number of options available for the dying person, as well as an intense effort to make the most of the person's relationships. Avery Weisman has summarized the work of the final phase of life as coping with disability, the maintenance of morale, and the search for meaning.[32] Although most understand "palliation" as aimed at physical comfort, this is gravely inadequate, and palliation of psychiatric, psychosocial, and spiritual suffering requires formal consideration and effort.

A Comprehensive Approach to Palliation of Psychiatric, Psychosocial, and Spiritual Suffering at the End of Life

Why have patients in the Netherlands requested euthanasia? The most frequent reasons are: loss of dignity, 57%; pain, 46% (but when pain is the only nociceptive number shrinks to 5%); unworthy dying, 46% dependence on others, 33%; tired of life, 23%.[33] These reasons are all ultimately psychosocial. Psychosocial suffering, as we see from this, is even worse than physical suffering, and requires in itself aggressive palliation. To cover all forms of psychosocial suffering, the multiaxial system of DSM-IV is useful,[34] and its categories are adapted here to describe what is required to make end of life care comprehensive.

Axis I

Axis I of DSM-IV includes all psychiatric disorders. Although every disorder involves some sort of suffering and therefore could be reviewed here, only a few obviously relevant examples will be discussed.

Major Depression.   The more seriously ill a person becomes, the more likely he is to develop major depression.[35] Because few forms of human suffering match or exceed major depression, careful vigilance for its appearance is necessary as is aggressive treatment when it appears. Suicidal ideation, rather than being accepted immediately as understandable, requires the same thoughtful examination that is demanded when it appears in any other circumstance. Avery Weisman (personal communication) formulated the wish to die as an existential signal that the person's conviction "that his potential for being someone who matters has been exhausted."

Depression is discussed in Chapter 2.

Anxiety.   Anxiety disorders may or may not intensify during a terminal illness but clearly require psychiatric attention when they do. Impending death can generate severe anxiety in the patients facing it, in their families and their friends, and in those who take care of them. When causes for panic, phobia, generalized anxiety, and other conditions have been sought by the consultant and not found, the four commonest fears associated with death are helplessness or loss of control, sense of being bad (guilt and punishment), physical injury or symbolic injury (castration), and abandonment.[36]

In the clinical examination, a severely anxious patient may not know what it is about death that is so frightening. Memories of someone who died of the same illness or associations to the illness

may produce specific material (e.g., it will be painful or disfiguring). Truly disruptive anxiety states may be related to the patient's developmental history: defective ability to trust or unresolved dependency conflicts, e.g., the fear of helplessness, and the loss of control. Conflicts over guilt and castration are lifelong. The worst anxiety encountered may be that associated with defective maternal bonding, where abandonment appears to be the object of fear. An example is the dying daughter, now overwhelmed by anxiety she cannot pinpoint or understand, for whom separation from mother has always been a major unresolved issue. Where the mother is available and willing, therapy of both simultaneously can be helpful, but since death's separation seems so irreversibly final, considerable discomfort may remain throughout the time left for treatment.

Increased anxiety may be associated with specific memories and associations to the death of parents or others one identifies with (as the woman whose family members died of breast cancer or the AIDS patient who tended a lover dying of it), where the patient pictures the same fate for herself, for example, agonizing pain or a violent scenario with excessive use of technology. Such stories may not come to light without explicit questions.

For further discussion on palliation of anxiety, see chapter 4.

Delirium and Dementia.   Cognitive difficulties are common. Concomitant confusion, wandering, sundowning, agitation, and belligerence add significant distress for everyone involved. Successful control of these difficulties (see chapters 6) makes an invaluable contribution to the care of the dying.

Axis II

Axis II in DSM-IV is used for reporting personality disorders (e.g., paranoid, schizoid, narcissistic, borderline, antisocial, dependent) and mental retardation. It may also be used for noting prominent maladaptive personality features and defense mechanisms. Because interpersonal relationships are the single most powerful supporting force at the end of life, these factors regularly complicate relationships, and during the last phase of life may pose obstacles to harmonious relations and quality of life. One skilled in handling traits like dependency, passive aggressiveness, hostility, and a histrionic style can provide for caregivers and family advice that lighten the burdens on everyone. When a personality disorder is severe, care may be disrupted unless professional intervention comes to the rescue.

Dependency on others is hard for many to tolerate. It was third on the list of reasons why those in the Netherlands requested euthanasia. One of the demands of maturity is to accept help from those we trust. Yet resolves like "If I have to be diapered by someone, that is where I draw the line" are not uncommon when persons think about the end of life. It is perhaps inevitable that we fear being a burden to others, especially those we love. Nevertheless, it may be helpful to ask patients who object to the work their illness imposes on family whether they feel that the work is an unacceptable burden or an opportunity to give something back to the dying person. Could the patient's accepting help give her children a chance to make a major contribution to a meaningful death and feel proud of this accomplishment and better about themselves, thereby creating a positive memory to hold onto the rest of their lives?

Among the most unfortunate of dying persons are those in the severely narcissistic or borderline range of personality, as well as some persons with a history of severe physical and sexual abuse. For such people, a fatal illness is but one more act of brutal victimization. Unfortunately, it may be difficult to believe that any physician, nurse, or caregiver will do anything but victimize them further. Help is therefore difficult if not impossible to accept and truth. Only a professional with psychodynamic diagnostic and treatment skills may be able to help such a person accept palliative care. See the discussion in chapters 6.

Axis III

Axis III in DSM-IV is used for reporting current general medical conditions that are potentially relevant to the understanding and management of the person's mental disorder. An illness that is threatening or actually taking a person's life is a major determinant of thought and feelings.

Palliation of the effects of the medical illness itself is the primary goal of palliative care and is a complex challenge requiring extensive expertise. Freedom from pain is basic to every care plan and should be achievable in 90% of cases. Pain

control for the cancer patient is described in detail in chapter 9. Unfortunately, palliation is often equated simply with pain control. Even though pain control in itself is so simple in concept that any medical student can master the principles in a few hours, physicians are repeatedly indicted for undertreatment of pain, whether for outpatients with metastatic cancer[37] or terminal AIDS,[38] or for patients dying in prominent academic center ICUs.[39] The same deficiencies are reported in house staff[40] and nurses,[41] although nurses with more education know significantly more.[41] In his presidential address to the twenty-fifth annual meeting of the Society of Critical Care Medicine, John Hoyt said that the ICU study "suggested that ICU physicians did not listen to families. They did not know when to stop treatment. They did not relieve pain and suffering."[42] Fear of addiction and harsh regulatory threats continue to be cited as reasons for this perplexing failure.[43,44] Guidelines for cancer pain management are widely publicized and available.[45,46]

Palliative care includes a vast number of problems more complicated than analgesia for nociceptive pain and is the subject of several texts.[1-6] The American Medical Association[11] and the American Board of Internal Medicine[45] have made available an educational resource documents on palliative care for all physicians.

Axis IV

In DSM-IV Axis IV is used to categorize psychosocial and environmental stressors that may be affecting the person's mental state. Here the caption is used for systematic review of all the potential psychosocial and environmental resources that may be available to help improve the quality of life.

Family.   For family and close friends, a fatal illness may be the only reality important enough to resolve long-standing conflicts. Comments such as "No mother wants to die with the thought that her children will never speak to one another again" may motivate individuals to rally to their mother and cooperate to ease her last months. Reconciliation may also result. Likewise, saying to the family gathered around the patient, "And I hope many years from now none of you will think 'If only I had told Dad/Jane this or that.'

You have time for this now." Making peace should be high on the agenda. Specific plans for the family are important: writing wills, clarifying the family history, reviewing the high points of family gatherings and achievements, undertaking family projects like trips or photo album reviews, and planning what sort of a funeral or memorial service to have.

The end of life is an opportunity to give a gift to the younger generation. When they are included in all the planning, the meetings, the discussions, the activities, the care, and final attendance at death, children learn that death need not be violent or terrifying and that the answer to mastering threat is contained in facing the loss itself, when all loved ones rally to put finishing touches on the relationships that are threatened. We face our losses best together.

Occupation and Work. Work has been critical for the self-esteem of many persons. The relationships made in the course of one's occupation should be activated so that self-esteem can be maintained and the sense given of a life lived meaningfully. But the dying person is often too disabled to get around easily; hence, mobilization of friends, especially friends who have been out of touch, needs deliberate attention. Many people begin to feel less valuable when work ceases or they retire. For them, the end of life may intensify a sense of failure. Seeing old friends can remind a dying person who he is, are, what he has accomplished, and that he is still remembered and respected despite the illness.

Recreational Activities. Old friends from athletic teams; bridge groups, and clubs devoted to books, vocal and musical performances, crafts, camping and hiking, political activism, travel, and similar pursuits represent a cadre of persons who knew the sick person as healthy or "complete." In their presence, no matter how changed by illness, one can often recapture old moments and remember former health, vigor, effectiveness, and normality, of which disease has deprived one. Having a serious illness is itself justification for forming new relationships, and self-help groups have been exceptionally helpful for all kinds of sufferers.

Interests, hobbies, and pastimes, even though pursued alone, represent a resource of pleasure. Family members should help the sick person list all the books, music, movies, and other forms of pleasure and entertainment that were high points or that brought regular pleasure. Not only can these be obtained for the person during this time of life, but long after the individual has lost the strength to read or use recording devices, a loved one can read to him, put on videotapes, and play musical favorites. What were the favorite passages from the Bible, poetry passages, history, or biography that were most comical, dramatic, uplifting, or inspiring? While visiting or attending the sick person, a family member or friend can sing or play a musical instrument, read the daily headlines, or reminisce about meaningful past events.

Role of Religious Faith and Value Systems. Lester[47] and Feifel[48] have reviewed much of the conflicting literature on the relationship between religious faith and fear of death. Other research has tried to clarify the way belief systems function within the individual. Allport[49] contrasted an extrinsic religious orientation, in which religion is mainly a means to social status, security, or relief from guilt, with an intrinsic religious orientation, in which the values appear to be internalized and subscribed to as ends in themselves. Feagin[50] provided a useful 21-item questionnaire for distinguishing these two types of believers. Experimental work[51] and clinical experience indicate that an extrinsic value system, without internalization, seems to offer no assistance in coping with a fatal illness. A religious commitment that is intrinsic, on the other hand, appears to offer considerable stability and strength to those who possess it.

Koenig et al.[52] have shown that, for depressed patients, stronger reliance on religion for coping significantly reduced cognitive, but not somatic, symptoms. Loss of interest, boredom, social withdrawal, feelings of being downhearted and blue, restlessness, a sense of failure or hopelessness, and a sense that other people are better off were rated as significantly less severe by religious patients.

One way of examining personal faith is to regard it as another personal relationship, this time with God. Although psychiatric training has often made practitioners suspicious of, hostile to, or uncomfortable with anything associated with religion, people who have a strong internalized faith possess a resource that helps significantly to negotiate a fatal illness. Exploration of this area is mandatory.[9,10]

Many patients are grateful for the chance to express their own thoughts about their faith. Faith is framed in psychological perspective simply as a relationship between the person and God. The patient is asked about God via the same questions used to assess the quality of relationship with a parent, friend, or any significant other. For you, what sort of a person is God? Do you picture God? Where? In what historical context was God introduced to you? Warm, secure, pleasant? Cold, scrutinizing, punitive? Does God regard you as a favorite? A black sheep? What sort of trust is there, you for God and vice versa? Does this sense of relationship give you confidence that God truly exists? What is the most powerful sense you have had of God's presence? Do you doubt? When you doubt, how is the sense of relationship affected? In general, the person's ability to tolerate doubt is a good index of the maturity of faith. If we *knew*, faith would be unnecessary. Doubt, as Gregory Baum said, is the shadow cast by faith.

Do you communicate with God? Pray? Do you feel heard? Is communication a two-way process? Do you have any sense of God speaking to you? How? Do you get answers or ever feel certain of getting a message in return? Do you (ever) feel "in touch"? Cared about? Do prayers ever feel like "dead letters" sent to an unoccupied address? What then?

Discussing the terminal illness provides an excellent chance to inquire about the patient's view of the age-old problem of evil. Given that you have such a severe or life-threatening illness, just where does God stand in this? Sympathetic? If all good and loving, how could God permit it to happen to you? Do you feel supported? Punished? Justly punished? Betrayed? Are you still able to pray? How has all this affected your prayer or dialogue with God?

When the conversation touches death, it is an opportunity to ask the patient's beliefs about an afterlife. Is there anything after? Do you ever picture it? Does this comfort you somehow or in any way ease some aspects of this illness? In general, those persons who possess a sense of a benign personal presence of God, of being cared for and watched over, will continue to do so, and it will help them maintain tranquility in their struggle with terminal illness. Firm religious convictions signal that a consultation with the chaplain should be discussed with the patient. The patient's own minister or rabbi, if available, usually can provide many valuable facts and insights about the patient and family and help uniquely to smooth the overall course before death.

Religious persons ordinarily are part of a community of believers who can be unusually thoughtful and generous in providing support. Again, they may not have been informed of the patient's plight and may need to be contacted. Does the person feel some need of reconciliation to God or to the community? Should the personal clergyperson be contacted?

For those without religious ties, strong convictions about life and values may be coded in a philosophy of life. What is important? What principles or guidelines have you tried to live by? Is there anything worth dying for? What are you proudest of? These issues are the material out of which a dying person may confirm a sense of a life lived well enough. If important persons have rallied to the patient, there may also be the sense of living on in their memories as an intact and valued person.

Society.   A dying person may be burdened by shame for actions censored or disapproved of by others. A person who has committed a crime, hurt a loved one, abandoned a family, or been disabled by a chronic disease may feel disowned by society. The intense work with caregivers and friends to get through the end of life with courage and graciousness can establish in such a person a sense of being respected as a worthwhile, even admirable human being.

Psychoeducational Group Treatment.   Cancer patients who participate in a psychoeducational treatment group gain significant advantages, including improved mood, reduced anxiety, and more adaptive coping skills. The most dramatic benefit demonstrated so far is the significant prolongation of life demonstrated for both breast cancer[53] and melanoma[54] patients. The Internet is also a potential source of information, advice, and electronic camaraderie.

Axis V

In DSM-IV, Axis V is used to report the clinician's overall estimate of the patient's global function. Here it is used as a reminder that maximizing function is a major goal of palliative care, namely that quality of life be maximized to the extent that a person can function as he or she wishes.

When things go well, care of the dying is a process of mutual growth. Just as the deterioration of another stricken by a fatal disease can be threatening (we feel both horrified at the prospect of the same happening to us and helpless to assist), the response of the dying person to the challenge may be not only edifying but an invaluable lesson in coping to everyone involved, including caregivers.

Nonabandonment is one of the most important principles in end-of-life care. Despite frustration, seemingly unsolvable problems, and relentless deterioration, one must learn that one's presence itself is of value. Near the end of life a patient may be too weak to communicate by speech, and sometimes consciousness itself is difficult to assess. Most patients who have lost the ability to communicate have a period when they can still hear or perceive those in attendance. Family feelings of helpless can be minimized by planning to read specially meaningful passages to the dying person, such as the daily headlines, favorite authors or columnists, poetry, passages from the Bible, the Dow Jones average, sports scores, letters new and old, and so on. Conversations should make natural reference to the person as if hearing and understanding were intact. Singing favorite songs, playing favorite music, or praying aloud may increase the sense of unity and purpose for the family. Although the patient may never be able to tell us how important that time is, an occasional incident will do so dramatically, as when a supposed "unconscious" person suddenly smiles appropriately, gestures, or even voices gratitude for the attention given her, which is very rewarding for loved ones in attendance.

One hopes that this mutual work at the end of life will have ratified the dying person's sense of self and given the family, friends, and caregivers a sense that they have provided good care and safe passage. The memory of the final phase of the sick person's life, though sad because of the loss, can be cherished with satisfaction and pride.

DIFFICULTIES FACING THOSE WHO CARE FOR THE DYING[10]

First in psychological importance among the caregiver's responsibility to the dying person is to understand. To do this, as Saunders[55] says, is "above all to listen." What is the experience like?

A suffering person often wants to communicate how awful a fatal illness is. Words are often irrelevant. "When no answers exist," says Saunders, "one can offer silent attention."

The best way to recognize and acknowledge the person's worth is to get to know those features of his history and nature that make him unique. The empathic effort takes its toll, most often by the insights the patients give us about ourselves. Their needs and vulnerabilities bring us face to face with our own. The relentless approach of death for a patient with cancer or AIDS may leave him with feelings of terror, hopelessness, and despair—which tend to be contagious, intensifying our feelings of impotence.

At this point our own helplessness and despair may endanger the patient, causing us to avoid him, retreat, neglect him, or even, feeling he would be better off dead, convey to him how burdensome he is to us. This can be devastating to the helpless person who looks to his doctor or nurse for some sense of hope. Hence, the greatest psychological challenge for caregivers is to learn to live with these negative feelings and to resist the urge to avoid the patients—actions that convey to the patient, not that it is difficult for us, but that he no longer matters. Fortunately, most patients, feeling that they are acceptable to their caregivers no matter how scared, disfigured, or miserable they are, find resources within and make what they can of each day. That sort of shared experience is an opportunity to grow for both persons.

Certain traits make these empathic difficulties hazardous for some caregivers. Dependent persons who expect patients to appreciate, thank, love, and nurture them are unconsciously prone to exhaust themselves regularly by "doing too much," a pattern that may be sustainable for a patient with the capacity to nurture the caregiver but has a disastrous outcome when the patient is completely depleted or intractably hostile. The harder the caregiver strives, the less rewarding the work. Exhaustion and demoralization follow. Some caregivers want to please every physician they consult and come to similar exhaustion because many of the patients cannot improve.

REFERENCES

1. Billings JA (ed). *The Outpatient Management of Advanced Cancer.* Philadelphia: J.B. Lippincott Company, 1985.

2. Cherny NI, Foley KM. *Pain and Palliative Care.* *Hematology/Oncology Clinics of North America.* Philadelphia: WB Saunders Company, 1996.

3. Doyle D, Hanks GWC, MacDonald N (eds): *Oxford Textbook of Palliative Medicine.* Oxford: Oxford University Press, 1993.

4. Walsh TD (ed). *Symptom Control.* Cambridge Mass: Blackwell Scientific Publications, 1989.

5. Woodruff R. *Palliative Medicine.* Melbourne, Australia: Asperula, 1993.

6. American Board of Internal Medicine. *Caring for the Dying. Identification and Promotion of Physician Competency* American Board of Internal Medicine, 1999.

7. Breitbart W, Holland JC (eds). *Psychiatric Aspects of Symptom Management in Cancer Patients.* Washington, DC: American Psychiatric Press, 1993: 173–230.

8. Breitbart W, Chochinov HM, Passik. S. Psychiatric aspects of palliative care. In: Doyle D, Hanks G, MacDonald N (eds), The Oxford Textbook of Palliative Medicine, 2nd ed. New York: Oxford Unviersity Press, 1997: 933–954.

9. Cassem NH. The Person confronting death. In: Nicholi AM Jr (ed), *The Harvard Guide to Psychiatry,* Cambridge, Mass: Harvard University Press, 1999: 699–734.

10. Cassem NH. The dying patient. In: Cassem NH, ed. *Massachusetts General Hospital Handbook of General Hospital Psychiatry,* 4th ed. St. Louis: Mosby YearBook, 1997: 605–636.

11. Council on Scientific Affairs, American Medical Association. Good care of the dying patient. *Journal of the American Medical Association,* 1996; 275:474–478.

12. Holland JC (ed). *Psycho-oncology,* New York: Oxford University Press, 1998.

13. Institute of Medicine. *Approaching Death. Improving Care at the End of Life.* Washington DC: National Academy Press, 1997.

14. Saunders C (ed). *The Management of Terminal Illness.* Chicago: Year Book Medical Publishers, 1978.

15. Kelly WD, Friesen SR. Do cancer patients want to be told? *Surgery* 1950; 27:822–826.

16. Gilbertsen VA, Wangensteen OH. Should the doctor tell the patient that the disease is cancer? Surgeon's recommendation, in American Cancer Society, *The Physician and the Total Care of the Cancer Patient.* New York: American Cancer Society, 1962:80–85.

17. Aitken-Swan J, Easson EC. Reactions of cancer patients on being told their diagnosis. *British Medical Journal,* 1959; 1:779–783.

18. Gerlé B, Lundgen G, Sandblom P. The patient with inoperable cancer from the psychiatric and social standpoints. *Cancer* 1960; 13:1206–1217.

19. Hackett TP, Weisman AD. The treatment of the dying. *Current Psychiatric Ther,* 1962;2:121–126.

20. Oken D. What to tell cancer patients: A study of medical attitudes. *Journal of the American Medical Association,* 1961; 175:1120–1128.

21. Novack DH, Plumer R, Smith RL, et al. Changes in physicians' attitudes toward telling the cancer patient. *Journal of the American Medical Association,* 1979; 241:897–900.

22. Croog SH, Shapiro SD, Levine S. Denial among male heart patients. *Psychosomatic Medicine,* 1971; 33:385–397.

23. Buckman R. *How to Break Bad News—A Guide for Health Care Professionals.* London: Macmillan Medical, 1993.

24. Saunders C. The moment of truth: Care of the dying person. In: Pearson L, ed. *Death and Dying.* Cleveland: Case Western Reserve University Press, 1969:49–78.

25. Kübler-Ross E. *On Death and Dying.* New York: Macmillan, 1969.

26. LeShan L, LeShan E. Psychotherapy and the patient with a limited life span. *Psychiatry,* 1961; 24:318–323.

27. LeShan L. Psychotherapy and the dying patient. In: Pearson L, ed. *Death and Dying.* Cleveland: Case Western Reserve University Press, 1969:28–48.

28. Weisman AD, Hackett TP. Predilection to death: Death and dying as a psychiatric problem. *Psychosomatic Medicine,* 1961; 23:232–256.

29. Cassell EJ. *The Nature of Suffering.* New York: Oxford University Press, 1991.

30. Bernardine J. *The Gift of Peace.* Chicago: Loyola Press, 1977.

31. World Health Organization. Cancer pain relief and palliative care: Report of a WHO Expert Committee. Geneva: World Health Organization, 1990.

32. Weisman AD. *The Vulnerable Self.* New York: Insight Books, 1993.

33. Van der Maas PJ, van Delden JJM, Pijnenborg L, Looman CWN. Euthanasia and other medical decisions concerning the end of life. *Lancet,* 1991; 338:669–674.

34. *Diagnostic and Statistical Manual of Mental Disorders,* 4th ed. DSM-IV. Washington DC: American Psychiatric Association, 1994.

35. Cassem NH. Depression and anxiety secondary to medical illness. *Psychiatric Clin North America,* 1990; 13(4):597–612.

36. Freud S. The ego and the id. In: Strachey J, transed, *Standard Edition,* vol. 19. London: Hogarth Press, 1961.

37. Cleeland CS, Gonin R, Hatfield AK, et al. Pain

and its treatment in outpatients with metastatic cancer. *New England Journal of Medicine*, 1994; 330:592–596.

38. Kimball LR, McCormick WC. The pharmacologic management of pain and discomfort in persons with AIDS near the end of life: Use of opioid analgesia in the hospice setting. *Journal of Pain Symptom Management*, 1996; 11:88–94.

39. The SUPPORT Principal Investigators: A controlled trial to improve care for seriously ill hospitalized patients. *Journal of the American Medical Association*, 1995; 274:1591–1598.

40. Sloan PA, Donnelly MB, Schwartz RW, Sloan DA. Cancer pain assessment and management by housestaff. *Pain*, 1996; 67:475–481.

41. Brunier G, Carson G, Harrison DE. What do nurses know and believe about patients with pain? Results of a hospital survey. *Journal of Pain and Symptom Management*, 1995; 10:436–445,

42. Hoyt JW. Critical care in 1996: Doing too much? Doing too little? Keeping the patient in focus during a time of smoke and fire. *Critical Care Medicine* 1996; 11:88–94.

43. Hill CS Jr. The barriers to adequate pain management with opioid analgesics. *Semin Oncology*, 1993; 20(suppl):1–5.

44. Reidenberg MM. Barriers to controlling pain in patients with cancer. *Lancet* 1996; 347:1278.

45. Jadad AR, Browman GP. The WHO analgesic ladder for cancer pain management: Stepping up the quality of its evaluation. *Journal of the American Medical Association*, 1995; 274:1874–1880.

46. Jacox A, Carr DB, Payne R, et al. *Management of cancer pain: Clinical practice guideline No. 9.* Rockville, Md: US Public Health Service, Agency for Health Care Policy and Research; March 1994. AHCPR publication 94-0592.

47. Lester D: Religious behaviors and attitudes toward death, in Godin A ed. *Death and Presence.* Brussels: Lumen Vitae, 1972:107–124.

48. Feifel H. Religious conviction and fear of death among the healthy and the terminally ill. *Journal of the Science Study Religion*, 1974; 13:353–360.

49. Allport G. *The Nature of Prejudice.* New York: Doubleday, 1958.

50. Feagin JR. Prejudice and religious types: Focused study, Southern Fundamentalists. *Journal of Science Study of Religion*, 1964; 4:3–13.

51. Magni KG: The fear of death. In: Godin A, ed. *Death and Presence.* Brussels: Lumen Vitae, 1972: 125–138.

52. Koenig HG, Cohen HJ, Blazer DG, et al. Religious coping and cognitive symptoms of depression in elderly medical patients. *Psychosomatics* 1995; 36:369–375.

53. Spiegel D, Bloom JR, Kraemer HC, Gottheil E. Effects of psychosocial treatment on survival of patients with metastatic breast cancer. *Lancet* 1989; 2:888–891.

54. Fawzy FI, Fawzy NW, Hun CS, et al. Malignant melanoma. Effects of an early structured psychiatric intervention, coping, and affective state on recurrence and survival 6 years later. *Archives of General Psychiatry*, 1993; 50:681–689.

55. Saunders C. Foreword. In Kearney M, *Mortally Wounded.* Dublin: Marino Books, 1996:11–12.

3

Diagnosis and Management of Depression in Palliative Care

Keith G. Wilson, Ph.D.
Harvey Max Chochinov, M.D., Ph.D., FRCPC
Barbara J. de Faye, M.A.
William Breitbart, M.D.

Depression is recognized as the most common mental health problem that arises in the palliative-care setting, yet it is also a construct that is widely misunderstood. The term "depressed" is so ubiquitous in colloquial expression that its specific clinical meaning, as a diagnostic term identifying a discrete and treatable syndrome, is often blurred. This blurring can be reinforced by the fact that depression does not occur with a clearly bimodal distribution separating patients who are depressed from those who are not. Rather, there is a continuum of severity for depressive symptoms, and somewhere along that continuum individual clinicians must make decisions about with whom to initiate treatment. In the case of patients with medical illness, these treatment decisions are apparently not being made as often as is warranted by the available data, because depression still tends to be underdiagnosed and undertreated.[1,2] For example, Goldberg and Mor[3] found that only 3% of patients with terminal cancer were being treated with antidepressant medications, despite a substantial body of evidence demonstrating that the prevalence of depressive disorders in this population is much higher than average.

The goal of this chapter is to provide an overview of the topic of depression in palliative care, with a specific emphasis on patients with advanced cancer. It addresses such issues as rea-sons for the underdiagnosis of depression, problems and options in diagnostic assessment, current knowledge about the prevalence and risk factors for depressive disorders, and treatment considerations for clinical management.

REASONS FOR THE UNDERDIAGNOSIS OF DEPRESSION

Massie[4] has discussed several reasons that clinicians tend to be hesitant in diagnosing and treating depression in patients with advanced cancer. First, many clinicians believe that depression, even if quite severe, is a completely appropriate reaction to the circumstances surrounding the patient's illness. In this event, clinicians may consider the initiation of treatment as interference with the process of coming to terms with death and dying. Second, clinicians may minimize the significance of depression and believe that almost all dying patients are "depressed," as manifested in expressions of sadness, fear, or occasional tearfulness.

Another issue for clinicians who do intend to initiate treatment is that they may be uncomfortable with their options. There is the concern that patients with severe medical illness will not be able to tolerate the side effects or drug interactions associated with the addition of an antidepressant to their regimen. Hence, these clinicians may take a very conservative approach when prescribing antidepressants, perhaps limiting their clinical effectiveness. The utility of psychotherapy, on the other hand, has been less well validated in this population, requires specialized training, and may not work quickly enough to be of primary therapeutic value for patients with a limited life expectancy.

Sometimes clinicians are also uncomfortable in probing too deeply into the psychological experiences of their patients. This may be due partly to a genuine sensitivity to the individual's care and a desire not to be intrusive regarding personal concerns that might get the patient upset.[5] Partly, it may also be due to clinicians' own discomfort in responding to the psychological issues of their dying patients. Whatever the reasons, it is common for clinicians to use various distancing tactics to contain the expression of emotional distress. These tactics include giving false reassurance to the patient with overly positive statements and selectively attending to patient disclosures of physical, rather than psychological concerns.[6] In general, professionals who work with the medically ill are not very accurate at estimating the level of psychological distress of their patients.[7–9] This is not simply a shortcoming on the part of caregivers, however; patients themselves can be quite sensitive to the possibility of causing discomfort among those around them. Hinton,[10] for example, found that 11% of patients in the final weeks of life completely concealed their feelings from others, while a further 35% were reticent about self-disclosure.

These are unfortunate barriers to the recognition and treatment of depression in palliative care, because, in fact, not all patients with terminal illness are depressed, and those who are can often be helped significantly with prompt diagnosis and well-managed intervention.[4,11] The consequences of failing to treat depression can include a reduction in the patient's quality of life and greater difficulty in managing the course of the patient's illness, resulting in earlier admission to inpatient or hospice care.[12,13]

COPING WITH CANCER

By the time patients approach the palliative stage of care, most will have gone through a process of investigation, physical diagnosis, and therapy with protocols that involve varying degrees of pain and trauma. Each of these phases has psychological consequences. For example, the investigative phase may be associated with considerable fear as one prepares for the possibility of a catastrophic diagnosis. After diagnosis, many patients experience a sense of numbing shock, punctuated by periods of anxiety and dysphoria.[4,11] Active treatment may entail disfiguring side effects and pain that tax one's psychological resources. Throughout these periods, the threat of loss of physical integrity, the possibility of deterioration in mental and functional capacities, changes in family and social roles, increasing dependence on the medical system, as well as the ultimate prospect of death, can all serve as sources of chronic mental strain. In general, patients may turn to a variety of strategies in order to cope with the distress associated with these events. Although their ways of coping may range from frank denial to stoic acceptance, some investigators have found that those who adopt more active strategies (e.g., seeking social support; constructive problem solving; focusing on the positive) may show better long-term adjustment than those who rely more often on passive-avoidant strategies (e.g., social withdrawal; rumination[14–17]). Nevertheless, the emotional consequences of coping with a life-threatening illness may include periods of anxiety, sadness, fatalism, and grief, all of which can be considered part of the normal adjustment process.[11,17] However, when the experience of depression becomes especially severe, pervasive, and prolonged to the point of interference with functional abilities, then the likelihood of a clinically significant depressive disorder is high.

ASSESSMENT OF DEPRESSION

There are two broad types of assessment procedures for depression that are in common use: criterion-based diagnostic systems and self-report measures.

Criterion-Based Diagnostic Systems

Criterion-based diagnostic systems include the Diagnostic and Statistical Manual of Mental Disorders, fourth edition (DSM-IV),[18] or its predecessors (DSM-III; DSM-III-R) and the Research Diagnostic Criteria (RDC[19]). These systems are based on the assumption that depression is a distinct syndromal disorder characterized by a constellation of symptoms, of a certain minimal level of severity and duration, that are associated with impairment in functional and social roles. The DSM-IV criteria for major depressive disorder, the most severe and well-documented diagnosis within the depression spectrum, are shown in Table 3.1. There are two core criterion symptoms for major depression in the DSM-IV—depressed mood and anhedonia, a marked loss of interest or pleasure in activities. In order to qualify for the diagnosis, a patient must exhibit 1 of these core symptoms, along with at least four other symptoms from the criterion list. In cases where the depressive syndrome is clearly caused by the direct physiological effect of a medication or other psychoactive substance, or by metabolic or neurochemical disturbances created by the disease process, then the diagnosis of mood syndrome secondary to the general medical condition would be more appropriately.

Issues in the Assessment of Depression in Palliative Care

The core criterion symptom of loss of interest or pleasure in activities merits some discussion when applied to patients in palliative care. Ultimately, all patients with advanced cancer experience a functional decline that restricts their physical ability to participate in activities. Furthermore, some disengagement from areas of interest that were of secondary importance are common among individuals who refocus their priorities to areas of deeper significance. When anhedonia is pervasive, however, and extends to a loss of interest or pleasure in almost all activities, including the social comforts of interaction with family and friends, then most authors consider it to be a valid criterion for the assessment of depression.[11,17]

In addition to major depression, there are other diagnoses that have depressed mood as a central presenting feature. Minor depression is similar to major depression but requires fewer symptoms in order to qualify for a diagnosis (two to four symptoms in total). Like major depression, minor depression is considered to be an episodic disorder. Dysthymia, in contrast, is defined as a chronic condition characterized by low-grade depressive symptoms that persist for at least two years. Adjustment disorder with depressed mood, on the other hand, describes a relatively short-lived maladaptive reaction to stress. This diagnosis requires that a patient's depressive response to the stressor must be "in excess of a normal and expectable reaction."

The diagnosis of adjustment disorder is a controversial one in palliative care.[4,17] It requires a

Table 3.1   DSM-IV Symptoms of Major Depressive Syndrome and Substitute Symptoms Recommended by Endicott (1984)

Symptom	Substitute
* Depressed mood most of the day	
* Markedly diminished interest or pleasure in all, or almost all, activities most of the day	
Weight loss or gain (e.g., more than 5% of body weight in a month) or decrease or increase in appetite	Depressed appearance
Insomnia or hypersomnia	Social withdrawal or decreased talkativeness
Psychomotor agitation or retardation	
Fatigue or loss of energy	Brooding, self-pity, or pessimism
Feelings of worthlessness or excessive or inappropriate guilt	
Diminished ability to think or concentrate, or indecisiveness	Lack of reactivity; cannot be cheered up
Recurrent thoughts of death, or suicidal ideation or planning, or a suicide attempt	

Note: One of the symptoms marked by an asterisk (*) must be present for a diagnosis of major depressive syndrome. Each symptom must also meet severity (e.g., "most of the day, nearly every day") and duration (greater than 2 weeks) criteria. Finally, the symptoms must be judged to cause clinically significant distress or impairment; they must not be due to the direct physiological effects of a medication or general medical condition; and they must not be better accounted for by bereavement.

subjective judgment as to what is a "normal and expectable response" to catastrophic medical circumstances. If applied loosely, it risks over-pathologizing the experience of some patients by applying a potentially stigmatizing psychiatric label to what may be a normal display of grief.

In addition to the controversy surrounding the diagnosis of adjustment disorder, a review of the criterion symptoms of depression shown in Table 2.1 reveals another obvious problem: Several of the defining symptoms are somatic in nature, and therefore their validity for patients with advanced medical illness can be questioned. Problems such as weight loss, fatigue, sleep disturbance, and poor concentration are common symptoms of the disease process in cancer, and they can also be associated with the side effects of treatment. In this context, should they be allowed contribute to a diagnosis of depression?

Several options have been proposed for handling the issue of confounding somatic symptoms.[20] The DSM-IV recommends that symptoms be excluded from consideration if they are caused directly by a medical condition. In practice, however, this distinction can be a difficult one to make. Technically, it also makes the standard for fulfilling diagnostic criteria more stringent.[21] For example, when all symptoms are included, a diagnosis of major depression requires that 5 of 9 criterion symptoms be present. If four symptoms are then excluded because of possible confounding with medical illness, then a patient must have all five of the remaining symptoms before the diagnostic criteria for major depression can be met. This is a very strict standard that would identify only the most severely depressed patients.

Cassem[22] has pointed out that the risks of failing to treat depression because of false negative diagnoses is greater, on balance, than the risks of initiating unnecessary therapy on the basis of a false positive. Hence, he suggests that it would be better for clinicians to err on the side of caution and include somatic symptoms in their diagnostic assessments of the medically ill. When this approach is used, however, there is the possibility that the prevalence rates of depressive disorders among medical patients will be exaggerated.

As an alternative position between these exclusive and inclusive approaches, Endicott[21] has proposed a substitutive method that removes somatic symptoms from the diagnostic criteria but

replaces them with different symptoms that address other nonsomatic features of depression. Endicott's proposed substitutions are presented in Table 2.1, alongside the DSM-IV somatic criterion symptoms that they are intended to replace.

Diagnostic Interviews

For research purposes, diagnostic assessments are usually conducted using structured interviews such as the Diagnostic Interview Schedule (DIS),[23] the Structured Clinical Interview for DSM-III-R (SCID),[24] or the Schedule for Affective Disorders and Schizophrenia (SADS).[25] These interviews differ with respect to their degree of structure and in the formats with which the interviewer codes the patient's verbal responses. The DIS is highly structured so that it can be used by lay interviewers in epidemiologic studies, whereas the SCID and SADS are semistructured and are intended for use by clinicians. With the DIS and the SCID, the interviewer is required to code specific symptoms as being either present or absent, whereas with the SADS, the interviewer rates the severity of symptoms on ordinal scales. All of these interview protocols have been subjected to extensive checks for reliability and validity.

If administered in their entirety, these interviews cover a broad range of common mental disorders. However, they can be very time-consuming, which seriously limits their use in palliative-care settings. More commonly, investigators may choose to administer only the modules within an interview that address the problem of depression. For example, Chochinov et al.[26] administered the depression module of the SADS to patients with advanced cancer in an inpatient palliative-care unit. They found that the inter-rater reliability for the RDC diagnoses of major or minor depression was kappa = .76, which reflects substantial agreement comparable to the levels found in studies of the general population or psychiatric patients.

Recently, Spitzer et al.[1] have developed a brief screening protocol for use by primary-care clinicians that seems to have good applicability to palliative care. The Primary Care Evaluation of Mental Disorders (PRIME-MD) uses a two-stage approach to review the DSM-IV criteria for major depression, minor depression, and dysthymia. In addition, it addresses the common anxiety syndromes of panic disorder and generalized anxiety disorder and provides a brief screen for alcohol abuse. In the first stage, the patient completes a one-page self-report checklist that covers only the most central symptoms of each disorder, using a simple yes/no response format. Using a structured interview guide, the clinician follows up on those symptoms acknowledged on the checklist (ensuring that they meet DSM-IV severity and duration criteria) and probes the remaining symptoms required to make a diagnosis. Spitzer et al. have found that the PRIME-MD shows good concordance with independent diagnoses made by mental health professionals and can be completed within 20 minutes for 95% of patients. Its brevity and comprehensiveness suggest that the PRIME-MD would be a suitable choice for both research and clinical use in palliative care, although the self-report component would have to be replaced with an interview administration for the most severely compromised patients.

Sometimes investigators have constructed their own semistructured interviews for use in palliative care, modifying the diagnostic criteria to account for the unique circumstances of this group of patients.[27,28] This approach has some disadvantages, however. The purpose of structured interviews is to enhance the reliability of clinical diagnostic assessments. When well-tested, psychometrically sound protocols are already widely available, new interviews must be tested rigorously for their reliability characteristics in order to represent an advance over existing measures. This has seldom been done in palliative-care research. Hence, an expert panel on the neuropsychiatric aspects of advanced cancer has recommended the utilization of existing validated tools in prevalence and intervention research.[29]

Self-Report Measures

In primary-care settings, nonpsychiatric clinicians fail to identify depressive disorders in 46% to 67% of the patients who qualify for a diagnosis on the basis of structured interview assessments.[1,2] This low rate of concordance suggests that any methods than can increase the accuracy of identification would be welcome additions to clinical care. Accordingly, a considerable body of research has examined the extent to which self-report mea-

sures can assist in this process, and some of this research has focused on cancer patients.

Among the measures that have been used in this context are the 11-item short form of the Beck Depression Inventory (BDI-SF);[30] the 14-item Hospital Anxiety and Depression Scale (HADS);[31] the 60-item General Health Questionnaire (GHQ);[32] the 8-item psychological symptoms subscale of the Rotterdam Symptom Checklist (RSCL);[33] and the 11-item short form of the Carroll Depression Rating Scale (CDRS),[34] which Golden et al.[35] validated for use with cancer patients. Although many other self-report measures of depressive symptoms are available in the literature, the advantages of these particular scales is that they have been developed or adapted for use with medical populations and have been tested in various groups of patients with cancer. Hence, information is available regarding the optimal cutoff scores for maximizing their concordance with the criterion standard of structured interview diagnoses administered by mental health professionals.

Table 3.2 provides an overview of studies with cancer patients that have used receiver-operating characteristics to determine the sensitivity (proportion of clinically diagnosed patients who score above the optimal cutoff on the questionnaire) and specificity (proportion of nondepressed patients who score below the cutoff) of different self-report measures. There are two main findings from these studies. First, even those that have used the same screening questionnaire (i.e., the HADS) have identified optimal cutoff scores that vary over a wide range. The discrepancies appear to be related to the characteristics of the patients and the type and stage of disease and, more important, to the range of depressive syndromes that are included in the criterion-standard diagnosis. For example, studies that include adjustment disorders identify much lower cutoff scores than those that screen only for the more severe major depressive episodes.

Second, none of the available questionnaires provides perfect concordance with structured interviews. Although some studies have reported marginally higher sensitivities associated with certain questionnaires,[35–40] the trade-off is a lower degree of specificity. In fact, the receiver-operating characteristics of each of the questionnaires appear to be roughly comparable, indicating similar empirical performance for screening depressed patients. Practically, therefore, considerations such as a scale's brevity, simplicity, and

Table 3.2   Screening for Depressive Disorders in Patients with Cancer: Sensitivity and Specificity of Common Self-Report Measures

Measure/ Study	Patients	N	Criterion for Standard Diagnosis	Cutoff Score	Sensitivity	Specificity
HADS						
Hopwood et al. (1991)[36]	Advanced breast cancer	81	DSM-III (depression or anxiety disorders)	≥18	.75	.74
Razavi et al. (1990)[37]	Mixed inpatients	210	Endicott criteria (major depression)	≥19	.70	.74
			DSM-III (major depression or adjustment disorder)	≥13	.75	.75
Razavi et al. (1992)[38]	Lymphoma outpatients	117	DSM-III-R (depression, anxiety or adjustment disorders)	≥10	.84	.66
RSCL						
Hopwood et al. (1991)[36]				≥11	.75	.80
CDRS						
Golden et al. (1991)[35]	Gynecologic cancer	65	DSM-III (major depression)	≥3	.87	.62
GHQ						
Hadman et al. (1989)[39]	Oncology inpatients	126	ICD (depression or anxiety disorders)	≥11	.79	.66
BDI-SF						
Chochinov et al. (1997)[40]	Mixed palliative care inpatients	197	RDC (major or minor depression)	≥8	.79	.71
VAS (100 mm)						
Chochinov et al. (1997)[40]				≤55 mm	.72	.50

Note: HADS = Hospital Anxiety and Depression Scale; RSCL = Rotterdam Symptom Checklist; CDRS = Carroll Depression Rating Scale; BDI-SF = Beck Depression Inventory, Short Form; VAS = Visual Analog Scale.

specific item content should factor into decisions about which ones to select for screening purposes. The average sensitivity (0.78) and specificity (0.71) values translate into estimates that about 22% of depressed patients will *not* score above the cutoff on any particular scale, while the false positive rate will be in the range of 29% of patients screened. Whether or not these error rates are ac-

ceptable depends on the purpose for which the screening is being done. For clinical purposes, a high false-positive rate is not necessarily a problem if screen-positive patients receive a follow-up interview to confirm the diagnosis. A high false-negative rate, on the other hand, presents a greater difficulty because a significant number of depressed patients will not be identified.

Many reasons underlie the lack of concordance between questionnaire assessments of depression and criterion-based diagnostic systems.[41] With questionnaires, for example, different patients can achieve similar summary scores from strongly endorsing only a few items or from weakly endorsing many items. The content of the specific items in a questionnaire is also important. With some questionnaires a patient can score above the scale cutoff without endorsing any individual symptoms that would actually contribute to the diagnosis of depression in a criterion-based system. Finally, most depression rating scales correlate highly with measures of anxiety as well as of depression. For these reasons, some investigators caution that the most common self-report measures of depression should really be used as indices of general distress. Distress in this sense may overlap with the construct of depression as a syndromal disorder, but it is not equivalent.[41]

In palliative care, questionnaires can also pose a burden for patients whose medical circumstances make it difficult for them to read. This limitation underscores the importance of simple measures for palliative case assessments, where depression is typically only one of several important symptom dimensions that must be reviewed. For this reason, visual analog scales have come into common use in palliative-care settings.[42] Chochinov et al.[40] have recently described the screening characteristics of a 100-mm visual analog scale of depressed mood (anchored at the endpoints with the descriptors 0 = "worst possible mood" and 1 = "best possible mood"), which was taken from the Memorial Pain Assessment Card.[43] The patients comprised a mixed group of inpatients with advanced cancer, and the criterion standard diagnoses were major and minor depressive episodes defined according to structured interviews. They found that the optimal cutoff score (55 mm) provided less accurate screening than the Beck Depression Inventory—Short Form. Thus, visual analog scales seem to provide a rather crude substitute for a careful diagnostic interview.

Interestingly, Chochinov et al.[40] also examined a brief interview-based screening for depression, which consisted simply of two questions addressing the core criterion symptoms of depressed mood and less of interest or pleasure in activities. They found that this method was actually quite accurate in identifying patients who qualified for a diagnosis on the basis of the administration of a full interview that covered all of the criterion symptoms of depression. Hence, they recommended that this type of brief screening be incorporated more routinely into clinical contacts.

In summary, then, the limitations of assessments with the more common self-report measures of depression should be recognized. Self-report and visual analog scales certainly have a role to play in providing gross assessments when direct interviews are not feasible, in providing additional information for difficult cases, in quantifying the severity of a depressive syndrome once it has been diagnosed, and in monitoring change over time. However, their efficiency as diagnostic aids in palliative-care settings is unlikely to approach that of a brief interview that directly addresses commonly accepted diagnostic criteria.

PREVALENCE OF DEPRESSION

Table 3.3 presents the results of 14 studies that have reported on the prevalence of depressive disorders in groups of patients receiving care for cancer. All of these studies have used an interview methodology in conjunction with a criterion-based diagnostic system, which should ensure some degree of methodological consistency across investigations. Perhaps the most striking aspect of the various results, therefore, is the degree of discrepancy that has been reported across studies. As is evident in Table 3.3, the prevalence of major depressive disorder has ranged from a low of 1% of patients to more than 40%.[44–50] This lack of consistency in the research literature has important implications for clinical practice. Is depression a common disorder that often goes undetected among patients with cancer,[51] or have clinicians tended to be overinclusive in their approach to diagnosis?[52,53] Unfortunately, this confusing situation probably does little to convince practitioners, who may already be reluctant to raise the issue of depression with their patients, to take a more aggressive stance in their management of this problem.

On the other hand, the reasons for the discrepancies across prevalence studies are beginning to become clear. Partly, they may be due to differences across settings. For example, Derogatis et al.[47] used the same interview protocol across three centers of a multisite study and found that

Table 3.3   Prevalence of Depressive Disorders Among Cancer Patients

Study	Population	N	Diagnostic Criteria	Prevalence
Alexander et al. (1993)[44]	Mixed inpatients	60	DSM-III-R	13% (major depression) 2% (dysthymia) 17% (adjustment disorder with depression)
Bukberg et al. (1984)[27]	Mixed inpatients	62	DSM-III (excluding somatic symptoms)	42% (major depression)
Chochinov et al. (1995)[45]	Mixed palliative-care inpatients	200	RDC	8% (major depression) 5% (minor depression)
Colón et al. (1991)[46]	Acute leukemia	100	DSM-III	1% (major depression) 8% (any adjustment disorder)
Derogatis et al. (1983)[47]	Mixed inpatients and outpatients	215	DSM-III	6% (major depression) 25% (adjustment disorder with depression)
Evans et al. (1986)[48]	Gynecology inpatients	83	DSM-III	23% (major depression) 5% (dysthymia) 13% (adjustment disorder with depression)
Golden et al. (1991)[35]	Gynecology inpatients	83	DSM-III	23% (major depression)
Lansky et al.[50]	Mixed female outpatients and inpatients	505	DSM-III	5% (major depression)
Power et al. (1993)[28]	Mixed palliative-care inpatients	81	DSM-III-R (excluding somatic symptoms)	26% (major depression)
Razavi et al. (1990)[38]	Mixed inpatients	122	Endicott Criteria/DSM-III	8% (major depression) 52% (any adjustment disorder)
Spiegel et al. (1994)[49]	Mixed outpatients	72	DSM-III	22% (major depression) 14% (adjustment disorder with depression)
Jenkins et al. (1991)[73]	Recurrent breast cancer	22	DSM-III	32% major depression
Fallowfied et al. (1986)[77]	Breast cancer	101	DSM-III	21% major depression
Dean (1987)[78]	Breast cancer	122	RDC	10% major depression 18% minor depression

one center had almost three times as many patients as another center who were diagnosed with psychiatric disorders. The authors concluded that the more advanced disease that also characterized patients at the high-diagnosis center probably accounted for this unexpected finding. There is also the possibility that the type of disease is related to the prevalence of depression. Of the studies shown in Table 2.3, the lowest prevalence was found among patients with leukemia who were about to be treated with bone marrow transplation,[46] whereas the highest prevalence was found in inpatients with mostly solid tumors and metastatic spread.[27]

In addition to patient-related factors, however, methodological issues represent a major source of inconsistency. These methodological factors include the diagnostic system that is used to define the depressive disorders of interest. Although the RDC and different versions of the DSM systems are quite similar, they are not identical. Kathol et al.[52] found that when the different systems were applied to the same group of patients, they differed significantly in the prevalence with which patients were diagnosed with major depressive disorder. In that study, the RDC resulted in a lower rate of diagnosis than the DSM-III, by about 13%.

Another methodological issue concerns the diagnosis of adjustment disorder. As noted earlier, this is a controversial diagnosis when applied to patients with life-threatening illnesses, and many prevalence studies have not attempted to address it. When it has been included, the prevalence with which these diagnoses are made is quite high. It is not unusual, for example, for fully 30% to 50% of all cancer patients to be given the diagnosis of adjustment disorder with depressed, anxious, or mixed features.[38,47]

It is also noteworthy that studies that include adjustment disorders as a separate diagnosis tend to report lower rates of the more severe major depressive disorder. In the six studies in Table 2.3 that addressed adjustment disorders, the average prevalence of major depression was 12.2%. Of the eight studies that did not consider adjustment disorders, the average prevalence of major depression was almost double that figure, at 20.9%. Evidently, then, patients are receiving different diagnoses in different studies.

Chochinov et al.[26] hypothesized that part of the discrepancy in prevalence rates across studies has to do with difficulties in agreeing on appropriate severity thresholds for specifying the boundary between "normal" distress and mental disorder. They also found that this distinction can be a very subtle one to make. These investigators administered SADS interviews, with ordinal ratings of symptom severity, to 130 palliative-care inpatients (a subject of the larger group described in Table 2.3). The goal of the study was to examine the impact on the rates of diagnosis of relatively minor differences in symptom severity ratings for the core criterion symptoms. A "high-threshold" diagnosis required a report of either depressed mood at a moderate level of severity (e.g., the patient feels depressed "most of the time") or a report that "almost all" activities are less interesting or pleasurable. These thresholds in fact correspond to those that are recommended in the DSM-IV. A "low-threshold" approach allowed slightly lower symptom severity levels to contribute to a diagnosis. These lower-level symptoms included reports of mild depression, in

which the patient "often feels somewhat depressed," "blue," or "downhearted" (but not "most of the time"), and less severe anhedonia (i.e., the patient finds "most" but not "almost all" activities less interesting or pleasurable).

These relatively minor distinctions had a substantial impact on the rates of diagnosis. Considering major and minor depression together, the high-threshold approach resulted in 13.0% of the patients receiving a diagnosis, compared to 26.1% with the low-threshold method. This type of methodological detail would typically not even be reported in an epidemiologic study, but it goes some way to explaining the diversity of findings in the empirical literature.

Another relevant issue concerns the extent to which the inclusion of somatic symptoms in the diagnostic criteria inflates the rate of diagnosis. This issue was also examined by Chochinov et al.,[26] who found that the problem of confounding by somatic symptoms interacted with the problem of identifying appropriate symptom-severity thresholds. Specifically, they compared the prevalence rates associated with the use of Endicott's substitutive criteria with those obtained with the more standard RDC. They found that with high symptom-severity thresholds, the Endicott and the RDC systems were comparable. When low thresholds were used, however, the Endicott criteria resulted in lower rates of diagnosis. Thus, it appears that the inclusion of somatic symptoms in the diagnostic criteria does not affect the identification of more severe presentations of depression. Patients with less severe presentations, on the other hand, are more likely to be diagnosed as depressed when an inclusive rather than a substitutive approach is used.

In summary, this analysis of the available prevalence literature suggests that the following conclusions can be drawn. First, it appears that about 5% to 15% of patients with cancer will meet criteria for major depression even when the most stringent criteria are used. In the general North American population, the rate of 1-month prevalence of major depression has been estimated at 1.6% to 4.9%.[53,54] Thus, it seems clear that the rate of depression is elevated among cancer patients. Furthermore, another 10% to 15% of patients present with symptoms that are somewhat less severe. In some studies, these patients are considered to be "subthreshold" for a clinical depressive disorder and are classified as not depressed. In other studies, they are apparently being diagnosed with major depression, whereas in yet other studies they are being given the diagnosis of adjustment disorder. Although there is currently a lack of consensus on how these patients should be classified in a criterion-based system, when they are considered together with the more severely depressed patients, there is good empirical support for Massie's[4] conclusion that at least one-quarter of patients with advanced cancer present with a significant degree of dysphoria. This general figure also corresponds well with family members' reports on the psychological well-being of their dying relatives.[55] Finally, many other patients have occasional, transient periods of distress or demoralization during the course of their struggle with cancer. Although they are usually not considered to be experiencing a mental disorder during these periods, some may qualify for a diagnosis of adjustment disorder using the criteria of a few of the studies presented in Table 2.3.

RISK FACTORS

If the overall prevalence of depressive syndromes is higher among cancer patients than among the general population, then the question arises as to whether the risk factors that are associated with depressive episodes in the population generally are also valid indicators of risk among patients with cancer. In addition, there are other risk factors that are specific to the circumstances of patients with cancer that have been investigated in different studies. Having an appreciation of the known risk factors for depression in this population may enable clinicians to initiate efforts at prevention and early intervention.[56]

Gender

One of the most consistent findings across epidemiologic studies within the general population has been that women have rates of major depressive disorder that are approximately double those of men.[57] This robust finding leads to the hypothesis that women might also be more likely to become depressed in the face of life-threatening illness. In fact, the available data are not so clear on this point.[58] Although some studies have indeed found higher levels of depressive symptoms and distress among female cancer pa-

tients,[59,60] including those at an advanced terminal stage,[61] other studies have found just the opposite. For example, both Plumb and Holland (1981) and Chochinov et al. (unpublished data) used interviews to assess depression in patients with advanced cancer and found that men were actually more likely to be classified as seriously depressed. These findings may be particularly significant for clinicians who work in palliative care. If assessments in this context are grounded in an appreciation of gender differences in depression based on the general population literature, they may be biased by assumptions that are inappropriate for this patient group.

Age

Epidemiologic studies suggest that depressive disorders are more common among younger adults (i.e., those under age 45) than older adults.[54,62,63] However, the expectation that this will translate into higher rates of depression among younger cancer patients must be tempered by the fact that cancer is a disease that, in the majority of cases, afflicts people in their older years. Nevertheless, a number of studies, although not all,[28,64] have identified the same trend and found that younger cancer patients do indeed show higher rates of diagnosed depressive disorders[52,65] or self-reported distress.[61,66,67] Factors that can contribute to the higher prevalence of depression in younger patients may include the feeling that life has been cut short and ambitions have not been realized, concerns about the welfare of one's dependants, and also methodological issues that are inherent in all age-related epidemiologic research, such as the possibility that younger people may be more willing to acknowledge psychological symptoms.

Prior History of Depression

There is a growing recognition that for some individuals, depression can be a chronic or recurrent disorder punctuated by periods of relative remission, relapse, and recurrence. In fact, within the general population, a prior episode of depression appears to be one of the stronger risk factors that predict the onset of new episodes.[68] A number of studies have also found that patients with cancer who are currently depressed are more likely to report prior episodes from earlier periods in their lives.[50,61,69,70] In this context, the struggle with life-threatening illness is clearly a major stressor that may precipitate an episode of depression in individuals who are particularly vulnerable.[15] Although the specific nature of the vulnerability remains unclear, personality factors such as pessimism, neuroticism, and low self-esteem have been implicated in some studies.[69–74]

Social Support

Supportive social ties are thought to be psychologically beneficial by fulfilling individuals' needs for security, belonging and self-esteem.[75] In studies of the general population, deficits in the adequacy of one's social support network have often been related to clinical depression; they have been associated with both the onset of first episodes[76] and poor recovery. The causal nature of this link is probably multifactorial, involving direct and indirect effects.[77–82] Theories about the direct effect posit that social resources have a positive impact on mental health, regardless of life stressors. According to this view, social attachment variables such as the size of the social network, good interpersonal relationships with friends, relatives, and confidants, and the degree of involvement in organizations help to promote a healthy sense of well-being. In addition, indirect effects may occur when an individual is under stress; the availability of an adequate support network is held to moderate or buffer the effect of exposure to stress on one's emotional state.

The experience of social support is also thought to play a role in the psychological adjustment of patients with serious medical illness. Emotional support, the provision of information, and instrumental help are three aspects of social support that have been discussed with regard to cancer patients in particular.[83] The physical and psychosocial stressors associated with cancer are likely to result in a greater need for all of these forms of support. In many cases, however, the provision of support may depend on family members who are under considerable strain themselves as they attempt to cope with the life-threatening illness of a loved one. In addition, the social stigma often associated with cancer can lead potentially supportive others to avoid a patient with this illness, thus increasing the risk of social isolation. Furthermore, many patients with good family relationships hesitate to add to their family's burden and avoid discussing their emotional

state, which can intensify their sense of isolation.[84] It has been proposed that this cycle of isolating events can cause the patient to withdraw and perhaps become depressed.[85]

In the context of cancer care, measures of social support have generally shown modest but statistically significant correlations with self-report measures of depression.[84,86] For example, in a study of older outpatients with metastatic disease reported by Hann et al.,[87] the correlations between a depression scale and the perceived adequacy of social support received from family and friends were $r = -.27$ and $r = -.30$, respectively. Similarly, Chochinov and Wilson[86] found a correlation of $r = -.25$ for a VAS rating of family support and scores on the BDI-SF.

It also appears likely that the association between social and support and depression in cancer patients is influenced by demographic and disease-related factors. In the largest study of this type, Noyes et al.[67] screened 438 patients with solid tumors using the Illness Distress Scale, which includes a measure of social isolation. They found that men actually reported greater social isolation overall, centered largely around concerns about their inability to work. Patients with more advanced illness also had higher social isolation scores than patients with local disease.

Although distress regarding social isolation may be more prominent among patients with advanced cancer, there is also evidence that the stress-buffering aspects of social support may be diminished at this stage of illness. Several studies have reported that measures of support (as opposed to measures of social isolation) show a stronger association with depression in patients with early stages of disease,[88] good prognosis,[84] or less physical disability.[27] Overall, this pattern suggests that patients receiving palliative care experience the greatest social deficits, but the buffering influence of supportive interpersonal relationships may hold only until a certain level of disability is reached.

Functional Status

Increasing physical disability has generally been found to be significantly correlated with measures of depression or distress.[27,50,89–91] Of course, functional disability is likely to increase with the progression of the disease, so patients with more advanced illness appear to have the greatest risk for a number of psychiatric disorders.[47] It also suggests that the association between functional status and depression will be more apparent in studies that sample patients from a broad range of disease stages and disability levels. The association may be less evident in studies of either newly diagnosed patients with generally high levels of function[92] or in studies of palliative-care inpatients with uniformly low levels.

Pain

Although not all studies of patients with cancer have found an association between increased pain and reports of depression,[28] there is now a considerable body of evidence indicating that such a link is indeed reliable across a range of settings and methods of assessment.[27,47,49,50,86,90–93] The magnitude of the correlations are not especially high; in studies with relatively large sample sizes, they have been on the order of $r = .25$ to $.36$.[86,89–93] However, the clinical implications are substantial. Spiegel et al.[49] compared prevalence rates for depressive disorders in patients identified as having relatively low pain levels and those with relatively high levels and found that interview-based diagnoses were two to four times more common in the high-pain group. For the diagnosis of major depression, this association was particularly pronounced among patients with metastases.

At this point, the research emphasis has begun to shift from merely demonstrating that there is an association between pain and depression to considering more precisely what the nature of the causal link might be. While it may seem straightforward that any dimension of psychological distress is likely to be elevated in patients with poorly controlled pain or other sources of physical discomfort, some investigators have speculated that depression may result in an amplication of the pain experience,[94] or at least a difficulty in tolerating the stress of physical symptoms.[95] Thus, the causal pathway may be bidirectional.[49]

It should also be noted that many of the same studies that have found correlations between depression and pain have also found correlations between depression and functional status, as well as between functional status and pain.[89–93] This had led some investigators to conduct studies addressed directly to unraveling the relative contributions of pain and functional status to the emergence of symptoms of depression or distress.

The results have been inconsistent, however. Williamson and Schulz[90] conducted a longitudinal study of outpatients with cancer and reported that activity limitations largely mediate the link between pain and depression. Lancee et al.,[89] on the other hand, used statistical modeling procedures on data collected from a large community sample of patients with cancer. They found that pain was the single most important factor related to distress. It had both a direct effect and an additional indirect effect mediated through impaired role performance.

Illness and Treatment-Related Factors

Tumors that originate in or metastasize to the central nervous system have the potential to cause depressive symptoms.[96,97] However, tumors with no direct neurological involvement can also result in organic mood disorders. For example, hypercortisolism or Cushing's syndrome due to pituitary tumors have been linked to depression.[98,99] Metabolic complications such as hypercalcemia, most often associated with cancer of the breast and lung, have also been associated with depression.[100] These remote effects may be due to several factors, including toxins secreted by the tumor, autoimmune reactions, viral infections, nutritional deficits, and enuroendocrine dysfunction.[101,102]

A number of authors have noted that depression appears to be more prevalent in patients with pancreatic cancer, relative to other comparably ill patients with intra-abdominal malignancies.[103–106] In separate reviews of the literature, Shakin and Holland,[103] Green and Austin,[104] and Passik and Breitbart[11] have concluded that depression symptoms are present in about 30% to 40% of patients, regardless of the method of assessment. Several etiological mechanisms are plausible. Reports that psychiatric symptoms may actually precede the physical symptoms of the disease in some cases[106] suggest that tumor-induced changes in the neuroendocrine system may be linked to the emergence of depression.[103,104] However, Shakin and Holland[103] point out that the etiology is confounded by the presence of pain, which is often present in patients with pancreatic cancer. Furthermore, the knowledge that this illness carries a particularly poor prognosis offers another possible explanation for the high prevalence of depression in this group.

When making a differential diagnosis that includes a consideration of the role of organic factors, it is also important to note various treatments for cancer, particularly those that produce toxic side effects[107,108] that can precipitate the onset of depressive symptoms. These treatments include corticosteroids,[109] as well as various chemotherapy medications (vincristine, vinblastine, asparagines, intrathecal methotrexate, interferon, interleukin)[110–114] and radiotherapy[115–118] protocols.

Existential Concerns

In North American practice, which emphasizes fully informed consent to care, it is uncommon for patients with cancer not to be told of their diagnosis. This has not always been the case, however; nor is it the case presently in some other societies. Recent reports from India[44] and Poland[119] show that patients who are unaware of the nature of their illness have substantially lower rates of psychiatric morbidity than do patients who have a more accurate appraisal of their circumstances. This raises the likelihood that the open recognition that one is facing a life-threatening crisis brings with it a greater focus on existential concerns regarding unfulfilled ambitions, past regrets, meaning in life, and the maintenance of dignity and self-control, as well as social concerns about the welfare of one's family. These are central considerations in palliative care. Interestingly, in their study of sources of distress among patients with cancer, Noyes et al.[67] found that items related to a loss of meaning showed higher correlation with scores on a depression inventory that did items pertaining to physical symptoms, medical treatment, or social isolation. Hence, the relationship of existential distress to depressive syndromes among patients who are terminally ill—whether as a cause, consequence, or correlate—is worthy of further investigation in future research.

MANAGEMENT OF DEPRESSION IN THE TERMINALLY ILL

General Principles

The relationship with the primary medical caregiver is the most important component of psychotherapeutic support for many patients with a serious illness. Optimally, these relationships are based on mutual trust, respect, and sensitivity. The ability to acknowledge patients as "whole persons" and to respond to them on the basis of their own individual personal styles and needs tends to work best. Perhaps, more than in any other clinical setting, maintaining ongoing contact with the depressed terminally ill patient is of critical importance. It not only ensures that patients will be continually reevaluated but also provides reassurance to patients that they will not be abandoned and that care will be forthcoming and available throughout their terminal course.

Supportive psychotherapy with the dying patient consists of active listening with supportive verbal interventions and the occasional interpretation.[120] Despite the seriousness of the patient's plight, it is not necessary for the psychiatrist or psychologist to appear overly solemn or emotionally restrained. Often it is only the psychotherapist, of all the patient's caregivers, who is comfortable enough to converse lightheartedly and allow the patient to talk about his life and experiences, rather than focus solely on impending death. The dying patient who wishes to talk or ask questions about death should be allowed to do so freely, with the therapist maintaining an interested, interactive stance.

Psychosocial Therapies

For patients with advanced cancer who are suffering from major depression, adjustment disorder, or dysthymia, there are a variety of psychosocial interventions with proven efficacy. These include individual psychotherapy, group psychotherapy, hypnotherapy, psychoeducation, relaxation training and biofeedback, and self-help groups.[121] Any treatment for major depression in the terminally ill will be less effective if given in a context devoid of psychotherapeutic support. Depression in cancer patients with advanced disease is optimally managed utilizing a combination of supportive psychotherapy, cognitive-behavioral techniques, and antidepressant medication.[122] Psychotherapy and cognitive behavioral techniques are useful in the management of psychological distress in cancer patients and have been applied to the treatment of depressive and anxious symptoms related to cancer and cancer pain. Psychotherapeutic interventions, in the form of either individual or group counseling, have been shown to effectively reduce psychological distress and depressive symptoms in cancer patients.[123–125] Cognitive-behavioral interventions, such as relaxation and distraction with pleasant imagery, have also been shown to decrease depressive symptoms in patients with mild to moderate levels of depression.[126] If these approaches are not successful or have only partial success, they should be used in combination with psychopharmacological interventions.

Pharmacological Treatment of Depression in the Terminally Ill

Although both psychotherapy and cognitive behavioral therapy have proven effective in reducing psychological distress and mild to moderate depressive symptomatology in the cancer setting, pharmacotherapy is the mainstay for treating terminally ill patients who meet the diagnostic criteria for major depression.[122] The efficacy of antidepressants in the treatment of depression in cancer patients has been well established.[122,127–130,133] (see Table 3.4). Factors such as prognosis and the time-frame for treatment may play an important role in determining the type of pharmacotherapy for depression. A depressed patient with several months of life expectancy can afford to wait the two–four weeks it may take to respond to a tricyclic antidepressant. The depressed dying patient with less than three weeks to live may do best with a rapid-acting psychostimulant.[131] Patients who are within hours or days of death and in distress are likely to benefit most from the use of sedatives or narcotic analgesic infusions.

Tricyclic Antidepressants

The application of tricyclic antidepressants (TCAs) specifically to the terminally ill requires a careful risk-benefit ratio analysis. Although nearly 70% of patients treated with a tricyclic for nonpsychotic depression can anticipate a positive response, these medications are associated with a side-effect profile that can be particularly troublesome for terminally ill patients.[132] They have multiple pharmacodynamic actions that account for these side effects, including blockade of muscarinic cholinergic receptors, alpha-adrenoceptor blockade, and H_1 histamine receptor blockade. The tertiary amines (amitriptyline, doxepin,

Table 3.4   Antidepressant Medications Used in Advanced Cancer Patients

Drug	Therapeutic Daily Dosage mg (PO)
Tricyclic antidepressants	
Amitriptyline	25–125
Doxepin	25–125
Imipramine	25–125
Desipramine	25–125
Nortriptyline	25–125
Clomipramine	25–125
Second-generation antidepressants	
Buproprion	200–450
Fluoxetine	10–40
Paroxetine	10–40
Fluvoxamine	50–300
Sertraline	50–200
Nefazodone	100–500
Venlafaxine	37.5–225
Trazodone	150–300
Heterocyclic antidepressants	
Maprotiline	50–75
Amoxapine	100–150
Monoamine oxidase inhibitors	
Isocarboxazid	20–40
Phenelzine	30–60
Tranylcypromine	20–40
Psychostimulants	
Dextroamphetamine	5–30
Methylphenidate	5–30
Pemoline	37.5–150
Benzodiazepines	
Alprazolam	0.75–6.00
Lithium carbonate	600–1200

Source: Adapted from Massie MJ, Holland JC. Depression and the cancer patient. *Journal of Clinical Psychiatry*, 1990; 51:12–17.

imipramine) have a greater propensity to cause side effects than do secondary amines (nortriptyline, desipramine).[133] The secondary amines are thus often a preferable choice for the terminally ill.

The anticholinergic side effects of TCAs can be particularly problematic for terminally ill patients. These may include constipation, dry mouth, and urinary retention. Those patients who are receiving medication with anticholinergic properties (such as pethidine, atropine, diphenhydramine, or the phenothiazines) are at risk for developing an anticholinergic delirium, and thus antidepressants that are potently anticholinergic should be avoided.[134] To avoid exacerbating symptoms associated with genitourinary outlet obstruction, decreased gastric motility, or stomatitis, a relatively nonanticholinergic tricyclic such as desipramine or nortriptyline is a reasonable choice. The anticholinergic actions of TCAs can also cause serious tachycardia, which can be problematic for terminally ill patients with cardiac insufficiency. The quinidine-like effects of TCAs can also lead to arrhythmias by virtue of their ability to delay conduction via the His-Purkinje system[135] (associated with nonspecific ST-T changes and T waves on the electrocardiograph). These effects are particularly concerning for those terminally ill patients with preexisting conduction defects, especially second- or third-degree heart block.

Dying patients are often exposed to a wide variety of potentially sedating agents. H_1 histamine receptor blockage is associated with sedation and drowsiness. For patients already exposed to various sedating medications (e.g., narcotic analgesics, antiemetics, anxiolytics, neuroleptics), TCAs such as amitriptyline and doxepin are the most likely to accentuate the overall cumulative sedating effects of these medications. Alpha$_1$-blockade is associated with postural hypotension and dizziness. This can be of particular concern for the frail, volume-depleted patient who, because of these side effects, is at risk for falls and possible fractures. Nortriptyline and protrip-tyline are the TCAs least associated with alpha$_1$-blockade.

Particularly among patients with advanced disease—and therefore a higher likelihood of drug intolerance—tricyclic antidepressants should be started at low doses (10–25 mg qhs) and increased in 10- to 25-mg increments every 2 to 4 days. These incremental increases can continue until a therapeutic dose is attained or side effects become a dose-limiting factor. Depressed cancer patients often achieve a therapeutic response at significantly lower doses of TCAs (25 to 125 mg) than are necessary in the physically well (150 to 300 g).[44] There is also evidence to suggest that patients with advanced cancer achieve higher serum tricyclic levels at modest doses.[136] In order to minimize drug toxicity and more carefully guide the process of drug titration, prescribing tricyclics (desipramine, nortriptyline, amitriptyline, imipramine) with well-established therapeutic plasma levels may be advantageous.[137]

The nature of the underlying terminal medical condition, the characteristics of the depressive episode, past responses to antidepressant therapy, and the specific drug side-effect profile are among the factors that will guide the choice of TCA in a given circumstances. Those patients who present with agitation and insomnia may respond favorably to more sedating tricyclics (amitriptyline, doxepin). In general, however, desipramine and nortriptyline are better tolerated in this population than amitriptyline or imipramine. For the terminally ill depressed patient, the choice of TCA is made on the basis of a side-effect profile that will be least incompatible with the patient's overall medical condition. Most tricyclics are available as rectal suppositories for patients who are no longer able to take medication orally. Outside the United States, certain tricyclics are given as intravenous infusion.[138] Although it is not very practical, amitriptyline, imipramine, and doxepin can also be given intramuscularly.[122,131]

It must be borne in mind that a therapeutic response to TCAs (as with all antidepressants) has a latency time of 3 to 6 weeks. For the terminally ill depressed patient whose life expectancy is anticipated to be less than this, psychostimulants may offer a more viable, rapid response alternative.

Second-Generation Antidepressants

Selective Serotonin Reuptake Inhibitors   The selective serotonin reuptake inhibitors (SSRIs) are a recent important addition to the available antidepressant medications and have a number of features that may be particularly advantageous for the terminally ill. They have been found to be as effective in the treatment of depression as the tricyclics[139,140] and have a very low affinity for adrenergic, cholinergic, and histamine receptors, thus accounting for negligible orthostatic hypotension, urinary retention, memory impairment, sedation, or reduced awareness.[141] They have not been found to cause clinically significant alterations in cardiac conduction, are generally favorably tolerated, and have a wider margin of safety than the TCAs in the event of an overdose. They do not therefore require therapeutic drug-level monitoring.

Most of the side effects of SSRIs result from their selective central and peripheral serotonin re-uptake. These include increased intestinal motility (loose stools, nausea, vomiting, insomnia, headaches, and sexual dysfunction). Some patients may experience anxiety, tremor, restlessness, and akathisia (the latter is relatively rare, but it can be problematic for the terminally ill patient with Parkinson's disease).[142] These side effects tend to be dose related and may be problematic for patients with advanced disease.

Five SSRIs are currently marketed, including sertraline, fluoxetine, paroxetine, nefazodone, and fluvoxamine. With the exception of fluoxetine, whose elimination half-life is 2 to 4 days, the SSRIs have an elimination half-life of about 24 hours. Fluoxetine is the only SSRI with a potent active metabolite—norfluoxetine—whose elimination half-life is 7 to 14 days. Fluoxetine can cause mild nausea and a brief period of increased anxiety, as well as appetite suppression that usually lasts for a period of several weeks. Some patients can experience transient weight loss, but weight usually returns to baseline level. The anorectic properties of fluoxetine have not been a limiting factor in the use of this drug in cancer patients. Fluoxetine and norfluoxetine do not reach a steady state for 5 to 6 weeks, compared with 4 to 14 days for paroxetine, fluvoxamine, and sertraline. These difference are important, especially for the terminally patient in whom a switch from an SSRI to another antidepressant is being considered. If a switch to a monamine oxidase inhibitor is required, the washout period for fluoxetine will be at least 5 weeks, given the potential drug interactions between these two agents. Since fluoxetine has entered the market, there have been several reports of significant drug-drug interactions.[143,144] Until it has been studied further in the medically ill, it should be used cautiously in the debilitated dying patient. Paroxetine, fluvoxamine, and sertraline, on the other hand, require considerably shorter washout periods (10 to 14 days) under similar circumstances.

All the SSRIs have the ability to inhibit the hepatic isoenzyme P450 11D6, with sertraline (and, according to some sources, Luvox) being least potent in this regard. This is important with respect to dose/plasma-level ratios and drug interactions, since the SSRIs are dependent upon hepatic metabolism. For the elderly patient with advanced disease, the dose-response curve for sertraline appears to be relatively linear. On the other hand, particularly for paroxetine (which appears to be the most potent inhibitor of cytochrome P450 11D6), small dosage increases can result in dramatic elevations in plasma levels. Paroxetine and, to a somewhat lesser extent, fluoxetine appear to inhibit the hepatic enzymes responsible for their own clearance.[145] The co-administration of these medications with other drugs that are dependent on this enzyme system for their catabolism (e.g., tricyclics, phenothiazines, type-IC antiarrhythmics, and quinidine) should be done cautiously. Luvox has been shown in some instances to elevate the blood levels of propranolol and warfarin by as much as 200%, and should thus not be prescribed together with these agents.

SSRIs can generally be started at their minimally effective doses. For the terminally ill, this usually means initiating therapy at approximately half the usual starting dose used in an otherwise healthy patient. For fluoxetine, patients can begin on 5 mg (available in liquid form) given once daily (preferably in the morning) with a range of 10 to 40 mg per day; given its long half-life, some patients may require this drug only every second day. Paroxetine can be started at 10 mg once daily (either morning or evening) for the patient with advanced disease and has a therapeutic range of 10 to 40 per day. Fluvoxamine, which tends to be somewhat more sedating, can be started at 25 mg (in the evenings) and has a therapeutic range of 50 to 300 mg. Sertraline can be initiated at 50 mg, morning or evening, and titrated within a range of 50 to 200 mg per day. Nefazodone can be started at 50 mg bid and titrated within a range of 100 to 500 mg per day. If patients experience activating effects on SSRIs, they should not be given at bedtime but rather moved earlier into the day. Gastrointestinal upset can be reduced by ensuring the patient does not take medication on an empty stomach.

Serotonin-Norephinephrine Reuptake Inhibitor (SNRI)   Venlaflaxine (Effexor) is the only antidepressant in this class and was just recently released on the market. It is a potent inhibitor of neuronal serotonin and norephinephrine reuptake and appears to have no significant affinity for muscarinic, histamine, or α_1-adrenergic receptors. Some patients may experience a modest sustained increase in blood pressure, especially at doses above the recommended initiating dose. Compared with the SSRIs, venlaflaxine's protein binding (<35%) is very low. Few protein-binding-induced drug interactions are thus expected. Like other antidepressants, venlaflaxine should not be used in patients receiving monamine oxidase inhibitors. Its side-effect profile tends to generally be well tolerated, with few discontinuations. While there are currently no data addressing its use in the terminally ill depressed patient, its pharmacokinetic properties and side-effect profile suggest it may have a role to play.

Trazodone If given in sufficient doses (100 to 300 mg/day), Trazodone can be an effective antidepressant. Although its anticholinergic profile is almost negligible, it has considerable affinity for alpha$_1$-adrenoceptors and may thus predispose patients to orthostatic hypotension and its problematic sequelae (i.e., falls, fractures, head injuries). Trazedone is very sedating and in low doses (100 mg qhs) is helpful in the treatment of the depressed cancer patient with insomnia. It is highly serotonergic, and its use should be considered when the patient requires adjunct analgesics effect in addition to antidepressant effects. Trazodone has little effect on cardiac conduction but can cause arrhythmias in patients with premorbid cardiac disease.[146] Trazodone has also been associated with priapism and should thus be used with caution in male patients.[147] It is highly sedating, with drowsiness being its most common adverse side effect. In smaller doses it can thus be used as an effective sedative hypnotic.

Bupropion Bupropion is a relatively new drug in the United States, and there has not been much experience with its use in the medically ill. At present, it is not the first drug of choice for depressed patients with cancer. However, one might consider prescribing bupropion if patients have a poor response to a reasonable trial of other antidepressants. Bupropion may have a role in the treatment of the psychomotor retarded depressed terminally ill patient, as it has energizing effects

similar to the stimulant drugs.[148] However, because of the increased incidence of seizures, bupropion has a limited role for patients with CNS disorders in the oncology population.[149]

Heterocyclic Antidepressants The heterocyclic antidepressants have side-effect profiles that are similar to those for the TCAs. Maprotiline should be avoided in patients with brain tumors and in those who are at risk for seizures, since the incidence of seizures is increased with this medication.[150] Amoxapine has mild dopamine-blocking activity. Hence, patients who are taking other dopamine blockers (e.g., antiemetics) have an increased risk of developing extrapyramidal symptoms and dyskinesias.[151] Mianserin (not available in the United States) is a serotonergic antidepressant with adjuvant analgesic properties that is used widely in Europe and Latin America. Costa and colleagues[130] showed mianserin to be a safe and effective drug for the treatment of depression in cancer.

Psychostimulants The psychostimulants (dextroamphetamine, methylphenidate, and pemoline) offer an alternative and effective pharmacologic approach to the treatment of depression in the terminally ill.[152–159] These drugs have a more rapid onset of action than the tricyclics and are often energizing. They are most helpful in the treatment of depression in cancer patients with advanced disease and in cases where dysphoric mood is associated with severe psychomotor slowing and even mild cognitive impairment. Psychostimulants have been shown to improve attention, concentration, and overall performance on neuropsychological testing in the medically ill.[160] In relatively low dose, psychostimulants stimulate appetite, promote a sense of well-being, and relieve feelings of weakness and fatigue in cancer patients. Treatment with dextroamphetamine or methylphenidate usually begins with a dose of 2.5 mg at 8:00 A.M. and at noon. The dosage is slowly increased over several days until a desired effect is achieved or side effects (overstimulation, anxiety, insomnia, paranoia, confusion) intervene. Typically, a dose greater than 30 mg per day is not necessary, although occasionally patients require up to 60 mg per day. Patients usually are maintained on methylphenidate for one to two months, and approximately two-thirds will be able to be withdrawn from methylphenidate without a recurrence of depressive symptoms. Those who do recur can be maintained on a psychostimulant for up to one year without significant abuse problems. Tolerance will develop, and adjustment of dose may be necessary. An additional benefit of stimulants such as methylphenidate and dextroamphetamine is that they have been shown to reduce sedation secondary to opioid analgesics and provide adjuvant analgesics in cancer patients.[161] Common side effects of stimulants include nervousness, overstimulation, mild increase in blood pressure and pulse rate, and tremor. More rare side effects include dyskinesias or motor tics, as well as paranoid psychosis or exacerbation of an underlying and unrecognized confusional state.

Pemoline is a unique psychostimulant that is chemically unrelated to amphetamine. It is a less potent stimulant with little abuse potential.[156] Advantages of pemoline as a psychostimulant in cancer patients include the lack of abuse potential, the lack of federal regulation through special triplicate prescriptions, the mild sympathomimetic effects, and the fact that it comes in a chewable tablet form that can be absorbed through the buccal mucosa and is easily used by cancer patients who have difficulty swallowing or have intestinal obstruction. Pemoline appears to be as effective as methylphenidate or dextroamphetamine in the treatment of depressive symptoms in terminally ill cancer patients.[162] Pemoline can be started at a dose of 18.75 mg in the morning and at noon and increased gradually over days. Typically, patients require 75 mg a day or less. Pemoline should be used with caution in patients with liver impairment, and liver function tests should be monitored periodically with longer-term treatment.[163]

Monamine Oxidase Inhibitors In general, monoamine oxidase inhibitors (MAOIs) have been considered a less desirable alternative for treating depression in the terminally ill. Patients who receive MAOIs must avoid foods rich in tyramine, sympathomimetic drugs (amphetamines, methylphenidate), and medications that contain phenylpropranolamine and pseudoephedrine.[142] The combination of these agents with MAOIs may cause hypertensive crisis, leading to strokes and fatalities. MAOIs in combination with opioid analgesics have also been reported to be associated with myoclonus and delirium and must

therefore be used together cautiously.[131] The use of meperidine while on MAOIs is absolutely contraindicated and can lead to hyperpyrexia, cardiovascular collapses, and death. MAOIs can also cause considerable orthostatic hypotension. Avoiding this minefield of adverse interactions can be particularly problematic for the terminally ill. It is not surprising that MAOIs tend to be reserved in this patient population for those who have shown past preferential responses to them for treatment of their depression.

The new reversible inhibitors of monoamine oxidase-A (RIMAs) may reduce some of the problems associated with the older MAOIs (tranylcypromine, isocarboxazide). There are no studies on the role of RIMAs in the depressed terminally ill, but there are interesting theoretical reasons to suggest that they may eventually have a larger role to play than the nonselective MAOIs. RIMAs selectively inhibit MAO-A enzyme, therefore leaving MAO-B enzyme available to deal with any tyramine challenge. Moclobemide, a RIMA recently introduced onto the Canadian market, appears to be loosely bound to the MAO-A receptor and is thus relatively easily displaced by tyramine from its binding site. It has a very short half-life, which further reduces the possibility of any prolonged adverse effects, such as hypertensive crisis. Dietary restrictions that include avoidant of tyramine-containing foods are thus not required. The side-effect profile of moclobemide is far more favorable than that for nonselective MAOIs and tends to be well tolerated. Although the risk of hypertensive crisis is significantly reduced, it is not entirely eliminated. Agents such as meperidine, procarbazine, dextromethorphan, or other ephedrine-containing agents are still best avoided. Its short half-life requires that moclobemide be administered two times daily, with a total dosage range of 150 to 600 mg daily. Co-administration with cimetidine will increase its plasma concentration, requiring appropriate dosage adjustments. While RIMAs may offer some advantages over tranylcypromine and isocarboxazid for the terminally ill depressed patient, they will likely remain a second-line choice compared to available non-MAOI antidepressants.

Lithium Carbonate Patients who have been receiving lithium carbonate prior to a cancer illness should be maintained on it throughout their cancer treatment, although close monitoring is necessary in the preoperative and postoperative periods, when fluids and salt may be restricted.[164] Maintenance doses of lithium may need reduction in seriously ill patients. Lithium should be prescribed with caution for patients receiving cisplatinum because of the potential nephrotoxicity of both drugs. Several authors have reported possible beneficial effects from the use of lithium in neutropenic cancer patients. However, the functional capabilities of these leukocytes have not been determined. The stimulation effect appears to be transient; no mood changes have been noted in these patients.[165]

Benzodiazepines   The triazolobenzodiazepine alprazolam has been shown to be a mildly effective antidepressant as well as an anxiolytic. Alprazolam is particularly useful in cancer patients who have mixed symptoms of anxiety and depression. Starting dose is 0.25 mg three times a day; effective doses are usually in the range of 4 to 6 mg daily.[166]

Electroconvulsive Therapy

Occasionally, it is necessary to consider electroconvulsive therapy (ECT) for depressed cancer patients who have depression with psychotic features or in whom treatment with antidepressants pose unacceptable side effects. The safe effective use of ECT in the medically ill has been reviewed by others.[122]

CONCLUSIONS

Depression remains a considerable source of remediable suffering among the terminally ill. Underdiagnosing and undertreating depression can impair the quality of life and add to the burden of suffering of dying patients. Care providers frequently dismiss depression and mood states as "normal reactions" to the illness, even in the face of severe affective disturbances. Yet, diagnostic approaches are available to assist clinicians identify mood disorders in this vulnerable patient population.

Both psychological and psychopharmacological treatments have proven effective in patients with major depression and should be undertaken hand in hand. Medication without ongoing contact is often experienced as abandonment and thus is never an acceptable approach. Most psychotherapeutic approaches in patients who are terminally ill combine promotion of active coping strategies and assistance in patients to understand, manage, and work through their feelings related to their disease. Patients who are treated for their depression often renew their ability to find meaning in their lives, in spite of their impending death. The issue ultimately is to help patients attain as much comfort as possible so that they may examine their own personal circumstances and shape their deaths—and live the remainder of their lives—with as much grace and meaning as possible.

References

1. Spitzer RL, Williams JBW, Kroenke K, Linzer M, de Gruy III, FV, Hahn SR, Brody D, Johnson JG. Utility of a new procedure for diagnosing mental disorders in primary care: the PRIME-MD 1000 study. *Journal of the American Medical Association*, 1994; 272:1749–1756.

2. Wells KB, Hays RD, Burnham MA, Rogers W, Greenfield S, Ware JE. Detection of depressive disorder for patients receiving prepaid or fee-for-service care: results from the medical outcomes study. *Journal of the American Medical Association*, 1989; 262:3298–3302.

3. Goldberg RJ, Mor V. A survey of psychotropic use in terminal cancer patients. *Psychosomatics*, 1985; 26:745–751.

4. Massie MJ. Depression. In: Holland JC, Rowland JH, eds, *Handbook of Psychooncology: Psychological Care of the Patient with Cancer*. New York: Oxford University Press, 1989:283–290.

5. Rosser JE, Maguire P. Dilemmas in general practice: the care of the cancer patient. *Social Science and Medicine*, 16:315–322.

6. Maguire P. Barriers to psychological care of the dying. *British Medical Journal* 1985; 291:1711–1713.

7. Derogatis LR, Abeloff MD, McBeth CD. Cancer patients and their physicians in the perception of psychological symptoms. *Psychosomatics*, 1976; 17:197–200.

8. Lampic C, Nordin K, Sjödén PO. Agreement between cancer patients and their physicians in the assessment of patient anxiety at follow-up visits. *Psycho-oncology*, 1995; 4:301–310.

9. Rathbone GV, Horsley S, Goacher J. A self-evaluated assessment suitable for seriously ill hospice patients. *Palliative Medicine*, 1994; 8:29–34.

10. Hinton J. Can home care maintain an acceptable quality of life for patients with terminal cancer and their relatives? *Palliative Medicine*, 1994; 8: 183–196.

11. Passik SD, Breitbart WS. Depression in patients with pancreatic carcinoma: diagnostic and treatment issues. *Cancer*, 1996; 78(suppl 3):615–626.

12. Christakis NA. Timing of referral of terminally ill patients to an outpatient hospice. *Journal of General Internal Medicine*, 1994; 9:314–320.

13. Hinton, J. Which patients with terminal cancer are admitted from home care? *Palliative Medicine*, 1994; 8:197–210.

14. Dunkel-Schetter C, Feinstein LG, Taylor SE, et al. Patterns of coping with cancer. *Health Psychology*, 1992; 11:79–87.

15. Harrison J, Maguire P. Predictors of psychiatric morbidity in cancer patients. *British Journal of Psychiatry*, 1994; 165:593–598.

16. Watson M, Green S, Rowden L, et al. Relationships between emotional control, adjustment to cancer and depression and anxiety in breast cancer in patients. *Psychological Medicine*, 1991; 21: 51–57.

17. Lynch ME. The assessment and prevalence of affective disorders in advanced cancer. *Journal of Palliative Care*, 1995; 11:10–18.

18. American Psychiatric Association. *Diagnostic and Statistical Manual of Mental Disorders.* 4th ed. Washington DC: Author, 1994.

19. Spitzer RL, Endicott J, Robins E. Research Diagnostic Criteria: rationale and reliability. *Archives of General Psychiatry*, 1978; 35:773–782.

20. Cohen-Cole SA, Stoudemire A. Major depression and physical illness: special considerations in diagnosis and biologic treatment. *Psychiatric Clinics of North America*, 1987; 10:1–17.

21. Endicott J. Measurement of depression in patients with cancer. *Cancer*, 1984; 53:2243–2248.

22. Cassem EH. Depression and anxiety secondary to medical illness. *Psychiatric Clinics of North America*, 1990; 13:597–612.

23. Robins LN, Helzer JE, Croughan J, Ratcliff KF. National Institute of Mental Health Diagnostic Interview Schedule: its history, characteristics, and validity. *Archives of General Psychiatry*, 1981; 38:381–389.

24. Spitzer RL, Williams JBW, Gibbon M, First MB. *Structured Clinical Interview for DSM-III-R.* Washington, DC: American Psychiatric Press, 1990.

25. Endicott J, Spitzer RL. A diagnostic interview: the Schedule for Affective Disorders and Schizophrenia. *Archives of General Psychiatry*, 1978; 35:837–844.

26. Chochinov HM, Wilson KG, Enns M, Lander S. Prevalence of depression in the terminally ill: effects of diagnostic criteria and symptom threshold judgements. *American Journal of Psychiatry*, 1994; 151:537–540.

27. Bukberg J, Penman D, Holland JC. Depression in hospitalized cancer patients. *Psychosomatic Medicine*, 1984; 46:199–212.

28. Power D, Kelly S, Gilsenan J, Kearney M, O'Mahony D, Walsh JB, Coakley D. Suitable screening tests for cognitive impairment and depression in the terminally ill—a prospective prevalence study. *Palliative Medicine*, 1993; 7:213–218.

29. Breitbart W, Bruera E, Chochinov H, Lynch M. Neuropsychiatric syndromes and psychological symptoms in patients with advanced cancer. *Journal of Pain and Symptom Management*, 1995; 10:131–141.

30. Beck AT, Beck RW. Screening depressed patients in family practice: a rapid technic. *Postgraduate Medicine*, 1972; 52:81–85.

31. Zigmond AS, Snaith RP. The Hospital Anxiety and Depression Scale. *Acta Psychiatrica Scandinavica*, 1983; 67:361–370.

32. Goldberg DP. *Manual of the General Health Questionnaire.* Windsor, England: NFER Publishing, 1978.

33. DeHaes JCJM, van Knippenberg FCE, Neijt JP. Measuring psychological and physical distress in cancer patients: structure and application of the Rotterdam Symptom Checklist. *British Journal of Cancer*, 1990; 62:1034.

34. Carroll BJ, Feinberg M, Smouse PE, Rawson SG, Greden JF. The Carroll Rating Scale for Depression I. Development, reliability and validation. *British Journal of Psychiatry*, 1981; 138:194–200.

35. Golden RN, McCartney CF, Haggerty JJ, Raft D, Nemeroff CB, Ekstrom D, Holmes V, Simon JS, Droba M, Quade D, Fowler WC, Evans DL. The detection of depression by patient self-report in women with gynecologic cancer. *International Journal of Psychiatry in Medicine*, 1991; 21:17–27.

36. Hopwood P, Howell A, Maguire P. Screening for psychiatric morbidity in patients with advanced breast cancer: validation of two self-report questionnaires. *British Journal of Cancer*, 1991; 64: 353–356.

37. Razavi D, Delvaux N, Bredart A, Paesman M, Debusscher L, Bron D, Stryckmans P. Screening for psychiatric disorders in a lymphoma outpatient population. *European Journal of Cancer*, 1992; 28:1869–1872.

38. Razavi D, Delvaux N, Farvacques C, Robaye E. Screening for adjustment disorders and major de-

pressive disorders in cancer in-patients. *British Journal of Psychiatry*, 1990; 156:79–83.

39. Hardman A, Maguire P, Crowther D. The recognition of psyciatric morbidity on a medical oncology ward. *Journal of Psychosomatic Research*, 1989; 33:235–239.

40. Chochinov HM, Wilson KG, Enns M, Lander S. "Are you depressed?" Screening for depression in the terminally ill. *American Journal of Psychiatry*, 1997; 154:674–676.

41. Fechner-Bates S, Coyne JC, Schwenk TL. The relationship of self-reported distress to depressive disorders and other psychopathology. *Journal of Consulting and Clinical Psychology*, 1994; 60:550–559.

42. Bruera E, Kuehn N, Miller MJ, Selmser P, MacMillan K. The Edmonton Symptom Assessment System (ESAS): a simple method for the assessment of palliative care patients. *Journal of Palliative Care*, 1991; 7:6–9.

43. Fishman B, Pasternak S, Wallenstein SI, Houde RW, Holland JC, Foley KM. The Memorial Pain Assessment Card: a valid instrument for the evaluation of cancer pain. *Cancer*, 1987; 60:1151–1158.

44. Alexander PJ, Dinesh N, Vidyasagar MS. Psychiatric morbidity among cancer patients and its relationship with awareness of illness and expectations about treatment outcome. *Acta Oncological*, 1993; 32:623–626.

45. Chochinov HM, Wilson KG, Enns M, Mowchun N, Lander S, Levitt M, Clinch JJ. Desire for death in the terminally ill. *American Journal of Psychiatry*, 1995; 152:1185–1191.

46. Colón EA, Callies AL, Popkin MK, McGlave PB. Depressed mood and other variables related to bone marrow transplantation survival in acute leukemia. *Psychosomatics*, 1991; 32:420–425.

47. Derogatis LR, Morrow GR, Fetting J, Penman D, Piasetsky S, Schmale AM, Heinrichs M, Carnicke CLM Jr. The prevalence of psychiatric disorders among cancer patients. *Journal of the American Medical Association*, 1983; 249:751–757.

48. Evans DL, McCartney CF, Nemeroff CB, Raft D, Quade D, Golden RN, Haggerty JJ, Holmes V, Simon JS, Droba M, Mason GA, Fowler WC. Depression in women treated for gynecological cancer: clinical and neuroendocrine assessment. *American Journal of Psychiatry*, 1986; 143:447–452.

49. Spiegel D, Sands S, Koopman C. Pain and depression in patients with cancer. *Cancer*, 1994; 74:2570–2578.

50. Lansky SB, List MA, Hermann CA, Ets-Hokin EG, DasGupta TK, Wilbanks GD, Hendrickson FR. Absence of major depressive disorder in female cancer patients. *Journal of Clinical Oncology*, 1985; 3:1553–1560.

51. Katon W, Sullivan MD. Depression and chronic medical illness. *Journal of Clinical Psychiatry*, 1990; 51:3–11.

52. Kathol RG, Noyes R Jr, Williams J, Mutgi A, Carroll B, Perry P. Diagnosing depression in patients with medical illness. *Psychosomatics*, 1990; 31:434–440.

53. Régis DA, Boyd JH, Burke JD Jr, Rae DS, Myers JK, Kramer M, Robins LN, George LK, Karno M, Locke BZ. One-month prevalence of mental disorders in the United States: based on five Epidemiologic Catchment Area sites. *Archives of General Psychiatry*, 1988; 45:977–986.

54. Blazer DG, Kessler RC, McGonagle KA, Swartz MS. The prevalence and distribution of major depression in a national community sample: the National Comorbidity Survey. *American Journal of Psychiatry*, 1994; 151:979–986.

55. Lynn J, Teno JM, Phillips RS, Wu AW, Desbiens M, Harrold J, Claessens MT, Wenger M, Kreling B, Connors AF, for the SUPPORT investigators. Perceptions by family members of the dying experience of older and seriously ill patients. *Annals of Internal Medicine*, 1997; 126:97–106.

56. Harrison J, Maguire P. Predictors of psychiatric morbidity in cancer patients. *British Journal of Psychiatry*, 1994; 165:593–598.

57. Weissman MM, Bland RC, Canino GJ, Faravelli C, Greenwald S, Hwu HG, Joyce PR, Karam EG, Lee CK, Lellouch J, Lépine JP, Newman SC, Rubio-Stipec M, Wells JE, Wickramaratne PJ, Wittchen HU, Yeh EK. Cross-national epidemiology of major depression and bipolar disorder. *Journal of the American Medical Association*, 1996; 276:293–299.

58. Rodin G, Craven J, Littlefield C. *Depression in the Medically Ill: an Integrated Approach*. New York: Brunner/Mazel, 1991.

59. Irwin PH, Kramer S, Diamond NH, Malone D, Zivin G. Sex differences in psychological distress during definitive radiation therapy for cancer. *Journal of Psychosocial Oncology*, 1986; 4:63–75.

60. Stommel M, Given BA, Given CW, Kalaian HA, Schulz R, McCorkle R. Gender bias in the measurement properties of the Center for Epidemiologic Studies Depression Scale (CES-D). *Psychiatry Research*, 1993; 49:239–250.

61. Plumb MM, Holland J. Comparative studies of psychological function in patients with advanced

cancer—II. Interviewer-rated current and past psychological symptoms. *Psychosomatic Medicine*, 1981; 42:243–254.

62. Fredman L, Weissman MM, Leaf PJ, Bruce ML. Social functioning in community residents with depression and other psychiatric disorders: results of the New Haven Epidemiologic Catchment Area study. *Journal of Affective Disorders*, 1988; 15:103–112.

63. Sorenson SB, Rutter CM, Aneshensel CS. Depression in the community: an investigation into age of onset. *Journal of Consulting and Clinical Psychology*, 1991; 59:541–546.

64. Carroll BT, Kathold RG, Noyes R, Wald TG, Clamon GH. Screening for depression and anxiety in cancer patients using the Hospital Anxiety and Depression Scale. *General Hospital Psychiatry*, 1993; 15:69–74.

65. Levine PM, Silberfarb PM, Lipowski ZJ. Mental disorders in cancer patients: a study of 100 psychiatric referrals. *Cancer*, 1978; 42:1385–1391.

66. Craig TJ, Abeloff MD. Psychiatric symptomatology among hospitalized cancer patients. *American Journal of Psychiatry*, 1974; 131:1323–1326.

67. Noyes R, Kathold RG, Debelius-Enemark P, Williams J, Mutgi A, Suelzer MT, Clamon GH. Distress associated with cancer as measured by the Illness Distress Scale. *Psychosomatics*, 1990; 31:321–330.

68. Belsher G, Costello CG. Relapse after recovery from unipolar depression: a critical review. *Psychological Bulletin*, 1988; 104:84–96.

69. Weisman AD. Early diagnosis of vulnerability in cancer patients. *American Journal of the Medical Sciences*, 1976; 271:187–196.

70. Hughes JE. Depressive illness and lung cancer. I. Depression before diagnosis. *European Journal of Surgical Oncology*, 1985; 11:15–20.

71. Thomas C, Madden F, Jehu D. Psychological effects of stomas—II. Factors influencing outcome. *Journal of Psychosomatic Research*, 1987; 31:317–323.

72. Fallowfield LJ, Baum M, Maguire GP. Effects of breast conservation on psychological morbidity associated with diagnosis and treatment of early breast cancer. *British Medical Journal*, 1986; 293:1331–334.

73. Curbow B, Somerfield M, Legro M, Sonnega J. Self-concept and cancer in adults: theoretical and methodological issues. *Social Science and Medicine*, 1990; 31:115–128.

74. Dean C. Psychiatric morbidity following mastectomy: preoperative predictors and types of illness. *Journal of Psychosomatic Research*, 1987; 31:385–392.

75. Thoits PA. Social support and psychological well-being: theoretical possibilities. In: Sarason IG, Sarason BR, eds, *Social Support: Theory, Research and Applications*. Dordrecht: Martinus Nijhoff, 1985:51–72.

76. Bruce ML, Hoff RA. Social and physical health risk factors for major depressive disorder in a community sample. *Social Psychiatry and Psychiatric Epidemiology*, 1994; 29:165–171.

77. Billings AG, Moss R. Psychosocial processes of remission in unipolar depression: comparing depressed patients with matched controls. *Journal of Consulting and Clinical Psychology*, 1985; 53:314–325.

78. Brugha TS, Bebbington PE, MacCarthy B, Sturt E, Wykes T, Potter J. Gender, social support and recovery from depression: a prospective clinical study. *Psychological Medicine*, 1990; 20:147–156.

79. George LK, Blazer DG, Hughes DC, Fowler N. Social support and the outcome of major depression. *British Journal of Psychiatry*, 1989; 154:478–485.

80. Sherbowne CD, Hays RD, Wells KB. Personal and psychosocial risk factors for physical and mental health outcomes and course of depression among depressed patients. *Journal of Consulting and Clinical Psychology*, 1995; 63:345–355.

81. Cohen S, Wills TA. Stress, social support, and the buffering hypothesis. *Psychological Bulletin*, 1985; 98:310–357.

82. Thoits PA. Social support functions and network structures: a supplemental view. In: Veiel HOF, Baumann U, eds. The Meaning and Measurement of Social Support. New York: Hemisphere, 1992:57–62.

83. Dunkel-Schetter C, Wortman CB. The interpersonal dynamics of cancer: problems in social relationships and their impact on the patient. In Friedman HS, DiMatteo MR eds, *Interpersonal Issues in Health Care*. New York: Academic Press, 1982:69–100.

84. Dunkel-Schetter, C. Social support and cancer: findings based on patient interviews and their implications. *Journal of Social Issues*, 1984; 40:77–98.

85. Goldberg RJ. Management of depression in the patient with advanced cancer. *Journal of the American Medical Association*, 1981; 246:373–376.

86. Chochinov HM, Wilson KG. The euthanasia debate: Attitudes, practices and psychiatric considerations. *Canadian Journal of Psychiatry*, 1995; 40:593–602.

87. Hann DM, Oxman TE, Ahles TA, Furstenberg

CT, Stake TA. Social support adequacy and depression in older patients with metastatic cancer. *Psycho-oncology*, 1995; 4:213–221.

88. Baile WF, Gibertini M, Scott L, Endicott J. Depression and tumour stage in cancer of the head and neck. *Psycho-oncology*, 1992; 1:15–24.

89. Lancee WJ, Vachon MLS, Ghadirian P, Adair W, Conway B, Dryer D. The impact of pain and impaired role performance on distress in persons with cancer. *Canadian Journal of Psychiatry*, 1994; 39:617–622.

90. Williamson GM, Schultz R. Activity restriction mediates the association between pain and depressed affect: a study of younger and older cancer patients. *Psychology and Aging*, 1995; 10:369–378.

91. Kaasa S, Malt U, Hagen S, Wist E, Moum T, Kvikstad A. Psychological distress in cancer patients with advanced disease. *Radiotherapy and Oncology*, 1993; 27:193–197.

92. Kelsen DP, Portenoy RK, Thaler HT, Niedzwiecki D, Passik SD, Tao Y, Banks W, Brennan MF, Foley KM. Pain and depression in patients with newly diagnosed pancreas cancer. *Journal of Clinical Oncology*, 1995; 13:748–755.

93. Glover J, Dibble SL, Dodd MJ, Miaskowski C. Mood states of oncology outpatients: does pain make a difference? *Journal of Pain and Symptom Management*, 1995; 10:120–128.

94. Spiegel D, Bloom JR. Pain in metastatic breast cancer. *Cancer*, 1983; 52:341–345.

95. Wilson KG, Chochinov HM. Physician-assisted suicide. *New England Journal of Medicine*, 1996; 335:518–519.

96. Brown JH, Paraskevas F. Cancer and depression. Cancer presenting with depressive illness: an autoimmune disease? *British Journal of Psychiatry*, 1982; 141:227–232.

97. Massie MJ, Gagnon P, Holland JC. Depression and suicide in patients with cancer. *Journal of Pain and Symptom Management*, 1994; 9:325–340.

98. Kelly WF, Checkley SA, Bender DA. Cushing's syndrome, tryptophan and depression. *British Journal of Psychiatry*, 1980; 136:125–132.

99. Kelly WF, Checkley SA, Bender DA, Mashiter K. Cushing's syndrome and depression: a prospective study of 26 patients. *British Journal of Psychiatry*, 1983; 142:16–19.

100. Breitbart W. Endocrine-related psychiatric disorders. In: Holland JC, Rowland JH, eds, *Handbook of Psychooncology: Psychological Care of the Patient with Cancer*. New York: Oxford University Press, 1989:356–366.

101. McDaniel JS, Musselman DL, Porter MR, Reed DA, Nemeroff CB. Depression in patients with cancer: diagnosis, biology, and treatment. *Archives of General Psychiatry*, 1995; 52:89–99.

102. Patchell RA, Posner JB. Cancer and the nervous system. In: Holland JC, Rowland JH, eds, *Handbook of Psychooncology: Psychological Care of the Patient with Cancer*. New York: Oxford University Press, 1989:327–341.

103. Shakin EJ, Holland JC. Depression and pancreatic cancer. *Journal of Pain and Symptom Management*, 1988; 3:194–198.

104. Green AI, Austin CP. Psychopathology of pancreatic cancer. *Psychosomatics*, 1993; 34:208–221.

105. Holland JC, Korzun AH, Tross S, Siberfarb P, Perry M, Comis R, Oster M. Comparative psychological disturbance in patients with pancreatic and gastric cancer. *American Journal of Psychiatry*, 1986; 143:982–986.

106. Fras I, Litin EM, Pearson JS. Comparison of psychiatric symptoms in carcinoma of the pancreas with those in some other intra-abdominal neoplasms. *American Journal of Psychiatry*, 1967; 123:1553–1562.

107. Devlen J, Maguire P, Phillips P, Crowther D, Chambers H. Psychological problems associated with diagnosis and treatment of lymphomas I. Retrospective study. *British Medical Journal*, 1987; 295:953–954.

108. Devlen J, Maguire P, Phillips P, Crowther D. Psychological problems associated with diagnosis and treatment of lymphomas II. Prospective study. *British Medical Journal*, 1987; 295:955–957.

109. Steifel FC, Breitbart W, Holland JC. Corticosteroids in cancer: neuropsychiatric complications. *Cancer Investigation*, 1989; 7:479–491.

110. Young DF. Neurological complications of cancer chemotherapy. In: Silverstein A, ed, *Neurological Complications of Therapy: Selected Topics*. New York: Futura Publishing, 1982:57–113.

111. Holland JC, Fassanellos OT. Psychiatric symptoms associated with L-asparagines administration. *Journal of Psychiatric Research*, 1974; 10:105–113.

112. Adams F, Quesada JR, Gutterman JN. Neuropsychiatric manifestations of human leukocyte interferon therapy in patients with cancer. *Journal of the American Medical Association*, 1984; 252:938–941.

113. Denicoff KD, Rubinow DR, Papa MZ. The neuropsychiatric effects of treatment with interleukin-w and lymphokine-activated killer cells. *Annals of Internal Medicine*, 1987; 107:293–300.

114. Weddington W.W. Delirium and depression associated with amphotericin B. *Psychosomatics*, 1982; 23:1076–1078.

115. Bisno B, Richardson JL. The relationship between depression and reinforcing events in cancer patients. *Journal of Psychosocial Oncology*, 1987; 5:63–71.

116. Forester B, Kornfeld DS, Fleiss J. Psychiatric aspects of radiotherapy. *American Journal of Psychiatry*, 1978; 135:960–962.

117. Irwin PH, Kramer S, Diamond NH, Malone D, Zivin G. Sex differences in psychological distress during definitive radiation therapy for cancer. *Journal of Psychosocial Oncology*, 1986; 4:63–75.

118. Peck A, Boland J. Emotional reactions to radiation treatment. *Cancer*, 1977; 40:180–184.

119. De Walden-Galuszko K. Prevalence of psychological morbidity in terminally ill cancer patients. *Psycho-oncology*, 1996; 5:45–49.

120. Cassem NH. The dying patient. In: Hackett TP, Cassem NH, eds, *Massachusetts General Hospital Handbook of General Hospital Psychiatry*. 2nd ed. Littleton, Mass: PSG Publishing Co. Inc., 1987; 332–352.

121. Newport DJ, Nemeroff CB. Assessment and treatment of depression in the cancer patient. *Journal of Psychosomatic Research*, 1998; 45:215–237.

122. Massie MJ, Holland JC. Depression and the cancer patient. *Journal of Clinical Psychiatry*, 1990; 51:12–17.

123. Spiegel D, Bloom JR, Yalom ID. Group support for patients with metastatic cancer: A randomized prospective outcome study. *Archives of General Psychiatry*, 1981; 38:527–533.

124. Spiegel D, Bloom JR. Group therapy and hypnosis reduce metastatic breast carcinoma pain. *Psychosomatic Medicine*, 1983; 4:333–339.

125. Massie MJ, Holland JC, Straker N. Psychotherapeutic interventions. In: Holland JC, Rowland JH, eds, *Handbook of Psychooncology: Psychological Care of the Patient with Cancer*. New York: Oxford University Press, 1989:455–469.

126. Holland JC, Morrow G, Schmale A, et al. Reduction of anxiety and depression in cancer patients by alprazolam or by a behavioral technique. *Proceedings of the American Society of Clinical Oncology* 1988; 6:258. Abstract.

127. Popkin MK, Callies AL, Mackenzie TB. The outcome of antidepressant use in the medically ill. *Archives of General Psychiatry* 1985; 42:1160–1163.

128. Rifkin A, Reardon G, Siris S, et al. Trimipramine in physical illness with depression. *Journal of Clinical Psychiatry* 1985; 46:4–8.

129. Purohit DR, Navlakha PL, Modi RS, et al. The role of antidepressants in hospitalized cancer patients. *Journal of the Association of Physicians of India* 1978; 26:245–248.

130. Costa D, Mogos I, Toma T. Efficacy and safety of mianserin in the treatment of depression of women with cancer. *Acta Psychiatr Scandinavica* 1985; 72:85–92.

131. Breitbart W. Psychiatric complications of cancer. In: Brain MC, Carbone PP, eds, *Current Therapy in Hematology Oncology-3*. Toronto and Philadelphia: BC Decker, 1988:268–274.

132. Davis JM, Glassman AH. Anti-depressant drugs. In: Kaplan HI, Sadock BJ, eds, *Comprehensive Textbook of Psychiatry*. 5th ed. Baltimore: Williams and Wilkins, 1989.

133. Preskorn SH. Recent pharmacologic advances in anti-depressant therapy for the elderly. *American Journal of Medicine*, 1993; 54 Supplement:14–34.

134. Breitbart W, Possick SD. Psychiatric aspects of palliative care. In: Doyle D, Hanks GW, MacDonald, eds, *Oxford Textbook of Palliative Medicine*. New York: Oxford University Press, 1993.

135. LeMelledo MJ, Bradweijn J. Pharmacotherapy of Depression. *Pharmanual* 1993:25–46.

136. Stoudemire A, Fogel BS. Psychopharmacolgy in the medically ill. In: Stoudemire A, Fogel BS, eds, *Principles of Medical Psychiatry*. Orlando Fla: Grune and Stratton, Inc. 1987:79–112.

137. Preskorn SH, Jerkovich GS. Central nervous system toxicity of tricyclic antidepressants: phenomenology, course, risk factors, and role of therapeutic drug monitoring. *Journal of Clinical Psychopharmacology*, 1990; 10:88–95.

138. Massie MJ, Holland JC. Diagnosis and treatment of depression in the cancer patient. *Journal of Clinical Psychiatry* 1984; 42:25–28.

139. Mendels J. Clinical experience with serotonin reuptake inhibiting antidepressants. *Journal of Clinical Psychiatry* 1987; 48(Supp):26–30.

140. Glassman AH. The newer antidepressant drugs and their cardiovascular effects. *Psychopharmacology Bulletin* 1984; 20:272–279.

141. Cooper GL. The safety of fluoxetine—an update. *British Journal of Psychiatry*, 1988; 153:77–86.

142. Preskorn S, Burke M. Somatic therapy for major depressive disorder: selection of an antidepressant. *Journal of Clinical Psychiatry*, 1992; 53(Suppl): 1–14.

143. Ciraulo DA, Shader RI. Fluoxetine drug-drug interactions: I. Antidepressants and antipsychotics. *Journal of Clinical Psychopharmacology* 1990; 10:48–50.

144. Pearson HJ. Interaction of fluoxetine with carbamazepine. *Journal of Clinical Psychiatry*, 1990; 51:126.

145. Preskorn SH. Recent pharmacologic advances in antidepressant therapy for the elderly. *American Journal of Medicine*, 1993; 94(Suppl 5A):

146. Rudorfer MV, Potter WZ. Anti-depressants. A comparative review of the clinical pharmacology and therapeutic use of the "newer" versus the "older" drugs. *Drugs*, 1989; 37:713–38.

147. Sher M, Krieger JN, Juergen S. Trazodone and priapism. *American Journal of Psychiatry*, 1983; 140:1362–1364.

148. Shopsin B: Buproprion: a new clinical profile in the psychobiology of depression. *Journal of Clinical Psychiatry*, 1983; 44:140–142.

149. Peck AW, Stern WC, Watkinson C. Incidence of seizures during treatment with tricyclic antidepressant drugs and buproprion. *Journal of Clinical Psychiatry*, 1983; 44:197–201.

150. Lloyd AH. Practical consideration in the use of maprotiline (ludiomil) in general practice. *Journal of International Medical Research*, 1977;5:122–125.

151. Ayd F. Amoxapine: a new tricyclic antidepressant. *International Drug Therapy Newsletter*, 1979; 14:33–40.

152. Fernandez F, Adams F, Holmes VF, et al. Methylphenidate for depressive disorders in cancer patietns. *Psychosomatics*, 1987; 28:455–461.

153. Katon W, Raskind M. Treatment of depressionin the medically ill elderly with methylphenidate. *American Journal of Psychiatry*, 1980; 137:963–965.

154. Kaufmann MW, Muarray GB, Cassem NH. Use of psychostimulants in medically ill depressed patients. *Psychosomatics* 1982; 23:817–819.

155. Fisch R. Metylphenidate for medical inpatients. *International Journal of Psychiatry in Medicine*, 1985–1986; 15:75–79.

156. Chiarillo RJ, Cole JO. The use of psychostimulants in general psychiatry. A reconsideration. *Archives of General Psychiatry*, 1987; 44:286–295.

157. Satel SL, Nelson CJ. Stimulants in the treatment of depression: a critical overview. *Journal of Clinical Psychiatry*, 1989; 50:241–249.

158. Woods SW, Tesar GE, Murray GB, Cessem NH. Psychostimulant treatment of depressive disorders secondary to medical illness. *Journal of Clinical Psychiatry*, 1986; 47:12–15.

159. Burns MM, Eisendrath SJ. Dextroamphetamine treatment for depression in terminally ill patients. *Psychosomatics*, January–February 1994; 35(11):80–82.

160. Fernandez F, Adams F, Levy J, et al. Cognitive impairment due to AIDS related complex and its response to psychostimulants. *Psychosomatics* 1988; 29:38–46.

161. Bruera E, Chadwick S, Brennels C, et al. Methylphenidate associated with narcotics for the treatment of cancer pain. *Cancer Treatment Reports*, 1987; 71:67–70.

162. Breitbart W, Mermelstein H. Pemoline: an alternative psychostimulant for the management of depressive disorders in cancer patients. *Psychosomatics*, 1992; 33:352–356.

163. Nehra A, et al. Pemoline-associated hepatic injury. *Gastroenterology*, 1990; 99:1517–1519.

164. Greenberg DB, Younger J, Kaufman SD. Management of lithium in patients with cancer. *Psychosomatics*, September–October 1993; 34(5): 388–394.

165. Stein RS, Flexner JH, Graber SE. Lithium and granulocytopenia during induction therapy of acute myelogenous leukemia: update of an ongoing trial. *Adv Exp Med Biol* 1980; 127:187–198.

166. Holland JC, Morrow G, Schmale A, et al. Reduction of anxiety and depression in cancer patients by alprazolam or by a behavioral technique. *Proceedings of the American Society of Clinical Oncologists*, 1988; 6:258. Abstract.

4

Suicide, Assisted Suicide, and Euthanasia in the Terminally Ill

Barry Rosenfeld, Ph.D.
Suzanne Krivo, M.D.
William Breitbart, M.D.
Harvey Max Chochinov, M.D., Ph.D., FRCPC

Jerzy Kosinski, the Polish novelist and Holo-caust survivor, committed suicide in May 1991. Like other individuals with chronic medical ill-nesses, he chose suicide as a means of controlling the course of his disease and the circumstances of his death. "I am not a suicide freak, but I want to be free," Kosinski told an interviewer in 1979. "If I ever have an accident or a terminal disease that would affect my mind or body, I will end it." Twelve years later, he did so. Similar sentiments are shared by a significant proportion of Ameri-cans. Advocates demanding autonomy for pa-tients who wish to choose how and when they die have been increasingly vocal during recent years, sparked by the highly publicized assisted-suicide deaths attended by Drs. Jack Kevorkian and Timothy Quill. These cases have focused at-tention on the plight of patients with terminal illnesses.

What has often been overlooked, however, in the political and legal machinations has been the importance of medical, social, and psychological factors that may contribute to suicidal ideation, requests for hastened death, or suicide in termi-nally ill patients. This chapter reviews the rele-vant research regarding factors that may influence suicidal ideation and requests for physician-assisted suicide (PAS hereafter). In addition, we discuss health-care provider obligations and sug-gest responses that are appropriate when patients verbalize requests for help in dying so that providers can respond in a manner that is both ethical and, one hopes, therapeutic.

DEFINITION OF EUTHANASIA AND ASSISTED SUICIDE

Euthanasia is defined as the administration of lethal medications to a patient, by a physician, with the intention of ending the patient's life. Physician-assisted suicide, on the other hand, is the provision, by a physician, of medications or advice that enable the patient to end his own life. While theoretical and/or ethical distinctions between euthanasia and assisted suicide may be subtle to some, the practical distinctions may be significant. Many terminally ill patients have ac-cess to potentially lethal medications, at times even request them from their physicians, yet do not use these medications to end their own lives (despite the widespread sale of publications such as *Final Exit*, which describes how to use such medications in a lethal, yet painless manner). Moreover, physicians are often more comfortable assisting the patient with advice and/or medica-tion than actually administering the lethal dose. While euthanasia is more commonly performed in the Netherlands than PAS, current U.S. policy debates have focused almost exclusively on PAS.

Both euthanasia and PAS have been distinguished, legally and ethically, from the administration of high-dose pain medication meant to relieve a patient's pain that may hasten death (often referred to as the rule of double effect), or even the withdrawal of life support (see Emmanuel[1] and New York State Task Force on Life and the Law[2] for a discussion of these legal and ethical distinctions). The distinction between euthanasia/PAS and the administration of high-dose pain medications that may hasten death is premised on the intent behind the act. In euthanasia/PAS, the intent is to end the patient's life, while in the administration of pain medications that may also hasten death, the intent is to relieve suffering. In practice, however, this distinction is often artificial, since many advocates for the legalization of euthanasia/PAS cite the relief of suffering as the basis for fulfilling patients' requests for help in dying and clinicians who administer potentially lethal pain medications do so with the awareness that death is likely to occur.

Distinctions between withdrawal of life support and euthanasia/PAS are, in many ways, considerably clearer. Long-standing civil case laws have supported the rights of patients to refuse any unwanted treatment, even though such treatment refusals may cause death.[3] On the other hand, patients have not had the right to demand treatments or interventions that they desire. This distinction has had the effect of allowing patients on life support to end their lives on request, whereas patients who are not dependent upon life support do not have such a right. In fact, this difference in perceived "rights" formed the basis of the arguments made to the Supreme Court in *Washington v. Glucksberg*[4] and *Quill v. Vacco*,[5] in which it was argued that this distinction violated the due process clause of the Fourteenth Amendment (the U.S. Supreme Court unanimously rejected this argument). Nevertheless, the Court's decision suggested that, while laws prohibiting assisted suicide were not unconstitutional, neither were laws permitting assisted suicide. Legal and ethical debates regarding the legalization of assisted suicide continue, despite the limited body of research in support of arguments about equity in rights.

THE DEBATE REGARDING LEGALIZATION OF PHYSICIAN-ASSISTED SUICIDE AND EUTHANASIA

Arguments in Support of Legalization of Physician-assisted Suicide/Euthanasia

The arguments in support of the legalization of euthanasia/physician-assisted suicide are substantial. Proponents perceive assisted suicide as an act of humanity toward the terminally ill patient. They believe the patient and the family should not be forced to suffer through a long and painful death, even if the only way to alleviate the suffering is through suicide. To the advocate for assisted suicide, legalization of assisted suicide is a natural extension of patient autonomy and the individual's right to determine what treatments he will accept or refuse. Since patients are allowed to refuse life-sustaining medical interventions (e.g., life support, artificial nutrition and hydration), they are effectively permitted to commit suicide by treatment refusal. Despite the refutation of this argument by the U.S. Supreme Court, advocates of legalization argue that no ethical difference exists between terminating life-sustaining care and administering lethal medication to the terminally ill patient. In both cases, the primary goal of the physician can be seen as the prevention of suffering at the end of life by hastening an inevitable death.

Arguments in favor of the legalization of assisted suicide are typically premised on the assumption that requests for assisted suicide are a "rational" decision, given the circumstances of terminal illness, pain and increased disability, and fears of becoming (or continuing to be) a burden to one's family and friends. Given the possibility that these symptoms and circumstances may not be relieved, even with aggressive palliative care and social services, the decision to hasten one's death may seem rational. Moreover, the desire to include one's physician in carrying out a decision to end one's life can be viewed as an extension of a terminally ill patient's natural reliance on his physician for help with most aspects of the illness, as well as a reasonable mechanism to ensure that one does not become even more disabled and burdensome to family or friends by attempting suicide unsuccessfully and possibly being left in a persistent vegetative state or with increased disability.

Another argument raised by proponents of legalization is that merely knowing that one can control the timing and manner of one's death serves as a form of "psychological insurance" for the dying patient. In other words, knowing there can be an escape from the suffering of illness in itself alleviates some of the stress associated with the dying process. It may be (as argued by some proponents of assisted suicide) that many individuals with terminal illnesses wish to have the option to end their lives if certain possible conditions arise, even though the likelihood that they will utilize this option is small.

Arguments in Opposition to Legalization of Physician-Assisted Suicide/Euthanasia

Opposition to legalization of assisted suicide and/or euthanasia has come from numerous different perspectives. As frequently noted in the editorial pages of various medical journals, the medical profession is guided by a desire to heal and extend life. This guideline is best exemplified in the Hippocratic Oath, which states, "I will prescribe regimen for the good of my patients according to my ability and my judgment and never do harm to anyone. To please no one will I prescribe a deadly drug, nor give advice that may cause his death." Thus, the possibility that physicians may directly hasten the life of patients whom they have presumably been treating in an effort to extend and improve life contradicts the central tenet of the medical profession.

From a mental health perspective, professional psychiatric and psychological training reinforces the view that suicide is a manifestation of psychological disturbance.[6] As such, mental health clinicians typically view suicide, regardless of the context, as an outcome that should be prevented at all costs. Several studies have supported this connection between mental disorder (e.g., depression) and interest in assisted suicide, suggesting that suicidal ideation in terminally ill patients is a manifestation of undiagnosed, untreated mental illness.[7,8] Consequently, physician compliance with a suffering patient's stated wish for assisted suicide may circumvent the provision of appropriate psychiatric care. Similar arguments have been made regarding pain and physical symptoms, suggesting that requests for PAS may be evidence of inadequate palliative care.[9] If assisted suicide is legalized, physicians may unknowingly participate in assisted suicide intended to alleviate symptoms that could perhaps be managed with better palliative care and improved medical management.

Opponents of assisted suicide also posit that individuals of lower socioeconomic classes or other disenfranchised groups will be "coerced," either directly or indirectly, into requesting PAS as a means of resolving the difficulties posed by their illness. Family members may subtly suggest that death, since inevitable, would be preferable if it occurred sooner rather than later because of the social and financial burdens involved in caring for the terminally ill person. Physicians may view assisted suicide, perhaps because of their own unrecognized feelings (countertransference), as the appropriate and preferable response to a terminal illness and the resulting disability. Thus, physicians may be particularly poor at recognizing "irrational" requests for assisted suicide because of their belief that they would not want to live in a condition similar to their patient's. An even more frightening possibility is that physicians or other health-care providers might recommend assisted suicide as an option because the alternative, providing adequate palliative care, is too expensive or difficult to obtain. Thus, patients with poor health insurance or limited financial resources may be "coerced" into requesting PAS because of poorly managed or untreated physical and psychological symptoms; they may perceive their only options to be continued suffering or death. Several studies have demonstrated the prevalence of inadequate recognition and treatment of both psychological and physical symptoms,[10] with symptoms such as depression and anxiety going largely unrecognized in many medically ill patients. Moreover, even when such symptoms are observed, undertreatment of symptoms such as pain is common.[11] According to a recent review of palliative care in Canada, only 5% of dying patients in Canada receive adequate palliative care.[12] These and related studies are often cited by opponents of legalization of assisted suicide/euthanasia as evidence that legalization is premature until all dying patients and their families have access to skilled and effective palliative-care services.

In response to these concerns, legislators who have proposed guidelines for assisted suicide have incorporated several mechanisms to minimize the risk that assisted suicide, if legalized, will be misused. These guidelines include a voluntarily request by the patient for assistance in dying, evidence of a terminal illness, and documentation by the primary physician of the reason for the request and efforts made to optimize the patient's care. Opponents, however, suggest that these limitations are more arbitrary than scientific and argue that the legal and medical communities will eventually end up on a "slippery slope" where euthanasia is ultimately legalized as acceptable practice for a wider patient population, including nonterminal, nonvoluntary patients.[13] Opponents point to a similar evolution of euthanasia use in the Netherlands (discussed later in this chapter), where regulations regarding assisted suicide have gradually weakened in the decade and a half since this practice was decriminalized. For example, in 1994 the Dutch Supreme Court accepted the argument that chronic diseases, even if not terminal, were an acceptable basis for euthanasia, and more recent cases have extended this "right" even to patients without a physical illness.

ATTITUDES TOWARD PHYSICIAN-ASSISTED SUICIDE/EUTHANASIA

Studies investigating attitudes toward assisted suicide and euthanasia have been conducted periodically for many years; both the frequency of such studies and the range of their subject populations have increased steadily in recent years. Because of the interesting differences in the findings, research conducted with physically healthy adults (the general public), with health-care professionals, and with medically ill patients is summarized separately.

The General Public

Blendon et al.[14] recently reviewed the literature on public attitudes toward euthanasia and assisted suicide as researched over the past 40 years. They observed that public support for legalization of euthanasia and assisted suicide has grown steadily over the past four decades, rising from 30–40% in the 1940s and 1950s to more than 60% dur-

ing the 1990s. In their own national survey of 2,000 adults, conducted in 1991, Blendon et al.[14] found that 63% of the American public supported legalization of euthanasia, and 64% supported legalization of physician-assisted suicide. As in the earlier studies they reviewed, Blendon and colleagues found that younger adults were more likely to support legalization of assisted suicide and euthanasia than were older adults, and Caucasians were more likely to support legalization than were minority respondents. Religious differences in this sample were also reported, with Protestants less likely to support legalization than Jewish and Catholic respondents.

A recent Canadian survey reported roughly comparable results, but with some differences. Suarez-Alomar and colleagues,[15] in their study of 1,200 Canadian adults, found that 52% supported legalization of assisted suicide, and 66% supported legalization of euthanasia. While they found no racial or religious differences (possibly because of differences between the Canadian and the American samples), they observed that level of education was significantly correlated with approval of legalization for assisted suicide. Better-educated respondents were more likely to support legalization of assisted suicide than were less-educated respondents. These studies, taken as a whole, demonstrate that, although assisted suicide has been legalized in only one state in the United States, the majority of American and Canadian people appear to support such legislation.

Health-Care Professionals

A growing number of opinion surveys have also focused on the attitudes of health-care professionals toward legalization of assisted suicide and euthanasia. These studies have included physicians from various disciplines, medical students, nurses, and social workers, and interesting differences have been observed among these groups. Chochinov and Wilson,[12] in their review of studies of physician attitudes toward PAS/euthanasia, found widely varying rates of support for legalization, ranging from 35% to 60%, depending on the methodology used in the study and on the subject group. For example, a recent study of oncologists found that only 45% of respondents considered euthanasia "appropriate" in response to a hypothetical vignette describing a terminally ill cancer patient who was suffering from un-remitting pain.[16] Rates of approval of euthanasia decreased substantially for other vignettes, with 35% approving of euthanasia in cases of func-tional disability, 23% approving in cases where the patient presents a burden to his family, and 18% approving in cases where the patient views his life as meaningless.

A study of psychiatrists conducted in Oregon, on other hand, found that two-thirds of respon-dents approved of legalization of assisted suicide.[17] As in the general public, physician attitudes to-ward assisted suicide and euthanasia vary accord-ing to the respondent's age and religious af-filiation, with older physicians more opposed to legalization than younger physicians and Catholic and Protestant physicians more opposed to legal-ization than Jewish and nonreligious physicians.[18] Interestingly, health-care professionals who have frequent contact with terminally ill patients are less likely to support legalization of assisted sui-cide or euthanasia.

Estimates of the proportion of physicians will-ing to participate in these practices, if legalized, however, have typically been lower still, ranging from 28% to 50%.[12] More important, in a study of Oregon psychiatrists conducted shortly after the voters approved the ballot initiative legaliz-ing assisted suicide, only 6% of the respondents indicated that they felt very confident about their ability to assess, in a single clinical evaluation, whether a psychiatric disorder was impairing a pa-tient's decision making.[17] This finding, coupled with provisions in the Oregon law that stipulate that mental health clinicians must provide expert evaluation whenever the competence of the pa-tient requesting assisted suicide is questioned, sug-gests that further training and research are neces-sary in this critical area of mental health law.

Medically Ill Patients

Despite the importance of understanding the at-titudes of terminally ill patients toward assisted suicide and euthanasia, relatively little empirical research has addressed this issue. Breitbart et al.[19] surveyed the attitudes of 378 ambulatory patients with AIDS regarding legalization of assisted sui-cide and euthanasia. These authors found rates of support for legalization that were roughly com-parable to those reported in published studies on the general population, with 63% supporting as-sisted suicide and 64% supporting euthanasia. Emanuel and colleagues,[16] in their study of can-cer patients, reported roughly comparable results, finding similar rates of support for euthanasia (roughly 66%) among cancer patients and the general public.

In addition to assessing the attitudes of med-ically ill patients toward legalization of assisted suicide, it is important to understand the pro-portion of patients who might consider this al-ternative. Published statistics, however, are sig-nificantly limited by a host of methodological problems, including the use of nonrandom sam-pling and imprecise questions. Thus, the reported percentage of subjects who consider these alter-natives has varied widely. Brown and colleagues[7] found that 23% of terminally ill patients at a palliative-care unit acknowledged some desire for hastened death; however, their sample of 44 pa-tients was culled from a several-hundred-bed hos-pital, with no detail provided on the sampling method. Breitbart et al.,[19] on the other hand, found that 55% of terminally ill AIDS patients indicated a possible interest in assisted suicide, were this option legalized.

Studies with more precise definitions of inter-est in assisted suicide, however, have produced more conservative estimates of the prevalence of these thoughts. Chochinov et al.,[8] for example, found that 8.5% of patients in a Winnepeg pal-liative-care unit expressed a "serious and perva-sive" desire for hastened death. Rosenfeld and col-leagues[20] found a slightly higher rate of desire for death among terminally ill patients with AIDS, with roughly 18% of patients obtaining elevated scores on a measure designed to assess desire for hastened death. In a 1996 study of oncology pa-tients,[16] 25% of cancer patients reported that they had thought seriously about euthanasia, and 12% had discussed this option with their physicians. Thus, despite the continued legal prohibitions against assisted suicide, a substantial number of patients think about and discuss this alternative with their physicians, family, or friends.

EUTHANASIA AND ASSISTED SUICIDE IN CLINICAL PRACTICE

A number of surveys have been published that document the practice of euthanasia and assisted suicide among health-care professionals. For example, an anonymous survey of Washington physicians conducted in 1995 found that 26% of responding physicians had received at least one request for assisted suicide, and two-thirds of those physicians had granted such requests.[21] Thus, roughly one in six Washington physicians acknowledged having granted a patient's request for assisted suicide or euthanasia. Of course, because of the survey nature of this study it is not possible to determine whether responding physicians were an accurate representation of all Washington physicians (e.g., physicians less interested in or more opposed to assisted suicide may have been less likely to return the surveys), let alone for the larger United States. Yet, these statistics suggest that assisted suicide is not a rare event, despite its illegal status. (It is also possible that, despite the anonymous nature of the survey, some physicians who had in fact carried out these requests were unwilling to acknowledge their actions for fear of repercussions.)

Even more striking results were reported in a survey of San Francisco–area AIDS physicians. Slome and colleagues[22] found that 98% of respondents had received requests for assisted suicide, and more than half of all responding physicians reported having granted at least one patient's request for assisted suicide. The average number of times that responding physicians had granted requests for assisted suicide was 4.2, with some physicians fulfilling dozens of such requests. Moreover, in response to a hypothetical vignette, nearly half of the sample (48%) indicated that they would be likely to grant a hypothetical patient's *initial* request for assisted suicide.

A more recent national survey sampled nearly 2,000 physicians from those disciplines most likely to receive requests for assisted suicide or euthanasia.[23] Meier and colleagues found that more than 18% of responding physicians reported having received at least one request for assisted suicide, and more than 11% had received requests for "lethal injection" (the author's definition of euthanasia). Only 6.4% of the total sample, however, reported having acceded to a request for hastened death (3.3% reported having prescribed medications to be used for this purpose, and 4.7% reported having provided lethal injection), roughly one-fourth of those who reported having received such a request. The most common reasons for the requests for hastened death, according to the physicians, included "discomfort other than pain" (present in 79% of cases), "loss of dignity" (53% of cases), "fear of uncontrollable symptoms" (52% of cases), pain (50% of cases), and "loss of meaning in their lives" (47% of cases). Although most physicians responded to requests for hastened death with either more aggressive palliative care (i.e., increased analgesic medications) or less aggressive life-prolonging treatments, 25% of physicians reported having prescribed antidepressant medications. Despite this seeming acknowledgment of the possible role of depression in patient requests for hastened death, only 2% of physicians reported having sought psychiatric consultation for their patients who requested assistance in dying.

Perhaps the most striking research to date regarding the use of assisted suicide and euthanasia is a study of critical-care nurses conducted by David Asch.[24] This study, based on the results of an anonymous survey, found that 17% of respondents reported having received at least one request for assisted suicide, and 11% had granted such a request. Aproximately 5% of responding nurses acknowledged having hastened a patient's death at the request of the physician but without the request of the patient or the family (termed "involuntary euthanasia" by some writers). Moreover, 4.7% percent of the sample indicated that they had hastened a patient's death without the knowledge of or a request by the physician. Respondents described having stopped oxygen therapy or increased pain medication in order to hasten death.[24] Asch suggested, on the basis of the reports of the respondent nurses, that these actions were done in order to ease the suffering of the patients, and he cited the traditional role of nursing in palliative care as the basis for these results. It should also be noted that Asch's controversial study generated considerable response, including many suggestions that methodological issues such as vague wording of questions may make these data unreliable.[25] Nevertheless, while these data may not accurately indicate the prevalence of assisted suicide or euthanasia in the United States, requests for assistance in dying are clearly not rare events, and physicians occasionally grant such requests despite legal prohibitions. Furthermore, because legal restrictions limit the ability of physicians to consult with colleagues regarding how to react to a request for assisted suicide, the appropriateness of patient requests and physician responses is unknown.

In the Netherlands, however, where physician-assisted suicide and euthanasia have been practiced regularly for more than 10 years, data regarding the frequency of requests for assistance in dying and the proportion of terminally ill patients whose lives end in this manner are available. Euthanasia was granted its current status in 1984 after a Dutch supreme court decision authorized this practice, provided a number of conditions are met. Specifically, the patient's request for assisted suicide must be considered free, conscious, explicit, and persistent. Both the physician and patient must agree that the patient's suffering is intolerable, and other measures for relief must have been exhausted. A second physician must be consulted and must concur with the decision to assist in ending the patient's life. Finally, all of these conditions must be adequately documented and reported to the governmental body that supervises the practice of euthanasia. Because of the availability of such records, several studies have documented the proportion of deaths in the Netherlands in which euthanasia or assisted suicide are implicated (these estimates have been adjusted to account for the underreporting of euthanasia acknowledged by many Dutch physicians). In reporting on euthanasia and assisted-suicide practices in the Netherlands from 1990 to 1995, van der Maas and colleagues[26] used both official reports of euthanasia and responses to anonymous surveys to estimate the rates of euthanasia and assisted suicide. They concluded that euthanasia and assisted suicide were involved in roughly 4.7% of all deaths in the Netherlands during 1995, a substantial increase over the 2.7% of deaths in 1991 that involved medical assistance.

Supporters of assisted suicide point to the Netherlands data as evidence that legalization has not led to widespread abuse or overuse of euthanasia/assisted suicide. Critics, however suggest that the 75% increase in deaths involving euthanasia or assisted suicide (from 2.7% to 4.7%) demonstrates a growing tendency toward their more frequent use, and therefore an increase in the number of potentially inappropriate uses. Such concerns are clearly reflected in a 1994 Dutch supreme court decision in which the right to euthanasia/assisted suicide was extended to include patients suffering from chronic illnesses that are not terminal, including mental disorders such as depression, provided the illness is refrac-

tory and causes intolerable suffering. Although the vast majority of requests for assisted suicide from mentally ill individuals have been denied, isolated cases have occurred in which mentally ill Dutch adults have been allowed to receive physician-assisted suicide or euthanasia as a result of this court ruling. This experience has been identified as evidence in favor of the "slippery slope" argument,[13] in which legalization of assisted suicide is presumed to lead to a gradual widening of the group of patients eligible for this "intervention," even though in many caes it may not be appropriate (e.g., for physically healthy but clinically depressed individuals).

REASONS THAT PATIENTS MAY SEEK HASTENED DEATH

A growing body of literature has emerged on the types of physical and psychological concerns that may give rise to a desire for hastened death and requests for assisted suicide. Although this literature has not always been consistent, a growing concensus has supported many of the assumptions put forth by the initial advocates and opponents of legalization. The issues that have received the broadest empirical support are pain, depression, social support, and cognitive dysfunction.

Pain

The relationship between pain and desire for death is often described as a relatively straightforward one: Intractable or severe pain is thought to lead to a desire for hastened death and, in particular, to thoughts of suicide.[9] While some research has supported this presumption, most studies have suggested that the relationship may be considerably more complex. For example, in their studies of ambulatory patients with AIDS, Breitbart and colleagues found that, while the presence and severity of pain appeared to heighten psychological distress and depression,[27] there was no direct relationship between pain and interest in assisted suicide.[19] Interest in assisted suicide appeared to be more a function of psychological and social factors (e.g., depression, social support, fears of becoming a burden to one's friends) than of physical factors (e.g., pain, symptom distress, disease status). Emanuel and colleagues[16] found similar results with regard to the link between pain and the desire for death in their sample of cancer patients. They found that patients who were in pain at the time of the survey were less likely to consider euthanasia appropriate than were patients without pain, even in response to a hypothetical vignette that described a patient with unremitting pain.[16] These studies, however, are limited by several factors, including the use of indirect measures of desire for hastened death (e.g., willingness to consider assisted suicide as an option or approval of euthanasia as a legitimate alternative) and their focus on the presence of pain rather than on the intensity of the pain or physical symptom distress more generally.

Studies that have employed more precise measures of desire for death and of severity of pain, on the other hand, have generally supported the hypothesis that severe pain can result in a heightened desire for death. Chochinov and colleagues,[8] in their study of terminally ill cancer patients, found that 76% of patients with moderate to severe pain had a "significant" desire for hastened death, compared to only 46% of patients with mild or no pain. More recently, Rosenfeld and colleagues[20] found that pain intensity contributed significantly to the prediction of desire for death (even after including measures of depression and social support) for patients who had pain. When the presence or absence of pain was included as a variable in these analyses, no such relationship was observed. Thus, the presence of severe pain is likely to add significantly to a patient's desire for a hastened death; however, this relationship may be masked when pain is studied as a dichotomous (present/absent) variable.

Depression

Several studies have demonstrated that depression plays a significant role in terminally ill patients' desire for hastened death . Although these studies often suffer from a host of methodological problems, the consistency of this finding across multiple studies, including several that demonstrated more careful attention to methodological issues, supports the apparent connection between depression and the desire for hastened death in terminally ill patients. Brown et al.,[7] for example, found that in their sample of palliative-care patients, all those patients who expressed a desire for death or suicidal ideation also met the diagnostic criteria for a major depressive episode.

Unfortunately, this study did not evaluate depression and suicidal ideation independently, leading to a confounding of these two classifications (i.e., patients who express suicidal ideation would be quite likely to be diagnosed as suffering from a depression, given that suicidal ideation is one of the diagnostic criteria).

More convincing evidence in support of the connection between depression and the desire for death was offered by Chochinov and colleagues,[8] who found that 58% of terminally ill cancer patients that were classified as having a "significant" desire for death were simultaneously diagnosed with a major depressive episode. They concluded that many, although not all, terminally ill patients who express interest in a hastened death may be suffering from a depressive disorder. These findings were replicated, with even stronger results, by Rosenfeld and colleagues,[20] who used multivariate models to assess the role of depression while simultaneously considering other variables, such as social support and pain. They found that, among terminally ill patients with AIDS, depression was the strongest predictor of desire for hastened death, although lack of social support, pain intensity, and symptom distress all provided independent contributions to this model. In their sample, nearly all patients who were classified as having an elevated desire for death were simultaneously diagnosed with a major depressive episode (although the reverse was not necessarily true; depressed patients did not necessarily report a high level of desire for death). Thus, while strong evidence exists that depression contributes significantly to a desire for death among terminally ill patients, the precise magnitude of this relationship is still unknown.

A related and similarly unresolved issue is whether treatment for depression affects desire for hastened death among terminally ill patients. In the only study to directly address the impact of treatment for depression on medical treatment decisions, Ganzini and colleagues[28] studied depressed geriatric patients' preferences for life-sustaining treatments. They found that, while treatment for depression did not result in a significant overall change in the preferences of depressed geriatric patients, several of the most severely depressed patients who responded positively to antidepressant therapy demonstrated a change in their preferences for life-sustaining treatments (i.e., having previously opted to refuse such treatment, they subsequently expressed a desire for these interventions). While this study suggests that interventions for depression may result in changed preferences among a subset of terminally ill patients who seek assisted suicide or euthanasia, no research to date has demonstrated such an effect. Breitbart and Rosenfeld are currently conducting an investigation in which terminally ill patients with AIDS who meet the criteria for a major depressive disorder are being treated and monitored with regard to their level of depression and their desire for hastened death. Such research may help elucidate the extent to which depression impedes rational end-of-life decision making in terminally ill patients.

Social Support

Although social factors were ignored in much of the early research on desire for death,[1,7,29] a growing body of research has demonstrated an important relationship between social support and desire for death. The importance of social factors in determining patient requests for assisted suicide or euthanasia was first evident in the results of a Dutch study described by van der Maas and colleagues,[26] in which the researchers found that social and psychological factors (e.g., concern regarding a loss of dignity, fears of becoming a burden to others) comstituted four of the five most frequently cited reasons for euthanasia requests. Chochinov and colleagues,[8] for example, found a significant correlation between social support and desire for death among their sample of terminally ill cancer patients, with patients with lower levels of social support having more desire for hastened death than patients with higher levels of social support. Similarly, Breitbart et al.[19] demonstrated a significant relationship between the quality of social support and interest in assisted suicide. In addition, a number of other social variables (e.g., fear of becoming a burden to family and friends; experience with the death of a friend or family member due to AIDS) were significant predictors of interest in assisted suicide among ambulatory patients with AIDS. More recently, Rosenfeld and colleagues[20] found that social support provided an independent contribution to the prediction of desire for death even after they controlled for the impact of depression, pain, and symptom distress. Thus, despite methodological differences, research studies have repeatedly shown the importance of social support as a factor in understanding patient requests for assisted suicide.

Cognitive Dysfunction and Delirium

Delirium has been increasingly recognized as a factor that may substantially increase the likelihood of suicidal ideation or attempts among medically ill individuals. Because delirium involves a general clouding of one's consciousness and ability to think rationally as a result of an underlying medical condition, the potential for impulsive or, at times, irrational acts such as a suicide attempt is considerable.[30] Although delirium may be less likely to influence patient requests for assisted suicide than actual suicide attempts (since the former are typically less impulsive), the potential impact of such cognitive deficits on decision making is substantial. For example, Rosenfeld et al.[31] found that even subthreshold levels of cognitive dysfunction appeared to adversely impact on HIV+ patients' ability to make rational treatment decisions. Similarly, Rosenfeld et al.[20] found that cognitive impairment was significantly associated with desire for death among a sample of hospitalized terminally ill patients with AIDS. Thus, cognitive impairments (which are common among terminally ill patients) may lead to a diminished ability to perceive long-term risks and benefits (in contrast to short-term ones) and therefore adversely influence end-of-life decision making and suicidal ideation.

CLINICAL RESPONSE TO SUICIDAL IDEATION OR REQUESTS FOR ASSISTED SUICIDE

The response of the clinician to a patient's expression of suicidal ideation or request for assisted suicide has obvious ramifications for the patient's quality of life as he or she approaches death. Several issues emerge in clinical settings when patients express a desire for hastened death, with or without the assistance of the physician. These issues, and appropriate clinical responses, are discussed in this seciton, along with the legal and ethical issues that exist in such situations.

As with any individual who expresses a desire for death, a terminally ill patient's expression of suicidal ideation or a request for assisted suicide must be addressed both rapidly and thoughtfully. Perhaps the single most important response a clinician can offer to his or her patients is a willingness to engage in this discussion. Clinician should not only allow their patients to discuss these thoughts and/or feelings openly but perhaps even facilitate an open discussion through direct questions and inquiries. Facilitating a free, open discussion of the patient's decision making is essential in order to ascertain the basis for the suicidal thoughts and the extent of any plans or intentions. Moreover, by expressing his willingness to discuss these issues in a nonjudgmental manner, the clinician conveys a willingness to keep such topics open, often providing significant relief to the patient.

Many experienced clinicians, however, are uncomfortable discussing suicide or death with their patients, and several fears often arise from situations. Among these is the thought that by allowing a patient to discuss his or her desire for hastened death, the physician is conveying approval or agreement with this decision. Although many physicians express concern that their inquiry into the patient's thoughts about suicide or death may give rise to suicidal thought or feelings when none existed previously, this belief is almost always unfounded. Rather, terminally ill patients often avoid discussing these thoughts with their physicians because they perceive that such discussions are off-limits or inappropriate, or they await a cue from the clinician that the topic is acceptable even thougyh they are tormented by dealing with the thoughts in isolation. The failure to allow an open dialogue regarding suicidal thoughts or desire for hastened death curtails an important avenue by which physicians can gain a more complete understanding of their patient's mental and physical state. Many patients also find discussions of suicidal thoughts therapeutic; at times they even relieve some of the urge to act on such thoughts. Even physicians who are opposed to suicide or assisted suicide on moral, ethical or religious grounds should be capable of engaging in a discussion of these thoughts or feelings without conveying a willingness to carry out such actions or a judgment of the appropriateness of such feelings.

Once an open dialogue has been established, a discussion of the patient's understanding of his illness and of the presence and severity of current symptoms is an essential second step. This type of discussion can enable the physician to assess both the degree to which the patient's beliefs or thoughts are rational and the extent to which untreated symptoms are driving the desire for a hastened death. The disclosure of untreated or undertreated physical and psychological symptoms can facilitate more effective treatment of those symptoms that may be resolvable with improved palliative care.

Another aspect of patient decision making that can be addressed once an open dialogue has been established is the extent of depression that is present in the patient. Not all terminally ill patients become severely depressed, nor are all terminally ill patients who desire a hastened death suffering from a major depression. On the other hand, many terminally ill patients are likely to be experiencing a depression that may be both treatable as well as temporary. Identifying when severe symptoms of depression exist and providing a referral to a trained psychologist or psychiatrist, preferably one with experience treating patients with terminal illnesses, can be crucial in optimizing the quality of life of these patients. Of course, even when a severe depression exists, a patient's ability to make rational treatment decisions is not always impaired as a result of this disorder. Thus, a referral to a mental health professional should likely also include an evaluation of the patient's decision-making competence.

Whenever potentially treatable disorders appear to underlie a patient's desire for hastened death, aggressive treatment for these symptoms or conditions is necessary. Many patients may be reluctant to pursue such treatments, particulary if the patient believes that treatment will be futile and/or painful. Thus, clinicians should assure the patient that initiating treatment does not imply a lack of willingness to continue to discuss other options (e.g., assisted suicide), merely a desire to exhaust all possible options to improve their existing quality of life. Therefore, clinicians should seek expert assistance in addressing whatever symptoms or problems have been identified, whether psychological (e.g., depression or despair), physical (e.g., pain, fatigue) or social (e.g., concern regarding becoming a burden to one's social supports).

Because assisted suicide and euthanasia (as well as suicide more broadly) are illegal in the United States (with the exception of Oregon), any clinician who learns of a patient's desire for assistance in dying is presented with several ethical and legal quandaries in addition to the clinical issues that arise. These quandaries are simplified somewhat by the physician's determination to resolve or reduce by available intervention any problems that appear amenable to such treatment. If the patient's desire for hastened death does not appear related to potentially resolvable problems and the patient has specifically requested assistance in committing suicide (or expressed a specific intent to kill himself), the clinician is faced with the uncomfortable burden of deciding how to respond to the patient's statements. This decision will no doubt rest on a number of factors, including the physician's personal beliefs regarding the appropriateness of suicide and assisted suicide. Although consultation with a colleague is certainly hindered by the illegal nature of assisted suicide, such consultation is nevertheless advisable whenever a patient's request for assisted suicide is being seriously considered. Consultation with a peer, even if done in a confidential and discreet manner, can reassure the clinician that his perception of the situation and condition of the patient is accurate, as well as provide a second opinion regarding the potential for, and the availability of, possible interventions. Unfortunately, we have no easy answer for facilitating clinical decision making in these difficult situations, other than to hope that if patients receive adequate interventions and clinical response, such requests will be relatively infrequent.

References

1. Emanuel EJ. Ethics of treatment: palliative and terminal care. In: Holland J, ed, *Psycho-oncology*. New York: Oxford University Press, 1998:1096–1111.
2. New York State Task Force on Life and the Law. *When Death Is Sought: Assisted Suicide and Euthanasia in the Medical Context.* Albany, NY: Health Research Inc., 1994.
3. *Cruzan v. Director, Missouri Dep't of Health* (1990). 497 U. S. 261.
4. *Washington v. Glucksburg*
5. *Quill v. Vacco*, 80F.3d716 (2nd Cir 1996).
6. Holland JC. Psychological aspects of cancer. In: Holland F, Frie E, eds, *Cancer Medicine*. 2nd ed. Philadelphia: Lea and Febiger, 1982.
7. Brown JH, Henteleff P, Barakat S, Rowe CJ. Is it normal for terminally ill patients to desire death? *American Journal Psychiatry*, 1986; 143:208–211.
8. Chochinov HM, Wilson KG, Enns M, Mowchun N, Lander S, Levitt M, Clinch JJ. Desire for death in the terminally ill. *American Journal of Psychiatry*, 1995; 152:1185–1191.
9. Foley K. Pain, physician-assisted suicide, and euthanasia. *Pain Forum*, 1995; 4:163–178.
10. Passik SD, Dugan W, McDonald MV, Rosenfeld B, Theobald D, Edgerton S. Oncologist's recognition of depression in their patients with cancer. *Journal of Clinical Oncology* 1998; 16:1594–1600.
11. Breitbart W, Rosenfeld B, Passik SD, McDonald MV, Thaler H, Portenoy RK. The undertreatment of pain in ambulatory AIDS patients. *Pain*, 1996; 65:243–249.
12. Chochinov HM, Wilson KG. The euthanasia debate: attitudes practices and psychiatric considerations. *Canadian Journal of Psychiatry*, 1995; 40: 593–602.
13. Hendin H, Rutenfrans C, Zylicz Z. Physician-assisted suicide in the Netherlands: lessons from the Dutch. *Journal of the American Medical Association*, 1997; 277:1720–1722.
14. Blendon RJ, Szalay US, Knox RA. Should physicians aid their patients in dying? *Journal of the American Medical Association*, 1992; 267:2658–2662.
15. Suarez-Almazor ME, Belize M, Bruera E. Euthanasia and physician-assisted suicide: a comparative survey of physicians, terminally ill cancer patients, and the general population. *Journal of Clinical Oncology*, 1997; 15:418–427.
16. Emanuel EJ, Fairclough DL, Daniels ER, Clarridge BR. Euthanasia and physician-assisted suicide: Attitudes and experiences of oncology patients, oncologists, and the public. *Lancet*, 1996; 347:1805–1810.
17. Ganzini L, Fenn DS, Lee MA, Heintz RT, Bloom JD. Attitudes of Oregon psychiatrists towards physician-assisted suicide. *American Journal of Psychiatry*, 1996; 153:1469–1475.
18. Portenoy RK, Coyle N, Kash KM, Brescia F, Scanlon C, O'Hare D, Misbin RI, Holland J, Foley K. Determinants of the willingness to endorse assisted suicide: a survey of physicians, nurses, and social workers. *Psychosomatics*, 1997; 38(30):277–287.
19. Breitbart W, Rosenfeld B, Passik SD. Interest in physician-assisted suicide among ambulatory HIV-infected patients. *American Journal of Psychiatry*, 1996; 153:238–242.
20. Rosenfeld B, Galieta M, Breitbart W, Krivo S. Interest in physician-assisted suicide among terminally ill AIDS patients: measuring and understanding desire for death. Paper presented at the biennial conference of the American Psychol-

ogy–Law Society; March 1998; Redondo Beach, Calif.

21. Back AL, Wallace JI, Starks HE, Pearlman RA. Physician-assisted suicide and euthanasia in Washington State. *Journal of the American Medical Association*, 1996; 275:919–925.

22. Slome LR, Mitchell TF, Charlebois E, Benevedes JM, Abrams DI. Physician-assisted suicide and patients with human immunodeficiency virus disease. *New England Journal of Medicine*, 1997; 336:417–421.

23. Meier DE, Emmons C, Wallenstein S, Quill T, Morrison RS, Cassel CK. A national survey of physician-assisted suicide and euthanasia in the United States. *New England Journal of Medicine*, 1998; 338:1193–1201.

24. Asch D. The role of critical care nurses in euthanasia and assisted suicide. *New England Journal of Medicine*, 1996; 334:1374–1379.

25. Scanlon C. Euthanasia and nursing practice: right question, wrong answer. *New England Journal of Medicine*, 1996; 324:1401–1402.

26. van der Maas PJ, van der Wal G, Haverkate I, et al. Euthanasia, physician-assisted suicide and other medical practices involving the end of life in the Netherlands, 1990–1995. *New England Journal of Medicine*, 1996; 335:1699–1705.

27. Rosenfeld B, Breitbart W, McDonald MV, Passik S, Portenoy R, Thaler H. Pain in ambulatory patients with AIDS. II: Impact on psychological functioning and quality of life. *Pain*, 1996; 68(3): 323–328.

28. Ganzini L, Lee MA, Heintz RT, Bloom JD, Fenn DS. The effect of depression treatment on elderly patients' preferences for life-sustaining medical therapy. *American Journal of Psychiatry*, 1994; 151: 1631–1636.

29. Owen C, Tennant C, Levi J, Jones M. Suicide and euthanasia: Patient attitudes in the context of cancer. *Psycho-oncology*, 1992; 1:79–88.

30. Breitbart W. Suicide in cancer patients. *Oncology*, 1987; 1:49–53.

31. Rosenfeld B, Passik S, White M. Treatment decision making with HIV: a pilot study of patient preferences. *Medical Decision Making*, 1997; 17(3): 307–314.

5

Anxiety in Palliative Care

David K. Payne, Ph.D.
Mary Jane Massie, M.D.

As patients enter the palliative or terminal phase of their illness, both physical and psychological burdens change. Anxiety commonly increases as patients become aware of both the relative ineffectiveness of medical treatments in halting the progress of their disease and, consequently, their limited life expectancy. Fears of death, disability, disfigurement, and dependency loom ever larger for patients who have been told that medical treatment will not, in all likelihood, lead to cure but will be palliative. The clinicians' awareness of the impact of the psychological and medical end-of-life issues on the development and persistence of anxiety will allow them to be more effective in helping patients manage their psychological distress.

PREVALENCE OF ANXIETY IN PATIENTS RECEIVING PALLIATIVE CARE

Throughout the span of the illness, cancer disrupts the social roles of patients, their interpersonal relationships, and the ways in which they view their future;[1] most people who have cancer are both fearful and sad. Although in the general population anxiety is associated with female gender, young age, and low socioeconomic status,[2] these patterns do not appear in cancer patients;

as cancer progresses, demographic factors may become less important. The evaluation of anxiety symptoms is a frequent reason for requesting a psychiatric consultation for cancer patients and accounted for 16% of requests for referrals in one study.[3] In that consultation study, 25% of patients were diagnosed as having either an anxiety (4%) or an adjustment disorder with anxious mood (21%), and 57% were diagnosed as having major depression (9%) or an adjustment disorder with depressed mood (48%). Most of the studies that have evaluated the presence of psychiatric symptoms in cancer patients have reported a higher prevalence of mixed anxiety and depressive symptoms than of anxiety alone.[4] Correlations between measures of depression and of anxiety on both clinician-rated[5] and self-report measures[6] are high, in all likelihood because these measures tap a common psychological trait: negative affect.[7] In the PSYCOG study of the prevalence of psychiatric disorders in cancer patients, about 21% of the sample had symptoms of anxiety.[4] In several controlled studies, cancer patients have been found to have higher levels of anxiety than healthy individuals. In looking at anxiety in the patient with advancing disease, Brandenberg[8] reported that 28% of advanced melanoma patients were anxious, in comparison to 15% of controls. Maguire et al. reported that anxiety increases with the diagnosis of cancer, peaks prior to surgical interventions, and frequently remains high, declining gradually during the first postoperative years.[9] Others have reported that anxiety increases as cancer progresses and that psychological health declines along with a decline in physical status.[6,10]

Patients who are receiving palliative chemotherapy may have a conditioned anticipatory response that arose from their past experience with chemotherapy and that may have persisted for years following the cessation of the original chemotherapy treatment.[11–13] Patients who are receiving palliative radiotherapy treatment may experience increased anxiety associated with concerns about increased bodily vulnerability and worries about whether the radiation will cause further body damage and may also experience claustrophobia, feeling that the radiation therapy suite is "tomb-like."[14] The anxiety experienced during chemotherapy and radiation therapy may paradoxically increase at the termination of treatment as patients feel "unprotected," see their physician(s) less often, and worry about the effectiveness of treatment. Patients with advanced disease frequently worry that they are losing their fight against cancer and that any cessation in chemotherapy or radiation therapy places them closer to the inevitability of death. Patients who are participating in clinical trials and who feel that they have been randomized to a less aggressive treatment modality may also experience increased anxiety.[15] Those patients who are receiving Phase I or Phase II trials may feel increased anxiety as they wonder if the treatment will either result in cure or "buy" them additional time.

DIAGNOSIS OF ANXIETY

Although by the time most patients enter the palliative-care phase they have likely had any anxiety disorders diagnosed, it is important to remember that prior to the palliative phase many patients may not have seen a mental health practitioner; therefore, the possibility of diagnosing anxiety disorder in patients with terminal illness should not be ruled out. Generally, however, only a small percentage of cancer patients have anxiety disorders that antedate the diagnosis of cancer and are exacerbated by the stress associated

with cancer diagnosis or treatment.[16] Although patients with anxiety usually report subjective feelings of foreboding, apprehension, or dread, these symptoms frequently intensify when patients perceive that death is imminent. Anxiety symptoms can be either cognitive or somatic; the most salient symptoms are usually somatic and include tachycardia, shortness of breath, diaphoresis, gastrointestinal distress, and nausea. Loss of appetite, diminished libido, and insomnia, symptoms also associated with depression, are common in patients with anxiety, as are feelings of hyperarousal and irritability. In patients with panic attacks, symptoms related to increased autonomic discharge increase dramatically.

In addition to somatic symptoms, anxious cancer patients facing death may often be plagued with recurrent unpleasant thoughts about cancer, including fears of death and of dependency on others. The thinking style of the anxious patient is characterized by overgeneralization and catastrophizing; negative outcomes seem inevitable, and patients view themselves as helpless in a hopeless situation. As their fears increase, patients may see their environment as threatening and often are motivated to flee, a reaction that commonly precipitates treatment refusals or demands for premature hospital discharge.[17]

The DSM-IV refers to anxiety resulting from uncontrolled pain, abnormal metabolic states, pulmonary emboli, and hormone-producing tumors as an anxiety disorder due to a general medical condition. Anxiety induced by medication (e.g., steroids, psychostimulants, sedatives, hypnotics, or anxiolytics) is called substance-induced anxiety disorder.[18]

In the palliative-care setting, a common cause of anxiety is uncontrolled pain. Although the hospice movement in this country and abroad has led the way in the understanding and treatment of pain in the terminal phase of illness, undermanaged pain remains a common cause of anxiety and diminished quality of life in the palliative setting. Understanding the specific nature of the patient's pain phenomenon may be helpful in determining the most appropriate treatment for pain and, consequently, anxiety. Patients with breakthrough pain (episodes of severe or excruciating pain superimposed on relatively stable, well-controlled baseline pain) reported significantly more anxiety and depression than did patients who did not report these episodes.[19] The undermanagement of patients' pain may result from a lack of understanding of the most appropriate pharmacological interventions. Rather than treating the patient's pain with short-acting opioids, such as oxymorphone, which may result in alternating periods of oversedation and periods of pain, the physician may prescribe longer-acting opioids, given around the clock and supplemented with shorter-acting opioids, that may provide more consistent pain relief. The consequence may be that not only does the patient receive more consistent pain relief, but also the patient's sense of control over the pain may alleviate his anxiety.

The presentation of the patient in acute pain is well known; the patient appears tense and is often restless and perspiring.[20] Agitation may ensue if adequate relief is not provided. Suicidal ideation is common with uncontrolled pain; no psychiatric diagnosis, however, can be made until the pain has been controlled.[21] If, after the pain has been adequately treated, the patient remains anxious, other medical or psychological factors should be considered.

A change in metabolic state or an impending medical catastrophe may be heralded by symptoms of anxiety. Suddenly occurring symptoms of anxiety with chest pain or respiratory distress may indicate a pulmonary embolus. Patients who are hypoxic often appear anxious and fear that they are suffocating or dying. Medications, such as bronchodilators and beta-adrenergic receptor stimulants that are commonly used for chronic respiratory conditions, may cause anxiety, irritability, and tremulousness. Patients who have a delirium often manifest symptoms of anxiety, restlessness, and agitation. These confusional states generally have multiple etiologies, including hypoglycemia, organ failure, electrolyte imbalance, nutritional failure, and infection.[22]

Although a less frequent cause of anxiety, hormone-secreting tumors may also produce symptoms of anxiety. Pheochromocytoma,[23] thyroid[24] and parathyroid[25] tumors, and adrenocorticotropic hormone (ACTH)-producing tumors[26] (most frequently associated with lung cancer and insulinoma) may be associated anxiety symptoms.

Among the medications used in palliative-care settings, corticosteroids are frequently a cause of anxiety symptoms such as motor restlessness and agitation. Dexamethasone may be given in high doses for the treatment of a spinal cord compression, and prednisone may be given as a premedication to reduce nausea for patients who are receiving palliative chemotherapy. The psychiatric symptoms associated with the use of steroids are dose-related and often persist even after the medications have been tapered. Akathisia, a common side effect of neuroleptic drugs (i.e., metoclopramide and prochlorperazine) used to control nausea and to treat the symptoms of a delirium, may often manifest as anxiety and restlessness.[27] The patient and the patient's family may be distressed by these symptoms and reluctant to report them for fear that they indicate that the patient is having a "nervous breakdown." Fortunately, these symptoms can be controlled by the addition of a benzodiazepine (e.g., lorazepam 0.5 to 2.0 mg po tid to qid), a beta blocker (e.g., propranolol 10 mg po tid), or an antiparkinsonian agent (e.g., diphenhydramine 25 to 50 mg po or iv). Patients and family members should be educated about the side effects of these medications and encouraged to report these easily managed symptoms when they occur.

Withdrawal states from alcohol, opioids, and benzodiazepines are often overlooked as causes of anxiety and agitation. Patients with head and neck cancers often have unreported or underreported histories of alcohol abuse. Consequently, with the presentation of increased anxiety and agitation, consideration of withdrawal states should be considered in these patients.[28] Patients in the palliative-care setting may have been prescribed shorter-acting benzodiazepines (e.g., lorazepam, alprazolam, and oxazepam) to control both anxiety and nausea. With inadequate dosing regimens, these patients often have rebound anxiety between doses. These patients may benefit from an increase in the dosing frequency of the short-acting benzodiazepine or a switch to a longer-acting benzodiazepine (e.g., clonazepam). Bronchodilators and beta-adrenergic stimulants, psychostimulants, and caffeine can all cause anxiety, irritability, and tremulousness.[29] Thyroid-replacement medication can produce symptoms of anxiety, especially when the dosage is being adjusted.[30]

Although patients in the palliative-care setting, in all likelihood, have had substantial experience with a variety of medical treatment modalities, chemotherapy and radiation therapy can be associated with increases in anxiety. Re-

peated exposures to highly emetogenic chemotherapeutic agents may have led to the development of anticipatory nausea and vomiting (ANV),
a conditioned response to environmental cues
(e.g., the sight of the hospital, smell of alcohol
preps) that surround the chemotherapy experience. There is evidence that ANV may be linked
to a preexisting anxiety diathesis and that it may
persist for years following the cessation of
chemotherapy.[13,31] Although newer antiemetic
regimens have led to a decrease in ANV, those
patients who are receiving palliative chemotherapy may have had past experiences with chemotherapy that may have led to the development of
persistent anxiety related to chemotherapy. In a
like manner, patients who are undergoing radiation therapy may feel apprehensive and anxious.[32] Anxiety associated with radiation therapy
may not decline as treatment progresses because
of the accumulated side effects and the fear associated with the cessation of treatment; the psychological distress associated with radiation therapy may exceed the physical distress that results
from the treatment itself.[33-35]

The diagnosis of anxiety usually is determined
by a clinical interview, and this remains the preferred assessment technique in the palliative-
care setting, where patients may be physically debilitated and/or may have cognitive deficits. In
patients who are less debilitated and who are cognitively intact, however, the use of assessment
instruments adds specificity to the diagnosis and
facilitates the monitoring of treatment progress.
Several instruments have been used to measure
anxiety: the Profile of Mood States,[36] the Brief
Symptom Inventory,[37] the Hospital Anxiety and
Depression Scale,[38] and the Rotterdam Symptoms Checklist.[39] The Hospital Anxiety and Depression Scale (HADS) is a self-report measure
that assesses the cognitive items associated with
depression and anxiety and thus avoids the confound of physical symptoms in medically ill patients.[38] The HADS has demonstrated validity
in assessing mood disturbances in cancer patients.[40] The Rotterdam Symptoms Checklist is
a self-report scale that measures both psychological and physical distress.[39] Although the Rotterdam Symptoms Checklist measures anxiety
and depression in its psychological distress scale
as a unitary phenomenon, the psychological distress scale does contain items associated with
anxiety.

The patient who appears anxious usually will
be determined to have "reactive" anxiety or an
adjustment disorder with anxious mood (described earlier); anxiety that is a manifestation of
a preexisting anxiety disorder; anxiety that is secondary to the exacerbation of the illness or related to medication side effects; or anxiety that
is a manifestation of another psychiatric disorder,
such as delirium or depression.

Phobia, Panic Disorders, Generalized Anxiety Disorder, and Posttraumatic Stress Disorder

Phobias, panic disorder, posttraumatic stress disorder, and generalized anxiety disorder may have
been treated in cancer patients for years prior to
the patient's cancer diagnosis. A small number of
patients are first diagnosed with these disorders
while undergoing cancer treatment. Although
the assumption is made (and is usually true) that
patients, throughout the course of disease and
treatment, will have had these anxiety disorders
addressed and treated, the possibility that these
disorders will appear for the first time when the
patient is in the palliative-care setting should not
be excluded from consideration. Because they
have the potential not only to cause extreme distress but also to interfere with adequate medical
management of the patient, it is important to accurately diagnose and treat these anxiety disorders.[41,42]

There is a range of phobias that can be exacerbated by exposure to the medical environment;
phobias relatd to needles, blood, hospitals, and
doctors are common. The common characteristic of all phobias is extreme anxiety on exposure
to a feared object(s) or situation(s) and a persistent anxiety in anticipation of these situations.
Agoraphobia, the most common phobia in the
general population, and claustrophobia may appear to present de novo in patients who are confined in the frightening hospital environment
without the usual environmental supports that
keep their anxiety symptoms manageable. Patients who require magnetic resonance imaging
or radiation therapy or who must be confined in
intensive-care or reverse-isolation settings frequently experience increased anxiety.[43]

In contrast to phobias, in which there is a
clearly defined situation or object of dread, panic
disorder often presents as a sudden, unpredictable

episode of intense discomfort and fear accompanied by shortness of breath, diaphoresis, tachycardia, feelings of choking or being smothered, and thoughts of impending doom. Symptoms of a preexisting panic disorder may intensify during the palliative-care phase when patients are confronting increasing physical symptoms and their own mortality; severe untreated symptoms may prevent the patient from participating in adequate symptom management. Generalized anxiety disorder is characterized by excessive worry, difficulty controlling the worry or apprehension, and the presence of symptoms of autonomic hyperactivity and hypervigilance.

In addition to heightened psychological distress associated with cancer treatment, cancer patients may experience the symptoms characteristic of posttraumatic stress disorder (PTSD), similar to those reported by individuals who have been subjected to other types of trauma (e.g., combat, rape, or natural disaster).[44,45] Alter et al. reported that almost half (48%) of a group of cancer survivors reported symptoms related to PTSD, with 4% meeting the criteria for current PTSD diagnosis and 22% meeting the criteria for a lifetime diagnosis of PTSD.[46] Patients with this disorder may repeatedly reexperience frightening events associated with their cancer diagnosis or treatment and have a chronic exaggerated startle response, nightmares, or autonomic hyperactivity.

Anxiety as a Manifestation of Other Psychiatric Disorders

In terminally ill patients, anxiety may be a manifestation of either depression or delirium. Increasingly, depression and anxiety are viewed as syndromes that exist along a continuum, and there is an overlap in the symptomatology of these two mood states. Depression may be distinguished from anxiety by the presence of the psychological symptoms of depression, such as hopelessness, anhedonia, worthlessness, and suicidal ideation. Delirium, a common diagnosis in patients who are receiving palliative care, frequently has anxiety or restlessness as a prominent feature but is distinguished from anxiety by the presence of disorientation; impaired memory and concentration; fluctuating level of consciousness; and altered perceptions, including hallucinations, delusions, or illusions.[47]

Case Example

A 66-year-old man with metastatic colon cancer was being followed in a home hospice program. Nausea had been a persistent problem, and the patient was prescribed metoclopramide, which he had been taking on an "as needed" basis. The patient began to report feeling general discomfort, jitteriness, and anxiety. Evaluation revealed that the patient had evidence of akathisia, likely from metoclopramide. Additionally, when asked whether he was experiencing pain, the patient stated that, although he was taking a long-acting opioid, he still experienced moderate to severe pain with episodes of breakthrough pain. He told the hospice physician that he thought that all patients who had cancer were supposed to experience pain. The patient, an independent and rather stoic individual, also worried about the impact that his illness was having on his wife and adult children and felt that "by complaining" he would make matters worse. The dose of metoclopramide was reduced, and, after the patient underwent a thorough mental status examination that was not suggestive of cognitive impairment, low doses of lorazepam (0.5 mg bid) were added to treat both nausea and anxiety. The patient was given information about the appropriate monitoring of pain and was instructed in how to supplement around-the-clock doses of morphine sulfate with doses as needed of oxycodone, a shorter-acting opioid. Finally, supportive therapy focused on the patient's anxieties about his increasing dependence on his family as well as on his fear of death allowed him to face the end of his life with reduced psychological distress.

TREATMENT OF ANXIETY

The most effective management of anxiety is multimodal and usually involves psychotherapy, behavioral therapy, and pharmacological management. During the initial evaluation of the patient's symptoms, both emotional support and information is given to the patient.[48] Exploration of the patient's fears and apprehensions about the progression of his disease, upcoming procedures, or psychosocial difficulties often serves to alleviate a substantial degree of the patient's anxiety. As the patient enters the palliative phase and increasingly becomes aware of the foreshortening of his life, his concerns may change or intensify. Patients may become increasingly focused on concerns about suffering and death. At this stage, worries about increased dependence, changes in marital, family, or social-role functioning, spiritual concerns, and financial issues may wax or wane, depending on the degree to which the patient has worked through issues concerning mortality.[49]

Psychological Treatment of Anxiety in Palliative Care

As patients enter the terminal phase of the disease process, the focus of psychotherapy often changes. Rather than helping patients understand the antecedents of their anxiety or change maladaptive styles of coping, psychotherapy is more often focused on helping patients to contain the anxiety associated with their impending death or to deal with practical concerns and fears around the issue of dying.

Death anxiety, the fear associated with death, is a phenomenon associated with being human. It is the fear of nonbeing, the ultimate existential concern. Although some patients may have convictions about the veracity of their spiritual belief systems that allow them to face this transition with diminished anxiety and depression,[50] is not uncommon for patients with seemingly well-established spiritual beliefs to become destabilized in the face of end-of-life issues. The clergy can frequently be helpful in shoring up the spiritual beliefs of some patients. The fears and anxiety associated with death vary across the life span, and the clinician's knowledge of these developmental differences allows for more effective therapeutic interventions.

There are specific characteristics that distinguish psychotherapy with the terminally ill from psychotherapy with less medically ill patients.[51] In the face of the patient's impending death, the goals of psychotherapy are much more finite; insight is not a essential therapeutic task. Therapy does not usually move toward a specific goal such as termination; the focus on providing a nurturing, supportive relationship with the dying patient becomes paramount. As the patient grapples with the practical fears and anxieties associated with dying (e.g., "How do I want my children reared?" "Who will take care of my mentally retarded sister?" "How can I resolve the problems that I am having with my family before I die?"), the therapist may need to be active on the patient's behalf by serving as an advocate or om-

budsman; maintaining a therapeutic facade or detachment may not be as essential in the work with the dying. In the psychotherapeutic treatment of anxiety in the terminally ill patient, the line between psychotherapy and a supportive relationship is blurred; the patient sets the pace, elements not generally present in traditional psychotherapy (e.g., normal conversation) may be present, and defenses such as denial, although acknowledged, may be considered a healthy and adaptive response to impending death and consequently may not be challenged. Ultimately, the goals of therapy with the dying patient are to increase the patient's sense of psychological as well as physical comfort. A number of therapeutic modalities help achieve this goal.

Frank discussions about patient's fears and anxieties concerning dying have been shown to be effective in alleviating patients' anxieties. Spiegel et al., in their group intervention for women with Stage IV breast cancer, have demonstrated that the process of detoxifying and demystifying the experience of death leads to reduced levels of anxiety and psychological distress.[52]

Relatively short-term psychological interventions have proven to be effective in reducing the distress associated with cancer.[53] The efficacy of psychological treatments without the use of drugs depends on the duration and severity of the patient's anxiety. For patients with mild to moderate anxiety, the use of psychological techniques alone may be sufficient to assist them in managing anxiety.[54]

Careful patient selection is important to the success of psychological approaches to managing anxiety. Those dying patients who are most likely to benefit from psychological interventions are those whose anxiety has not been controlled by other means; those who have a need for self-control and are reluctant to take medication; and those who have experienced or acknowledge the efficacy of such approaches. Individuals who are poor candidates for psychological approaches to the management of distress are those who have delirium or dementia; those who are disinterested or demonstrate noncompliance in learning to use psychological techniques; and those who have a history of serious psychiatric illness.[55] Psychological interventions for anxiety in cancer patients fall into four categories: psychoeducational, behavioral, cognitive-behavioral, and group interventions.[56]

Psychoeducational interventions are particularly useful for anxious patients who have difficulty understanding medical information about their prognoses and planned procedures and treatments. Although many patients will be quite knowledgeable about the sequelae of particular treatment modalities, providing information about predictable side effects of palliative chemotherapy or radiotherapy helps to normalize the experience for them and to reduce their anxiety.[57,58] Similarly, explaining the predictable emotional phases through which patients pass as they face new and frightening information may also alleviate their anxiety. Providing information to patients' families enables them to cope more effectively, which in turn enhances patients' sense of support.[59,60]

The rationale for all behavioral techniques is the substitution of more adaptive behavior (i.e., increased coping ability) for less adaptive behavior (i.e., anxiety). Behavioral approaches to the management of anxiety are more useful than standard psychodynamic approaches for children and for adults who are not psychologically minded. Progressive muscle relaxation has been demonstrated in a number of studies to be effective in the management of anxiety.[61,62] In a study comparing the efficacy of relaxation and alprazolam in cancer patients, both treatments were shown to be effective for mild to moderate anxiety, with alprazolam having a slight advantage over relaxation training alone.[63] Progressive relaxation involves instructing the patient to relax different parts of the body sequentially by either tensing and relaxing the muscle groups (active muscle relaxation) or by concentrating on relaxing parts of the body without tensing the muscles (passive muscle relaxation). Both approaches are effective in reducing anxiety, although in medically debilitated patients passive relaxation may prove to be more manageable.[64] Frequently, guided imagery is a component of a progressive relaxation training program; a behavioral treatment that includes both guided imagery and relaxation has been demonstrated to be more effective in lowering distress level than use of either component alone.[65,66] In addition to progressive muscle relaxation, hypnosis has proven to be effective in the management of psychological distress associated with procedures,[67] as well as in the management of treatment-related side effects such as anticipatory nausea and vomiting and pain. Desensitization, response prevention, thought stopping, modeling, and distraction are other behavioral techniques that may be useful in the management of anxiety and phobias.[55]

Behavioral techniques have also been demonstrated to be effective in the treatment of anticipatory nausea and vomiting. A conditioned response to chemotherapy, anticipatory nausea and vomiting appears to be correlated with preexisting trait anxiety[31] and with state anxiety at the time of the chemotherapy infusions.[68] Progressive muscle relaxation has been shown to decrease both nausea and vomiting, as well as anxiety, in patients who are receiving emetogenic chemotherapy.[61,65,69]

Individual psychotherapy in general[56] and cognitive-behavioral approaches in particular[70] have been demonstrated to reduce psychological distress. Accordingly to the cognitive-behavioral model, emotional distress arises or continues because of maladaptive beliefs and thinking patterns. Patients are encouraged to identify these maladaptive thoughts, reconsider them more logically, and experiment with alternative viewpoints and behaviors that give them greater control over their situation. Using this model to develop an intervention designed to address issues associated with cancer, Moorey and Greer[70] teach patients to identify negative thoughts; rehearse impending stressful events; implement ways of handling them more effectively; plan and carry out practical activities that create a sense of mastery; express feelings openly to their partners; and increase both their self-esteem and their "fighting spirit" by identifying and fostering personal strengths. Follow-up studies of this intervention have consistently demonstrated that patients who have had behavioral-cognitive therapy receive significantly lower scores on anxiety and psychological distress than do controls.[71,72] Although these interventions were conducted with patients who were receiving active treatment, the principles are applicable to patients receiving palliative care. Approaching the fear of death, concluding unfinished business, and restructuring one's expectations for life to include finding pleasure in short-term goals rather than in long-term projects are appropriate foci for cognitive-behavioral therapy with terminally ill patients.

Group interventions have also been shown to reduced psychological distress in cancer patients[56] and have demonstrated effectiveness for individuals with a variety of cancer diagnoses[73] and in varying stages of cancer.[74] In one study, patients who participated in support groups for at least a year reported less tension than did controls.[52] The techniques employed in these groups included fostering a sense of supportive commonality among the members; providing education, emotional support, and instruction in stress management and coping strategies; and behavioral training.

Case Example

A 59-year-old professional woman with Stage IV breast cancer was told by her physician that palliative chemotherapy was the "best option." The patient was terrified about her deteriorating physical condition and tearfully described her growing understanding of the reality of her death. Her medical course was complicated by a spinal cord compression that had resulted in paraplegia. As she was given increasing doses of dexamethasone for her cord compression, she became progressively anxious and tearful. Although the patient indicated that she had dealt with anxiety throughout the course of her illness "by strength of character," she felt that her anxiety level at this point was much more intense and no longer manageable. The psychiatric consultant believed that her anxiety was in part exacerbated by the dexamethasone and prescribed the neuroleptic haloperidol (0.5 mg po), which reduced her level of anxiety. The patient had been reluctant to use any psychotropic medications during the course of her illness, but she did indicate that she had in the past utilized meditation techniques for controlling stress. The patient was reintroduced to behavioral techniques for managing her anxiety, and she assisted her therapist in making an audiotape of a progressive relaxation exercise. The patient's growing control over her anxiety allowed her to deal more effectively with the debilitation associated with cord compression, as well as with her impending death.

Pharmacological Management of Anxiety

A variety of anxiolytic drugs are prescribed for cancer patients; one-quarter to one-third of patients with advanced cancer receive antianxiety medication during their hospitalizations.[74] In deciding whether a pharmacological approach to

the management of anxiety may be useful, the severity of the patient's symptoms that is the most reliable guide. Patients with mild "reactive" anxiety may benefit from either supportive measures or behavioral measures alone. Given the likelihood of decreased hepatic and renal functioning, as well as increased sensitivity to pharmacological interventions, in patients receiving palliative care, if drugs are to be used, the rubric of starting with lower doses than would be used with physically healthy patients and increasing these doses more cautiously will lead to more manageable side-effects. Table 5.1 lists the drugs normally used to treat anxiety.

For the patient who has felt persistently apprehensive and anxious, the first-line antianxiety drugs are the benzodiazepines. In the palliative-care setting, however, the excessive use of benzodiazepines may result in mental-status changes such as confusion, impaired concentration, memory, or confusion. These changes are more often seen in elderly patients, those with advanced disease, and those with impaired hepatic function. For patients with compromised hepatic function, the use of shorter-acting benzodiazepines, such as lorazepam, oxazepam, and temazepam, is preferred, since these drugs are metabolized by conjugation with glucuronic acid and have no active metabolites. Lorazepam (0.25 to 2 mg qid) and alprazolam (0.25 to 0.5 mg tid) are useful not only for anxiety but also as antiemetic (lorazepam) and antipanic (alprazolam) drugs. Lorazepam has demonstrated antiemetic properties; both lorazepam and alprazolam have been shown in controlled trials to reduce both anticipatory nausea and vomiting associated with both chemotherapy and postchemotherapy.[75,76] Lorazepam also has amnestic properties and when given prior to chemotherapy or a procedure may produce amnesia for the event, thus reducing the likelihood that a conditioned aversion will develop.[77] A longer-acting benzodiazepine, such as clonazepam (0.5 to 2 mg bid), may provide more consistent relief of anxiety symptoms and may have mood-stabilizing effects as well. For insomnia, the benzodiazepines temazepam (15 to 30 mg qhs) and triazolam (0.25 to 0.5 mg qhs), as well as the nonbenzodiazepine hypnotic zolpidem (10 to 20 mg qhs), may be effective. A relatively nonsedating neuroleptic such as haloperidol (5 mg qhs) or a sedating neuroleptic such as thioridazine (25 to 50 mg tid) may be more effective for the pa-

Table 5.1 Drugs Used To Treat Anxiety

Drug (Trade Name)	Approximate Dose Equivalent	Initial Dosage	Adsorption	Metabolites
Benzodiazepines				
Alprazolam (Xanax)	0.5	.25–5 tid	Intermediate	Yes
Oxazepam (Serax)	10.0	10–15 tid	Slow-intermediate	No
Lorazepam (Ativan)	1.0	.5–2.0 tid	Intermediate	No
Chlordiazepoxide (Librium)	10.0	10–25 tid	Intermediate	Yes
Diazepam (Valium)	5.0	5–10 bid	Fast	Yes
Chlorazepate (Tranxene)	7.5	7.5–15 bid	Fast	Yes
Clonazepam (Klonopin)	0.25	.25–1 bid	Intermediate	Yes
Temazepam (Restoril)	30.0	15–30 qhs	Intermediate	No
Triazolam (Halcion)	0.25	.25–.50 qhs	Intermediate	No
Antihistamines				
Hydroxyzine (Vistaril)	10	10–50 mg tid		
Diphenhydramine (Benadryl)	25	25–75 mg bid		
Neuroleptics				
Haloperidol (Haldol)	0.5	.5–1 mg bid		
Thioridazine (Mellaril)	10	10–50 mg tid		
Other				
Zolpidem (Ambien)	10	10–20 mg qhs		

tient who is both anxious and confused. Neuroleptics may also be useful for the patient whose anxiety is substance-induced (e.g., steroids). Drowsiness and somnolence are the most common adverse effects of benzodiazepines; reductions in dose and the passage of time eliminates these effects. Structurally unlike other anxiolytics, buspirone (5 to 20 mg tid) is useful for patients with generalized anxiety disorder and for those in whom there is the potential for abuse. Buspirone is not effective on a prn ("as needed") basis, and its effects are not apparent for 1 to 2 weeks. Additionally, patients who have been prescribed benzodiazepines in the past may find that buspirone does not alleviate their anxiety as effectively as benzodiazepines.

For the treatment of panic disorder and agoraphobia, the benzodiazepine alprazolam and antidepressant medications (i.e., serotonin reuptake inhibitors, tricyclic antidepressants, and monoamine oxidase inhibitors) have demonstrated effectiveness. Alprazolam rapidly blocks panic attacks. The tricyclic antidepressant imipramine is effective in the management of panic disorder; its anticholinergic side effects, however, are not well tolerated by debilitated cancer patients. In the oncology setting, the serotonin reuptake inhibitors sertraline and paroxetine, which have fewer side effects than the tricyclic antidepressants, are effective in the management of both depression and panic disorder. Antidepressants tend to require from 1 to 4 weeks to reach therapeutic levels and therefore may be less useful in the palliative-care setting. Although monoamine oxidase inhibitors are effective in the management of panic disorder and depression, the risk of hypertensive crisis from concomitant ingestion of sympathomimetics (e.g., amphetamines and meperidine) commonly used in the oncology setting, coupled with the need for a low-tyramine diet, make these medications less desirable for cancer patients.

In anxious patients with severely compromised pulmonary function, the use of benzodiazepines that suppress central respiratory mechanisms may be unsafe. A low dose of an antihistamine (e.g., hydroxyzine 10 to 50 mg tid or diphenhydramine 25 to 75 mg bid) can be useful for these individuals. The anticholinergic effects of these medications must be monitored carefully in the debilitated patient who is prone to develop a delirium.

SUMMARY

The palliative phase of terminal illness brings new challenges in the management of psychological distress in general and anxiety in particular.[29,78] The clinician's understanding of the medical and psychological precipitants of anxiety, coupled with an appreciation of the multimodal treatments options, offers patients receiving primarily palliative care the possibility of comprehensive treatment for anxiety.

References

1. Derogatis L, Wise T. *Anxiety and Depressive Disorders in the Medical Patient.* Washington, DC: American Psychiatric Press, 1989.
2. Kessler R, McGonagle K, Zhao S, Nelson CB, Hughes M, Eshelman S, Wittchen HV, Kendler KS. Lifetime and 12 month prevalence of DSMIII-R psychiatric disorders in the United States. *Archives of General Psychiatry,* 1994; 51:8–19.
3. Massie MJ, Holland JC. Consultation and liaison issues in cancer care. *Psychiatric Medicine,* 1987; 5:343–359.
4. Derogatis LR, Morrow GR, Fetting J, et al. The prevalence of psychiatric disorders among cancer patients. *Journal of the American Medical Association,* 1983; 249:751–757.
5. Moorey S, Greer S, Watson M, et al. The factor structure and factor stability of the Hospital Anxiety and Depression Scale in patients with cancer. *British Journal of Psychiatry,* 1991; 158:255–259.
6. Cassileth BR, Lusk E, Huter R, Strouse T, Brown L. Concordance of depression and anxiety in patients with cancer. *Psychology Report,* 1984; 54: 588–590.
7. Zinberg R, Barlow D. Mixed anxiety-depression. A new diagnostic category. In: Rapee R, Barlow D, eds, *Chronic Anxiety: Generalized Anxiety Disorder and Mixed Anxiety-Depression.* New York: Gilford Press, 1991:136.
8. Brandenberg Y, Bolund C, Sigurdardottir V. Anxiety and depressive symptoms at different stages of malignant melanoma. *Psycho-oncology,* 1992; 1: 71–78.
9. Maguire GP, Lee E, Bevington D, Kuchman C, Crabtree R, Cornell C. Psychiatric problems in the first year after mastectomy. *British Medical Journal,* 1978; 1:963–965.
10. Weisman A, Worden J. The emotional impact of recurrent cancer. *Journal of Psychosocial Oncology,* 1986; 3:5–16.
11. Olafsdottir M, Sjoder P, Westling B. Prevalence and prediction of chemotherapy-related anxiety, nausea and vomiting in cancer patients. *Behavioral Research Therapy,* 1986; 24:59–66.
12. Holland J. Anxiety and cancer: The patient and the family. *Journal of Clinical Psychiatry,* 1989; 50:20–25.
13. Kvale G, Glimelius B, Hoffman K, Sjoden P. Prechemotherapy nervousness as a marker for anticipatory nausea: a case of a non-causal predictor. *Psycho-oncology,* 1993; 2:33–41.
14. Peck A, Boland J. Emotional reactions to radiation treatment. *Cancer,* 1977; 40:180–184.
15. Cassileth B, Knuiman M, Abeloff G, et al: Anxiety levels in patients randomized to adjuvant therapy versus observation for early breast cancer. *Journal of Clinical Oncology,* 1986; 4:972–974.
16. Shalev A, Schreiber S, Galai T, McLoud R. Posttraumatic stress disorder following medical events. *British Journal of Clinical Psychology,* 1993; 32:247–253.
17. Braun P, Greenberg D, Dasberg H, Lerer B. Core symptoms of PTSD improved by alprazolam treatment. *Journal of Clinical Psychiatry,* 1990; 51:236–238.
18. American Psychatric Association. *Diagnostic and Statistical Manual of Mental Disorders,* 4th ed. Washington, DC: Author, 1994.
19. Payne, D. Cognitive factors in breakthrough pain. Ph.D. dissertation, University of Louisville, 1995.
20. Sternbach R. *Pain Patients: Traits and Treatments.* New York: Academic Press, 1974.
21. Massie MJ, Gagnon P, Holland JC. Depression and suicide in patients with cancer. *Journal of Pain and Symptom Management,* 1994; 9:325–340.
22. Massie MJ, Holland JC, Glass E. Delirium in terminally ill cancer patients. *American Journal of Psychiatry,* 1983; 140:1048–1050.
23. Starkman M, Zelnik T, Nesse R, et al. Anxiety in patients with pheochromocytomas. *Archives of Internal Medicine,* 1985; 145:248–252.
24. Kathol R, Dalahunt J. The relationship of anxiety and depression to symptoms of hyperthyroidism using operational criteria. *General Hospital Psychiatry,* 1986; 8:23–28.
25. Lawlor B. Hypocalcemia, hypoarathyroidism, and organic anxiety syndrome. *Journal of Clinical Psychiatry,* 1988; 49:317–318.

26. Breitbart W. Endocrine-related psychiatric disorders. In: Holland JC, Rowland JH, eds. *Handbook of Psychooncology: Psychological Care of the Patient with Cancer.* New York: Oxford University Press, 1989:356–366.

27. Fleishman S, Lavin M, Sattler M, Szarka H. Antiemetic-induced akathisia in cancer patients. *American Journal of Psychiatry,* 1994; 151:763–765.

28. Lundberg JC, Passik SD. Alcoholism and cancer. In: Holland JH, Breitbart WS, Jacobsen PJ, Lederberg MS, Loscalzo M, Massie MJ, McCorkle R, eds, *Textbook of Psycho-oncology.* New York: Oxford University Press, 1998; 45–48.

29. Levy MH, Catalino RB. Control of common physical symptoms other than pain in patients with terminal disease. *Seminars in Oncology,* 1985; 12:411–430.

30. Hall R. Psychiatric effects of thyroid hormone disturbance. *Psychosomatics,* 1983; 27:7–18.

31. Jacobsen P, Bovberg D, Redd W. Anticipatory anxiety in women receiving chemotherapy for breast cancer. *Health Psychology,* 1993; 12:469–475.

32. Forester B, Kornfeld D, Fleiss J. Psychiatric aspects of radiotherapy. *American Journal of Psychiatry,* 1978; 135:960–963.

33. Anderson B, Karlson J, Anderson B, Tewfik H. Anxiety and cancer treatment: response to stressful radiotherapy. *Health Psychology,* 1984; 3:535–551.

34. Holland J, Rowland J, Lebovitz A, et al. Reactions to cancer treatment: assessment of emotional response to adjuvant radiotherapy as a guide to planned intervention. *Psychiatric Clinics of North America,* 1979; 2:347–358.

35. Munro A, Biruls R, Griffin A, Thomas H, Vallis K. Distress associated with radiotherapy for malignant disease: a quantitative analysis based on patients perceptions. *British Journal of Cancer,* 1989; 60:370–374.

36. Cella D, Jacobsen P, Orav E, Holland J, Silberfarb P, Rafla S. A brief POMS measure of distress in cancer patients. *Journal of Chronic Disease,* 1987; 40:939–942.

37. Derogatis LR, Melisaratos N. The brief symptom inventory: an introductory report. *Psychological Medicine,* 1983, 13:595–605.

38. Zigmond A, Snaith R. The Hospital Anxiety and Depression Scale. *Acta Psychiatrica Scandinavia,* 1983; 67:361–370.

39. de Haes J, van Knippenberg F, Neijut J. Measuring psychological and physical distress in cancer patients: structure and application of the Rotterdam Symptom Checklist. *British Journal of Cancer,* 1990; 62:1034–1038.

40. Ibbotson T, Maguire P, Selby T, Priestman T, Wallace L. Screening for anxiety and depression in cancer patients: the effects of disease and treatment. *European Journal of Cancer,* 1994; 30A: 37–40.

41. Massie MJ. Anxiety, panic and phobias. In: Holland JC, Rowland JH, eds, *Handbook of Psychooncology: Psychological Care of the Patient with Cancer.* New York: Oxford University Press, 1989: 300–309.

42. Noyes R, Holt CS, Massie MJ. Anxiety disorders. In: Holland JH, Breitbart WS, Jacobsen PJ, Lederberg MS, Loscalzo M, Massie MJ, McCorkle R, eds, *Textbook of Psycho-oncology.* New York: Oxford University Press, 1998; 548–563.

43. Brennan S, Redd W, Jacobsen P, et al. Anxiety and panic during magnetic resonance scans. *Lancet,* 1988; 2:512.

44. Hamner M. Exacerbation of posttraumatic stress disorder symptoms with medical illness. *General Hospital Psychiatry,* 1994; 16:135–137.

45. Passik SD, Grummon KL. Post-traumatic Stress Disorder. In: Holland JH, Breitbart WS, Jacobsen PJ, Lederberg MS, Loscalzo M, Massie MJ, McCorkle R, eds, *Textbook of Psycho-oncology.* New York: Oxford University Press, 1998; 595–607.

46. Alter CL, Pelcovitz D, Axelrod A, et al. The identification of PTSD in cancer survivors. *Psychosomatics,* 1996; 37:137–143.

47. Wise M, Rieck S. Diagnostic considerations approaches to underlying anxiety in the medically ill. *Journal of Clinical Psychiatry,* 1993; 54:22–26.

48. Massie MJ, Shakin E. Management of depression and anxiety in cancer patients. In: Breitbart W, Holland J, eds. *Psychiatric Aspects of Symptom Management in Cancer Patients.* Washington, DC: American Psychiatric Press, 1993:1–21.

49. Maguire P, Faulkner A, Regnard C. Eliciting the current problems of the patient with cancer. *Palliative Medicine,* 1993; 7:151–156.

50. Alvarado DA, Templer DI, Bresler C, Thomas-Dobson S. The relationship of religious variables to death, depression and death anxiety. *Journal of Clinical Psychology,* 1995; 51: 202–204.

51. Feigenberg L, Shneidman E. Clinical thanatology and psychotherapy: some reflections on caring for the dying person. *Omega,* 1979; 10:1–8.

52. Spiegel D, Bloom J, Yalom I. Group support for patients with metastatic cancer. *Archives of General Psychiatry,* 1981; 38:527–533.

53. Trijsburg R, Van Knippenbert F, Rijpma W. Effects of psychological treatment on cancer patients: a critical review. *Psychosomatic Medicine,* 1992; 54:489–517.

54. Maguire P, Faulkner A, Regnard C. Managing the anxious patient with advancing disease: a flow diagram. *Palliative Medicine*, 1993; 7:239–244.

55. Mastrovito R. Behavioral techniques. In: Holland JC, Rowland JH, eds. *Handbook of Psychooncology: Psychological Care of the Patient with Cancer.* New York: Oxford University Press, 1989:492–501.

56. Fawzy F, Fawzy N, Arndt L, Pasnau R. Critical review of psychosocial interventions in cancer care. *Archives of General Psychiatry*, 1995; 52:100–113.

57. Ali N, Khalil H. Effect of psychoeducational intervention on anxiety among Egyptian bladder cancer patients. *Cancer Nursing*, 1989; 12:236–242.

58. Jacobs C, Ross R, Walker I, Stockdale F. Behavior of cancer patients: a randomized study of the effects of education and peer support groups. *American Journal of Clinical Oncology*, 1983; 6:347–353.

59. Massie MJ, Holland JC. Overview of normal reactions and prevalence of psychiatric disorders. In: Holland JC, Rowland JH, eds, *Handbook of Psychooncology: Psychological Care of the Patient with Cancer.* New York: Oxford University Press, 1989: 273–283.

60. Wellisch D, Moster M, Van Scoy C. Management of family emotional stress: family group therapy in a private oncology practice. *International Journal of Group Psychotherapy*, 1978; 28:225–231.

61. Burish T, Tope D. Psychological techniques for controlling adverse side effects of cancer chemotherapy: findings from a decade of research. *Journal of Pain Symptom Management*, 1992; 7:287–301.

62. Fleming U. Relaxation therapy for far-advanced cancer. *Practitioner*, 1985; 229:471–475.

63. Holland J, Morrow G, Schmale A, et al. A randomized clinical trial of alprazolam versus progressive muscle relaxation in cancer patients with anxiety and depressive symptoms. *Journal of Clinical Oncology*, 1991; 9:1004–1011.

64. Ferguson J, Marquis J, Taylor C. A script for deep muscle relaxation. *Diseases of the Nervous System*, 1977; 38:703–708.

65. Burish T, Carey M, Krozely M, Grego F. Conditioned side effects induced by cancer chemotherapy prevention through behavioral treatment. *Journal of Consulting Clinical Psychologists*, 1987; 55:42–48.

66. Gruber B, Hersh S, Hall N, et al. Immunological responses of breast cancer patients to behavioral interventions. *Biofeedback Self Regulation*, 1993; 18:1–22.

67. Wilson-Barnet, J. Psychological reaction to medical procedures. *Psychotherapy and Psychosomatics*, 1992; 57:118–127.

68. Andrykowski, M. The role of anxiety in the development of anticipatory nausea in cancer chemotherapy: a review and synthesis. *Psychosomatic Medicine*, 1990; 52:458–475.

69. Vasterling J, Jenkins R, Tope D, Burish T. Cognitive distraction and relaxation training for the control of side effects due to cancer chemotherapy. *Journal of Behavioral Medicine*, 1993; 16:65–80.

70. Moorey S, Greer S. *Psychological Therapy for Patients with Cancer: A New Approach.* Oxford: Heinemann, 1989.

71. Greer S, Moorey S, Baruch J, et al. Adjuvant psychological therapy for patients with cancer: a prospective randomized trial. *British Medical Journal*, 1992; 304:675–680.

72. Moorey S, Greer S, Watson M, et al. Adjuvant psychological therapy for patients with cancer: outcome at one year. *Psycho-oncology*, 1994; 3:39–46.

73. Cain D, Kohorn E, Quinlan D, Latimer K, Schwartz P. Psychosocial benefits of a cancer support group. *Cancer*, 1986; 57:183–189.

74. Stiefel FC, Kornblith A, Holland J. Changes in the prescription patterns of psychotrophic drugs for cancer patients during a 10 year period. *Cancer*, 1990; 65:1048–1053.

75. Triozzi PL, Goldstein D, Laszlo J. Contributions of benzodiazepines to cancer therapy. *Cancer Investigation*, 1988; 6:103–111.

76. Greenberg D, Surman O, Clarke J, et al. Alprazolam for phobic nausea and vomiting related to cancer chemotherapy. *Cancer Treatment Reports*, 1987; 71:549–550.

77. Klein D: Prevention of claustrophobia induced by MR imaging: use of alprazolam. *American Journal of Roentgenology*, 1991; 156:633.

78. Payne DK, Massie MJ. Anxiety and depression. In: Berger A, Levy MH, Portenoy RK, Weissman DE, eds, *Principles and Practice of Supportive Oncology.* Philadelphia: Lippincott, 1997:497–511.

6

Delirium in the Terminally Ill

William Breitbart, MD
Kenneth Cohen, M.D.

Delirium is extremely common in cancer and AIDS patients with advanced disease, particularly in the last weeks of life. Delirium is associated with increased morbidity in the terminally ill, causing distress in patients, family members, and staff.[1–3] Delirium can interfere dramatically with the recognition and control of other physical and psychological symptoms, such as pain,[4–6] in the later stages of illness. Sometimes a preterminal event, delirium is a sign of significant physiologic disturbance, usually involving multiple medical etiologies, including infection, organ failure, and medication side effects (including opioids), as well as extremely rare paraneoplastic syndromes.[7–11] Unfortunately, delirium is often underrecognized or misdiagnosed and inappropriately treated or untreated in terminally ill patients. Impediments to progress in the recognition and treatment of delirium have included confusion regarding terminology and lack of consistency in the use of diagnostic classification systems. In addition, the signs and symptoms of delirium can be diverse and are sometimes mistaken for other psychiatric disorders, such as mood or anxiety disorders. Practitioners who care for patients with life-threatening illnesses must be able to diagnose delirium accurately, undertake appropriate assessment of etiologies, and understand the benefits and the risks of the pharmacologic and nonpharmacologic interventions currently available for managing delirium among the terminally ill.

PREVALENCE OF DELIRIUM IN THE TERMINALLY ILL

Delirium is one of the most prevalent mental disorders in general hospital practice. At greater risk for delirium are the elderly, the postoperative, and cancer and AIDS patients.[12–20] Knight and Folstein[21] estimated that 33% of hospitalized medically ill patients have serious cognitive impairments. Approximately 30% to 40% of medically hospitalized AIDS patients develop delirium,[20] and as many as 65% to 80% develop some type of organic mental disorder.[22] Massie and coworkers found delirium in 85% (11 of 13) of terminal cancer patients.[12] Pereira and coworkers found the prevalence of cognitive impairment in cancer inpatients to be 44%; just prior to the patients' deaths, the prevalence rose to 62.1%.[13] Delirium also occurs in up to 51% of postoperative patients.[14,23] The incidence of delirium is currently increasing, which reflects the growing numbers of elderly, who are particularly susceptible.[15] Studies of elderly patients admitted to medical wards estimate that 30% to 50% of patients age 70 years or older showed symptoms of delirium at some point during hospitalization.[16,17] A study using the SCID to measure psychiatric morbidity in terminally ill cancer patients found delirium to account for 52% of all diagnoses in subjects who met the DSM-IV criteria for a psychiatric disorder. In addition, patients with dementia are at even greater risk; thus, as the prevalence of dementia increases with the aging of the population, so the incidence of delirium may also be expected to rise.

CLINICAL FEATURES

The clinical features of delirium are quite numerous and include a variety of neuropsychiatric symptoms that are also common to other psychiatric disorders, such as depression, dementia, and psychosis.[24] Clinical features of delirium include prodromal symptoms (restlessness, anxiety, sleep disturbance, and irritability); rapidly fluctuating course; reduced attention (distractibility); altered arousal; increased or decreased psychomotor activity; disturbance of sleep-wake cycle; affective symptoms (emotional lability, sadness, anger, or euphoria); altered perceptions (misperceptions, illusions, poorly formed delusions, and hallucinations); disorganized thinking and incoherent speech; disorientation to time, place, or person; and memory impairment (inability to register new material). Neurologic abnormalities can also be present during delirium, including cortical abnormalities (dysgraphia, constructional apraxia, dysnomic aphasia); motor abnormalities (tremor, asterixis, myoclonus, and reflex and tone changes); and electroencephalogram (EEG) abnormalities (usually global slowing). It is the protean nature of delirious symptoms, the variability and fluctuation of clinical findings, and the unclear and often contradictory definitions of the syndrome that have made delirium so difficult to diagnose and treat.

The definitions and descriptions (including diagnostic criteria) of delirium over the years have reflected the evolution of our understanding of delirium, moving from purely descriptive symptomatology toward pathophysiologic concepts. From the wide array of neuropsychiatric symptoms, certain clinical criteria have been recognized as being essential to and most specific to delirium diagnosis: (a) chronological features, that is, acute or subacute onset, as well as the transient and re-

versible nature of the disorder, and (b) pathognomonic clinical features. Lipowski emphasized certain clinical symptoms as pathognomonic of delirium: disordered attention and cognition, accompanied by disturbances of psychomotor behavior and the sleep-wake cycle. The essential clinical features of delirium as described in the American Psychiatric Association's (APA) Diagnostic and Statistical Manual of Mental Disorders (DSM-III), in 1980,[25] were (1) clouding of consciousness and impaired attention, (2) impaired cognition (disorientation and memory disorders), and (3) two of the following: (a) psychomotor behavior disturbance, (b) sleep-wake cycle (arousal systems?) anomalies, (c) perceptual disturbances, and (d) incoherent speech, in the context of acute onset and transitory duration. The DSM-III-R[26] further added disorganized thinking. The DSM-IV diagnostic criteria are described in a later section.

Pathophysiology

Although very little is known about the neuropathogenesis of delirium, the symptoms of delirium suggest that it is a dysfunction of multiple regions of the brain. Delirium has been characterized as an etiologically nonspecific, global, cerebral dysfunction characterized by concurrent disturbances of level of consciousness, attention, thinking, perception, memory, psychomotor behavior, emotion, and the sleep-wake cycle. Disorientation, fluctuation, and waxing and waning of these symptoms, as well as acute or abrupt onset of such disturbances, are other critical features of delirium. Delirium, in contrast with dementia, is conceptualized as a reversible process, even in the patient with advanced illness; however it may not be reversible in the last 24 to 48 hours of life.

Our current understanding of delirium is that it involves a reversible disruption of cerebral attentional processes due to metabolic anomalies that affect certain neurotransmitters. Wise and Brandt[24] describe delirium as a "transient, essentially reversible dysfunction in cerebral metabolism that has an acute or subacute onset and is manifest clinically by a wide array of neuropsychiatric abnormalities." Although delirium involves widespread metabolic cerebral dysfunction, recent work in the pathophysiology of delirium has suggested several discrete etiologic models for this dysfunction.

Another view of delirium focuses on the extent of brain dysfunction: "Delirium is often considered a global and nonspecific disorder of brain function. This characterization may be appropriate for delirium caused by such widespread systemic processes as hypoxia, hypothermia, and acid-base disorders. However, several important etiologies of delirium may be associated with more limited and specific brain pathophysiology."[27] In other words, delirium can be seen as either (1) a global and nonspecific disorder of brain function that implies a generalized dysfunction in cerebral metabolism or (2) a more limited and specific brain pathology that is initially caused by the derangement of a specific neurotransmitter or set of neurotransmitters. Evidence is growing to support the contention that delirium is a heterogeneous group of different disorders with different symptomatologies. As examples, according to Ross,[27] perturbations of certain neurotransmitters produce specific pathophysiologic changes, resulting in delirious symptoms:

1. Anticholinergic drugs produce delirium through suppression of cholinergic systems.
2. Some hallucinatory drugs such as D-lysergic acid dimethylamide (LSD) involve antagonism of the serotonin system.
3. Phencyclidine (PCP) produces delirium by blocking glutamate-sensitive NMDA receptors in the central nervous system (CNS).
4. Hepatic encephalopathy and benzodiazepine intoxication both produce delirium through overstimulation of GABA systems.
5. Benzodiazepine withdrawal states, as well as alcoholic withdrawal, produce delirium through acute understimulation of GABA systems.
6. In a variety of etiologies, such as the anticholinergic-induced type, delirium symptoms such as hallucinations seem to involve a further perturbation: a relative overactivation of the dopaminergic mesocortical system responsible for many of the features of hyperactive delirium.

The global dysfunction model, however, seems to apply more readily to deliria where multiple neurotransmitter systems or a cascade of interacting neurotransmitter systems are involved, such as in infection or hypoxia. This global model may also be interpreted as a final end pathway common to the different specific etiologies of delirium. The metabolic basis of the final common pathway, however, is open to question. On the basis of studies in Alzheimer's disease, researchers have suggested perturbations in second-messenger systems: "The diversity of the changes in neurotransmitters suggests that alterations in second-messenger systems may be the more fundamental change. Results clearly implicate second-messenger systems such as calcium, cyclic GMP, and the phosphatidylinosital cascade."[28]

Subtypes of Delirium

Lipowski[23] clinically describes two subtypes of delirium, based on psychomotor behavior and arousal levels. The subtypes included the hyperactive (or agitated, or hyperalert) subtype and the hypoactive (or lethargic, or hypoalert) subtype (Table 6.1). Other researchers have proposed a "mixed" subtype,[24] with alternating features of each. Ross[27] suggests that the hyperactive form is most often characterized by hallucinations, delusions, agitation, and disorientation, while the hypoactive form is characterized by confusion and sedation but is rarely accompanied by hallucinations, delusions, or illusions. Ross further suggests that specific delirium subtypes are related to specific etiologies of delirium and have unique pathophysiologies; he posits that hyperactive forms are typical of withdrawal syndromes and anticholinergic-induced delirium, whereas the hypoactive forms are typical of hepatic or metabolic encephalopathies, acute intoxications from sedatives, or hypoxia. The pathophysiology of a hyperactive delirium due to benzodiazepine withdrawal is characterized by elevated or normal cerebral metabolism, fast or normal EEG, and reduced activity in (γ-aminobutyric acid (GABA) systems, while the pathophysiology of a hypoactive delirium due to benzodiazepine intoxication is characterized by decreased global cerebral metabolism, diffuse slowing of the EEG, and overstimulation of GABA systems.

Diagnostic Criteria

These criteria are from DSM-IV.[29] The essential feature of a delirium is a disturbance of consciousness (or arousal) that is accompanied by a change in cognition that cannot be better accounted for by a preexisting or evolving dementia. The disturbance develops over a short period of time, usually hours to days, and tends to fluctuate during the course of the day. There is evi-

Table 6.1   Contrasting Features of Subtypes of Delirium

	Hyperactive	Hypoactive
Type	Hyperalert Agitated	Hypoalert Lethargic
Symptoms	Hallucinations Delusions Hyperarousal	Sleepy Withdrawn Slowed
Examples	Withdrawal syndromes (benziodiazepines, alcohol)	Encephalopathies (hepatic, metabolic) Benzodiazepine intoxication
Pathophysiology	Elevated or normal cerebral metabolism EEG: fast or normal Reduced activity in GABA systems	Decreased global cerebral metabolism EEG: diffuse slowing Overstimulation of GAMA systems

dence from the history, physical examination, or laboratory tests that the delirium is a direct physiological consequence of a general medical condition, substance intoxication or withdrawal, use of a medication, or toxin exposure, or a combination of these factors (Table 6.2).

The disturbance in consciousness (or arousal) is manifested by a reduced clarity of awareness of the environment. The ability to focus, sustain, or shift attention is impaired (Criterion A). Questions must be repeated because the individual's attention wanders, or the individual may perseverate with an answer to a previous question rather than appropriately shift attention. The person is easily distracted by irrelevant stimuli. Because of these problems, it may be difficult (or impossible) to engage the person in conversation.

There is an accompanying change in cognition (which may include memory impairment,

TABLE 6.2   DSM-IV Criteria for Delirium

293.00 Delirium due to a general medical condition
  A. Disturbance of consciousness (that is, reduced clarity of awareness of the environment) with reduced ability to focus, sustain, or shift attention.
  B. Change in cognition (such as memory deficit, disorientation, language disturbance, or perceptual disturbance) that is not better accounted for by a preexisting, established, or evolving dementia.
  C. The disturbance develops over a short period of time (usually hours to days) and tends to fluctuate during the course of the day.
  D. There is evidence from the history, physical examination, or laboratory findings of a general medical condition judged to be etiologically related to the disturbance.

disorientation, or language disturbance) or development of a perceptual disturbance (Criterion B). Memory impairment is most commonly evident in recent memory and can be tested by asking the person to remember several unrelated objects or a brief sentence and then to repeat them after a few minutes of distraction. Disorientation is usually manifested by the individual's disorientation to time (e.g., thinking it is morning in the middle of the night) or to place (e.g., thinking he or she is home, rather than in a hospital). In mild delirium, disorientation to time may be the first symptom to appear. Disorientation to self is less common. Language disturbance may be evident as dysnomia (i.e., the impaired ability to name objects) or dysgraphia (i.e., the impaired ability to write). In some cases, speech is rambling and irrelevant, in others pressured and incoherent, with unpredictable switching from subject to subject. It may difficult for the clinician to assess changes in cognitive function because the individual may be inattentive and incoherent. Under these circumstances, it is helpful to review carefully the individual's history and to obtain information from other informants, particularly family members.

Perceptual disturbances may include misinterpretations, illusions, or hallucinations. For example, the banging of a door may be mistaken for a gunshot (misinterpretation); the folds of the bedclothes may appear to be animate objects (illusion); or the person may "see" a group of people hovering over the bed when no one is actually there (hallucination). Although sensory misperceptions are most commonly visual, they may occur in other sensory modalities as well.

Misperceptions range from simple and uniform to highly complex. The individual may have a delusional conviction of the reality of the hallucinations and exhibit emotional and behavioral responses in keeping with their content.

The disturbance develops over a short period of time and tends to fluctuate during the course of the day (Criterion C). For example, the person may be coherent and cooperative during the morning hospital rounds, but at night insist on pulling out intravenous lines and going home to parents who died years ago.

DSM-IV places less diagnostic emphasis on incoherent speech, disturbance of sleep-wake cycle, and increased or decreased psychomotor activity. As a result of these progressive changes in DSM criteria for delirium, the different versions are more or less sensitive in diagnosing the condition.[30]

Arousal and Cognition

The emphasis in defining delirium in recent years has thus shifted from an extensive list of symptoms to a focus on the two essential concepts of disordered attention (arousal) and cognition, while continuing to recognize the importance of acute onset and organic etiology. Ross[27] now defines delirium simply as "a disorder of cognition and alteration in arousal and attention," in contrast to dementia, which is a disorder primarily of cognition. Because the disorder of arousal/attention is pathognomonic to delirium, the pathophysiology of alterations in central nervous system arousal/attention has become paramount in delirium research. New models that use neural network theory have suggested that selective attention involves modulation of different neural systems; competing perceptions of internal and external origin are held in relative abeyance, allowing one to be selectively analyzed. In this view, delirium could involve an absence of modulation of competing perceptions so that the patient is uncontrollably and randomly dominated by them, probably with internal rather than external perceptions dominant, especially for patients with hallucinations.[30]

ASSESSMENT OF DELIRIUM

Historically, the major objective of clinical evaluation in the area of delirium has been the identification of delirious patients through the use of screening questionnaires, instruments that are rapid and easily administered by minimally trained raters. More recently, with the development of the standardized diagnostic classification criteria of the DSM and the International Classification of Diseases (ICD) systems, formally confirming the diagnosis of delirium for research purposes has become important. Emphasis has shifted to more sophisticated diagnostic instruments that maximize diagnostic precision and can be used by trained clinician and nonclinician raters. Measuring the severity of delirium once it has been diagnosed, differentiating subtypes, describing delirium in children, and identifying new specific etiologic subtypes (for example, opioid-induced delirium) are some of the new challenges in this field.[31]

Instruments for the evaluation of delirium have been grouped into five categories: (1) tests that measure cognitive impairment, which are usually used to screen for delirium [such as the Mini-Mental-Status Exam (MMSE)]; (2) delirium diagnostic instruments based on DSM or ICD criteria, which are used to make a yes/no judgment on the presence or absence of delirium (such as the Confusion-Assessment Method); (3) delirium-specific numerical rating scales, whose scores can be used to evaluate the likelihood of diagnosis or to estimate the severity of the delirium (such as the Delirium-Rating Scale); (4) delirium severity rating scales (such as the Memorial Delirium Assessment Scale); and (5) laboratory and paraclinical exams for the physiologic correlates of delirium (the precise role of these tests in screening, diagnosis, and severity evaluation has yet to be fully determined). (Please refer to Table 6.3 on assessment methods for diagnosing delirium].

The MMSE, while not a screening tool specifically for delirium, has become one of the most frequently used neuropsychological tests in the clinical evaluation of delirium and thus has become a de facto reference against which other instruments are judged.[32] It was originally conceived as a brief (5 to 10 minutes) practical clinical instrument for distinguishing functional from organic mental status impairment. It includes 11 simple questions, including 2 with written answers, and yields a score that is a weighted sum of the items, with a maximum of 30 and a cutoff for cognitive impairment of 24. It assesses

Table 6.3   Methods of Assessing Delirium in
Cancer Patients

Diagnostic classification systems

  DSM-IV[29]
  ICD-9, ICD-10

Diagnostic interviews/instruments

  Delirium Symptom Interview[93] (DSI)
  Confusion Assessment Method[94] (CAM)

Delirium rating scales

  Delirium Rating Scale[38] (DRS)
  Confusion Rating Scale[95] (CRS)
  Saskatoon Delirium Checklist[96] (SDC)
  Memorial Delirium Assessment Scale[39] (MDAS)

Cognitive impairment screening instruments

  Mini-Mental State Exam[34] (MMSE)
  Short Portable Mental Status Questionnaire[97] (SPMSQ)
  Cognitive Capacity Screening Examination[98] (CCSE)
  Blessed Orientation Memory Concentration Test[99]
  (BOMC)

---

the subject's orientation to time and place, in-stantaneous recall, short-term memory, serial sub-tractions or reverse spelling, constructional ca-pacities, and use of language. Although a score of 23 or less has generally been considered an indi-cation of cognitive impairment, a three-tiered system is now becoming popular on the basis of the results of new epidemiologic data, and scores are now interpreted as follows: 24 to 30, no im-pairment; 18 to 23, mild impairment; and 0 to 17, severe impairment.[32] The MMSE has the ad-vantage of being able to be administered by lay interviewers.[33–36] Precise instructions for admin-istering and scoring the exam have been pro-vided,[37] and useful suggestions such as using the three words "apple, penny, table" for the mem-ory task as well as commonly used variations in administration have been published.[32]

The Delirium-Rating Scale (DRS) is a nu-merical rating scale that specifically integrates DSM-III criteria. It is a 10-item scale, with items scored from 0 to 3 or 0 to 4 in the following do-mains: (1) temporal onset, (2) perceptual distur-bance, (3) hallucinations, (4) delusions, (5) psy-chomotor behavior, (6) cognitive status, (7) physical disorder, (8) sleep-wake cycle distur-bance, (9) lability of mood, and (10) variability of symptoms.[38] A single validation study on a rather small clinical sample (20 delirious patients, 9 schizophrenic patients, 9 demented patients, and 9 medical patients used as controls) offered some evidence of validation, but with certain methodologic shortcomings. A limitation of the DRS is that it was created and then validated us-ing items more pertinent for diagnosing delirium than for rating its severity. Thus, although it is proposed as a severity rating scale, it actually mea-sures diagnostic certainty.

Because of the shortcomings of existing delir-ium assessment instruments, faculty in the De-partment of Psychiatry and Behavioral Sciences at Memorial Sloan-Kettering Cancer Center de-veloped a measure specifically designed to quan-tify the severity of delirium symptoms for use in clinical intervention trials. The Memorial Delir-ium Assessment Scale (MDAS) was designed to be administered repeatedly within the same day, in order to allow for objective measurement of changes in delirium severity in response to med-ical changes or clinical interventions. Potential items were developed by the principal investiga-tors and were reviewed with regard to content va-lidity by a group of experienced consultation-li-aison psychiatrists.

The MDAS is a 10-item, 4-point clinician-rated scale (possible range: 0 to 30) designed to quantify the severity of delirium in medically ill patients. Items included in the MDAS reflect the diagnostic criteria for delirium in the DSM-IV, as well as symptoms of delirium from earlier or alternative classification systems (e.g., DSM-III, DSM-III-R, ICD-9). Scale items assess distur-bances in arousal and level of consciousness, as well as in several areas of cognitive functioning (memory, attention, orientation, disturbances in thinking) and psychomotor activity. Items were anchored with statements reflecting the severity or intensity of the symptom and were reviewed by experienced clinicians to ensure ease of ad-ministration and ability to generate accurate (re-liable) ratings. The resulting scale, which requires approximately 10 minutes to administer (not in-cluding the additional time necessary to establish rapport, review chart records, and speak to staff or family members), integrates behavioral obser-vations and objective cognitive testing. When items cannot be administered, scores can be pro-rated from the remaining items to an equivalent

10-item score; however, this process was never necessary in the studies reported.[39]

When confronted with a delirium in the terminally ill or dying patient, the clinician should always formulate a differential diagnosis as to the likely etiology(ies). There is an ongoing debate as to the appropriate extent of diagnostic evaluation that should be pursued in a dying patient with a terminal delirium.[4,40–42] Most palliative-care clinicians would undertake diagnostic studies only when a clinically suspected etiology can be identified easily, with minimal use of invasive procedures, and treated effectively with simple, interventions that carry minimal burden or risk of causing further distress. Diagnostic workup in pursuit of an etiology for delirium may be limited by either practical constraints such as the setting (home, hospice) or the focus on patient comfort so that unpleasant or painful diagnostics may be avoided. Most often, however, the etiology of terminal delirium is multifactorial or may not be determined. Bruera et al.[42] report that an etiology is discovered in fewer than 50% of terminally ill patients with delirium. When a distinct cause is found for delirium in the terminally ill, it is often irreversible or difficult to treat. However, studies in patients with earlier stages of advanced cancer have demonstrated the potential utility of a thorough diagnostic assessment[42,43] When such diagnostic information is available, specific therapy may be able to reverse delirium. One study found that 68% of delirious cancer patients could be improved, despite a 30-day mortality of 31%.[43] Another found that one-third of the episodes of cognitive failure improved following evaluation that yielded a cause for these episodes in 43% of the paients in the study.[42]

The diagnostic workup should include an assessment of potentially reversible causes of delirium. A full physical examination should assess for evidence of sepsis, dehydration, or major organic failure. Medications that could contribute to delirium should be reviewed. A screen of laboratory parameters will allow assessment of the possible role of metabolic abnormalities, such as hypercalcemia, and other problems, such as hypoxia or disseminated intravascular coagulation. Imaging studies of the brain and assessment of the cerebrospinal fluid may be appropriate in some instances.

Delirium can have multiple potential etiologies. In patients with advanced cancer, for instance, delirium can result either from the direct effects of cancer on the central nervous system (CNS) or from indirect CNS effects of the disease or treatments (medications, electrolyte imbalance, failure of a vital organ or system, infection, vascular complications, and preexisting cognitive impairment or dementia).[43] Given the large numbers of drugs cancer patients require and the fragile state of their physiologic functioning, even routinely ordered hypnotics are enough to tip patients into a delirium. Narcotic analgesics such as levorphanol, morphine sulfate, and meperidine are common causes of confusional states, particularly in the elderly and the terminally ill. Chemotherapeutic agents known to cause delirium include methotrexate, fluorouracil, vincristine, vinblastine, bleomycin, BCNU, cis-platinum, asparaginase, procarbazine, and the glucocorticosteroids.[44–49] Except for steroids, most patients who receive these agents will not develop prominent CNS effects. The spectrum of mental disturbances related to steroids includes minor mood lability, affective disorders (mania or depression), cognitive impairment (reversible dementia), and delirium (steroid psychosis). The incidence of these disorders range from 3% to 57% in noncancer populations, and they occur most commonly at higher doses. Symptoms usually develop within the first 2 weeks on steroids but in fact can occur at any time, on any dose, even during the tapering phase.[44] These disorders are often rapidly reversible after dose reduction or discontinuation.[44]

Differential Diagnosis

Many of the clinical features and symptoms of delirium can be also be associated with other psychiatric disorders, such as depression, mania, psychosis, and dementia. For instance, delirious patients not uncommonly exhibit emotional (mood) disturbances such as anxiety, fear, depression, irritability, anger, euphoria, apathy, and mood lability. Delirium, particularly the "hypoactive" subtype, is often initially misdiagnosed as depression. Symptoms of major depression, including altered level of activity (hypoactivity), insomnia, reduced ability to concentrate, depressed mood, and even suicidal ideation, can overlap with symptoms of delirium, making accurate diagnosis more difficult. In distinguishing delirium from depression, particularly in the context of advanced disease, an evaluation of the onset and the temporal sequencing of depressive and cognitive symptoms is particularly helpful. It is important to note that the degree of cognitive impairment is much more severe and pervasive in delirium than in depression, with a more abrupt temporal onset. Also, in delirium the characteristic disturbance in arousal or consciousness is present, while it is usually not a feature of depression. Similarly, a manic episode may share some features of delirium, particularly a "hyperactive" or "mixed" subtype of delirium. Again, the temporal onset and course of symptoms, the presence of a disturbance of consciousness (arousal) as well as cognition, and the identification of a presumed medical etiology for delirium are helpful in differentiating these disorders. Delirium that is characterized by vivid hallucinations and delusions must be distinguished from a variety of psychotic disorders. In delirium, such psychotic symptoms occur in the context of a disturbance in consciousness or arousal, accompanied also by memory impairment and disorientation, which is not the case in other psychotic disorders. Delusions in delirium tend to be poorly organized and of abrupt onset, and hallucinations are predominantly visual or tactile, rather than auditory, as is typical of schizophrenia. Finally, the development of these psychotic symptoms in the context of advanced medical illness makes delirium a more likely diagnosis.

The most common differential diagnostic issue is whether the patient has delirium, dementia, or a delirium superimposed on a preexisting dementia. Both delirium and dementia are cognitive impairment disorders and so share such common clinical features as impaired memory, thinking, judgment, and disorientation. The patient with dementia is alert and does not have the disturbance of consciousness or arousal that is characteristic of delirium. The temporal onset of symptoms in dementia is more subacute and chronically progressive, and one's sleep-wake cycle seems less impaired. Most prominent in dementia are difficulties in short- and long-term memory, impaired judgment, and abstract thinking, as well as disturbed higher cortical functions (such as aphasia and apraxia). Occasionally, one encounters delirium superimposed on an underlying dementia, such as in the case of an elderly patient, an AIDS patient, or a patient with a paraneoplastic syndrome. Delirium, in contrast with dementia, is conceptualized as a reversible process. Reversibility of the process of delirium is often possible even in the patient with advanced

illness; however, it may not be reversible in the last 24 to 48 hours of life, probably because irreversible processes such as multiple organ failure are occurring in the final hours of life. Delirium that occurs in these last days of life is sometimes referred to as "terminal delirium" in the palliative-care literature.

MANAGEMENT OF DELIRIUM IN THE TERMINALLY ILL

The standard approach to the managing delirium in the medically ill, even in those with advanced disease, includes a search for underlying causes, correction of those factors, and management of the symptoms of delirium.[31,50] The desired and often achievable outcome is a patient who is awake, alert, calm, cognitively intact, not psychotic, and communicating coherently with family and staff. In the terminally ill patient who develops delirium in the last days of life (terminal delirium), the management of delirium is in fact unique, presenting a number of dilemmas, and the desired clinical outcome may be significantly altered by the dying process (See Figure 6.1.).

Nonpharmacologic Interventions

In addition to seeking out and potentially correcting underlying causes for delirium, symptomatic and supportive therapies are important.[4,31,40–42] In fact, in the dying patient they may be the only steps taken. Maintaining fluid and electrolyte balance, adequate nutrition vitamin intake, taking steps to help reduce anxiety and disorientation, and fostering interactions with and educating family members may be useful. Measures to help reduce anxiety and disorientation (i.e., structure and familiarity) may include providing a quiet, well-lit room with familiar objects, a visible clock or calendar, and the presence of family. Judicious use of physical restraints, along with one-to-one nursing observation, may also be necessary and useful.

Pharmacologic Interventions in Delirium

Supportive techniques alone are often not effective in controlling the symptoms of delirium, and symptomatic treatment with neuroleptics or seda-

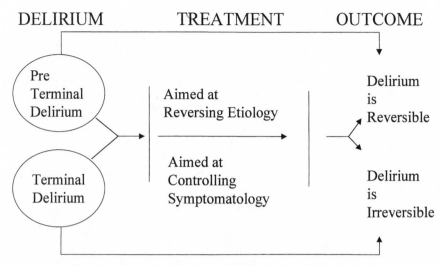

Figure 6.1. Overview of Management of Delirium in Pre-Terminal and Terminally Ill Patients

tive medications may be necessary (Table 6.4). Neuroleptic drugs (dopamine-blocking drugs), such as as haloperidol, are utilized frequently as antiemetics in the medical setting; however, only 0.5% to 2% of hospitalized cancer patients, for instance, receive haloperidol for the management of the symptoms of delirium.[51,52] As many as 17% of terminally ill patients receive antipsychotic drugs for agitation or psychological distress, despite an estimated prevalence of delirium that ranges from 25% in the hospitalized cancer patient to 85% in the terminally ill.[53,54]

Haloperidol, a neuroleptic drug that is a potent dopamine blocker, is often the drug of choice in the treatment of delirium in the medically ill and in patients with advanced disease.[31,55–64] Haloperidol in low doses, 1 to 3 mg per day, is usually effective in targeting agitation, paranoia, and fear. Typically 0.5 to 1.0 mg haloperidol (PO, IV, IM, SC) is administered, with repeat doses every 45 to 60 minutes titrated against target symptoms.[12,65–66] An intravenous route can facilitate rapid onset of medication effects. If intravenous access is unavailable, one can start with intramuscular or subcutaneous administration and switch to the oral route when possible. The majority of delirious patients can be managed with oral haloperidol. Parenteral doses are approximately twice as potent as oral doses. Delivery of haloperidol by the subcutaneous route is utilized by many palliative-care practitioners.[67,68] In general, doses need not exceed 20 mg of haloperidol in a 24-hour

period; however, some clinicians advocate high doses (up to 250 mg per 24 hours of haloperidol, usually intravenously) in selected cases.[69]

A common strategy in the management of symptoms related to delirium is to add parenteral

Table 6.4   Medications for Managing Delirium in Terminally Ill Patients

Generic Name	Approximate Daily Dosage Range Route
Neuroleptics	
Haloperidol	0.5–5 mg every 2–12 hr PO, IV, SC, IM
Thiorodazine	10–75 mg every 4–8 hr PO
Chlorpromazine	12.5–50 mg every 4–12 hr PO, IV, IM
Methotrimeprazine	12.5–50 mg every 4–8 hr IV, SC, PO
Molindone	10–50 mg every 8–12 hr PO
Olanzipine	2.5–10 mg every 12 hr PO
Risperidone	1–3 mg every 12 hr PO
Benzodiazepines	
Lorazepam	0.5–2.0 mg every 1–4 hr PO, IV, IM
Midazolam	30–100 mg every 24 hr IV, SC
Anesthetics	
Propofol	10–70 mg every hr IV, titrated up to 200–400mg/hour

lorazepam to a regimen of haloperidol.[2,7,62,63,67,69] Lorazepam (0.5 to 1.0 mg q1–2 h PO or IV) along with haloperidol may be more effective in rapidly sedating the agitated delirious patient and may help minimize the extrapyramidal side effects associated with haloperidol.[70] In a double-blind, randomized comparison trial of haloperidol, chlorpromazine, and lorazepam, Breitbart and colleagues demonstrated that lorazepam alone, in doses up to 8 mg in a 12-hour period, was ineffective in the treatment of delirium and in fact contributed to worsening delirium and cognitive impairment.[71] Both neuroleptic drugs, however, in low doses (approximately 2 mg of haloperidol equivalent per 24 hours) were highly effective in controlling the symptoms of delirium (measured by DRS scores) and in improving cognitive function (shown by dramatic improvement in MMSE scores). In addition, both haloperidol and chlorpromazine were demonstrated to significantly improve the symptoms of delirium in both the hypoactive and the hyperactive subtypes of delirium.[72] Methotrimeprazine, a phenothiazine neuroleptic with properties similar to those of chlorpromazine, is often utilized parenterally (intravenously or by subcutaneous infusion) to control confusion and agitation in terminal delirium.[73] Dosages range from 12.5 to 50 mg every 4 to 8 hours up to 300 mg per 24 hours for most patients. Side effects such as hypotension and excessive sedation are potential limitations on the use of this drug. However, methotrimeprazine has the advantage of also being an analgesic, equipotent to morphine, through nonopioid mechanisms.[73] Several new antipsychotic agents with less or more specific dopamine-blocking efects (reduced risk of extrapyramidal side effects or tardive dyskinesia) are now available and include such agents as clozaril, risperidone, and olanzapine.[74,75] Risperidone has been useful in the treatment of dementia and psychosis in AIDS patients at doses of 1 to 6 mg per day, suggesting that it is safe to use in patients with delirium.[75] At Memorial Sloan-Kettering Cancer Center, we have had substantial clinical experience with olanzepine in doses ranging from 2.5 to 20 mg per day and have found it to be a useful agent in the management of delirium. There are no published studies of the use of these agents in the treatment of delirium; however, some palliative-care clinicians are using olanzaprine or risperidone in low doses (e.g., 0.5 to 1.0 mg bid, orally) in the management of delir-ium in terminally ill patients who have a demonstrated intolerance to the extrapyramidal side effects of the classic neuroleptics.[76] Currently, a limitation on the use of these new agents is their unavailablity in parenteral formulations.

While neuroleptic drugs such as haloperidol are most effective in diminishing agitation, clearing the sensorium, and improving cognition in the delirious patient, this is not always possible in terminal delirium. Processes that cause delirium may be ongoing and irreversible during the active dying phase (see Figure 6.1). Ventafridda et al.[77] and Fainsinger et al.[78] have reported that a significant number (10% to 20%) of terminally ill patients experience delirium that can be controlled only by sedation to the point of a significantly decreased level of consciousness. The goal of treatment with such agents as midazolam, propofol, and, to some extent, methotrimeprazine is quiet sedation only. Midazolam, given by subcutaneous or intravenous infusion in doses ranging from 30 to 100 mg per 24 hours, can be used to control agitation related to delirium in the terminal stages.[79,80] Propofol, a short-acting anesthetic agent, is also utilized primarily as a sedating agent for the control of agitated patients with terminal delirium. In several case reports of propofol's use in terminal care, an intravenous loading dose of 20 mg of propofol was followed by a continuous infusion of propofol, with initial doses ranging from 10 to 70 mg per hour and with titration of doses up to as high as 400 mg/hour over a period of hours to days in severely agitated patients.[81,82] Propofol has an advantage over midazolam in that it allows the level of sedation to be controlled more easily and recovery is rapid when the rate of infusion is decreased.[81]

Controversies in the Management of Terminal Delirium

Several aspects of the use of neuroleptics and other pharmacologic agents in the management of delirium in the dying patient remain controversial in some circles. Some researchers have argued that pharmacologic interventions with neuroleptics or benzodiazepines are inappropriate in the dying patient. Delirium is viewed by some as a natural part of the dying process that should not be altered. In particular, some clinicians who care for the dying view hallucinations and delusions that involve dead relatives communicating with or in fact welcoming dying patients to heaven as an important element in the transition from life to death. Clearly, there are many patients who experience hallucinations and delusions during delirium that are pleasant and in fact comforting, and many clinicians question the appropriateness of intervening pharmacologically in such instances. Another concern is that these patients are so close to death that aggressive treatment is unnecessary, and parenteral neuroleptics or sedatives may be mistakenly avoided because of exaggerated fears that they might hasten death through hypotension or respiratory depression. Many clinicians are unnecessarily pessimistic about the possible results of neuroleptic treatment for delirium. They argue that since the underlying pathophysiologic process often continues unabated (such as hepatic or renal failure), no improvement can be expected in the patient's mental status. There is concern that neuroleptics or sedatives may worsen a delirium by making the patient more confused or sedated.

Clinical experience in managing delirium in dying patients suggests that the use of neuroleptics in the management of agitation, paranoia, hallucinations, and altered sensorium is safe, effective, and often quite appropriate.[71] Management of delirium on a case-by-case basis seems wisest. The agitated, delirious dying patient should probably be given neuroleptics to help restore calm. A "wait-and-see" approach may be appropriate with some patients who have a lethargic or somnolent presentation of delirium or who are having frankly pleasant or comforting hallucinations. Such a wait-and-see approach must, however, be tempered by the knowledge that a lethargic or hypoactive delirium may very quickly and unexpectedly become an agitated or hyperactive delirium that can threaten the serenity and safety of the patient, family, and staff. An additional rationale for intervening pharmacologically with patients who have a lethargic or hypoactive delirium is recent evidence that neuroleptics (i.e., haloperidol, chlorpromazine) are effective in controlling the symptoms of delirium in both hyperactive and hypoactive deliria.[72] In fact, neuroleptics improved both the arousal function and cognitive functioning in patients with hypoactive delirium. Also, some clinicians suggest that hypoactive delirium may respond to psychostimulants or combinations of neuroleptics and stimulants.[83] Similarly, hallucinations and

delusions during a delirium that are pleasant and comforting can quickly become menacing and terrifying. It is important to remember that, by their nature, the symptoms of delirium are unstable and fluctuate over time.

Perhaps the most challenging clinical problem is the management of the dying patient with a terminal delirium that is unresponsive to standard neuroleptic interventions and that falls into that 10% to 20% of patients, described by Ventafridda et al.[77] and Fainsinger et al.,[78] whose symptoms can be controlled only by sedation to the point of a significantly decreased level of consciousness. Before undertaking interventions, such as midazolam or propofol infusions, where the best achievable goal is a calm, comfortable, but sedated and unresponsive patient, the clinician must first take several steps. The clinician must have a discussion with the family (and the patient if there are lucid moments when the patient appears to have capacity), eliciting their concerns and wishes for the type of care that can best honor their desire to provide comfort and symptom control during the dying process. The clinician should describe the optimal achievable goals of therapy as they currently exist. Family members should be informed that the goal of sedation is to provide comfort and symptom control and not to hasten death. They should also be told to anticipate that sedation may result in a premature sense of loss and that they may feel their loved one is in some sort of limbo state, not yet dead but yet no longer alive in the vital sense. The distress and confusion that family members can experience during such a period can be ameliorated by including the family in the decision making and by emphasizing the shared goals of care. Sedation in such patients is not always complete or irreversible; some patients have periods of wakefulness despite sedation, and many clinicians periodically lighten sedation to reassess the patient's condition. Ultimately, the clinician must always keep in mind the goals of care and communicate these goals to the staff, patients, and family members. The clinician must weigh each of the issues outlined here in making decisions on how to best manage the dying patient who presents with delirium that preserves and respects the dignity and values of that individual and family.

Several interesting clinical questions in this area exist, and more research could help inform clinical management. Must we always treat delirium in the terminally ill or dying patient? What are appropriate goals for treatment? What is the impact of delirium on patients, family, and staff? What are effective pharmacologic and nonpharmacologic interventions? An interesting, currently important topic is that of differential therapeutics. Hypoactive and hyperactive subtypes of delirium seem to have distinct phenomenologies and etiologies[84] and therefore may require different treatment strategies.

Pain Assessment and Delirium

Delirium often impacts on the assessment of other symptomatology in terminally ill patients. For example, assessment of pain intensity in patients during an episode of cognitive failure was significantly higher than before and after the episode, when similar intensities suggested a stable pain syndrome. It is recognized that success in the treatment of cancer pain is highly dependent on proper assessment.[85,86] Unfortunately, the assessment of pain intensity becomes very difficult in patients with cognitive failure (CF). Fainsinger and Bruera[67] report that 40% of patients required treatment for delirium in the last week of life, and they and Ventafridda and colleagues[77] report that about 10% of terminally ill patients are sedated to control this symptom. Assessing the intensity of pain when patients develop agitated CF is, therefore, a frequent problem. It may be speculated that delirium can increase pain through associated emotional lability and affective disinhibition, that is, increased anxiety (distress), or through distortion in the patient's ability to report pain accurately. Accurate pain reporting depends on the ability to perceive the pain normally and to communicate the experience appropriately. Delirium may both impair the ability to perceive and report pain accurately.

Morphine and Alternative Opioids

Delirium is a well-recognized side effect of opioid administration.[7,87,88] Much of the literature that discusses this problem suggests that the effect usually is short-lived. Ellison[89] notes that euphoria and dysphoria are acute and usually evanescent problems and that tolerance usually develops rapidly. Bruera et al.[9] suggests that it is escalation of the morphine dosage that leads to confusion and

that this confusion resolves quite quickly. The specific causes of acute confusional states in patients with advanced cancer are not determined in up to 75% of cases, and management usually focuses on the appropriate use of psychotropic agents.[22,67]

Rotation of opioid has been shown previously to improve delirium,[90] and in one study 73% of patients in whom confusion was regarded as troublesome experienced improvement after a change in opioid.[91] Experience in Finland[92] has previously suggested that oxycodone is less likely to cause delirium than morphine, but this has not previously been confirmed in prolonged use or in palliative-care patients. Fentanyl, the opioid that is often used as an alternative, has a short duration of action. Consequently, it is suitable only for transcutaneous, continuous infusion or epidural use. Oxycodone, an opioid equipotent to morphine in the oral form, has been shown to be far less likely to cause delirium in an unpublished study by Maddocks et al. The improvement was progressive over the course of several days following a change from morphine, suggesting that a long-acting metabolite of morphine may be responsible for causing delirium. This study suggests that the ready availability of oxycodone in a wider range of formulations and administration routes would provide a major benefit for the great majority of patients who require palliative care, particularly those who are unable to tolerate parenteral morphine.

SUMMARY

The physician who cares for patients with life-threatening illness is likely to encounter delirium as a common major psychiatric complication of advancing illness, particularly in the last weeks of life, when up to 85% of patients may develop a delirium. Proper assessment, diagnosis, and management are important in minimizing morbidity and in improving the quality of life and often the quality of death.

References

1. Lichter I, Hunt E. The last 24 hours of life. *Journal of Palliative Care*, 1990; 6(4):7–15.
2. Stiefel F, Holland J. Delirium in cancer patients. *International Psychogeriatrics*, 1991; 3:333–336.
3. Trzepacz PT, Teague GB, Lipowski ZJ. Delirium

and other organic mental disorders in a general hospital. *General Hospital Psychiatry*, 1985; 7:101–106.

4. Fainsinger RL, MacEachern T, Bruera E, et al. Symptom control during the last week of life in a palliative-care unit. *Journal of Palliative Care*, 1991; 7(1):5–11.

5. Bruera E, Fainsinger R, Miller MJ, Kuehn N. The assessment of pain intensity in patients with cognitive failure: a preliminary report. *Journal of Pain and Symptom Management*, 1992; 7(5):267–270.

6. Coyle N, Breitbart W, Weaver S, Portenoy R. Delirium as a contributing factor to "crescendo" pain: three case reports. *Journal of Pain and Symptom Management*, 1994; 9:44–47.

7. Stiefel F, Fainsinger R, Bruera E. Acute confusional states in patients with advanced cancer. *Journal of Pain and Symptom Management*, 1992; 7:94–98.

8. Silberfarb PM. Chemotherapy and cognitive defects in cancer patients. *Annual Review of Medicine*, 1983; 34:35–46.

9. Bruera E, Macmillan K, Hanson J, MacDonald RN. The cognitive effects of the administration of narcotic analgesics in patients with cancer pain. *Pain*, 1989; 39:13–16.

10. Stiefel F, Breitbart WS, Holland JC. Corticosteroids in cancer: Neuropsychiatric complications. *Cancer Investigation*, 1989; 7:479–491.

11. Posner JB. Delirium and exogenous metabolic brain disease. In: Beeson PB, McDermott W, and Wyngaarden JB (eds), *Cecil Textbook of Medicine*. Philadelphia: WB Saunders, 1979:644–651.

12. Massie MJ, Holland J, Glass E. Delirium in terminally ill cancer patients. *American Journal of Psychiatry*, 1983; 140:1048–1050.

13. Pereira J, Hanson J, Bruera E. The frequency and clinical course of cognitive impairment in patients with terminal cancer. *Cancer*, 1997; 835–841.

14. Tune LE. Post-operative delirium. *International Psychogeriatrics*, 1991; 3:325–332.

15. Lipowski ZJ. Transient cognitive disorders (delirium, acute confusional states) in the elderly. *American Journal of Psychiatry*, 1983; 140:1426–1436.

16. Gillick MR, Serrel NA, Gillick LS. Adverse consequences of hospitalization in the elderly. *Social Sciences and Medicine*, 1982; 16:1033–1038.

17. Warsaw GA, Moore J., Friedman SW, et al. Functional disability in the hospitalized elderly. *Journal of the American Medical Association*, 1982; 248:847–850.

18. Berman K, Eastham EJ. Psychogeriatric ascertainment and assessment for treatment in an acute medical ward setting. *Age and Aging*, 1974; 3:174–188.

19. Seymour DJ, Henschke PJ, Cape RDT, et al. Acute confusional states and dementia in the elderly: the role of dehydration/volume depletion, physical illness and age. *Age and Aging*, 1980; 9:137–146.

20. Hodkinson HM. Mental impairment in the elderly. *Journal of the Royal College of Physicians*, 1973; 7:305–317.

21. Knight EB, Folstein MF. Unsuspected emotional and cognitive disturbance in medical patients. *Annals of Internal Medicine*, 1977; 87:723–724.

22. Lipowski, ZJ. *Delirium: Acute Brain Failure in Man*. Springfield, IL: Charles C Thomas, 1980.

23. Lipowski ZJ. *Delirium: Acute Confusional States*. New York: Oxford University Press, 1990.

24. Wise MG, Brandt GT. Delirium. In: Yudofsky SC, Hales RE, eds., *Textbook of Neuropsychiatry*. 2nd ed. Washington, DC: American Psychiatric Association, 1992.

25. American Psychiatric Association (APA). *Diagnostic and Statistical Manual of Mental Disorders*. 3rd ed. Washington, DC: American Psychiatric Association, 1980.

26. American Psychiatric Association (APA). *Diagnostic and Statistical Manual of Mental Disorders*. 3rd ed. Washington, DC: American Psychiatric Association, 1987.

27. Ross CA. CNS arousal systems: possible role in delirium. *International Psychogeriatrics*, 1991; 3:353–371.

28. Gibson GE, Blass JP, Huang H-M, Freemen GB. The cellular basis of delirium and its relevance to age-related disorders including Alzheimer's disease. *International Psychogeriatrics*, 1991; 3:373–395.

29. American Psychiatric Association (APA). *Diagnostic and Statistical Manual of Mental Disorders*. 4th ed. Washington, DC: Author, 1994.

30. Liptzin B, Levkoff S, Cleary P, et al. An empirical study of diagnostic criteria for delirium. *American Journal of Psychiatry*, 1991; 148:454–457.

31. Smith M, Breitbart W, Platt M. A critique of instruments and methods to detect, diagnose, and rate delirium. *Journal of Pain and Symptom Management*, 1994; 10:35–77.

32. Tombaugh TN, McIntyre NJ. The mini-mental state examination: a comprehensive review. *Journal of the American Geriatric Society*, 1992; 40:922–935.

33. Anthony JC, Leresche LA, Niaz U, Von Korff MR, Folstein MF. Limits of the "mini mental state" as a screening test for dementia and delirium among hospital patients. *Psychological Medicine*, 1982; 12:397–408.

34. Folstein MF, Folstein SE, McHugh PR. "Mini

mental state": a practical method of grading the cognitive state of patients for the clinician. *Journal of Psychiatric Research*, 1975; 12:189–198.

35. Folstein MF, McHugh PR. Psychopathology of dementia: implications for neuropathology. In: Katzman R, ed., *Congenital and Acquired Cognitive Disorders.* New York: Raven, 1979:17–30.

36. Dick JPR, Guiloff RJ, Stewart A, et al. Mini mental state examination in neurological patients. *Journal of Neurology and Neurosurgical Psychiatry*, 1984; 47:496–499.

37. Spencer MP, Folstein MF. The mini mental state examination. In: Keller PA, Ritt LG, eds, *Innovations in Clinical Practice: A Source Book.* Sarasota, FL. Professional Resource Exchange, 1985:305–310.

38. Trzepacz PT, Baker RW, Greenhouse J. A symptom rating scale for delirium. *Psychiatry Research*, 1988; 23:89–97.

39. Breitbart W, Rosenfeld B, Roth A, Smith M, Cohen K, Passik S. The Memorial Delirium Assessment Scale. *Journal of Pain and Symptom Management*, 1997; 13:128–137.

40. Fainsinger R, Young C. Cognitive failure in a terminally ill patient. *Journal of Pain and Symptom Management*, 1991; 6:492–494.

41. Bruera E. Case Report. Severe organic brain syndrome. *Journal of Palliative Care* 1991; 7(1):36–38.

42. Bruera E, Miller L, McCallion J, MacMillan K, Krefting L, Hanson J. Cognitive failure in paients with terminal cancer: a prospective study. *Journal of Pain and Symptom Management*, 1992; 7(4): 192–195.

43. Tuma R, DeAngelis L. Acute encephalopathy in patients with systemic cancer. *Annals of Neurology*, 1992:32:288.

44. Bruera E, MacMillan K, Kuehn N, et al. The cognitive effects of the administration of narcotics. *Pain*, 1989; 39:13–16.

45. Young DF. Neurological complications of cancer chemotherapy. In: Silverstein A, ed, *Neurological Complications of Therapy: Selected Topics.* New York: Futura Publishing, 1982:57–113.

46. Holland JC, Fassanellows, Ohnuma T. Psychiatric symptoms associated with L-asparaginase administration. *Journal of the Psychiatric Research*, 1974:10: 165.

47. Adams F, Wuesada JR, Gutterman JU. Neuropsychiatric manifestations of human leukocyte interferon therapy in patients with cancer. *Journal of the American Medical Association*, 1984; 252:938–941.

48. Denicoff KD, Rubinow Dr, Papa MZ, et al. The neuropsychiatric effects of treatment with interleukin-w and lymphokine-activated killer cells. *Annals of Internal Medicine*, 1987; 107(3):293–300.

49. Weddington WW. Delirium and depression associated with amphotericin B. *Psychosomatics*, 1982; 23:1076–1078.

50. Stiefel F, Holland J. Delirium in cancer patients. *International Psychogeriatrics*, 1991; 3:333–336.

51. Derogatis LR, Feldstein M, Morrow G, et al. A survey of psychotropic drug prescriptions in an oncology population. *Cancer*, 1979; 44:1919–1929.

52. Steifel F, Kornblith A, Holland J. Changes in prescription patterns of psychotropic drugs for cancer patients during a 10-year period. *Cancer*, 1990; 1048–1053.

53. Jaeger H, Morrow G, Brescia F. A survey of psychotropic drug utilization by patients with advanced neoplastic disease. *General Hospital Psychiatry*, 1985; 7:353–360.

54. Goldberg G, Mor V. A survey of psychotropic use in terminal cancer patients. *Psychosomatics*, 1985; 26:745–751.

55. Smith GR, Taylor CW, Linkons P. Haloperidol versus thioridazine for the treatment of psychogeriatric patients: a double-blind clinical trial. *Psychosomatics*, 1974; 15:134–138.

56. Fernandez F, Holmes VF, Adams F, Kavanaugh JJ. Treatment of severe refractory agitation with a haldol drip. *Journal of Clinical Psychiatry*, 1988;49: 239–241.

57. Tsuang MM, Lu LM, Stotsky BA, Cole JO. Haloperidol versus thioridazine for hsopitalized psychogeriatrics patients: double-blind study. *Journal of the American Geriatrics Society*, 1971;19:593–600.

58. Rosen JH. Double-blind comparison of haloperidol and thioridazine in geriatric outpatients. *Journal of Clinical Psychiatry*, 1979; 40:17–20.

59. Thomas H, Schwartz E, Petrilli R. Droperidol versus haloperidol for chemical restraint of agitated and combative patients. *Annals of Emergency Medicine*, 1992; 21:407–413.

60. Fernandez F, Levy JF, Mansell PWA. Management of delirium in terminally ill AIDS patients. *International Journal of Psychiatry in Medicine*, 1989; 19:165–172.

61. Akechi T, Uchitomi Y Okamura H, et al., Usage of haloperidol for delirium in cancer patients. *Supportive Care Cancer*, 1996; 4:390–392.

62. Adams F, Fernandez F, Andersson BS. Emergency pharmacotherapy of delirium in the critically ill cancer patient. *Psychosomatics*, 1986; 27:33–37.

63. Murray GB. Confusion, delirium, and dementia. In: Hackett TP, Cassem NH, eds, *Massachusetts General Hospital Handbook of General Hospital Psychiatry.* 2nd ed. Littleton, Mass: PSG Publishing Company, 1987:84–115.

64. Fernandez F, Holmes VF, Adams F, Kavanaugh JJ.

Treatment of severe refractory agitation with a haloperidol drip. *Journal of Clinical Psychiatry*, 1988; 49:239–241.

65. Breitbart W. Psychiatric management of cancer pain. *Cancer* 1989; 63:2336–2342.

66. Breitbart W. Psychiatric complications of cancer. In: Brain MC, Carbone PP, eds, *Current Therapy in Hematology Oncology-3*. Toronto and Philadelphia: BC Decker, 1988:268–274.

67. Fainsinger R, Bruera E. Treatment of delirium in a terminally ill patient. *Journal of Pain and Symptom Management*, 1992; 7:54–56.

68. Twycross RG, Lack SA. *Symptom Control in Far Advanced Cancer: Pain Relief*. London: Pitman Brooks, 1983.

69. Fernandez F, Levy JK, Mansell PWA. Management of delirium in terminally ill AIDS patients. *International of Journal of Psychiatry in Medicine*, 1989; 19:165–172.

70. Menza M, Murray G, Holmes V. Controlled study of extrapyramidal reactions in the management of delirious medically ill patients: Intravenous haloperidol versus intravenous haloperidol plus benzodiazepines. *Heart/Lung* 1988: 17:238–241.

71. Breitbart W, Marotta R, Platt M, et al. A double-blind trial of halperidol, chlorpormazine, and lorazepan in the treatment of delirium in hospitalized AIDS patients. *American Journal of Psychiatry*, 1996:231–237.

72. Platt M, Breitbart W, Smith M, Marotta R, Weisman H, Jacobsen P. Efficacy of neuroleptics for hypoactive delirium. *Journal of Neuropsychiatry and Clinical Neurosciences*, 1994; 6:66–67. Letter.

73. Oliver DJ. The use of methotrimeprazine in terminal care. *British Journal of Clinical Practice*, 1985; 39:339–340.

74. Baldessarini R, Frankenburg F. Clozapine: a novel antipsychotic agent. *New England Journal of Medicine*, 1991; 324:746–752.

75. Singh A. Safety of risperidone in patients with HIV and AIDS, and Belzie L. Risperidone for AIDS—associated dementia: a case series. In: Proceedings of the 149th annual meeting, American Psychiatric Association, May 1996, New York, NY; 4–9:1–126. Abstracts.

76. Breitbart W, Chochinov HM, Passik S. Psychiatric aspects of palliative care. In: Doyle D, Hanks GEC, MacDonald N, eds, *Oxford Textbook of Palliative Medicine*. 2nd ed. New York: Oxford University Press, 1998:933–954.

77. Ventafridda V, Ripamonti C, DeConno F, et al. Symptom prevalence and control during cancer patients' last days of life. *Journal of Palliative Care*, 1990; 6:7–11.

78. Fainsinger R, MacEachern T, Hanson J, et al. Symptom control during the last week of life in a palliative care unit. *Journal of Palliative Care*, 1991; 7:5–11.

79. Bottomley DM, Hanks GW. Subcutaneous midazolam infusion in palliative care. *Journal of Pain and Symptom Management*, 1990; 5:259–261.

80. De Sousa E, Jepson A. Midazolam in terminal care. *Lancet* 1988; 1:67–68.

81. Moyle J. The use of propofol in palliative medicine. *Journal of Pain and Symptom Management*, 1995; 10:643–646.

82. Mercadante S, DeConno F, Ripamonti. Propofol in terminal care. *Journal of Pain and Symptom Management*, 1995; 10:639–642.

83. Stiefel F, Bruera E. Psychostimulants for hypoactive hypoalert delirium? *Journal of Palliative Care*, 1991; 3:25–26.

84. Ross CA, Peyser CE, Shapiro I, Folstein MF. Delirium: Phenomenologic and etiologic subtypes. *Internal Psychogeriatrics*, 1991, 3:135–147.

85. Foley K. The treatment of cancer pain. *New England Journal of Medicine*, 1984; 313:84–95.

86. Foley K. Pain syndromes in patients with cancer. *Medicine Clinics of North America*, 1987; 169–184.

87. Kalso E, Vainio A. Hallucinations during morphine but not during oxycodone treatment. *Lancet* 1988:56:912. Letter.

88. Caraceni A, Martini C, DeConno F, Ventafridda V. Organic brain syndromes and opioid analgesia for cancer pain. *Journal of Pain and Symptom Management*, 1994; 9:527–533.

89. Ellison NM. Opioid analgesics for cancer pain: toxicities and their treatment. In: Patt R, ed, *Cancer Pain*. Philadelphia: JB Lippincott, 1993:185–194.

90. McDonald N, Der L, Allen S, Champion F. Opioid hyperexcitability: the application of an alternate opioid therapy. *Pain* 1993; 53:353–355.

91. DeStoutz ND, Bruera E, Suarez-Almazor M. Opiate rotation (OR) for toxicity reduction in terminal cancer patients. In: *Abstracts of the Seventh World Congress on Pain*. Paris: IASP, 1993:331. Abstract.

92. Kalso E, Vainio A, Manri J, Rosenberg P, Seppala T. Morphine and oxycodone in the management of cancer pain: plasma levels determined by chemical and radioreceptor assays. *Pharmacological Toxicology*, 1990; 67:322–328.

93. Albert MS, Levkoff SE, Reilly C, et al. The delirium symptom interview: an interview for the detection of delirium symptoms in hospitalized patients. *Journal of Geriatrics, Psychiatry and Neurology*, 1991; 5:14–21.

94. Inouye SK, Vandyck CH, Alessi CA, et al. Clarifying confusion: the confusion assessment method, a new method for detection of delirium. *Annals of Internal Medicine*, 1990; 113:941–948.

95. Williams MA. Delirium/acute confusional states: evaluation devices in nursing. *International Psychogeriatrics*, 1991; 3:301–308.

96. Miller PS, Richardson JS, Jyu CA. Association of low serum anticholinergic levels and cognitive impairment by elderly presurgical patients. *American Journal of Psychiatry*, 1988; 145:342–345.

97. Wolber G, Romaniuk M, Eastman E, Robinson C. Validity of the short Portable Mental Status Questionnaire with elderly psychiatric patients. *Journal of Consultation and Clinical Psychology*, 1984;52: 712–713.

98. Jacobs JC, Bernhard MR, Delgado A, Strain JJ. Screening for organic mental syndromes in the medically ill. *Annals of Internal Medicine*, 1977; 86:40–46.

99. Katzman R, Brown T, Fuld P, et al. Validation of a short orientation-memory-concentration test of cognitive impairment. *American Journal of Psychiatry*, 1983; 140:734–739.

Palliative Care in the Chronically Mentally Ill

David Goldenberg, M.D.
Jimmie Holland, M.D.
Sherry Schachter, R.N., M.A.

The medical management of the patient with a chronic psychiatric illness can be complicated. Often, chronic mentally ill patient's psychiatric symptoms and clinical staff's feelings about and attitudes toward mental illness create an expectancy of dysfunction and poor coping, especially with life-threatening illness. Difficulties are likely to be exacerbated when the patient with a chronic psychiatric illness requires palliative care near the end of life. In this chapter we discuss the challenges of providing palliative care to the individual with a chronic, major mental illness. We specifically use schizophrenia and bipolar disorder as illustrative, prototypical examples. We briefly describe these illnesses, their basic mental and behavioral manifestations, and their treatments, and we discuss complicating factors and offer suggestions and recommendations on how to address these patients to try to avoid complications and what to do when they arise.

PREVALENCE

Not surprisingly, the prevalence of palliative-care patients with major mental illness has not been studied, nor are there data on the numbers of mentally ill who require palliative care. However, psychiatric disorders among medically ill patients appear to be relatively common. Rates of DSM-III psychiatric disorders observed in 215 cancer patients from three cancer centers showed that 6% of the consults were for major affective disorders; in a study of 546 patients referred to the Psychiatry Service at Memorial Sloan-Kettering Cancer Center, 9% were for major depression, and 5% were for either schizophrenia or manic-depression.[1] The prevalence of psychiatric disorders in a study of an outpatient primary-care clinic population ranged from 15% for patients with a medical explanation for their presenting symptoms to 45% for patients with ill-explained symptoms.[2] High prevalence rates of psychiatric disorders have been described in the primary-care population[3] and in general hospital patients.[4]

The prevalence of medical illness in psychiatric patients has also been studied and has traditionally been high. In a screening of 2,090 patients in a psychiatric clinic, 43% had one or more physical illnesses.[5] In a study of a group of chronic mentally ill patients, 53% had undiagnosed medical problems, and 36% had known medical illnesses requiring treatment.[6] In one study, 88% of chronic mentally ill outpatients had a significant medical illness.[7] This topic is also extensively reviewed in a recent review article.[8]

The complications of psychiatric disorders (e.g., self-harm or suicide) can be serious, and psychiatric consultation is appropriate. We discuss the potential role(s) of the psychiatric consultant, when to consult, and ways the psychiatrist may be helpful. In addition, we provide some basic information on pharmacologic recommendations.

SCHIZOPHRENIA

Schizophrenia is a psychotic disorder with a lifetime prevalence estimated to range from 0.5% to 1.0%.[9] Its symptoms include a disorder of thought processes and content, including hallucinations and or/delusions, along with significant impairment in interpersonal relationships. People with this disorder often manifest disorganized speech and behavior, and their odd appearance often leads others to perceive them as threatening. The particular symptom picture varies according to the subtype of the illness and among individual patients; one patient may appear docile, withdrawn, and catatonic, while another may be agitated and belligerent.

Symptoms of schizophrenia are often the cause of a significant delay in diagnosis and treatment of medical illnesses, and thus palliative care becomes the treatment from the time of detection and diagnosis of an illness.[10–13] For example, the Memorial group has seen several women who have appeared with fungating, ulcerating breast cancer for which they never sought treatment. It is thought that the pain that would bring psychologically healthy persons to the doctor appears either muted or highly tolerated in many people with schizophrenia. Talbott and Linn[12] studied this issue and explored some schizophrenic patients' lack of verbalization of pain and discomfort, toleration and exhibition of loathsome and fungating lesions, and inability or unwillingness to tolerate medical care. They found that patients did not verbalize pain or discomfort from acute illnesses including myocardial infarction, major fractures, third-degree burns, perforated peptic ulcers, and gangrenous extremities. They concluded that this lack of responses was multifactorial and related to biological, social, and psychological issues. We observe that this failure to respond may be a manifestation of the negative symptoms of schizophrenia (affective flattening, alogia, avolition), or the patient may incorporate the pain and its believed source into a delusional system, thus distorting the understanding and recognition of pain as a symptom.[14]

Case Example

C.B., a 55-year-old divorced woman, was diagnosed with metastatic ovarian cancer. Her family described a history of schizophrenia over 30 years characterized by paranoid delusions that isolated her socially from family and friends. She moved often and was poorly compliant with neuroleptic medications, including long-acting parenteral haloperidol decanoate. Her family brought her to the hospital when they noticed her shortness of breath.

Diagnostic workup revealed the presence of multiple metastases with significant disease in her lungs. A treatment plan for palliative radiation to relieve the shortness of breath was undertaken. The patient was compliant with her outpatient radiation appointments, but a psychiatric consultation was requested because of her increasing agitation and erratic behavior characterized by complaints that staff were trying to hurt her. At times, she believed they had threatened to kill her. She repeatedly refused psychiatric interventions as well as physical examinations. Nevertheless, during one outpatient visit when she was accompanied by her son, she agreed to a limited psychiatric consultation. Efforts were made to hospitalize her to treat her psychiatric illness, but she refused. Risperidone 0.5 mg po bid was prescribed, and, although the patient agreed to take it, she did not. She began to call her doctors and nurses more and more frequently, expressing fears that the staff were trying to hurt her. She often refused to come for treatment but would be coaxed in by a favorite nurse. At one visit, the patient reluctantly consented to psychiatric follow-up and subsequent intramuscular injection of haloperidol 5 mg. Again, she left with a prescription for risperidone 0.5 mg po bid, and her son agreed to strongly assist in compliance.

The patient's palliative radiation treatments were rescheduled to give the total dose over a shorter period, and she took pain medications as scheduled: morphine sulfate 5 mg po q4h prn. She could not be persuaded, however, to take psychotropic medications, fearing she was being "tricked" and that she would be "locked up." She allowed her son to help with general hygiene and daily activities. As her illness progressed, the patient was admitted to the hospital and treated with haloperidol 10 mg po bid. Her agitation and paranoia significantly decreased. However, her physical status deteriorated, and she was transferred to hospice where she died quietly with her son in attendance.

Discussion

The psychiatrist's role in the management of this case was to assist in the patient's palliative treatment by assessing her competency, assisting in compliance with her cancer treatment, and helping staff to understand the source of her uncooperative behavior and to recognize the limits of treating her long-standing psychiatric disorder. Through discussions with her son, the psychiatrist confirmed the diagnosis and explored the treatment options for the patient's psychiatric illness, including appropriateness and potential benefits of psychiatric hospitalization. She had a history of responding well to psychotropic medications while hospitalized, but she refused hospitalization and she did not meet criteria for involuntary hospitalization. It was important to weigh the benefits of psychiatric hospitalization and stabilization against the risk of delaying her treatment for palliation. A psychiatric unit that could have ensured access to daily radiation treatment, such as a med-psych unit in a general hospital, would have been ideal. A psychiatric unit in a psychiatric hospital is generally not an appropriate place for caring for the dying patient because the expert emphasis is on treatment and management of psychotic symptoms and secondary behavioral problems, not on pain management and palliative care. Additional concerns include the effect of a dying medically ill person on the severely psychotic and suicidal patients who lack the ability to adaptively defend themselves psychologically. For medical staff, it is often extremely helpful to be reminded that the patient's behaviors are not expressions of the patient's desire or right to be difficult but rather are driven by symptoms from which the patient suffers uncomfortably, even if those symptoms seem to be preferred or sought by the patient; psychosis is an uncomfortable state.

This patient refused both psychiatric and medical hospitalization. She also refused psychotropic medications, which she incorporated into her paranoid delusions. The psychiatrist suggested that her compliance would be better if the staff member whom the patient most trusted saw her at clinic visits and other contacts were minimized. This strategy helped the patient by enabling her to develop a modicum of trust in a clinical nurse specialist, who helped decrease the patient's agitation and encouraged her to take an intramuscular injection of haloperidol.

With this patient, palliative care included primarily radiation therapy and narcotic pain medications. In other patients, it often includes chemotherapy and surgical procedures as well. Intravenous lines, feeding tubes, monitoring equipment, and even surgical wounds are fodder for paranoid delusions and agitation, which can disrupt palliative measures. Psychiatric intervention may be necessary in these patients to control symptoms, decrease agitation, and improve compliance and cooperation. As with any agitated patient, restraints, such as a Posey or finger restraints, are at times necessary to avoid having the patient remove intravenous lines. Careful monitoring on an hourly basis is important when restraints are used. (Every hospital or care facility has its own rules and regulations regarding agitated patients and restraints, and staff should be familiar with the specifics of their institution.)

Intravenous neuroleptics, specifically haloperidol and chlorpromazine in doses equivalent to the patient's usual oral medications, are particularly useful in patients who are physically unable to take medications by mouth or who refuse medications because of delusions or agitation (see Table 7.1).

Atypical neuroleptics, such as risperidone, are also useful in patients able or willing to take oral medications. The risk of extrapyramidal symptoms (stiffness, rigidity) or akathisia is less with these medications. Akathisia is a particularly uncomfortable symptom that is often mistaken for

Table 7.1 Neuroleptics Useful in Treating Delirium and Agitation in the Medically Ill

Name	Route of Administration	Starting Dose
Haloperidol (Haldol)	po/iv/im	0.5 mg tid
Chlorpromazine (Thorazine)	po/iv	50 mg
Thioridazine (Mellaril)	po	10–20 mg bid
Risperidone (Risperdal)	po	0.5 mg bid
Olanzapine (Zyprexa)	po	2.5 mg qhs

Table 7.2   Medications to Treat Akathisia

Name	Dose
Benztropine (Cogentin)	0.5 mg po bid–2 mg po tid
Lorazepam (Ativan)	0.5–1 mg bid–q4hr
Propranolol	10 mg bid–30 mg tid

anxiety or agitation. It consists of a sensation of needing to move, and patients often appear fidgety, constantly moving their hands or feet, shifting or bouncing from one foot to the other, pacing, or rocking from the waist. Treatment (see Table 7.2) consists of lowering or changing the neuroleptic or using anticholinergics, propranolol, or lorazepam. Benztropine, an anticholinergic that is particularly effective against extrapyramidal side effects and is frequently used to treat akathisia, is generally less effective than lorazepam or propranolol in treating akathisia.[15]

Another important point to derive from this case is the importance of family or trusted staff in helping to treat agitation. One patient with chronic paranoid schizophrenia was helped through the recovery from a Whipple procedure by the constant companionship of his father, whom the patient trusted and relied on in his daily life. This patient was fortunate to have his father available and also not to have incorporated his father into his paranoid delusions.

BIPOLAR DISORDER

Of the affective disorders, manic symptoms of bipolar disorder present a particularly difficult problem in the context of palliative care. Lifetime prevalence of Bipolar I is about 0.4% to 1.6%.[9] Manifestations of mania include elevated, expansive, or irritable mood; grandiosity; increased energy and decreased need for sleep; pressured speech; racing thoughts; impulsivity; and possible psychosis. Judgment is often impaired. Mood stabilizers, such as lithium and valproic acid, are the mainstay of pharmacologic treatment, and while these medications are very effective, patients may experience breakthrough manic episodes.

Case Example

M.R. was a 68-year-old married lawyer with a long history of chronic lymphocytic leukemia (CLL) and a long history of bipolar disorder with episodes of depression and mania. Her manic episodes were characterized by increased energy, decreased sleep, racing disorganized thoughts, and, sometimes, psychotic, delusional thinking. Her bipolar symptoms were well controlled on lithium carbonate at therapeutic blood levels. She had been successfully treated for CLL with chemotherapy and radiation, and for many years it had been in remission. She had twice-yearly checkups. At one of these visits, the patient's oncologist noticed she had difficulty walking and that she had an unusual affect with manic behavior. A workup revealed a fractured hip sustained from a fall. Because the patient was beginning a manic episode, she had not acknowledged pain or decreased function, which was brought to her attention by her oncologist. She was admitted and her fracture surgically treated. A psychiatric consultation was requested to treat her mania. Intravenous benzodiazepines (lorazepam 1 mg iv q6h) and neuroleptics (haloperidol 2 mg iv q6h) were successfully used to control her symptoms of racing, disorganized thoughts, and hyperactivity. As her mania cleared, her awareness of her pain increased, and morphine sulfate was initiated. The doses of benzodiazepine and neuroleptic were reduced, and she was stabilized on lithium. Despite successful treatment of her hip fracture and her mania, she did not have a successful convalescence. She was extremely resistant to continuing narcotic medications at home because of her experience with substance addiction in her husband and her son. She suffered with her pain and was thus less mobile than would be desirable for a full recovery. Her mood was "down," possibly a depressive phase of her bipolar disorder, but it was not as low as during previous episodes, and she exhibited existential signs of depression (hopelessness, helplessness, a pervasive sense of futility, pervasive thoughts of death or suicide). She developed pneumonia and then a manic breakthrough in which she stopped sleeping and began cleaning and reorganizing her house in a manic, disorganized manner. She agreed to a medical hospitalization so that she could be treated for pneumonia and mania. Hospital staff viewed her as an "affable, enjoyable" manic patient, and there were no problems relating to her. Her mania was treated with thioridazine 50 mg po qam, 100 mg po qhs, and valproic acid 250 mg po bid, which was eventually increased to 500 mg po bid. Thioridazine was discontinued after a week, and the patient was discharged with extensive home nursing. She recovered from both the pneumonia and the mania, but the episode weakened her substantially. She never recovered her full strength, and she grew increasingly debilitated. Her family was unable to care for her, and she was admitted to a nursing care facility where she died several months later.

Discussion

In this case, the patient's preexisting psychiatric disorder led to neglect of a serious medical problem common in the elderly: hip fracture.[16,17] Her chronic leukemia was in remission, but she developed a medical problem because of her psychiatric disorder and then had complications because of psychological factors associated with her long-standing family problems. (Many relatives of substance abusers, as well as recovering addicts or alcoholics, are often resistant to pain medications. They fear addiction and its disastrous results.) The consultant psychiatrist's role in this case was to control the patient's manic symptoms and to integrate the treatment for mania with appropriate pain management. During the second bout of mania, the psychiatrist chose not to use benzodiazepines because the concomitant presence of an infection probably increases the risk of serious delirium.

In palliative-care patients, a mixed picture of delirium and mania may develop in patients with a bipolar history who receive steroids. In the presence of mania without any symptoms of delirium or cognitive changes, a mood stabilizer such as valproic acid has been effective. Treatment should begin with a low dose, 250 mg qd, and the physician must follow blood levels to avoid toxicity. In the presence of delirium and mania, a neuroleptic such as haloperidol is helpful. Higher doses, such as 5 mg bid, are frequently necessary for agitated delirious and manic patients with psychotic features, but initial treatment should be at a low dose, such as 0.5 mg po/iv q8h with frequent prn doses. Sometimes a more sedating neuroleptic, like thioridazine initiated at 20 mg bid, is helpful.

In addition to controlling symptoms, the psychiatrist in this case worked as part of a team. The doctors involved were initially treating the problems related to their own specialties, but collaboration was necessary. The internist who initially noted the patient's difficulty walking involved the psychiatrist in the patient's care early on, and the team was able to follow the patient's needs as her care evolved into palliative treatment. Team members often include internists, psychiatrists, nurse clinicians or clinical nurse specialists, and social workers. Each discipline has a particular area of expertise, and effective team members can communicate with team members from other disciplines.

SUMMARY

The terminally ill patient with a chronic psychiatric disorder presents special challenges to the palliative health-care team, primarily challenges relating to compliance and behavioral problems. These problems usually arise from symptoms that interfere with the patient's ability to perceive his or her clinical picture correctly and to make decisions free from the influence of perceptual and cognitive distortions. All too often, staff do not appreciate the degree to which symptoms of mental illness influence behaviors and decisions, and this misperception leads to frustration and angry feelings. All too often, a frustrated but well-meaning staff member will ask, "Why can't he just make the appointment and take his medications? I've explained it to him a hundred times!" Increased familiarity with the nature of chronic and severe psychiatric illness can help reduce the staff's frustration.

There are many resources to call on to help with the psychiatric patient. We have discussed a small range of medications that can be used for psychiatric symptom management during palliative care. It is useful to remember that it may be best to try to continue an individual patient's medication regimen if it has been successful but that this regimen may need to be altered as a result of the patient's medical status and other medications. Additionally, as we have illustrated, interpersonal supports can be effective interventions. The effect of a trusting relationship should not be underestimated. A trusted staff person or family member can be very helpful and influential not only in aiding compliance but also in decreasing the fear, anxiety, and tension that often occur in a terminally ill and dying patient. It should be noted, however, that in the course of severe symptom expression (e.g., florid paranoid delusions), even the most long-standing, stable relationship can be torn apart. In the event of such a rift, it is important for staff members not to view the patient's actions as a personal rejection. Again, it is an expression of symptoms of severe mental illness with which the individual suffers. The role of the team can be particularly important when dealing with a difficult patient. These patients trigger a wide range of emotional responses among caregivers, and team members can serve to help support each other and share the work when treating a particularly difficult patient.

Finally, it is never too early to involve the consultant psychiatrist in palliative care of the psychiatric patient. The two cases presented reflect a small but important part of the work of the consultation psychiatrist. Too few psychiatrists choose to consult in hospice and palliative-care settings, yet the complex issues intrinsic to these settings are among the most challenging in consultation psychiatry today.

References

1. Massie MJ, Holland JC. The cancer patient with pain: psychiatric complications and their management. *Medical Clinics of North America*, 1987; 71: 243–258.
2. vanHemert AM, Hengeveld MW, Bolk JH, Rooijmans HG, Vandenbroucke JP. Psychiatric disorders in relation to medical illness among patients of a general medical outpatient clinic. *Psychological Medicine*, 1993; 23(1):167–173.
3. Burvill PW, Knuiman MW. The influence of minor psychiatric morbidity on consulting rates to general practitioners. *Psychological Medicine*, 1983; 13:635–643.
4. Feldman E, Mayou R, Hawton K, Ardern M, Smith EBO. Psychiatric disorders in medical inpatients. *Quarterly Journal of Medicine*, 1987; 63: 405–412.
5. Koranyi IK. Morbidity and rate of undiagnosed physical illness in a psychiatric clinic population. *Archives of General Psychiatry*, 1979; 36:414–419.
6. Farmer S. Medical problems of chronic patients in a community support program. *Hospital and Community Psychiatry*, 1987; 38(7):745–749.
7. Maricle RA, Hoffman WF, Bloom JD, Faulkner LR, Keepers GA. The prevalence and significance of medical illness among chronically mentally ill outpatients. *Community Mental Health Journal*, 1987; 23(2):81–90.
8. Felker B, Yazel JJ, Short D. Mortality and medical comorbidity among psychiatric patients: a review. *Psychiatric Services*, 1996; 47:1356–1363.
9. American Psychiatric Association. *Diagnostic and Statistical Manual of Mental Disorders*. 4th ed., Washington, DC: American Psychiatric Association, 1994.
10. Massie MJ. Schizophrenia. In: Holland JC, Rowland JH, eds, *Handbook of Psychooncology: Psychological Care of the Patient with Cancer*. New York: Oxford University Press, 1989:320–323.
11. Shuster JL. Schizophrenia. In: Holland J, ed, *Psycho-oncology*. Oxford University Press, 1998: 614–618.
12. Talbott JA, Linn L. Reactions of schizophrenics to life-threatening disease. *Psychological Quarterly*, 1987; 50:218–227.
13. Solomon S, McCartney JR, Saravay SM, Katz E. Postoperative hospital course of patients with history of severe psychiatric illness. *General Hospital Psychiatry*, 1987; 9:376–382.
14. Karasu TB, Waltzman SA, Lindermayer JP, Buckley PJ. The medical care of patients with psychiatric illness. *Hospital and Community Psychiatry*, 1980; 31:463–472.
15. Halstead SM, Barnes TRE, Speller JC. Akathisia: prevalence and associated dysphoria in an inpatient population with chronic schizophrenia. *British Journal of Psychiatry*, 1994; 164:177–183.
16. Tsuang MT, Perkins K, Simpson JC. Physical diseases in schizophrenia and affective disorder. *Journal of Clinical Psychiatry*, 1983; 44:42–46.
17. Fava GA, Molnar G, Zielezny M. Health attitudes of psychiatric inpatients. *Psychopathology*, 1987; 20:180–186.

PART II
Symptom Management

8

Physical Symptom Management in the Terminally Ill

An Overview for Mental Health Professionals

Russell K. Portenoy, M.D.

Patients with progressive diseases present complex symptomatology that evolves unpredictably over time. Although the degree to which suffering is determined by unrelieved symptoms varies from patient to patient and from time to time, clinicians often observe dramatic improvement in quality of life after adequate symptom control is achieved. All clinicians who care for such patients should have the skills necessary to assess common physical and psychological symptoms and to implement routine management strategies within the limits defined by the overall goals of care.

Somewhat arbitrarily, symptoms are conventionally divided into the physical and the psychological. Although this division is heuristic in one sense, encouraging an appropriate emphasis on the role of disease-related factors, it should not be taken to imply a lack of interaction between the physical and the psychological determinants of symptoms. For some symptoms, such as pain and dyspnea, physical factors may offer a sufficient etiologic explanation, but intensity or distress may be more closely tied to anxiety or cognitions concerning the symptom than to any physiological perturbation. For others, such as fatigue, the predominating pathophysiology can be related to an overt physical factor, such as anemia, or to a psychiatric disorder, such as depression. These interactions indicate that the assessment and management of common physical symptoms must always consider psychosocial context and associations.

SYMPTOM MANAGEMENT AND PALLIATIVE CARE

Symptoms are usually only one aspect of the suffering experienced by patients with incurable progressive diseases. As a result, symptomatic therapies are usually pursued within a broader model of palliative care, which attempts to address many other concerns concurrently. The nature of this palliative care is exemplified in the definition promulgated by the World Health Organization:

> Palliative care is the active total care of patients whose disease is not responsive to curative treatment. Control of pain, of other symptoms, and of psychological, social and spiritual problems is paramount. The goal of palliative care is the achievement of the best possible quality of life for patients and their families.[1]

Palliative-care interventions aim to improve the physical, psychosocial, and spiritual condition that define both the quality of life and the quality of death for patients throughout the course of life-threatening disorders. Thus, palliative care is the "parallel universe" to life-prolonging treatment and is continually addressed by clinicians in diverse disciplines. Although the focus of palliative care intensifies at the end of life, the core issues—comfort and function, defined broadly and evaluated within the context of the family—are salient for all clinicians during and after the period of active disease-oriented treatment.

A palliative-care model recognizes the need to address symptom distress, physical impairments, and psychosocial disturbances even during the period of aggressive primary therapy, the avowed goal of which may be cure or prolongation of life. The importance of symptom management is evident in all palliative care, but the degree to which symptoms are the major concern varies with the particular issues expressed by the patient and family. During a period of active life-prolonging therapy, which can extend to years in many disorders, symptom management may be integrated into a broader approach to palliative care that also emphasizes psychological support and a range of function-oriented therapies that may grade into the discipline of cancer rehabilitation. For the dying patient, symptom control may be an intensive focus in a comprehensive approach that fulfills the needs for practical support, attempts to address spiritual or existential concerns in addition to physical and psychosocial concerns, and assists in advance care planning.

The evolving perspective on palliative care has encouraged the gradual acceptance of medical specialization in this area. The publication of a major textbook devoted to palliative medicine was a milestone in this process.[2] Although most dying patients continue to have no access to specialists in palliative care, these opportunities are growing. The involvement of specialists is usually most helpful during the management of distressed patients with far-advanced medical diseases, including those who are dying from cancer, AIDS, neurodegenerative diseases, and other incurable progressive diseases. Palliative-care specialists also may be helpful early in the course of an incurable disease by assisting in symptom control and providing an assessment that may be able to project future needs.

PREVALENCE OF PHYSICAL SYMPTOMS

The importance of physical symptoms as determinants of quality of life is suggested by their prevalence in populations with advanced diseases. In the cancer population, pain, fatigue, somnolence or mental clouding, and gastrointestinal symptoms are extremely prevalent (Table 8.1), and most patients experience multiple physical and psychological symptoms.[3–21] In one recent survey, for ex-

Table 8.1   Prevalence Rates (%) for Some Common Physical Symptoms in Four Large Surveys

	Curtis et al. (1991) N = 100	Reuben et al. (1988) N = 1592	Portenoy et al. (1994) N = 243	Ventafridda et al. (1990) N = 115
Fatigue	40		74	
Pain	89	51	64	59
Somnolence			60	13
Dyspnea	41	53	24	10
Cough			28	6
Anorexia	55	79	44	30
Nausea	32	44	44	6
Vomiting	25		21	4
Constipation	40	54	35	23
Weight loss		75	27	

Note: All surveys were in populations with advanced cancer, with the exception of Portenoy et al. (1994), which included a minority of patients with earlier disease. All surveys were performed in a palliative-care or hospice program, again with the exception of Portenoy et al. (1994), which was conducted on an inpatient and outpatient population at a large cancer hospital.

ample, outpatients with cancer who completed a symptom assessment questionnaire averaged more than 9 concurrent symptoms, and inpatients averaged more than 13 symptoms.[18]

SYMPTOM ASSESSMENT

Symptom management depends on a detailed knowledge of presentation, pathogenesis, and impact within the larger set of phenomena that enhance or undermine well-being. In contrast to the traditional medical model, which encourages an approach to the patient that focuses on the chief complaint in relative isolation, the model of palliative care requires this broader perspective.

Symptom Characteristics

Each symptom can be described in terms of multiple dimensions (Table 8.2). A detailed evaluation of a symptom should identify the involved site or sites, intensity, temporal features, quality, and factors that provoke or relieve it. Each of these aspects, in turn, can be depicted with varying detail. For example, the temporal description can include onset, duration, and daily pattern.

The measurement of symptom intensity is an essential component of symptom assessment. Intensity relates to distress and often determines the urgency of evaluation and treatment. In the case of some symptoms, such as pain, fatigue, and dyspnea, measurement of intensity can be performed using validated scales.[22] These scales vary in complexity and may be unidimensional or multidimensional. In some cases, including pain and dyspnea measurement, simple verbal rating scales

(e.g., none, mild, moderate, severe) or numeric scales have been validated, and these usually suffice in the clinical setting. More sophisticated instruments may be preferable in clinical investigation. Other common symptoms, such as itch, have not been systematically studied and can be measured only using a nonvalidated approach. In such cases, a verbal rating scale or a 10-point numeric scale can be constructed at the bedside.

The measurement of pain intensity exemplifies the salience of this aspect of the assessment. Guidelines for cancer pain management emphasize the necessity of repeated pain measurement as a foundation for therapy,[23] and the use of simple intensity scales has been considered the linchpin of hospital-based quality improvement programs.[24,25] Although the measurement of intensity cannot substitute for a comprehensive assessment, it increases the visibility of the symptom for the staff and encourages salutary adjustments in therapy. The routine measurement of symptoms other than pain has been explored little,[4] but is likely to favorably influence management in a similar manner. Clinicians who are working toward system changes that will improve the palliative care offered patients with advanced medical disease should consider the potential benefits of such routine measurements.

Although the subjective characteristics of symptoms provide essential information, they often offer an insufficient basis for therapy. Further information about the nature of the symptom and the disease is usually required, particularly when the symptom is presenting anew or has changed. In such cases, the assessment must include a physical examination and a review of available laboratory and radiographic studies. Even these data

Table 8.2   Characteristics and Constructs in Symptom Assessment

Characteristics	Symptom-Related Constructs	Illness-Related Constructs
Subjective	Syndrome	Extent of disease
Temporal features	Etiology	Quality of life
Severity	Inferred pathophysiology	Goals of care
Quality		
Locations		
Provocative and palliative factors		
Objective		
Physical findings		
Laboratory and imaging studies		

sometimes allow only a provisional understanding and must be followed by additional studies to elaborate or confirm the first impression.

The importance of physical assessment in the evaluation of symptoms in the medically ill has been highlighted by a survey of new referrals to a pain service at a cancer center.[26] The comprehensive pain assessment performed by the service led to the discovery of a previously unrecognized lesion that could account for the pain in approximately two-thirds of patients; almost 20% of these patients could receive a new primary therapy—either antineoplastic or antibiotic—as a result of this discovery. The comprehensive assessment of a symptom, therefore, has important implications for disease management that extend beyond symptomatic therapies alone.

Symptom-Related Constructs

The information about symptom and disease status that can be acquired from the history, examination, and review of laboratory and imaging studies may clarify the existence of a recognized syndrome and facilitate inferences about the likely etiology and pathophysiology (see Table 8.2). This integration may be relevant diagnostically or therapeutically.

A syndrome represents a constellation of symptoms and signs that define a recognizable clinical entity and may offer clues about etiology or response to therapy. For some symptoms, such as pain in the cancer population, well-defined syndromes have been described,[27] and the designation of a syndrome may have important clinical implications. For example, the syndrome of back pain in patients with metastatic cancer may be managed using an algorithm based on the known threat of epidural spinal cord or cauda equina compression.[28] Knowledge of the common syndromes associated with the symptoms reported by patients with advanced disease is one foundation for effective palliative care.

Information about the likely etiology of a symptom and inferences about its pathophysiology are also therapeutically relevant. This information may allow the selection of a primary treatment for an underlying disorder, which may be a very effective approach to symptom control. For example, fatigue that worsens in parallel with a decline in hemoglobin suggests the potential utility of primary interventions for anemia. Similarly,

dyspnea associated with wheezing on examination suggests the existence of bronchospasm, which may be evaluated to identify the proximate cause (e.g., heart failure) or treated directly with bronchodilators.

Illness-Related Constructs

The comprehensive assessment should also provide the information necessary to define the extent of disease, other quality of life concerns, and the goals of care (Table 8.2). These considerations are essential in developing an approach to therapy that can address the varied sources of the patient's suffering and offer interventions that are appropriate to both the medical status and the expressed wishes of the patient.

Consideration of the goals of care is especially important in the treatment of patients with advanced medical disease. These goals may emphasize prolongation of life, maintenance of function, or comfort. Although these goals are not mutually exclusive, one or another usually predominates at any given time, and the selection of therapies is continually influenced by the overriding goal. During the course of the disease, goals may evolve with information about progression or prognosis, the availability of treatments and the responses expected, changes in symptoms or functional outcomes associated with the disease or its therapy, and other factors that contribute to physical and psychosocial adaptation.

Confusion about the goals of care or divergence in goals among patient, family, and caregivers can complicate management and pose challenging ethical issues. Although clinicians are usually explicit about the immediate aims of therapy, larger goals may not be overtly expressed or may be obscured by the complexity and acuity of the immediate clinical problem. Patients may fail to express their true desires because of denial or fear, family concerns, or other reasons. Whatever the causes, lack of clarity about the goals of care can lead to miscommunication and inappropriate interventions, both of which can contribute to the distress of the patient or family.

Conflict is also possible when the goals are clearly expressed. There is ample opportunity for discordant views in a dynamic clinical situation. In developed countries, for example, many patients undergo aggressive life-prolonging therapy with little realistic hope that a cure or long-term remission may result. The administration of such therapies may actually undermine quality of life in some patients or appear to "medicalize" the dying process to such an extent that both patient and family suffer more.

Given the stakes involved, assessment of the goals of care and communication with the patient and family about these goals must be considered among the most important and challenging aspects of patient care. In the setting of advanced medical disease, symptom assessment must repeatedly clarify these goals to ensure that treatment decisions remain appropriate and consistent with the needs and desires of the patient. This process, in turn, requires an ongoing evaluation of the patient's medical and psychosocial status and a broad knowledge of both the available primary therapies and the options that exist in the domain of palliative care. Both the patient and caregivers are better served if the clinician has successfully communicated from the start that palliative care, with its focus on quality of life, functionality, and symptom control, is as central to treatment as interventions for the disease itself.

MANAGEMENT OF COMMON PHYSICAL SYMPTOMS

The assessment and management of physical symptoms is a fundamental component of palliative care in populations with advanced medical diseases. All clinicians should be comfortable with the routine therapeutic approach to the most common symptoms.

Pain

Cancer pain is the model for the first-line use of opioid pharmacotherapy in the treatment of pain related to medical illness.[29-32] An enormous clinical experience convincingly demonstrates the potential for favorable outcomes associated with long-term opioid treatment. Indeed, surveys suggest that 70% to 90% of patients with cancer pain can achieve adequate analgesia with this approach.[23,32,33-36]

Although a consensus statement on the management of cancer pain has also recommended opioid therapy for pain associated with AIDS,[23]

there have actually been very few publications focused on pain related to advanced medical diseases other than cancer. Notwithstanding, the extremely favorable experience in the cancer population should encourage clinicians to consider opioid therapy for all such populations.

In many cases, opioid therapy is integrated with other analgesic approaches, including primary treatments for the underlying etiology of the pain, if appropriate. As discussed previously, therapeutic decision making should be guided by a comprehensive assessment that places pain in the context of other quality of life concerns and defines the extent of disease and goals of care.

Role of Primary Treatments

Primary therapy directed against the underlying etiology of the pain can have analgesic consequences. This is particularly relevant in the treatment of pain associated with cancer or other advanced medical diseases because of the high probability that an underlying structural abnormality can be identified as the source of the pain. These structural abnormalities may be amenable to a variety of primary therapies. Radiotherapy to tumors, for example, can provide pain relief to more than half the patients treated,[37] and other primary therapies, such as surgical resection of neoplastic lesions and chemotherapy, can also have analgesic consequences.[38] Recently, several chemotherapies have been specifically studied, and approved for commercial use, as interventions primarily directed toward the palliation of symptoms, including pain.[39,40]

Occasional patients may also be candidates for primary therapies that are not antineoplastic. For example, empirical antibiotic therapy has been found to have profound analgesic effects in some patients.[41] This response, which presumably indicates that occult infection contributes to the pain, suggests that a trial of an antibiotic may be indicated in patients with refractory or progressive pain who are predisposed to the development of local infection.

Pharmacologic Approaches

The pharmacologic management of pain requires expertise in the use of three broad groups of analgesics: nonsteroidal antiinflammatory drugs (NSAIDs), opioid analgesics, and the so-called

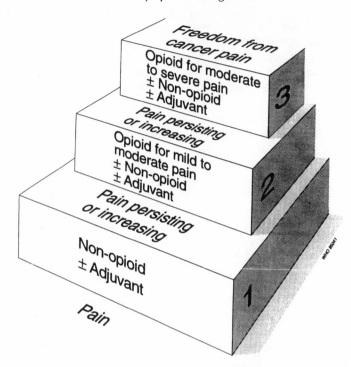

Figure 8.1. The "Analgesic Ladder" Approach to the Selection of Drug Therapies for Cancer Pain.*
*See text for a description of opioids used conventionally for moderate or severe pain. The term "adjuvant" in this context refers to both those drugs added to analgesics to treat side effects, such as laxatives for opioid-induced constipation, and the so-called adjuvant analgesics, which are drugs that have primary indications other than pain but can be analgesic in selected circumstances.
Reprinted with permission from *Cancer Pain Relief, With a Guide to Opioid Availability*. 2nd ed. Geneva: World Health Organization, 1996.

adjuvant analgesics. The latter are a diverse group of unrelated agents that have other primary indications but may be analgesic in selected circumstances.

An approach to the selection of analgesic drugs for cancer pain has been developed by the Cancer Pain Relief and Palliative Care Program of the World Health Organization.[32] Known as the "analgesic ladder" approach, this technique employs stepwise selection of analgesics based on the usual severity of pain (Figure 8.1). Patients with mild to moderate pain are typically first offered an NSAID. This drug is combined with one or more adjuvant drugs if a specific indication for one exists. These adjuvant drugs include those selected to treat a side effect of the analgesic (e.g., a laxative) and those with analgesic effects (the so-called adjuvant analgesics). Patients who present with moderate to severe pain or who fail to achieve adequate relief after a trial of a NSAID are treated with an opioid conventionally used

for pain of this severity. This opioid is usually combined with a NSAID and may be co-administered with an adjuvant drug, if indicated. Patients who present with severe pain or who fail to achieve adequate relief following appropriate administration of drugs on the second rung of the analgesic ladder should receive an opioid conventionally selected for severe pain. This treatment may also be combined with a NSAID or an adjuvant drug, as indicated.

Although drugs on the second and third rungs of the analgesic ladder have also been labeled "weak" and "strong" opioids, respectively, this designation misrepresents their pharmacology and should not be used. The drugs that are used for moderate pain, such as codeine, do not have a ceiling dose for analgesia, which would justify their description as "weak." Rather, these drugs are generally used in a limited dose range for reasons of convenience or convention. In many countries, for example, moderate pain is typically treated with a commercial formulation that contains an opioid and a nonopioid analgesic (aspirin or acetaminophen). The dose of this compound can be increased only until the recognized limits of the nonopioid component (for example, 4 to 6 g of acetaminophen for long-term dosing). If pain cannot be relieved with this maximum dose, the drug must be switched to one conventionally used to treat severe pain.

Thus, the division of opioid drugs into groups conventionally used for moderate or severe pain reflects only common practice, not optimal pharmacology. In some countries, limited availability of combination products has encouraged the use of an approach that incorporates two steps, a nonopioid analgesic for mild pain and a single entity opioid, such as morphine, for moderate or severe pain. In this approach, the opioid is initially administered at low doses appropriate for the treatment of moderate pain in the opioid-naive patient. These doses are then gradually increased, if needed, as the pain becomes more severe. The opioid regimen may still be co-administered with a nonopioid analgesic, which is provided as separate therapy.

Nonsteroidal Anti-inflammatory Drugs and Acetaminophen.   The NSAIDs (Table 8.3) and acetaminophen are characterized by a ceiling dose and analgesia that is additive to that of the opioids.[42,43] Anecdotal data suggest that they may be particularly effective for malignant bone pain.

NSAIDs should be used cautiously in patients with renal disease, history of peptic ulceration, history of a bleeding diathesis, congestive heart failure or volume overload of any other cause, and encephalopathy. Significant renal disease, active upper gastrointestinal ulceration, and coagulopathy are usually absolute contraindications. Acetaminophen is contraindicated in the setting of severe hepatic dysfunction and should also be used cautiously in patients with renal disease.[44]

There is great intraindividual variability in the response to different NSAIDs, and clinicians should be prepared to switch from one drug to another if desired effects are not achieved. To some extent, differences in toxicity can guide the selection of specific drugs. For example, the pyrazole class, specifically phenylbutazone, has a substantially greater risk of toxicity and has been supplanted by newer drugs. Acetaminophen is widely regarded to be the safest nonopioid analgesic, but

its minimal anti-inflammatory effects may limit its utility in some pain syndromes. Some salicylates, such as choline magnesium trisalicylate and salsalate, have less platelet toxicity and ulcerogenic effects at usually prescribed doses.[45] The ulcerogenic effects of several other NSAIDs have been assessed in epidemiologic studies,[46,47] which generally support the view that ibuprofen and diclofenac are relatively safer than aspirin and piroxicam is relatively less safe. Some surveys suggest that nabumetone is also relatively less likely to cause serious gastrointestinal toxicity and that ketorolac and some of the older NSAIDs, such as mefenamic acid, are relatively more so.

Given the frailty of patients with advanced medical diseases, NSAID therapy should usually be initiated at a relatively low dose. Upward dose titration can then be implemented to identify a minimal effective dose, the ceiling dose, and dose-related toxicity. The dose should be increased, usually on a weekly basis, until side effects develop, no further analgesia occurs with an increment in dose, or an arbitrary limit of approximately $1^1/_2$ to 2 times the usual starting dose is reached.

Opioid Analgesics.   The key principles of opioid pharmacotherapy are widely accepted.[23,30,32] They may be summarized as follows.

Select an appropriate drug. Several factors should be considered in the decision to use one opioid drug rather than another. First is the distinction between the pure agonist subclass and the agonist-antagonist subclass. The pure agonist opioids bind to one or more of the opioid receptors and demonstrate no antagonist activity. Morphine is the prototypic drug in this class, but numerous others are available in the United States, including hydromorphone, oxycodone, levorphanol, and methadone (Table 8.4). The agonist-antagonist opioids comprise two subtypes, a mixed agonist-antagonist type (e.g., pentazocine, nalbuphine, butorphanol, and dezocine) and a partial agonist type (e.g., buprenorphine). These agonist-antagonist opioids are not preferred for the management of chronic pain because of several properties, including a ceiling effect for analgesia, the capacity to reverse favorable effects and precipitate an abstinence syndrome in patients who are physically dependent on pure agonist opioids, and, in some cases, a likelihood of psychotomimetic effects substantially greater than that of the agonist drugs.[48]

Table 8.3 Nonsteroidal Antiinflammatory Drugs

Chemical Class	Generic Name	Approximate Half-Life (hr)	Dosing Schedule	Recommended Starting Dose (mg/day)	Maximum Recommended Dose (mg/day)	Comment
p-aminophenol	Acetaminophen[b]	2–4	q 4–6 h	2600	6000	Overdosage produces hepatic toxicity. Not anti-inflammatory. Lack of GI and platelet toxicity may be important.
Salicylates	Aspirin[b]	3–12[c]	q 4–6 h	2600	6000	Standard for comparison. May not be tolerated as well as some of the newer NSAIDs.[d]
	Diflunisal[b]	8–12	q 12 h	1000 × 1 then 500 q 12 h	1500	Less GI toxicity than aspirin.[d]
	Choline magnesium trisalicylate[b]	8–12	q 12 h	1500 × 1 then 1000 q12h	4000	Believed to have less GI toxicity than other NSAIDs. No effect on platelet aggregation, despite potent anti-inflammatory effects.[d]
	Salsalate	8–12	q 12 h	1500 × 1 then 1000 q 12 h	4000	
Propionic acids	Ibuprofen[b]	3–4	q 4–8 h	1600	4200	Available over the counter.[d]
	Naproxen[b]	13	q 12 h	500	1500	Available over the counter and as a suspension.[d]
	Naproxen sodium[b]	13	q 12 h	550	1375	—[d]
	Fenoprofen	2–3	q 6 h	800	3200	—[d]
	Ketoprofen	2–3	q 6–8 h	100	300	Available over the counter[d]
	Flurbiprofen[b]	5–6	q 8–12 h	100	300	Experience too limited to evaluate higher doses, though it is likely that some patients would benefit.[d]
	Oxaprozin	40	q24h	600	1800	Once-daily dosing may be useful.[d]

Class	Drug	Half-life (h)[c]	Dosing interval	Dose (mg)	Maximum dose (mg)	Comments
Acetic Acids	Indomethacin	4–5	q 8–12 h	75	200	Available in sustained-release and rectal formulations. Higher incidence of side effects, particularly GI and CNS, than propionic acids.[d]
	Tolmetin	1	q 6–8 h	600	2000	—[d]
	Sulindac	14	q 12 h	300	400	—[d]
	Diclofenac	2	q 6 h	75	200	—[d]
	Ketorolac (IM)	4–7	q 4–6 h	30 (loading), then 15 q6h	60	Parenteral formulation available. Long-term use not recommended[d]
	Etodolac	7	q 8 h	600	1200	—[d]
Oxicams	Piroxicam	45	q 24 h	20	40	Administration of 40 mg for >3 weeks is associated with a high incidence of peptic ulcer, particularly in the elderly.[d]
Naphthyl-alkanones	Nabumetone	24	q24	1000	1000–2000	Appears to have a relatively low risk of GI toxicity; once-daily dosing may be useful.
Fenamates	Mefenamic acid[b]	2	q 6 h	500 × 1 then 250 q6h	1000	Not recommended for use longer than 1 week and therefore not indicated in cancer pain therapy.[d]
	Meclofenamic acid	2–4	q 6–8 h	150	400	—[d]
Pyrazoles	Phenylbutazone	50–100	q 6–8 h	300	400	More toxic than other NSAIDs. Not preferred for cancer pain therapy.

[a]Starting dose should be one-half to two-thirds recommended dose in the elderly, those on multiple drugs, and those with renal insufficiency. Doses must be individualized. Studies of NSAIDs in the cancer population are meager; dosing guidelines are thus empiric.

[b]Pain is approved indication.

[c]Half-life of aspirin increases with dose.

[d]At high doses, stool guaiac, liver function tests, BUN, creatinine, and urinalysis should be checked periodically.

Table 8.4   Opioid Analgesics (Pure μ agonists) Used for the Treatment of Chronic Pain

	Equianalgesic Doses[a]	Half-life (hr)	Peak Effect (hr)	Duration (hr)	Toxicity	Comments
Morphine	10 i.m. 20–60 p.o.[b]	2–3 2–3	0.5–1 1.5–2	3–6 4–7	Constipation, nausea, sedation most common; respiratory depression rare in cancer patients.	Standard comparison for opioids; multiple routes available
Controlled-release morphine	20–60 p.o.[b]	2–3	3–4	8–12		
Sustained-release morphine	20–60 p.o.[b]	2–3	4–6	24		Once-a-day morphine recently approved in the U.S.
Hydromorphone	1.5 i.m. 7.5 p.o.	2–3 2–3	0.5–1 1–2	3–4 3–4	Same as morphine	Used for multiple routes
Oxycodone	20–30	2–3	1	3–6	Same as morphine	Combined with aspirin or acetaminophen, for moderate pain; available orally without coanalgesic for severe pain
Controlled-release oxycodone	20–30	2–3	3–4	8–12		
Oxymorphone	1 i.m. 10 p.r.	— —	0.5–1 1.5–3	3–6 4–6	Same as morphine	No oral formulation
Meperidine	75 i.m. 300 p.o.	2–3 2–3	0.5–1 1–2	3–4 3–6	Same as morphine + CNS excitation; contraindicated in those on MAO inhibitors	Not preferred for cancer pain due to potential toxicity
Heroin	5 i.m.	0.5	0.5–1	4–5	Same as morphine	Analgesic action due to metabolites, predominantly morphine; not available in U.S.

Drug					Toxicity	Comments
Levorphanol	2 i.m. 4 p.o.	12–15	0.5–1	3–6	Same as morphine	With long half-life, accumulation occurs after beginning or increasing dose
Methadone	10 i.m. 20 p.o.	12–>150	0.5–1.5	4–8	Same as morphine	Risk of delays toxicity due to accumulation; useful to start dosing on p.r.n. basis, with close monitoring
Codeine	130 i.m. 200 p.o.	2–3	1.5–2	3–6	Same as morphine	Usually combined with nonopioid
Propoxyphene HCl	—	12	1.5–2	3–6	Same as morphine plus seizures with overdose	Toxic metabolite accumulates but not significant at doses used clinically; often combined with Nonopioid
Propoxyphene napsylate	—	12	1.5–2	3–6	Same as hydrochloride	Same as hydrochloride
Hydrocodone	—	2–4	0.5–1	3–4	Same as morphine	Available only combined with acetaminophen
Dihydrocodeine	—	2–4	0.5–1	3–4	Same as morphine	Available only combined with acetaminophen or aspirin

[a]Dose that provides analgesia equivalent to 10 mg i.m. morphine. These ratios are useful guides when switching drugs or routes of administration. When switching drugs, reduce the equianalgesic dose of the new drug by 25–50% to account for incomplete cross-tolerance. The only exception to this is methadone, which appears to manifest a greater degree of incomplete cross-tolerance than other opioids; when switching to methadone, reduce the equianalgesic dose by 90%.

[b]Extensive survey data suggest that the relative potency of i.m.:p.o. morphine of 1:6 changes to 1:2–3 with chronic dosing.

[c]Approximate equianalgesic dose suggested from meta-analysis of available comparative studies.

A second consideration in the selection of an opioid drug relates to the distinction between those opioids conventionally used to treat moderate pain and those used to treat severe pain. In the United States, the former group includes codeine and oxycodone (administered with acetaminophen or aspirin in a combination product), hydrocodone and dihydrocodeine (available only with acetaminophen in a combination product), and propoxyphene (either alone or in combination products). Other drugs, such as oral meperidine, are also occasionally used. As discussed previously, conventional practice in some countries includes the treatment of moderate pain in the opioid-naive patient, using a combination product that contains one of these opioids and either aspirin or acetaminophen. The specific drug selected is usually a matter of convenience or experience. Meperidine is generally not preferred for chronic dosing because of the risk of toxicity, including dysphoria, tremulousness, hyperreflexia, and seizures; this risk relates to accumulation of a metabolite, normeperidine.[49]

The pure agonist drugs available in the United States that are conventionally used for severe pain comprise morphine, hydromorphone, fentanyl, oxycodone (when not combined with a co-analgesic), levorphanol, oxymorphone, and methadone. Morphine is usually the first-line drug; this choice is based on extensive clinical experience, the drug's relative ease of oral titration, and the availability of numerous formulations, including a controlled release formulation that allows dosing at 12-hour intervals and a sustained release formulation that is effective with once-daily dosing. Individual variability in the response to different opioids is very substantial, however, and an opioid other than morphine may yield a better therapeutic outcome.[50] Sequential trials of different opioid drugs may be needed to identify the drug with the most favorable balance between analgesia and side effects.[50,51]

The role of morphine in the management of chronic pain has also evolved with recognition of its active metabolites.[52] Recent studies have established that morphine 6-glucuronide is an active opioid compound that may contribute to the analgesia and side effects observed during morphine therapy.[53–55] Although the metabolite accumulates in patients with renal insufficiency and has been associated with toxicity in some renally impaired patients, a recent survey suggests that its impact overall is insufficient to recommend a change in routine dosing guidelines.[56] Similarly, high concentrations of another metabolite, morphine-3-glucuronide, have been speculated to cause toxicity, such as myoclonus and worsening pain, but the empirical evidence that this outcome is clinically relevant is meager.[52] Nonetheless, occasional patients who develop morphine toxicity, particularly in the setting of renal insufficiency, should be offered a trial of an alternative opioid, such as hydromorphone or fentanyl, in the hope that lesser metabolite accumulation may contribute to a better response.

The selection of a pure agonist drug as an alternative to morphine is largely empiric. Clinical experience suggests that patients with very severe pain, who require rapid dose titration, are best treated with drugs that approach steady state soon after the dose is changed. Controlled release drugs, including the long-acting morphine and oxycodone preparations and the transdermal fentanyl system, require several days to approach steady-state concentrations and are usually not preferred in this setting. Methadone can also be problematic because of its long and highly variable half-life, which ranges from less than 24 hours in some patients to more than 150 hours in others.[57] This long half-life implies that methadone can accumulate for relatively prolonged periods after a period of rapid titration to an effective dose. This potential for accumulation, which mandates careful observation for prolonged periods after dose changes, suggests that methadone should be considered a second-line drug for those who are difficult to monitor (e.g., noncompliant patients or those who live alone or at a distance) and those predisposed to opioid side effects (e.g., the elderly and those with encephalopathy or major organ dysfunction).

Select the route of administration. The oral route is preferred for chronic opioid therapy due to its simplicity, economy, and acceptability. A substantial proportion of patients, however, will require an alternative route at some point during the course of the disease. A large number of alternative routes are available (Table 8.5). In the setting of advanced disease, nonoral administration is usually implemented using the transdermal fentanyl system[58,59] or parenteral infusion, either subcutaneous infusion via ambulatory pump[60] or intravenous infusion.[61] Rectal admin-

Table 8.5   Routes of Opioid Administration Used for Chronic Pain

Route	Comment
Oral	Preferred in cancer pain management.
Sublingual	Buprenorphine effective but not available in U.S. Efficacy of highly lipid soluble drugs, such as fentanyl, is likely, but no studies and very little clinical experience. Efficacy of morphine controversial.
Rectal	Available for morphine, oxymorphone, and hydromorphone. Customarily used as if dose is equianalgesic to oral dose. Absorption is variable, however, and relative potency may be higher than expected.
Transdermal	Available for fentanyl. Dosing interval is 2–3 days. Empirical indications include problems with oral drug, desire to offer trial of fentanyl, compliance problems with oral dosing, or possibility of improved quality of life if oral therapy is avoided.
Oral transmucosal	Formulation using fentanyl currently undergoing trials for breakthrough pain.

Subcutaneous
  Repetitive bolus
  Continuous infusion
  Continuous infusion with
    with patient-controlled
	Ambulatory infusion pumps can provide continuous infusion with any parenteral opioid formulation. More advanced pumps can also provide patient-controlled analgesia. Clearest indication is inability to tolerate oral route.

Intravenous
  Repetitive bolus
  Continuous infusion
  Continuous infusion with
  patient-controlled analgesia
	Continuous infusion possible if permanent venous access device available.

Epidural
  Repetitive bolus
  Continuous infusion using
    percutaneous or
    implanted system
	Clearest indication is pain below arms and dose-limiting side effects from systemic opioid. Often co-administered with local anesthetic.

Intrathecal	Usually administered via a totally implanted infusion pump. May be cost-effective for those patients with clear indication for intraspinal therapy and long life expectancy.
Intracerebroventricular	Rarely indicated. Experience is limited.

istration is sometimes used when the opioid requirement is relatively low and the duration of therapy is anticipated to be short.[62] The rectal administration of a controlled-release oral morphine preparation can be effective and can increase the acceptability of therapy by allowing reduced dosing frequency. Although a very small proportion of patients will be considered candidates for invasive routes of administration, usually long-term epidural or intrathecal administration, the availability of these approaches can be extremely helpful in carefully selected cases.[63,64]

Apply appropriate dosing guidelines. Specific dosing guidelines for opioid therapy are based on an extensive clinical experience. Adherence to these guidelines is as strong a determinant of suc-

cessful therapy as is appropriate selection of a particular drug or route. The most important principles are as follows:

- *Dose "by the clock."* Fixed-scheduled dosing has replaced "as needed" dosing in the treatment of continuous or frequently recurring pain because of the observation that it is more effective to prevent the recurrence of severe pain than to abort it once it appears. "As needed" shall still be considered, however, in the relatively opioid-naive patient during the initiation of therapy (given the risk of gradual accumulation, methadone is often started with 1 to 2 weeks of "as needed" dosing), in the patient with rapidly changing pain (such as may follow radiotherapy to a painful bony lesion), and in patients with intermittent pains separated by pain-free intervals.

Additionally, clinical experience strongly supports the use of an "as needed" dose (so-called rescue dose) in combination with a fixed dosing schedule to treat "breakthrough" pains.[65]

• *Titrate the dose.* Once an opioid and the route of administration are selected, the dose should be increased until adequate analgesia occurs or intolerable and unmanageable side effects supervene. The objective during this process is to identify a favorable balance between analgesia and side effects. There is no ceiling dose for analgesia among the pure agonist opioids, and dose escalation is limited only by the occurrence of opioid side effects. If side effects do not occur or can be effectively treated, doses can become very high as stepwise increments are undertaken. Doses equivalent to more than 35 g morphine per day have been reported in highly tolerant patients with refractory cancer pain.[5]

Most patients do achieve a favorable balance between analgesia and side effects and stabilize for prolonged periods. Nonetheless, patients with pain due to progressive medical diseases usually require periodic dose escalation during long-term opioid therapy. In such patients, the need for a dose increase usually can be explained by some change in clinical status, typically worsening of a pain-producing structural lesion. Although tolerance to the analgesic effects of the opioid is an alternative explanation and may be contributing to declining effects at any time, the need for dose increases cannot be ascribed primarily to tolerance unless an alternative cause for progressive pain is not found. This is rarely the case. The changing opioid requirement over time underscores the need for repeated assessment and dose adjustment. An ongoing effort to individualize the opioid dose is essential to maintain favorable effects over time.

Use appropriate dosing intervals. With the exception of controlled-release oral morphine preparations (administered every 8 to 12 hours), sustained-release oral morphine formulations (administered every 24 hours), transdermal fentanyl system (administered every 48 to 72 hours), and methadone (usually effective with dosing every 6 to 8 hours), all other pure agonist opioid drugs must be administered every 3 to 4 hours to provide continuous analgesia. Methadone is the most variable of the drugs that may be administered less frequently. Although some clinicians find that methadone can provide analgesia at intervals as long as 12 hours, most observe a need for more frequent dosing. The reason for this counterintuitive need for frequent dosing with a long half-life drug is not clear, but the empirical basis has been established by a controlled trial that demonstrated such a short duration of effect following a dose.[66]

Be aware of relative potencies. Using morphine as a standard, relative potencies have been determined for most pure agonist opioid drugs in single-dose analgesic studies (see Table 8.4).[67] An equianalgesic dose table derived from these relative potency estimates should be consulted when switching from one drug or route of administration to another. The ratios in this table should be viewed as broad guidelines, the use of which must be tempered by clinical judgment. In most cases, a switch from one drug to another should be accompanied by a reduction in the equianalgesic dose of at least one-third, in recognition that incomplete cross-tolerance between opioids may result in a potency greater than anticipated for the newly initiated drug. The equianalgesic dose should be further reduced when patients are predisposed to opioid side effects (e.g., in the elderly or those with encephalopathy) and when the new drug is methadone. Although there is presently no confirmed explanation for the large degree of incomplete cross-tolerance observed when switching to methadone from another opioid, the phenomenon occurs commonly and is most likely when the dose of the starting drug is relatively high. To ensure safety, therefore, a switch to methadone from a high-dose therapy with morphine or any other opioid should always be accompanied by a 90% reduction in the equianalgesic dose.

Treat side effects. Although respiratory depression is the most feared adverse effect of opioid drugs, tolerance to this effect appears to develop rapidly with repeated dosing, and it is a rare occurrence during the long-term treatment of pain. If respiratory depression occurs during a period of stable dosing, it is invariably related to the development of some intercurrent cardiopulmonary disorder. In this setting, partial or even complete reversal of the respiratory depression with the specific opioid antagonist naloxone implies only that the opioid is contributing; the inciting cardiopulmonary event must still be sought. It is important to note that opioid-induced respiratory depression is always accompanied by slowed respirations and obtundation and is never associated with breathlessness. The occurrence of anxiety and tachypnea associated with breathlessness is not evidence of opioid overdose.

The common side effects of opioid therapy during long-term treatment include constipation, sedation, and mental clouding. Treatment of these effects is an integral part of opioid therapy for chronic pain.[68] Successful treatment enhances patients' comfort and allows continued upward dose titration of the opioid drug, if this is necessary to improve analgesia. The management of these side effects parallels their treatment when they occur unrelated to opioid therapy (see discussion later in this chapter).

When side effects are intolerable and cannot be managed, a trial of an alternative analgesic approach is indicated. One such approach is a trial of an alternative opioid. The pattern of side effects produced by one drug does not reliably predict the response to another, and sequential trials may be able to identify a more favorable drug.[50,51] Alternatively, any of a variety of other analgesic approaches may be considered, including the use of nonopioid analgesics.

Adjuvant Analgesics. Adjuvant analgesics are drugs that have primary indications other than pain but that can be analgesic in selected circumstances. This category is extremely diverse, representing numerous drugs in many classes (Table 8.6).[69] When used in the management of pain due to progressive medical disease, such as cancer pain, they are typically added to an optimally titrated opioid regimen.

Some adjuvant analgesics are particularly important in this setting. Corticosteroids, for example, may be administered to patients with cancer pain in an effort to manage refractory bone pain, neuropathic pain, headache due to intracranial hypertension, pain related to bowel obstruction, and other indications. In those with advanced disease, treatment with one of these drugs may also improve mood and appetite and reduce malaise.[70] Dexamethasone is the steroid most often selected, but there have been no comparative trials among the different agents; the best drug and dosing regimen remains uncertain, and the durability of effects is unknown.

Like the corticosteroids, other adjuvant analgesics may be administered in an effort to manage symptoms other than pain, while concur-

Table 8.6   Adjuvant Analgesics Used in the Medically Ill

Class	Comment
I. Drugs Typically used for Neuropathic Pain	

Antidepressants
  Tricyclic antidepressants
    Tertiary amines (e.g., amitriptyline)
    Secondary amines (e.g., desipramine)
  Serotonin selective reuptake
    inhibitors (SSRI) (e.g., paroxetine)
	Although these drugs are best considered nonspecific analgesics, they are used primarily for neuropathic pain in the medically ill. They are preferred for continuous dysesthesias. Select drug based on risk vs. expected efficacy; best evidence of efficacy: tertiary amine tricyclic > secondary amine tricyclic > SSRI, and risk of toxicity: SSRI > secondary amine tricyclic > tertiary amine tricyclic.

Oral Local Anesthetics
  Mexiletine
  Tocainide
	Used for any type of neuropathic pain; mexiletine often preferred on the basis of safety.

Anticonvulsants
  Carbamazepine
  Phenytoin
  Valproate
  Clonazepam
	Preferred for the management of lancinating or paroxysmal neuropathic pains.

GABAergic Drugs
  Baclofen
  Gabapentin
	Baclofen preferred for the management of lancinating or paroxysmal pain. Gabapentin is a gabaergic anticonvulsant with strong anecdotal support for analgesic efficacy in all types of neuropathic pain.

continued

Table 8.6   Adjuvant Analgesics Used in the Medically Ill (*continued*)

Class	Comment

N-Methyl-D-Aspartate Blockers
  Dextromethorphan
  Ketamine
	Limited evidence of analgesic efficacy; tried in refractory neuropathic pain.

Alpha-2 Adrenergic Agonists Clonidine	Another nonspecific analgesic; occasionally used for cancer-related neuropathic pain.

Neuroleptics
  Methotrimeprazine
  Fluphenazine
  Haloperidol
  Pimozide
	Methotrimeprazine is a nonspecific analgesic usually used to manage terminal agitation, particularly when associated with pain. Other neuroleptics sometimes tried for refractory neuropathic pain.

Calcitonin	Evidence of analgesic efficacy in phantom pain and reflex sympathetic dystrophy; occasionally tried for neuropathic pain

Corticosteroids
  Dexamethasone
  Methylprednisolone
	Short-term high-dose therapy used for crescendo pain; long-term low-dose therapy used for a variety of pains, including neuropathic pains, and many other symptoms

Topical Agents
  Capsaicin
  Local anesthetics
	Often tried in neuropathic pains with strong peripheral component; local anesthetics may be particularly useful if hyperalgesia

Drugs for Sympathetically Maintained Pain
  Phenoxybenzamine
  Nifedipine
  Prazocin
  Propranolol
	Patients suspected to have sympathetically maintained pain (suggested by coexistence of pain and local autonomic dysregulation) who cannot undergo sympathetic nerve blocks are sometimes treated with these drugs, with clonidine, or with a corticosteroid

II. Drugs used for Bone Pain	
Corticosteroids	Anecdotal reports of efficacy in bone pain

Bisphosphonates
  Alendronate
  Pamidronate
  Clodronate
	Reduces malignant bone pain and risk of skeletal morbidity

Calcitonin	Reduces bone pain; now available in an intranasal formulation
Radiopharmaceuticals (e.g., strontium-89)	Slow onset of effect; reduces marrow reserve and should be used only if no further chemotherapy is contemplated
III. Drugs used for Pain due to Bowel Obstruction	

Anticholinergics
  Scopolamine
  Atropine
  Glycopyrrolate
	Reduces peristalsis and secretions; anecdotal reports of analgesic effects

Octreotide	Reduces peristalsis and secretions; anecdotal reports of analgesic effects
Corticosteroids	Anecdotal reports of analgesic effects
IV. Drugs used for Muscle Spasm	
Benzodiazepine Diazepam	Although other drugs have been designated muscle relaxants, including orphenadrine, carisoprodol, methocarbamol, chlorzoxazone, and cyclobenzaprine, none have been shown to actually relax skeletal muscle. Their use in the medically ill is limited.

rently improving pain relief. The potential for dual benefits from the antidepressant analgesics is most evident.

The largest number of adjuvant analgesics are used in the setting of neuropathic pain. These syndromes are believed to be relatively less responsive to opioid drugs than pain syndromes sustained by persistent injury to pain-sensitive tissues.[71] Antidepressants, anticonvulsants, oral local anesthetics, and others are commonly administered to patients who continue to experience inadequate analgesia despite opioid dose titration.

Nonpharmacologic Approaches

As noted previously, the inability to identify a favorable balance between analgesia and side effects during routine opioid dose titration should be followed by selection of an alternative analgesic approach. In addition to pharmacologic interventions, such as a switch to an alternative opioid or trials with adjuvant analgesics, there are numerous nonpharmacologic therapies, which can be broadly categorized into anesthetic, surgical, rehabilitive, and psychologic approaches (Table 8.7). There have been no comparative tri-

als of these approaches, and the decision to implement one or another is based on best clinical judgment. Many of the most commonly used approaches are invasive,[72] and the attendant risks mandate a careful reassessment of the patient before any action is taken. Illness-related considerations, such as life expectancy and extent of disease, and other issues, including the goals of care, must be clearly understood before a well-informed recommendation can be offered.

Fatigue

Fatigue is among the most common symptoms experienced by patients with cancer.[6,18] The epidemiology is less well characterized in other populations, but clinical experience affirms that it is common and frequently distressing. Like pain, it is a complex symptom, which may be influenced by a broad range of disturbances and which may interact with other factors that impair quality of life.

The complexity inherent in the complaint of fatigue derives from both the varying phenomena to which the term is applied and the diverse pathophysiologic processes that may contribute.[73,74] Patients may describe fatigue in terms

Table 8.7 Alternative Analgesic Approaches for Patients Who Fail a Conventional Opioid Therapy

Approach	Examples	Comment
Anesthetic approaches	Intra-axial infusion with opioids and/or local anesthetics	Many techniques available. Usually require localized or regional pains. Neurolytic procedures require short life expectancy and have limitations related to the desire to retain motor and autonomic functions. Stimulation procedures, such as dorsal column stimulation, rarely performed in the medically ill.
	Temporary or neurolytic nerve blocks	
	Stimulation approaches	
Surgical approaches	Neurolysis possible at every level of the neuraxis. Cordotomy is the most widely used procedure.	Neurolysis requires short life expectancy. Stimulation procedures, such as deep brain stimulation, rarely performed in the medically ill.
Rehabilitative approaches	Bracing; physical therapy	Orthotocis may be useful to reduce breakthrough pain induced by motion of the spine or a limb. Physical therapy may reduce myofascial pains and prevent secondary painful complications, such as joint ankylosis.
Psychologic approaches	Cognitive therapies	May be useful adjunct to reduce predictable pain, lessen pain-related anxiety, and improve function.

that relate to lack of energy or vitality, muscular weakness, dysphoric mood, or somnolence. There is an association between fatigue and cognitive functioning, and patients may also describe fatigue in language that suggests difficulty in concentrating or focusing attention. None of these phenomena occur exclusive of the others, and, in the clinical effort to clarify the nature of the symptom, it is common to identify several of these phenomena at the same time. The development of multidimensional assessment instruments reflects this interaction among the diverse characteristics that contribute to the symptom of fatigue.[75–77]

Role of Primary Treatments

Given this complexity, the first step in the management of fatigue is an assessment that attempts to define the characteristics of the symptom and to infer from this description the existence of specific, potentially reversible, etiologic factors. If primary treatment for the underlying disorder can be offered, fatigue may remit.

Numerous factors may contribute to the experience of fatigue (Table 8.8). These factors may directly or indirectly relate to the underlying disease, to treatments for the disease, or to disturbances unrelated to the disease or its treatment. Neoplasms are associated with a fatigue syndrome that presumably involves metabolic dysfunction induced by compounds produced by the tumor or the immune response to the tumor. These factors have not been empirically confirmed but could involve disturbances in cytokine levels that interfere with energy metabolism or neuromuscular functioning. Such a pathogenesis may also be involved in the fatigue experienced by patients with AIDS or other systemic infections and the fatigue associated with chemotherapy and radiation therapy.

The involvement of such factors in the genesis of fatigue is suggested by the observation that the symptom may improve if effective treatment for the underlying disease can be provided. If antineoplastic therapy reduces tumor burden, antiviral approaches diminish HIV levels, or other antibiotic therapy eliminates a systemic bacterial infection, patients may experience a rebound in energy. Nonetheless, the reliability of these primary approaches in reducing fatigue is not known, and, as noted, some of these treatments can actually cause fatigue. The existence of fa-

Table 8.8   Possible Etiologies of Fatigue in the Medically Ill

I. Medical/Physical Conditions

   Associated with the underlying disease itself
   Associated with treatment for the disease
      Chemotherapy
      Radiotherapy
      Surgery
      Biological response modifiers
   Associated with intercurrent systemic disorders
      Anemia
      Infection
      Pulmonary disorders
      Hepatic failure
      Heart failure
      Renal insufficiency
      Malnutrition
      Neuromuscular disorders
   Associated with sleep disorders
   Associated with immobility and lack of exercise
   Associated with chronic pain
   Associated with the use of centrally acting drugs
      (e.g., opioids)

II. Psychosocial Factors

   Associated with anxiety disorders
   Associated with depressive disorders
   Stress related
   Related to environmental reinforcers

tigue does not usually influence the decision to implement or withhold a primary therapy of this type.

Other metabolic and biochemical abnormalities may also be associated with fatigue. Anemia is a well-recognized precipitant, which could presumably induce fatigue as a result of impaired energy metabolism related to a decline in the oxygen-carrying capacity of the blood. Similar mechanisms may be involved when fatigue is associated with the hypoxia that may accompany severe cardiopulmonary diseases.

Other metabolic abnormalities are associated with fatigue for reasons that are entirely unknown. Major organ dysfunction, such as renal failure, hepatic failure, and pulmonary insufficiency (even if characterized only by mild CO_2 retention and no hypoxia) can each be associated with fatigue. Hypothyroidism and adrenal insufficiency, even if relatively mild, may also be etiologically important. Clinicians often observe that postchemotherapy leukopenia appears to correlate with the onset of fatigue, and this phenomenon may indicate a role for other immune system processes in the genesis of fatigue.

Recognition of these abnormalities offers several important opportunities for treatment. Although the degree of anemia required to produce fatigue has not been studied empirically, any moderate to severe anemia might be considered a target for treatment in the patient with disabling fatigue. Treatment may be offered by transfusion or via administration of erythropoetin. Similarly, hypoxia may be improved through oxygen therapy, and salutary interventions may be possible to lessen the impact of renal or hepatic insufficiency. Hormone repletion can reverse the fatigue caused by thyroid or adrenal insufficiency.

In some cases, fatigue appears to be related to a disorder that directly affects neuromuscular function. Diseases such as multiple sclerosis, amytrophic lateral sclerosis, neuromuscular junction disorders (including Eaton Lambert syndrome, myasthenia gravis, and myasthenic syndromes produced by drugs), and myopathies and polyneuropathies of diverse cause may be associated with the complaint of fatigue. The more common problem of fatigue associated with physical inactivity may also relate to inefficiency in neuromuscular functioning. This association between neuromuscular disorders and fatigue underscores the potential utility of a neurological evaluation of the patient whose complaint of fatigue is related to a sense of muscular weakness.

Sleep disorders appear to be common among the medically ill and may also be an important contributor to fatigue. On the basis of clinical observation, it is likely that the clinical entities related to disturbed sleep are variable. Some patients appear to experience excessive daytime somnolence but relatively little fatigue when awake, whereas others report substantial fatigue with relatively modest somnolence. The sleep disorder itself may be described as insomnia, frequent awakening, or a lack of refreshing sleep. Improved sleep hygiene and hypnotic therapy may offer an effective approach to the treatment of fatigue related to these sleep disorders. Appropriate patients whose fatigue appears to be related to a sleep problem but who fail to improve with simple measures should be considered for normal evaluation using polysomnography.

Many patients link their experience of fatigue to the drugs they receive to treat other problems. Some patients report fatigue as a side effect of opioid therapy for pain, for example; this symptom can occur without somnolence in some cases. Some patients experience similar side effects from other centrally acting drugs, including anticonvulsants and antidepressants. Again, however, these responses appear to be variable.

Fatigue is a well-recognized accompaniment of depression, and antidepressant therapy is an important primary treatment that may ameliorate this symptom as the underlying disorder remits. Fatigue also commonly associates with unrelieved pain, and effective analgesic therapy can sometimes yield dramatic improvement in energy levels.

The diversity of the primary therapies that may influence the complaint of fatigue reflects the many potential causes of this symptom. Multiple etiologies commonly coexist and it is often impossible to distinguish the more important ones from those less important. Accordingly, the decision to intervene in an effort to reduce or eliminate one or more of these etiologies is often difficult. The clinician cannot know in advance if the treatable factor is a powerful enough influence to warrant intervention, and the intervention itself may have risks. For example, the patient who is receiving an opioid for pain and reports more fatigue as the dose is increased could be developing fatigue as a side effect of opioid therapy, as a secondary manifestation of the pain, as a result of a worsening depression linked to unrelieved pain, or as a consequence of another factor related to the progressive disease or other treatments. The decision to change the opioid or offer a nonopioid analgesic approach obviously carries some risk; the new intervention may be less tolerable than the old, and pain can flare as a new approach is implemented. This complexity places a great burden on the clinician, who must perform careful reassessments and repeatedly judge the likelihood that a potential etiology is in fact relevant and that the risks involved in implementing a primary therapy for this etiology are outweighed by the likelihood of benefit.

Pharmacologic Approaches

Although pharmacologic therapy for fatigue associated with medical illness has not been evaluated in controlled studies, there is evidence to support the use of several drug classes for this indication. The utility of the psychostimulants has been suggested in studies of methylphenidate and pemoline.[78,79] There is a substantial clinical experience with these drugs in the treatment of opioid-related cognitive impairment[80] and of depression in the elderly and medically ill.[81–84] A favorable anecdotal experience supports a therapeutic trial for the treatment of fatigue.

In the cancer population, the largest experience is with methylphenidate. In medically fragile patients, the initial dose is usually 2.5 to 5 mg once or twice daily. This dose is then gradually escalated until favorable effects occur or toxicity supervenes. Most patients require low doses; doses above 60 mg per day are very uncommon. Effects sometimes wane over time, a change that could reflect tolerance or progression of the underlying cause of the fatigue, and dose escalation may be needed to maintain effects. The risk of toxicity increases with the dose, however, and the ability to regain lost efficacy is usually limited.

The potential toxicities associated with methylphenidate, like other psychostimulants, include anorexia, insomnia, anxiety and confusion, tremor, and tachycardia. These effects can be particularly problematic in the medically ill, who may be predisposed to the same symptoms for other reasons. To ensure safety, dose escalation of the psychostimulants should be undertaken cautiously and at intervals long enough to evaluate the full gamut of potential toxicities.

Dextroamphetamine and pemoline have also been used anecdotally for the treatment of fatigue. There have been no controlled comparisons of these drugs, and clinical experience suggests that the response to one does not necessary predict responses to the others. Sequential trials may be valuable to identify the most useful drug. Pemoline is a novel psychostimulant with relatively less sympathomimetic activity. A controlled trial demonstrated efficacy in the treatment of fatigue associated with multiple sclerosis,[79] and there has been anecdotal use as an antidepressant in the medically ill.[81] In the United States, this drug is available in a chewable formulation that can be absorbed through the buccal mucosa; this may be useful in patients with advanced disease who are unable to swallow or absorb oral drugs. There is a very small risk of severe hepatotoxicity from pemoline that has not been reported with the other psychostimulants.

The use of low-dose corticosteroids in the treatment of fatigue has also been supported empirically[70,85] and may be particularly helpful in the population with advanced disease and multiple symptoms. This therapy is usually undertaken with dexamethasone 1 to 2 mg twice daily or prednisone 5 to 10 mg twice daily; there have been no comparative studies.

Amantadine has been used for the treatment of fatigue due to multiple sclerosis for many years. There is no experience with this drug in populations with other diseases. Nonetheless, amantadine has relatively low toxicity, and an empirical trial may be warranted in selected patients with refractory fatigue associated with other diseases.

A trial of an antidepressant drug is clearly appropriate if fatigue is related to a clinical depression. Theoretically, an antidepressant that is relatively more likely to be activating, such as one of the serotonin-specific reuptake inhibitors or buproprion, would be preferred. There have been no clinical trials of these drugs with fatigue as an endpoint, however, and the utility of one drug class over another and the potential benefit of these drugs in nondepressed patients remains to be studied.

Nonpharmacologic Approaches

Nonpharmacologic interventions may be very useful in the symptomatic management of fatigue. All patients who are distressed by this symptom can potentially benefit from information and reassurance. Many patients assume that the problem reflects worsening of the disease, and information about alternative factors, if any can be identified, can also be very reassuring. Some patients take solace from the knowledge that the fatigue is expected to be transitory, if it can indeed be ascribed to an event with a defined time course, such as radiation therapy, or to a treatable disorder. Patients should also be told to avoid complete physical inactivity in the mistaken belief that more rest will eliminate the fatigue.

Some nonpharmacologic interventions may ameliorate the symptom or improve the patient's functional capacity.[74] On the basis of details provided by the patient and family, interventions might include organization of activities so that essential functions can be performed in the morning, a scheduled afternoon nap, and acceptance of help (from family members or others) for some tasks that had previously been performed by the patient. Well-defined rest periods during the day may allow the patient to function more efficiently overall. If debilitation from the disease is not limiting, a modest exercise schedule may be useful. The exercise should be daily and aerobic and should gradually increase from a level that is not experienced as exhausting. If the fatigue is related to a sleep disturbance, instructions to improve sleep hygiene may be salutary. This may involve the use of a set bedtime, more efficient use of a hypnotic, or other maneuvers.

Common Gastrointestinal Symptoms

The most common gastrointestinal symptoms experienced by patients with advanced disease are constipation, nausea and vomiting, and anorexia. These symptoms can often be greatly improved with simple interventions. Clinicians should be prepared to offer such recommendations to any patient troubled by these symptoms.

Constipation

Constipation, which may be defined as diminished frequency of defecation associated with difficulty or discomfort, is associated with a constellation of symptoms, including abdominal pain, bloating, distention, anorexia, and nausea.[86–88] It rarely contributes to life-threatening complications, such as bowel obstruction or perforation.[89]

The pathophysiology of constipation is complex and may involve processes that relate primarily to central or peripheral effects of drugs, bowel dysmotility or obstruction, impaired fluid regulation, or psychological factors (Table 8.9). Patients with advanced diseases commonly present a combination of potential etiologies. The assessment of constipation must clarify these contributing factors, determine their treatability, and elucidate their relationship to the underlying disease or its treatment.

Role of Primary Treatments. Many of the etiologies that contribute to constipation in the medically ill are amenable to primary treatment. The chronic administration of opioid drugs is often the most obvious etiology. Dehydration and other metabolic disturbances can potentially be corrected, and drugs with constipating effects can be minimized or discontinued. These interventions seldom eliminate the problem but may contribute

Table 8.9   Common Causes of Constipation in the Medically Ill

Physiologic and Psychosocial Factors

   Advanced age
   Inactivity
   Change in diet
   Physical or social impediments to defecation
   Rectal or abdominal pain
   Depression

Metabolic Disturbances

   Dehydration
   Hypercalcaemia
   Hypokalemia
   Hypothyroidism

Structural Factors

   Intraluminal or extraluminal masses, adhesions or
     fibrosis

Drugs

   Opioids
   Drugs with anticholinergic actions
   Antacids
   Diuretics
   Anticonvulsants
   Iron
   Antihypertensives

Neurologic Disorders

   Damage from any cause to sacral plexus, cauda
     equina, or spinal cord
   Autonomic neuropathy from any cause

to the success of a well-tolerated laxative therapy.

Other etiologies cannot be easily managed. Neurological disorders, particularly autonomic neuropathy, are common and often refractory to treatment. Autonomic neuropathy, for example, can occur as a direct consequence of the disease (such as a paraneoplastic syndrome caused by a cancer), disease-related therapy (such as chemotherapy-induced neuropathy), or an unrelated disorder (such as diabetes). There is no reliable primary therapy for any of these types. Even physical inactivity and dehydration, which might be treatable during the earlier stages of disease, can become unremitting problems as the disease progresses.

Constipating drugs can be withdrawn only if their benefits are outweighed by the adverse effect. This is seldom the case with opioid drugs, despite the marked constipating effects that characterize this class. Opioids have both central and peripheral actions that together decrease peristalsis, impair the defecation reflex, and dessicate intraluminal contents through increased absorption of fluid and electrolytes. In contrast to other side effects produced by these drugs, tolerance appears to develop slowly to these constipating effects, particularly in the setting of multiple concurrent etiologies for constipation.

Pharmacologic Approaches. Routine laxative therapy should not be initiated in patients with severe constipation until serious problems, such as fecal impaction, have been excluded. Low impaction can be assessed by examination of the rectum; suspicion of a high impaction or another cause of bowel obstruction requires abdominal imaging for evaluation. The management of impaction may require physical disimpaction, repeated enemas, and a combination of rectal and oral laxatives. Routine laxative therapy can begin after impaction is cleared.

Therapeutic interventions for constipation may be administered rectally or orally.[86,88] Although enemas and rectal suppositories are used commonly, they are generally preferred for the intermittent management of severe constipation and not for day-to-day treatment. Some patients do prefer rectal laxatives on a regular basis, however, and these measures should be available to patients who do not have contraindications to their use.

Systematic long-term therapy with oral laxatives is the usual approach to chronic constipation in the medically ill. The administration of this therapy is complicated by a lack of information from clinical trials. There are no data from which to judge comparative safety or efficacy, drug-dependent effects, or the utility of combination therapy.

There has also been no systematic evaluation of prophylactic therapy. Although many specialists in palliative medicine believe that prophylaxis is warranted in opioid-treated patients and in others with strong predisposing factors, the risks and benefits of this approach must be considered on a case-by-case basis. It is apparent that some patients can manage constipation with simple dietary approaches, and others undergo spontaneous improvement over time. The use of laxatives can be costly and burdensome, and it may be reasonable to manage constipation expectantly in those patients, such as younger ambulatory patients with relatively early disease, who are probably at the lowest risk of this disorder.

The available therapies for the treatment of chronic constipation comprise bulk agents, osmotic compounds and agents for colonic lavage, lubricants, contact cathartics, prokinetic drugs, and oral naloxone. A rational approach to the selection and administration of these agents can be developed on the basis of extensive clinical experience (Table 8.10).

Bulk laxatives. Bulk agents typically use cellulose or psyllium seeds to supplement the con-

Table 8.10   Strategies for the Management of Constipation in the Medically Ill

---

Approaches for All Patients

Increase fluid intake.
Increase dietary fiber (unless patient is debilitated or bowel obstruction is suspected).
Ensure comfort, privacy, and convenience for defecation.
Ensure that impaction has not complicated constipation.

Discuss Approaches with the Patient and Select One or More

Intermittent (every 2–3 days) osmotic laxative
Trial of a daily softening agent alone
Intermittent (every 2–3 days) use of a contact cathartic
Daily contact cathartic (with or without softening agent)
Daily lactulose or sorbitol

Optimize Selected Therapy

Adjust dose and dosing schedule.
Consider combining approaches if the initial therapy is inadequate.
Switch approaches if needed.

Consider Alternative Approaches in Refractory Cases

Rectal approaches, including suppositories or intermittent enemas
Intermittent or daily use of colonic lavage
Daily treatment with a prokinetic drug
Daily treatment with oral naloxone in opioid-treated patients

sumption of fiber in the food. These products are generally safe, but anecdotal experience suggests that they can worsen some symptoms, such as flatulence, distension, or abdominal pain, in patients with dysmotility or structural intra-abdominal disease. They are best avoided in patients who are severely debilitated and in those with partial bowel obstruction from any cause.

Osmotic laxatives. Osmotic laxatives include magnesium salts (magnesium hydroxide and magnesium citrate) and sodium salts (for example, sodium phosphate). These agents draw fluid into the intestinal lumen. Although they are usually administered for acute bowel cleansing prior to medical procedures, some patients find that intermittent administration (usually every 2 to 3 days) is an effective long-term therapy. The risks associated with these agents are generally minor. If diarrhea occurs, electrolyte disorders or dehydration is possible. More important, rare patients develop problems related to the absorption of the therapeutic electrolyte, such as magnesium or sodium. Osmotic laxatives should be used cautiously by patients who may be predisposed to these problems, such as those with renal insufficiency or cardiac failure.

Lactulose and sorbitol are poorly absorbed sugars that act as osmotic laxatives, liquefying the intraluminal contents and increasing its bulk. Although lactulose is used more often, sorbitol is equally effective[90] and far less costly. Most patients consume a dose once or twice daily following a period of dose adjustment.

A rarely used approach to severe constipation involves the intermittent use of an agent for colonic lavage. Colonic lavage using a large volume of a nonabsorbable fluid (such as Go-Lytely®) is typically administered for bowel cleansing prior to procedures. Consumption of a smaller volume, such as 250 to 500 ml, every few days or more frequently can be used to reverse chronic constipation.[91]

Lubricating oil. Mineral oil may be an effective laxative in some patients, but the long-term use of this approach is limited by concerns related to perianal irritation, poor absorption of fat-soluble vitamins, and the potential for serious lipoid pneumonia should aspiration occur. This approach is not recommended for chronic laxation in debilitated patients.

Contact cathartics. The contact cathartics comprise diverse drugs in two major classes, the anthraquinones and the diphenylmethanes. The former group includes cascara, senna, and dantron, and the latter includes phenolphthalein and bisacodyl. All these drugs act by increasing peristalsis and reducing absorption of water and electrolytes. Although there have been no systematic studies of these drugs in the medically ill, clinical experience suggests that patients may respond differently to the various agents and that all these drugs potentially have dose-dependent effects. Therapy is usually initiated with a low daily dose (such as one senna tablet twice daily), then increased as needed until constipation is relieved, the patient reports side effects, or the therapy becomes too burdensome or costly to continue. Failure with one drug can be followed by a trial of another. Some patients prefer to use a contact cathartic on an intermittent basis, such as every 3 to 4 days if needed.

The risks associated with the contact cathartics are minimal. Long-term ingestion may result in so-called laxative bowel, a condition characterized by dependence on laxatives for bowel function. This syndrome is not a contraindication to therapy in the setting of advanced disease but should be considered a potential problem for patients with long life expectancies. It may be reasonable to consider alternative laxatives in such patients.

Castor oil is the only contact cathartic with a mechanism of action mediated in the small bowel. Cramping and diarrhea are common with this agent, and it is not generally used in medically ill populations.

Sodium docusate is a contact cathartic at high doses but is typically used at doses sufficient to produce a surfactant effect that allows water and fats to mix with feces. This softening effect may provide adequate laxation for some patients. Most clinicians, however, combine docusate with a contact cathartic in an effort to improve the overall outcome. The risk of this combination therapy appear to be minimal, and clinical experience has been favorable.

Prokinetic drugs. There is evidence that the use of a prokinetic agent may improve colonic transit.[92] On this basis, cisapride or metoclopramide can be considered for a therapeutic trial in patients with severe constipation. Theoretically, metoclopramide is the preferred agent because its action is exerted throughout the gastrointestinal tract. The doses that have been used empirically have been identical to those administered for chronic nausea.

Oral naloxone. The recent demonstration that oral naloxone can reverse constipation, including opioid-induced constipation,[93,94] confirms the importance of local opioid receptors in gastrointestinal motility. Naloxone is very poorly absorbed systemically and can potentially reverse opioid-induced constipation without causing systemic withdrawal. Some patients, however, absorb sufficient naloxone to develop uncomfortable signs of abstinence,[93] and this possibility suggests that naloxone therapy should not be used until conventional therapies have failed. A reasonable approach begins with a dose of 0.8 mg twice daily and doubles the dose every two to three days until favorable effects occur or side effects are experienced.

Nonpharmacologic Approaches. Constipation can be worsened by lack of privacy and other psychological concerns, enforced use of a bedpan, or inconvenient timing of institutional routines. To the extent possible, these factors should be addressed in the overall management of this symptom. Patients should be given adequate privacy at appropriate times, and, if possible, the use of a bathroom or bedside commode should be encouraged.

Nausea and Vomiting

Chronic nausea is a prevalent but poorly recognized symptom in populations with advanced diseases. The potential etiologies for chronic or recurrent nausea are diverse (Table 8.11). Similar to other symptoms, evaluation may be needed to clarify the most likely contributing factors. If the course or features are atypical for the obvious predisposing factors, additional assessment is needed.

The pathophysiology of nausea and vomiting is complex,[95,96] and there are presumably multiple contributing mechanisms in many cases. On the basis of the connections that have been identified in experimental models, it may be speculated that nausea and vomiting in humans may be precipitated by input to the so-called emetic center in the medulla from any of several regions, including the gastrointestinal tract, the labyrinthine-vestibular system, other brainstem sites (the best characterized of which is the chemoreceptor trigger zone in the area postrema of the medulla), and the cerebral cortex.

Table 8.11   Causes of Chronic Nausea in the Medically Ill

Drugs

   Opioids
   Nonsteroidal anti-inflammatory drugs
   Other centrally acting drugs

Intra-abdominal Neoplasm

Antineoplastic Therapy

   Abdominal radiotherapy
   Chemotherapy

Autonomic Neuropathy of Any Cause

Metabolic Disturbances

   Hepatic failure
   Renal failure
   Electrolyte abnormalities

Constipation

Intracranial Neoplasm or Other Lesions

Psychological Processes

   Conditioned responses
   Anxiety disorder

This conceptualization suggests that the predominating mechanism for nausea may be inferred on the basis of its description. Nausea caused by direct activation of the chemoreceptor trigger zone or irritation of receptors in the gastrointestinal tract often has a clear precipitant and symptom severity that fluctuates in parallel with the intensity of the inciting stimulus. Nausea produced by a drug, for example, should peak at the time of highest concentration or soon thereafter. Nausea that relates to stimulation or sensitization of the vestibular system can be imputed by the occurrence of vertigo or marked exacerbation of symptoms with movement. Gastroparesis may be involved in the pathogenesis of nausea when patients report prominent postprandial symptoms, including vomiting, early satiety, and abdominal bloating. Finally, a prominent role for conditioned nausea may be suggested by the repeated occurrence of the symptom following specific stimuli.

Role of Primary Treatments. Similar to other symptoms, elimination of a precipitating etiology can be a highly effective strategy for the treatment of chronic nausea. Correction of metabolic disturbances, elimination of emetogenic drugs, and effective management of constipation are the most viable interventions that may be undertaken with this objective.

Some patients with nausea related to opioid therapy appear to benefit from a change in the route of administration. For example, the patient who becomes intensely nauseated at the start of opioid therapy may obtain some relief and acclimate to the drug more easily if parenteral therapy is used as a prelude to oral treatment.

Pharmacologic Approaches. Numerous drugs in many classes may be useful antiemetics in the medically ill (Table 8.12). Although there have been no comparative trials, it may be reasonable to select drugs for initial therapy on the basis of the inferences about predominating mechanism. Patients who do not have prominent symptoms consistent with vestibular dysfunction or gastroparesis are usually administered a drug that is primarily active at the chemoreceptor trigger zone, specifically a neuroleptic or metoclopramide. Although the dose-response relationship of these drugs during long-term administration has not been investigated and the safety of relatively high doses for prolonged periods is unknown, it is rea-

sonable to increase the dose above the standard starting dose if benefits are not promptly observed. On the basis of clinical experience, most practitioners will increase the dose to as high as two to three times the standard starting dose before considering the drug a failure. Sequential trials of the various drugs is justified by the observation of intraindividual variability in the response to different agents, including those that presumably act through similar mechanisms.

Patients who experience nausea associated with vertigo or who report the nausea is markedly worsened by movement may be considered for a trial of an antivertiginous drug. Drugs that presumably damp activity in the labyrinthine-vestibular system include anticholinergic drugs (such as scopolamine), antihistamines (such as meclizine), and benzodiazepines (such as lorazepam). Again, the selection of a specific drug is by trial and error, and dose escalation is warranted within a range defined by conventional clinical practice.

Patients who report prominent abdominal distension with postprandial nausea should be considered for a pharmacologic treatment that enhances gastric emptying. Both metoclopramide and cisapride improve gastrointestinal transit time. Metoclopramide also acts as the chemoreceptor trigger zone and may be preferred on this basis.

Other pharmacologic approaches to the patient with refractory nausea are similarly empirical. The antiemetic efficacy of corticosteroids is unexplained, but some patients clearly benefit from these drugs.[70] Occasional patients who have responded poorly to previous trials obtain substantial relief from the use of a cannabinoid, such as delta-9-tetracannabinol (dronabinol). Rare patients with refractory symptoms are considered for a trial of a 5-HT3 antagonists, such as ondansetron or granisetron. Although the latter drugs are relatively safe and are extremely effective in the short-term treatment of chemotherapy-induced emesis, their use in the setting of chronic nausea is limited by their cost and a lack of data demonstrating long-term benefit in this setting.

Trials of combination therapy using drugs with different mechanisms can also be justified in patients with refractory nausea. In the absence of studies that have assessed the safety and efficacy of combination therapy, however, this approach must be undertaken cautiously.

Table 8.12 Antiemetic Drugs for Chronic Nausea in the Medically Ill

Class	Examples
Neuroleptics	
Phenothiazines	Prochlorperazine
	Chlorpromazine
	Methotrimeprazine
Butyrophenones	Haloperidol
	Droperidol
Anticholinergic Drugs	Scopolamine
	Atropine
Antihistamines	Promethazine
	Meclizine
Prokinetic Drugs	Metoclopramide
	Cisapride
Corticosteroids	Prednisone
	Methylprednisolone
	Dexamethasone
Benzodiazepines	Lorazepam
Cannabinoids	Tetrahydrocannabinol
5-HT Antagonists	Ondansetron
	Granisetron

Nonpharmacologic Approaches. Dietary changes (such as smaller, more frequent meals or the use of fewer spices) and changes in some environmental cues (such as eating in a different room) may be helpful to some patients with chronic nausea. Cognitive therapy, which has established efficacy in the treatment of chemotherapy-induced emesis,[97] should be considered for patients whose histories suggest that there may be a prominent conditioned component to the nausea.

Anorexia

Anorexia is also a highly prevalent symptom, which may coexist with progressive weight loss (anorexia-cachexia syndrome) or present as a separate problem. If weight loss is not occurring, symptomatic improvement in appetite may be targeted to reduce associated distress. If cachexia is also developing, the syndrome is more complex and is often associated with both other symptoms, most notably fatigue (asthenia), and laboratory abnormalities, such as anemia and hypoglycemia.

In the syndrome of anorexia-cachexia, weight loss is not merely the result of reduced calorie intake, and repletion of calories does not produce any substantial weight gain in many affected patients.[98] Metabolic abnormalities may include increased protein turnover, skeletal muscle catabolism, and lipolysis with loss of lipid stores.[99] The etiology is unknown and may involve a variety of processes, including excessive release of a cytokine, tumor necrosis factor/cachectin, that induces catabolism.[100]

Given the variable relationship between anorexia and weight loss, the goals of therapy must be carefully defined. Patients usually seek both improved appetite and weight gain. There is no definitive evidence, however, that weight gain is needed to yield improvement in well-being. Studies in the cancer population also demonstrate that efforts to maintain weight using oral or parenteral nutrition do not reliably improve survival, tumor response, or treatment-related toxicity.[101] Accordingly, treatment for anorexia associated with advanced disease generally has symptom control and improved well-being, rather than maintenance or restoration of weight, as the primary objectives. The perception that appetite has improved may be sufficient reason to continue a therapy, particularly if linked to the con-

clusion that weight loss would be worse if treatment were discontinued.

Role of Primary Treatment. The assessment of anorexia should evaluate the possibility of contributing factors that may be amenable to primary treatment. Appetite may be impaired by change in taste, nausea, dysphagia, pain in the head or neck, psychological distress (particularly depression), and other disorders. Like other gastrointestinal symptoms, anorexia may respond, at least to an extent, if these contributing factors can be lessened.

The role of oral or parenteral nutritional support as a primary therapy for weight loss and malnutrition is limited in populations with advanced disease. As noted, studies in patients with cancer have not revealed substantial benefits from such support.[101] Parenteral nutritional support is very rarely indicated due to its cost and potential morbidity, and nutritional support via the gastrointestinal tract is best viewed as a means to provide symptom control and improve well-being. For some patients, the psychological need to intervene in an effort to stop weight loss is profound and justifies an aggressive approach, including a feeding tube. For others, the quality-of-life issues surrounding anorexia and weight loss are less prominent, and the decision to proceed with nutritional support must be very carefully considered.

Pharmacologic Approaches. The pharmacologic approaches for anorexia and weight loss include corticosteroid drugs, progestational drugs, cannabinoids, and miscellaneous agents. There have been no comparative studies, and sequential trials may be needed to identify the most favorable agent.

The value of relatively low-dose corticosteroid therapy for appetite stimulation has been suggested in surveys[102] and confirmed in controlled trials of methylprednisolone and prednisolone.[70,103] Although side effects, such as oral candidiasis, can occur during long-term therapy, an extensive clinical experience supports a favorable risk:benefit ratio for these drugs in the setting of advanced disease. There have been no comparative studies of the different corticosteroids, and there is no information about minimum effective dose, dose dependence, or the possibility of a ceiling dose. The use of dexamethasone might be preferred on the basis of the relatively low mineralocorticoid effect that characterizes this drug; the usual dose administered for long-term therapy is 2 to 8 mg per day.

Recent controlled trials of megestrol acetate, a progesterone derivative, have demonstrated favorable effects on appetite, caloric intake, weight, and quality of life.[104–108] Although this drug can produce a variety of dose-related side effects, including edema, hot flashes, glucose intolerance, and coagulation disturbances, clinical experience has been generally favorable. Dose-ranging studies have demonstrated the existence of dose-dependent effects for both the desired effect on appetite and side effects;[105] a relatively low dose, 160 mg/day or lower, may optimize the balance between favorable effects and side effects for most patients.

The cannabinoid delta-9-tetrahydrocannabinol (dronabinol) is also an effective appetite stimulant.[109] A placebo-controlled trial of 2.5 mg twice daily in patients with acquired immunodeficiency syndrome demonstrated improved appetite, maintenance of weight or weight gain, and reduced nausea in the treated group.[110] At this dose, the drug is well tolerated.

Other drugs may also stimulate appetite. A controlled trial of the antihistamine cyproheptadine suggested a modest benefit for anorexia, without weight gain.[111] The potential for sedation from this drug limits its utility in the population with advanced cancer. Early controlled trials of hydrazine sulfate yielded mixed results in terms of appetite and weight,[112,113] but more recent controlled studies have clearly demonstrated no benefit from this compound.[114–116]

Nonpharmacologic Approaches. Some patients are able to increase food intake if the diet is changed or food is made more or less pungent. If early satiety is a problem, smaller and more frequent meals can be helpful. These dietary changes may be facilitated by referral to a dietician.

Some patients appear to benefit from the social aspects of meal time. Patients can be encouraged to take meals with the family, even if food consumption is minimal. Families often require education and support to place anorexia in context. In the setting of advanced disease, it may be necessary to gently enjoin members of the family and other caregivers from contributing to the patient's distress by focusing on the need to eat as a primary goal.

CONCLUSION

Physical symptoms are highly prevalent among patients with advanced medical illnesses. Symptom management is a fundamental component of the comprehensive palliative care that should be provided throughout the course of disease. Effective symptom control increases the likelihood that the patient can cope adequately with the rigors of the disease and its therapy, maintain physical and psychosocial functioning as long as possible, and ultimately experience a comfortable death.

References

1. World Health Organization. Technical Report Series 804, Cancer Pain and Palliative Care. Geneva: World Health Organization, 1990:11.
2. Doyle D, Hanks GWC, MacDonald N, eds. *Oxford Textbook of Palliative Medicine.* Oxford: Oxford University Press, 1993.
3. Brescia FJ, Adler D, Gray G, Ryan MA, Cimino J, Mamtani R. Hospitalized advanced cancer patients: a profile. *Journal of Pain and Symptom Management,* 1990; 5(4):221–227.
4. Bruera E, Kuehn N, Miller MJ, Selmser P, Macmillan K. The Edmonton Symptom Assessment System (ESAS): a simple method for the assessment of palliative care patients. *Journal of Palliative Care,* 1991; 7(2):6–9.
5. Coyle N, Adelhardt J, Foley KM, Portenoy RK. Character of terminal illness in the advanced cancer patient: pain and other symptoms during the last 4 weeks of life. *Journal of Pain and Symptom Management,* 1990; 4:83–93.
6. Curtis EB, Kretch R, Walsh TD. Common symptoms in patients with advanced cancer. *Journal of Palliative Care,* 1991; 7:25–29.
7. De Haes JCJM, Van Knippenberg FCE, Neijt JP. Measuring psychological and physical distress in cancer patients: structure and application of the Rotterdam Symptom Checklist. *British Journal of Cancer,* 1990; 62:1034–1038
8. Dunlop GM. A study of the relative frequency and importance of gastrointestinal symptoms and weakness in patients with far-advanced cancer: student paper. *Palliative Medicine,* 1989; 4:37–43.
9. Dunphy KP, and Amesbury BDW. A comparison

of hospice and home care patients: patterns of referral, patient characteristics and predictors of place of death. *Palliative Medicine*, 1990; 4:105–XXX.

10. Fainsinger R, Miller MJ, Bruera E, Hanson J, Maceachern T. Symptom control during the last week of life on a palliative care unit. *Journal of Palliative Care*, 1991; 7(1):5–11.

11. Greer DS, Mor V, Morris JN, Sherwood S, Kidder D, Birnbaum H. An alternative in terminal care: Results of the National Hospice Study. *J Chronic Disease* 1986; 39(1):9–26.

12. Grosvenor M, Bulcavage L, Chlebowski RT. Symptoms potentially influencing weight loss in a cancer population. Correlations with primary site, nutritional status, and chemotherapy administration. *Cancer*, 1989; 63(2):330–334.

13. Hockley JM, Dunlop R, Davies RJ. Survey of distressing symptoms in dying patients and their families in hospital and the response to a symptom control team. *British Medical Journal*, 1988; 296:1715–1717.

14. Kornblith AB, Herr HW, Ofman US, Scher HI, Holland JC. Quality of life of patients with prostate cancer and their spouses: the value of a data base in clinical care. *Cancer*, 1994; 73:2791–2802.

15. McCorkle R, Young K. Development of a symptom distress scale. *Cancer Nurs* 1978; 1:373–378.

16. Mor V, Masterson-Allen S. A comparison of hospice vs conventional care of the terminally ill cancer patient. *Oncology*, 1990; 4(7):85–91.

17. Morris JN, Suissa S, Sherwood S, Wright SM, Greer D. Last days: A study of the quality of life of terminally ill cancer patients. *Journal of Chronic Disease*, 1986; 39(1):47–62.

18. Portenoy RK, Thaler HT, Kornblith AB, et al. Symptom prevalence, characteristics and distress in a cancer population. *Qual Life Res*, 1994; 3:183–189.

19. Reuben DB, Mor V. Dyspnea in terminally ill cancer patients. *Chest*, 1986; 89(2):234–236.

20. Reuben DB, Mor V, Hiris J. Clinical symptoms and length of survival in patients with terminal cancer. *Archives of Internal Medicine*, 1988; 148:1586–1591.

21. Ventafridda V, Deconno F, Ripamonti AC, Gamba A, Tamburini M. Quality-of-life assessment during a palliative care programme. *Annals of Oncology*, 1990; 1(6):415–420.

22. Ingham JM, Portenoy RK. Symptom assessment. *Hematol/Oncol Clin N Amer* 1996; 10:21–40.

23. Jacox A, Carr DB, Payne R, et al. Management of Cancer Pain. Clinical Practice Guideline No.

9. AHCPR Publication No. 94-0592. Rockville, MD. Agency for Health Care Policy and Research, U.S. Department of Health and Human Services, Public Health Service.

24. American Pain Society Quality of Care Committee. Quality improvement guidelines for the treatment of acute pain and cancer pain. *Journal of the American Medical Association*, 1995; 274:1875–1880.

25. Bookbinder M, Coyle N, Kiss M, et al. Implementing national standards for cancer pain management: program model and evaluation. *Journal of Pain and Symptom Management*, 1996; 12:334–347.

26. Gonzales GR, Elliot KJ, Portenoy RK, Foley KM. The impact of a comprehensive evaluation in the management of cancer pain. *Pain*, 1991; 47:141–144.

27. Caraceni A. Clinicopathologic correlates of common cancer pain syndromes. *Hematology/Oncology Clinical NA*, 1996; 10:57–78.

28. Weinstein S, Portenoy RK (in press). Back pain in cancer patients. In: Vinken PJ, Bruyn GW, eds, *Handbook of Clinical Neurology*. Amsterdam: Elsevier Science.

29. American College of Physicians Health and Public Policy Committee. Drug therapy for severe chronic pain in terminal illness. *Annual of Internal Medicine*, 1997; 99:870–873.

30. American Pain Society. *Principles of Analgesic Use in the Treatment of Acute Pain and Cancer Pain*. Skokie, Ill: American Pain Society, 1992.

31. American Society of Clinical Oncology Ad Hoc Committee on Cancer Pain. Cancer pain assessment and treatment curriculum guidelines. *Journal of Clinical Oncology*, 1992; 10:1976–1982.

32. World Health Organization. Cancer Pain Relief, 2nd ed. (with a Guide to Opioid Availability). Geneva: World Health Organization.

33. Schug SA, Zech D, and Dorr U. Cancer pain management according to WHO analgesic guidelines. *Journal of Pain Symptom Management*, 5:27–32.

34. Schug SA, Zech D, Grond S, Jung H, Meurser T, Stobbe B. A long-term survey of morphine in cancer pain patients. *Journal of Pain and Symptom Management*, 1992; 7:259–266.

35. Ventafridda V, Tamburini M, Caraceni A, et al. A validation study of the WHO method for cancer pain relief. *Cancer*, 1990; 59:850–856.

36. Walker VA, Hoskin PJ, Hanks GW, White ID. Evaluation of WHO analgesic guidelines for cancer pain in a hospital-based palliative care unit. *Journal of Pain and Symptom Management*, 1988; 3:145–149.

37. Tong D, Gillick L, Hendrickson FR. The palliation of symptomatic osseous metastases: final results of the study by the Radiation Therapy Oncology Group. *Cancer*, 1982; 50:893–899.

38. Macdonald N. The role of medical and surgical oncology in the management of cancer pain. In: Foley KM, Bonica JJ, Ventafridda V, eds, *Advances in Pain Research and Therapy*. Vol 16. New York: Raven Press, 1990:27–40.

39. Burris HA, Moorer MJ, Andersen J, et al. Improvements in survival and clinical benefit with gemcitabine as first-line therapy for patients with advanced pancreas cancer: a randomized trial. *Journal of Clinical Oncology*, 199X; .

40. Tannock IF, Osoba D, Stockler MR, et al. Chemotherapy with mitoxantrone plus prednison or prednisone alone for symptomatic hormone-resistant prostate cancer: a Canadian randomized trial with palliative endpoints. *Journal of Clinical Oncology*, 1996; 14:1756–1764.

41. Bruera E, MacDonald RN. Intractable pain in patients with advanced head and neck tumors: a possible role of local infection. *Cancer Treatment Reports*, 1986; 70:691–692.

42. Portenoy RK, Kanner RM. Nonopioid and adjuvant analgesics. In: Portenoy RK, Kanner RM, eds. *Pain Management: Theory and Practice*. Philadelphia: FA Davis, 1996:219–247.

43. Sunshine A, Olson NZ. Nonnarcotic analgesics. In: Wall PD, Melzack R, eds, *Textbook of Pain*. 3rd ed. Edinburgh: Churchill Livingstone, 1994:923–942.

44. Sandler DP, Smith JC, Weinberg CR, et al. Analgesic use and chronic renal disease. *New England Journal of Medicine*, 1989; 320:1238–1243.

45. Cohen A, Thomas GB, Coen EE. Serum concentration, safety and tolerance of oral doses of choline magnesium trisalicylate. *Current Therapy Research*, 1978; 23:358–364.

46. Langman MJS, Well J, Wainwright P, et al. Risks of bleeding peptic ulcer associated with individual nonsteroidal anti-inflammatory drugs. *Lancet*, 1994; 343:1075–1078.

47. Savage RL, Moller PW, Ballantyne CL, et al. Variation in the risk of peptic ulcer complications with nonsteroidal anti-inflammatory drug therapy. Arthritis Rheum, 1993; 36:84–90.

48. Hoskin PJ, Hanks GW. Opioid agonist-antagonist drugs in acute and chronic pain patients. *Drugs*, 1991; 41:329–344.

49. Kaiko RF, Foley KM, Grabinski PY, et al. Central nervous system excitatory effects of meperidine in cancer patients. Ann Neurol, 1983;13: 180–185.

50. Galer BS, Coyle N, Pasternak GW, Portenoy RK. Individual variability in the response to different opioids. Report of five cases. *Pain*, 1992; 49:87–91.

51. De Stoutz ND, Bruera E, Suarez-Almazor M. Opioid rotation for toxicity reduction in terminal cancer patients. *Journal of Pain and Symptom Management*, 1995; 10:378–384.

52. Sjogren P. Clinical implications of morphine metabolites. In: Portenoy, RK, Bruera, EB, eds, *Topics in Palliative Care*. Vol 1. New York: Oxford University Press, 1997:163–176.

53. Hagen NA, Foley KM, Cerbone DJ, Portenoy RK, Inturrisi CE. Chronic nausea and morphine-6-glucuronide. *Journal of Pain Symptom Management* 1991; 6:125–128.

54. Osborne JR, Joel SP, Slevin ML. Morphine intoxication in renal failure: the role of morphine-6-glucuronide. *British Medical Journal*, 1986; 292:1548–1549.

55. Portenoy RK, Thaler HT, Inturrisi CE, et al. The metabolite, morphine-6-glucuronide, contributes to the analgesia produced by morphine infusion in pain patients with normal renal function. *Clin Pharmacol Ther* 1992; 51:422–431.

56. Tiseo PJ, Thaler HT, Lapin J, et al. Morphine-6-glucuronide concentrations and opioid-related side effects: a survey in cancer patients. *Pain*, 1995; 61:47–54.

57. Plummer JL, Gourlay GK, Cherry DA, Cousins MJ. Estimation of methadone clearance: application in the management of cancer pain. *Pain*, 1988; 33:313–322.

58. Donner B, Zenz M, Tryba M, Strumpf M. Direct conversion from oral morphine to transdermal fentanyl: a multicenter study in patients with cancer pain. *Pain*, 1996; 64:527–534.

59. Portenoy RK, Southam M, Gupta SK, et al. Transdermal fentanyl for cancer pain: repeated dose pharmacokinetics. *Anesthesiology*, 1993; 28: 36–43.

60. Swanson G, Smith J, Bulich R, et al. Patient-controlled analgesia for chronic cancer pain in the ambulatory setting: a report of 117 cases. *Journal of Clinical Oncology*, 1989; 7:1903–1906.

61. Portenoy RK, Moulin DE, Rogers A, Inturrisi CE, Foley KM. Continuous intravenous infusion of opioids in cancer pain: review of 46 cases and guidelines for use. *Cancer Treatment Reports*, 1986; 70:575–581.

62. Cole L, Hanning CD. Review of the rectal use of opioids. *Journal of Pain and Symptom Management*, 1990; 5:118–126.

63. Arner S, Rawal N, Gustafson LL. Clinical expe-

rience of long-term treatment with epidural and intrathecal opioids: a nationwide survey. *Acta Anaesthesioliga Scandinavia*, 1988; 32:253–259.

64. Plummer JL, Cherry DA, Cousins MJ, et al. Long-term spinal administration of morphine in cancer and non-cancer pain: a retrospective study. *Pain*, 1991; 44:215–220.

65. Portenoy RK, Hagen NA. Breakthrough pain: definition, prevalence and characteristics. *Pain*, 1990; 41:273–282.

66. Grochow L, Sheidler V, Grossman S, Green L, Enterline J. Does intravenous methadone provide longer lasting analgesia than intravenous morphine? A randomized, double blind study. *Pain*, 1989; 38:151–157.

67. Houde RW. Misinformation: side effects and drug interactions. In: Hill CS, Fields WS, eds, *Advances in Pain Research and Therapy*. Vol 11. New York: Raven Press, 1989:145–161.

68. Portenoy RK. Management of opioid side effects. *Singapore Medical Journal*, 1994; 23:160–170.

69. Portenoy RK. Adjuvant analgesics. In: Cherny NI, Foley KM, eds, Hematology/Oncology Clinics of North America. Philadelphia: W.B. Saunders, Co. 1996; Vol 10:103–119.

70. Bruera E, Roca E, Cedaro L, Carraro S, Chacon R. Action of oral methylprednisolone in terminal cancer patients: a prospective randomized double-blind study. *Cancer Treatment Reports*, 1985; 69:751–754.

71. Portenoy RK, Foley KM, Inturrisi CE. The nature of opioid responsiveness and its implications for neuropathic pain: new hypotheses derived from studies of opioid infusions. *Pain*, 1990; 43:273–286.

72. Cherny NI, Arbit E, Jain S. Invasive techniques in the management of cancer pain. *Hematology/Oncology Clinical NA*, 1996; 10:121–138.

73. Smets EM, Garssen B, Schuster-Uitterhoeve AL, De Haes JCJM. Fatigue in cancer patients. *British Journal of Cancer*, 1993; 68:220–224.

74. Winningham ML, Nail LM, Burke MB, et al. Fatigue and the cancer experience: the state of the knowledge. *Oncol Nurs Forum* 1994; 21:23–36.

75. Glaus A. Assessment of fatigue in cancer and non-cancer patients and in healthy individuals. *Support Care Cancer* 1993; 1:305–315.

76. Irvine DM, Vincent L, Bubela N, Thompson L, Graydon J. A critical appraisal of the research literature investigating fatigue in the individual with cancer. *Canc Nurs*, 1991; 14:188–199.

77. Piper B, Lindsey A, Dodd M. Fatigue mechanisms in cancer patients: developing nursing theory. *Oncol Nurs Forum* 1987; 14:17–21.

78. Bruera E, Chadwick S, Brenneis C, Hanson J, Macdonald RN. Methylphenidate associated with narcotics for the treatment of cancer pain. *Cancer Treatment Reports*, 1987; 71:67–70.

79. Krupp LB, Coyle PK, Cross AH, Scheinberg LC. Amelioration of fatigue with pemoline in patients with multiple sclerosis. Ann Neurol 1989; 26:155–XXX.

80. Bruera E, Brenneis C, Paterson AH, Macdonald RN. Use of methylphenidate as an adjuvant to narcotic analgesics in patients with advanced cancer. *Journal of Pain and Symptom Management*, 1989; 4:3–6.

81. Breitbart W, Mermelstein H. Pemoline: An alternative psychostimulant for the management of depressive disorders in cancer patients. *Psychosomatics* 1992; 33:352–356.

82. Fernandez F, Adams F, Levy JK. Cognitive impairment due to AIDS-related complex and its response to psychostimulants. *Psychosomatics*, 1988; 29:38–46.

83. Katon W, Raskind M. Treatment of depression in the medically ill elderly with methylphenidate. *American Journal of Psychiatry*, 1980; 137:963–965.

84. Kaufmann MW, Murray GB, Cassem NH. Use of psychostimulants in medically ill depressed patients. *Psychosomatics*, 1982; 23:817–819.

85. Tannock I, Gospodarowicz M, Meakin W, et al. Treatment of metastatic prostatic cancer with low-dose prednisone: evaluation of pain and quality of life as pragmatic indices of response. *Journal of Clinical Oncology*, 1989; 7:590–597.

86. Derby S, Portenoy RK. Assessment and management of constipation. In: Portenoy RK, Bruera EB, eds, *Topics in Palliative Care*. Vol 1. New York: Oxford University Press, 1997:95–112.

87. Levy MH. Constipation and diarrhea in cancer patients. *Cancer Bulletin* 1991; 43:412–414.

88. Sykes NP. Constipation and diarrhoea. In: Doyle D, Hanks GW, MacDonald N, eds, *Oxford Textbook of Palliative Medicine*. New York: Oxford University Press, 1993:299–310.

89. Fadul CE, Lemann W, Thaler HT, Posner JB. Perforation of the gastrointestinal tract in patients receiving steroids for neurologic disease. *Neurology*, 1988; 38:348–352.

90. Lederle FA, Busch DL, Mattox KM, West MJ, Aske DM. Cost-effective treatment of constipation in the elderly: a randomized double-blind comparison of sorbitol and lactulose. *American Journal of Medicine*, 1990; 89:597–601.

91. Andorsky RI, Goldner F. Colonic lavage solution (polyethylene glycol electrolyte lavage solution)

as a treatment for chronic constipation: a double-blind, placebo-controlled study. *American Journal of Gastroenterology*, 1990; 85:261–265.

92. Krevsky B, Maurer AH, Malmud LS, Fisher RS. Cisapride accelerates colonic transit in constipated patients with colonic inertia. *American Journal of Gastroenterology*, 1989; 84:882–887.

93. Culpepper-Morgan JA, Inturrisi CE, Portenoy RK, et al. Treatment of opioid-induced constipation with oral naloxone: a pilot study. *Clinical Pharmacology Therapy*, 1992; 52:90.

94. Sykes NP. Oral naloxone in opioid associated constipation. *Lancet* 1991; 337:1475.

95. Allan SG. Nausea and vomiting. In: Doyle D, Hanks GW, MacDonald N, eds, *Oxford Textbook of Palliative Medicine*. New York: Oxford University Press, 1993:282–290.

96. Naylor RJ, Rudd JA. Emesis and anti-emesis. In: Hanks GW, ed, *Palliative Medicine: Problem Areas in Pain and Symptom Management*. Plainview, N.Y.: Cold Spring Harbor Laboratory Press, 1994:117–135.

97. Burish TG, Tope DM. Psychological techniques for controlling the adverse side effects of cancer chemotherapy: findings from a decade of research. *Journal of Pain and Symptom Management*, 1992; 7:287–301.

98. Bruera E, MacDonald N. Nutrition in patients with advanced cancer: an update and review of our experience. *Journal of Pain and Symptom Management*, 1988; 3:133–140.

99. Alexander HR, Norton JA. Pathophysiology of cancer cachexia. In: Doyle D, Hanks GW, MacDonald N, eds, *Oxford Textbook of Palliative Medicine*. New York: Oxford University Press, 1993:316–329.

100. Mahony SM, Beck SA, Tisdale MJ. Comparison of weight loss induced by recombinant tumor necrosis factor with that produced by a cachexia-induced tumor. *British Journal of Cancer*, 1988; 57:385–389.

101. Vigano A, Watanabe S, Bruera E. Anorexia and cachexia in advanced cancer patients. In: Hanks GW, ed, *Palliative Medicine: Problem Areas in Pain and Symptom Management*. Plainview, N.Y.: Cold Spring Harbor Laboratory Press, 1994:99–115.

102. Schell H. Adrenal corticosteroid therapy in far-advanced cancer. *Geriatrics*, 1972; 27:131–141.

103. Willox JC, Corr J, Shaw J, et al. Prednisolone as an appetite stimulant in patients with cancer. *British Medical Journal*, 1984; 200:37–288.

104. Bruera E, MacMillan K, Kuehn N, Hanson J, MacDonald RN. A controlled trial of megestrol acetate on appetite, caloric intake, nutritional status, and other symptoms in patients with advanced cancer. *Cancer* 1990; 66:1279–1282.

105. Kornblith AB, Hollis DR, Zuckerman E, et al. Effect of megestrol acetate on quality of life in a dose-response trial in women with advanced breast cancer. *Journal of Clinical Oncology*, 1993; 11:2081–2089.

106. Loprinzi CL, Ellison NM, Schaid DJ, et al. A controlled trial of megestrol acetate treatment of cancer anorexia and cachexia. *Journal of the National Cancer Institute*, 1990; 82:1127–1132.

107. Loprinzi CL, Michalak JC, Schaid DJ, et al. Phase III evaluation of four doses of megestrol acetate as therapy for patients with anorexia and/or cachexia. *Journal of Clinical Oncology*, 1993; 11:762–767.

108. Tchekmedyian NS, Tait N, Moody M, et al. High dose megestrol acetate: a possible treatment for cachexia. *Journal of the American Medical Association*, 1987; 257:1195–1198.

109. Nelson K, Walsh D, Deeter P, et al. A phase II study of delta-9-tetrahydrocannabinol for appetite stimulation in cancer-associated anorexia. *Journal of Palliative Care*, 1994; 10:14–18.

110. Beal JE, Olson R, Laubenstein L, et al. Long-term efficacy and safety of dronabinol for AIDS-associated anorexia. *Journal of Pain and Symptom Management*, 1997; 14:7–14.

111. Kardinal CG, Loprinzi C, Schaid DJ, et al. A controlled trial of cyproheptadine in cancer patients with anorexia. *Cancer* 1990; 65:2657–2662.

112. Chlebowski RT, Bulcavage L, Grosvenor M, et al. Hydrazine sulfate in cancer patients with weight loss: a placebo-controlled clinical experience. *Cancer*, 1987; 59:406–410.

113. Chlebowski RT, Bulcavage L, Grosvenor M, et al. Hydrazine sulfate influence on nutritional status and survival in non-small cell lung cancer. *Journal of Clinical Oncology*, 1990; 8:9–15.

114. Kosty MP, Fleischman SB, Herndon JE, et al. Cisplatin, vinblastine and hydrazine sulfate in advanced non-small-cell lung cancer: a randomized placebo-controlled, double-blind Phase III study of the Cancer and Leukemia Group B. *Journal of Clinical Oncology*, 1994; 12:1113–1120.

115. Loprinzi CL, Goldberg RM, Su JO, et al. Placebo-controlled trial of hydrazine sulfate in patients with newly diagnosed non-small-cell lung cancer. *Journal of Clinical Oncology*, 1994; 12:1126–1129.

116. Loprinzi CL, Kuross SA, O'Fallon JR, et al. Randomized placebo-controlled evaluation of hydrazine sulfate in patients with advanced colorectal cancer. *Journal of Clinical Oncology*, 1994; 12:1121–1125.

9

Psychiatric Aspects of Pain Management in Patients with Advanced Cancer and AIDS

William Breitbart, M.D.
David Payne, Ph.D.

Pain is perhaps among the most prevalent and distressing symptoms encountered in patients with advanced disease. Psychiatric and psychological consultation in the palliative-care setting must take into account the important relationships between pain and psychological and psychiatric morbidity. Uncontrolled pain can mimic psychiatric disorders, so mental health clinicians must be knowledgeable about pain and its appropriate management in order to recognize the undertreatment of pain when it is present. In addition, psychiatrists and psychologist can play a vital role in the multidisciplinary approach to managing pain at the end of life.[1–3] This chapter reviews the prevalence of pain in cancer and AIDS, pain syndromes, and pain assessment issues, as well as pharmacologic and nonpharmacologic interventions for pain. Psychiatric interventions in the treatment of cancer and AIDS pain have now become an integral part of a comprehensive approach to pain management and are highlighted in this review.[4–6]

PREVALENCE OF PAIN IN CANCER AND AIDS

Pain is a common problem for cancer patients, with approximately 70% of patients experiencing severe pain at some time in the course of their illness.[2] It has been suggested that nearly 75% of patients with advanced cancer have pain[7] and that 25% of cancer patients die in severe pain.[8] There is considerable variability in the prevalence of pain among different types of cancer. For example, approximately 5% of leukemia patients experience pain during the course of their illness, compared to 50% to 75% of patients with tumors of the lung, gastrointestinal tract, or genitourinary system. Patients with cancers of the bone or cervix have been found to have the highest prevalence of pain, with as many as 85% of patients experiencing significant pain during the course of their illness.[1] Yet, despite the prevalence of pain, studies have shown that it is frequently underdiagnosed and inadequately treated.[2,9] It is important to remember that pain is frequently only one of several symptoms present in cancer patients. In addition to pain, patients were found, in a survey of symptoms, to suffer from an average of three additional troubling physical symptoms.[10] A global evaluation of the symptom burden allows for a more complete understanding of the impact of pain for the cancer pain. (Tables 9.1 and 9.2)

The prevalence of pain in HIV-infected individuals varies depending on stage of disease, care setting and study methodology. Estimates of the prevalence of pain in HIV-infected individuals generally range from 30% to 80% with prevalence of pain increasing as the disease progresses.[11-14] The studies cited suggest that approximately 25% to 30% of ambulatory HIV-infected patients with early HIV disease (pre-AIDS; Category A or B disease) experience clinically significant pain. A study of pain in hospitalized patients with AIDS revealed that more than 50% of patients required treatment for pain, with pain being the presenting complaint in 30% (second only to fever[14]). A recent review of pain in ambulatory HIV-infected men[15] reported that 80% of those with AIDS experienced one or more painful symptoms over a six-month period. Schofferman and Brody[13] reported that 53% of patients with far-advanced AIDS cared for in a hospice setting had pain, while Kimball and McCormick[15] reported that up to 93% of AIDS patients in their hospice experienced at least one 48-hour period of pain during the final 2 weeks of life. Larue and colleagues,[16] in a national study in France, demonstrated that patients with AIDS being cared for by hospice at home had prevalence rates and intensity ratings for pain that were comparable to, and even exceeded, those of cancer patients. AIDS patients with pain, like their counterparts with cancer pain, typically describe an average of two to three concurrent pains at a time.

PAIN SYNDROMES IN CANCER AND HIV/AIDS

A number of well-defined pain syndromes have been identified in cancer patients. Most are directly related to tumor involvement; this accounted for 78% of inpatient and 62% of outpatient pain complaints.[1] Tumor invasion of the bone, compression or infiltration of nerves, and obstruction of hollow viscus are the most common causes. Stretching of fascia or periosteum, tumor infiltration or occlusion of blood vessels, and damage to mucous membranes or other soft tissues is a less common cause of pain. The second pain syndrome, occurring in 19% of inpatients and 25% of outpatients, is related to cancer treatment.[1] Surgery, chemotherapy, and radiation therapy each can have painful sequelae. Postsurgical syndromes include postthoracotomy syndrome, postmastectomy syndrome, postradical neck syndrome, and phantom limb. Chemother-

apy can result in peripheral neuropathy, aseptic necrosis or femoral head, steroid pseudorheumatism, and postherpetic neuralgia. Finally, radiation therapy can result in radiation fibrosis or brachial and lumbar plexus, radiation myelopathy, radiation-induced second primary tumors, and radiation-induced necrosis or the bone.

Fewer than 10% of cancer patients have pain syndromes that are unrelated to the disease or therapy. These syndromes include cervical or lumbar osteoarthritis, thoracic and abdominal aneurysms, and diabetic neuropathy.

Pain syndromes encountered in AIDS are diverse in nature and etiology. The most common pain syndromes reported in studies to date include painful sensory peripheral neuropathy, pain due to extensive Kaposi's sarcoma, headache, oral and pharyngeal pain, esophageal pain, abdominal pain, chest pain, and arthralgias and myalgias, as well as painful dermatologic conditions.[11,12,14-19] Aside from these more common syndromes, however, others exist, including esophageal pain, such as dysphagia or odynophagia and biliary tract and pancreatic pain, and anorectal pain. [17-22]

Similar to the pain syndromes found in cancer pain, pain syndromes seen in HIV disease can be categorized into three types: those directly related to HIV infection or consequences of immunosuppression; those due to AIDS therapies; and those unrelated to AIDS or AIDS therapies.[23] In studies to date, approximately 50% of pain syndromes encountered are directly related to HIV infection or consequences of immunosuppression; 30% are due to therapies for HIV- or AIDS-related conditions, as well as diagnostic procedures; and the remaining 20% are unrelated to HIV or its therapies.

MULTIDIMENSIONAL CONCEPT OF PAIN IN CANCER AND AIDS

Pain, and especially pain in cancer and AIDS, is not a purely nociceptive or physical experience but involves complex aspects of human functioning, including personality, affect, cognition, behavior, and social relations.[24] A more enlightened description of the pain resulting from a terminal illness coined by Cecily Saunders[25] is "total pain," a label that attempts to describe the all-encompassing nature of this type of pain. It is important to note that the use of analgesic drugs alone does not always lead to pain relief.[26] In a recent study,[27] it has been demonstrated that psychological factors play a modest but important role in pain intensity. The interaction of cognitive, emotional, socioenvironmental and nociceptive aspects of pain shows the multidimensional nature of pain in terminal illness and suggests a model for multimodal intervention.[3] The challenge of untangling and addressing both the physical and the psychological issues involved in pain is essential to developing rational and effective management strategies. Psychosocial therapies directed primarily at psychological variables have profound impact on nociception, while somatic therapies directed at nociception have beneficial effects on the psychological aspects of pain. Ideally, such somatic and psychosocial therapies are used simultaneously in a multidisciplinary approach to pain management in the terminally ill.[4]

ASSESSMENT ISSUES

The initial step in pain management is a comprehensive assessment of pain symptoms. The health professional working in the cancer or AIDS setting must have a working knowledge of the etiology and treatment of pain in cancer and AIDS. This includes an understanding of the different types of cancer or AIDS pain syndromes, as well as a familiarity with the parameters of appropriate pharmacologic treatment. A close collaboration of the entire health-care team is optimal when attempting to adequately manage pain in the cancer or AIDS patient.

A careful history and physical examination may disclose an identifiable syndrome (e.g., herpes zoster, bacterial infection, or neuropathy) that can be treated in a standard fashion.[28,29] A standard pain history[30,31] may provide valuable clues to the nature of the underlying process and, indeed, may disclose other treatable disorders. A description of the qualitative features of the pain, its time course, and any maneuvers that increase or decrease pain intensity should be obtained. Pain intensity (current, average, at best, at worst) should be assessed to determine the need for weak versus potent analgesics and as a means to serially evaluate the effectiveness of ongoing treatment. Pain descriptors (e.g., burning, shooting, dull, or sharp) help determine the mechanism of

pain (somatic, nociceptive, visceral nociceptive, or neuropathic) and may suggest the likelihood of response to various classes of traditional and adjuvant analgesics (e.g., nonsteroidal antiinflammatory drugs, opioids, antidepressants, anticonvulsants, oral local anesthetics, and corticosteroids).[32–35] Additionally, detailed medical, neurological and psychosocial assessments (including a history of substance use or abuse) must be conducted. Where possible, family members or partners should be interviewed. During the assessment phase, pain should be aggressively treated while pain complaints and psychosocial issues are subject to an ongoing process of reevaluation.[30]

An important element in assessment of pain is the concept that assessment is continuous and needs to be repeated over the course of pain treatment. There are essentially four aspects of pain experience in cancer and AIDS that require ongoing evaluation, and they include: pain intensity, pain relief, pain-related functional interference (e.g., mood state, general and specific activities), and monitoring of intervention effects (analgesic drug side effects, abuse).[36] The Memorial Pain Assessment Card (MPAC)[37] is a helpful clinical tool that allows patients to report their pain experience. The MPAC consists of visual analog scales that measure pain intensity, pain relief, and mood. Patients can complete the MPAC in less than 30 seconds. Patients' reports of pain intensity, pain relief, and present mood state provide the essential information required to help guide their pain management. The Brief Pain Inventory[38] is another pain assessment tool that has useful clinical and research applications.

These principles of pain assessment have been described by Foley[2] and include the following:

1. Believe the patient's complaint of pain.
2. Take a detailed history.
3. Assess the psychosocial status of the patient.
4. Perform a careful medical and neurological examination.
5. Order and personally review the appropriate diagnostic procedures.
6. Evaluate the patient's extent of pain.
7. Treat the pain to facilitate the diagnostic workup.
8. Consider alternative methods of pain control during the initial evaluation.
9. Reassess the pain complaint during the prescribed therapy.

Inadequate Pain Management: Assessment Issues in the Treatment of Pain

While recent studies suggest that pain in cancer is still being undertreated,[39] pain in AIDS is dramatically undertreated.[16,40,41] Reports of marked undertreatment of pain in AIDS are appearing in the literature.[16,40,41] These studies suggest that opioid analgesics are underused in the treatment of pain in AIDS. Our group has reported[41] that, in our cohort of AIDS patients, only 6% of individuals reporting pain in the severe range (8 to 10 on a numerical rating scale) received a strong opioid, such as morphine, as recommended in the WHO Analgesic Ladder. This degree of undermedication far exceeds published reports of undermedication of pain in cancer populations.[39] As with cancer, we have found that factors that influence undertreatment of pain in AIDS include gender (women are more undertreated), education, substance abuse history, and a variety of patient-related and clinician-related barriers.[41,42,43] While opioid analgesics are underused, it is also clear from our work and the work of others that adjuvant agents such as antidepressants are also dramatically underused.[16,39–43] Only 6% of subjects in a sample of AIDS patients reporting pain received an adjuvant analgesic drug (i.e., an antidepressant). This class of analgesic agents is a critical part of the WHO Analgesic Ladder and is vastly underused.

Inadequate management of pain is often a result of the inability to properly assess pain in all its dimensions.[2,4,8] All too frequently, psychological variables are proposed to explain continued pain or lack of response to therapy, when in fact medical factors have not been adequately appreciated. Other causes of inadequate pain management include lack of knowledge of current pharmaco- or psychotherapeutic approaches; focus on prolonging life rather than alleviating suffering; lack of communication between doctor and patient; limited expectations of patients regarding pain relief; limited communication capacity in patients impaired by organic mental disorders; unavailability of opioids; doctors' fear of causing respiratory depression; and, most important, doctors' fear of amplifying addiction and substance abuse. In advanced cancer, several factors have been noted to predict the undermanagement of pain, including a discrepancy between physician and patient in judging the severity of pain; the presence of pain that physicians do not attribute to cancer; better performance status; age of 70 years or more; and female sex.[39]

Fear of addiction affects both patient compliance and physician management of narcotic analgesics, leading to undermedication of pain in cancer and AIDS patients.[2,41,44–46] Studies of the patterns of chronic narcotic analgesic use in patients with cancer have demonstrated that, although tolerance and physical dependence commonly occur, addiction (psychological dependence) is rare and almost never occurs in individuals without a history of drug abuse prior to cancer illness.[46] Escalation of narcotic analgesic use by cancer patients is usually a result of progression of cancer or the development of tolerance. Tolerance means that a larger dose of narcotic analgesic is required to maintain an original analgesic effect. Physical dependence is characterized by the onset of signs and symptoms of withdrawal if the opioid is suddenly stopped or a opioid antagonist is administered. Tolerance usually occurs in association with physical dependence but does not imply psychological dependence; psychological dependence or addiction is not equivalent to physical dependence or tolerance and is a behavioral pattern of compulsive drug abuse characterized by a craving for the drug and overwhelming involvement in obtaining and using it for effects other than pain relief. The cancer-pain patient with a history of intravenous opioid abuse presents an often unnecessarily difficult management problem. Macaluso et al.[45] reported on their experience in managing cancer pain in such a population. Of 468 inpatient cancer-pain consultations, only eight patients (1.7%) had a history of intravenous drug abuse, but none had been actively abusing drugs in the previous year. All eight of these patients had inadequate pain control, and more than half were intentionally undermedicated because of staff concern that drug abuse was active or would recur. Adequate pain control was ultimately achieved in these patients by using appropriate analgesic dosages and intensive staff education.

More problematic, however, is the management of pain in the growing segment of the AIDS population that is actively abusing intravenous drugs.[47] Such active drug use, in particular intravenous opiate abuse, poses several pain treatment difficulties, including high tolerance to narcotic analgesics, drug-seeking and manipulative behavior, lack of compliance or unreliable patient history, and the risk of spreading HIV while the patient is high and disinhibited. Unfortunately, the patient's subjective report is often the best or only indication of the presence and intensity of pain, as well as the degree of pain relief achieved by an intervention. Physicians who believe they are being manipulated by drug-seeking individuals are hesitant to use opioids in appropriate dosages for adequate control of pain, often leading to undermedication. Most clinicians experienced in working with this population of AIDS patients recommend clear and direct limit setting. While that is an important aspect of the care of IV-drug-using AIDS patients, it is by no means the whole answer. As much as possible, clinicians should attempt to eliminate the issue of drug abuse as an obstacle to pain management by dealing directly with the problems of opiate withdrawal and drug abuse treatment. Often, specialized substance abuse consultation services are available to help manage such patients and to initiate drug rehabilitation. One should avoid making the analgesic drugs the focus of a battle for control between the patient and the physician, especially in the terminal stages of illness. Clinicians are advised to err on the side of believing patients when they complain of pain and to utilize their knowledge of the specific pain syndrome seen in AIDS patients to corroborate the patient's report if they feel it is unreliable.

The risk of inducing respiratory depression is too often overestimated and can limit appropriate use of narcotic analgesics for pain and symptom control. Bruera, et al.[48] demonstrated that, in a population of terminally ill cancer patients with respiratory failure and dyspnea, administration of subcutaneous morphine actually improved dyspnea without causing a significant deterioration in respiratory function. The adequacy of cancer pain management can be influenced by the lack of concordance between patient ratings or complaints of their pain and those made by caregivers. Persistent cancer pain is often ascribed to a psychological cause when it does not respond to treatment attempts. In our clinical experience, we have noted that patients who report their pain as severe are quite likely to be viewed as having a psychological contribution to their complaints. Staff members' ability to empathize with a patient's pain complaint may be limited by the intensity of the pain complaint. Grossman et al.[49] found that, while there is a high degree of concordance between patient and caregiver ratings of patient pain intensity at the low and moderate levels, this concordance breaks down at high levels. Thus, a clinician's ability to assess a patient's level of pain becomes unreliable once a patient's report of pain intensity rises above 7 on a visual analogue rating scale of 0 to 10. Physicians must be educated as to the limitations of their ability to objectively assess the severity of a subjective pain experience. Additionally, patient education is often a useful intervention in such cases. Patients are more likely to be believed and adequately treated if they are taught to request pain relief in a nonhysterical, businesslike fashion.

Psychological Factors in Pain Experience

The patient with cancer or AIDS faces many stressors during the course of illness, including dependency, disability, and fear of painful death. Such fears are universal; however, the level of psychological distress is variable and depends on medical factors, social supports, coping capacities, and personality. Pain has profound effects on psychological distress in cancer patients, and psychological factors such as anxiety, depression, and the meaning of pain for the patient can intensify cancer pain experience. Daut and Cleeland[50] showed that cancer patients who attribute a new pain to an unrelated benign cause report less interference with their activity and pleasure than cancer patients who believe their pain represents progression of disease. Spiegel and Bloom[51] found that women with metastatic breast cancer experience more intense pain if they believe their pain represents spread of their cancer and if they are depressed. Beliefs about the meaning of pain and the presence of a mood disturbance are better predictors of level of pain than is the site of metastasis.

In an attempt to define the potential relationships between pain and psychosocial variables, Padilla et al.[52] found that there were pain-related quality of life variables in three domains: physical well-being; psychological well-being, consisting of affective factors, cognitive factors, spiritual factors, communication skills, coping skills, and meaning attributed to pain or cancer;

and interpersonal well-being, focusing on social support or role functioning. The perception of marked impairment in activities of daily living has been shown to be associated with increased pain intensity.[53-54] Measures of emotional disturbance have been reported to be predictors of pain in the late stages of cancer, and cancer patients with less anxiety and depression are less likely to report pain.[55-56] Cancer and AIDS patients who report negative thoughts about their personal or social competence report increased pain intensity and emotional distress.[51,52] In a prospective study of cancer patients, it was found that maladaptive coping strategies, lower levels of self-efficacy, and distress specific to the treatment or disease progression were modest but significant predictors of reports of pain intensity.[57]

Psychological variables, such as the amount of control people believe they have over pain, emotional associations and memories of pain, fear of death, depression, anxiety, and hopelessness, contribute to the experience of pain in people with AIDS and can increase suffering.[58] We recently reported[53] that negative thoughts related to pain are associated with greater pain intensity, psychological distress, and disability in ambulatory patients with AIDS. Pain appears to have a profound impact on levels of emotional distress and disability. In a pilot study of the impact of pain on ambulatory HIV-infected patients,[58] depression was significantly correlated with the presence of pain. In addition to being significantly more distressed and depressed, those with pain were twice as likely to have suicidal ideation (40%) as those without pain (20%). HIV-infected patients with pain were more functionally impaired. Such functional interference was highly correlated to levels of pain intensity and depression. Those who felt that pain represented a threat to their health reported more intense pain than those who did not see pain as a threat. Patients with pain were more likely to be unemployed or disabled, and they reported less social support. Singer and colleagues[14] also reported an association among the frequency of multiple pains, increased disability, and higher levels of depression.

All too frequently, psychological variables are proposed to explain continued pain or lack of response to therapy when in fact medical factors have not been adequately appreciated. Often, the psychiatrist is the last physician to consult on a cancer or AIDS patient with pain. In that role, one must be vigilant that an accurate pain diagnosis is made and be able to assess the adequacy of the medical analgesic management provided. Psychological distress in terminally ill patients with pain must initially be assumed to be the consequence of uncontrolled pain. Personality factors may be quite distorted by the presence of pain, and relief of pain often results in the disappearance of a perceived psychiatric disorder.[5,59]

Psychiatric Disorders and Pain in Cancer and AIDS

Psychiatric disorders are found with increased frequency in cancer patients with pain. In the Psychosocial Collaborative Oncology Group Study[60] on the prevalence of psychiatric disorders in cancer patients, of the patients who received a psychiatric diagnosis, 39% reported significant pain, while only 19% of patients without a psychiatric diagnosis had significant pain. The psychiatric disorders seen in cancer patients with pain include primarily adjustment disorder with depressed or anxious mood (69%) and major depression (15%). This finding of increased frequency of psychiatric disturbance in cancer pain patients has been reported.[61,62] Tables 9.1 and 9.2 show the relevant pain syndromes for AIDS and cancer, respectively.

Epidural spinal cord compression (ESCC) is a common neurological complication of systemic

Table 9.1. Pain Syndromes in AIDS Patients

I. Pain Related to HIV/AIDS
    HIV neuropathy
    HIV myelopathy
    Kaposi's sarcoma
    Secondary infections (intestines, skin)
    Organolmegaly
    Arthritis/vasculitis
    Myopathy/myositis
II. Pain Related to HIV/AIDS Therapy
    Antiretrovirals, Antivirals
    Antimyocobacterials, PCP prophylaxis
    Chemotherapy (Vincristine)
    Radiation
    Surgery
    Procedures (bronchoscopy, biopsies)
III. Pain Unrelated to AIDS
    Disc Disease
    Diabetic Neuropathy

Table 9.2 Pain Syndromes in Patients with Cancer

I. Pain Associated with Direct Tumor Involvement
    Tumor infiltration of bone
    Tumor infiltration of nerve, plexus, and meninges
II. Pain Associated with Cancer Therapy
    Postsurgical pain syndromes
    Postchemotherapy pain syndromes
    Postradiation therapy pain syndromes
III. Pain Unrelated to the Cancer or the Cancer Therapy

---

cancer that occurs in 5% to 10% of patients with cancer and can often present with severe pain. These patients are routinely treated with a combination of high-dose dexamethasone and radiotherapy. Patients who receive this high-dose regimen are exposed in some centers to as much as 96 mg a day of dexamethasone for up to 1 week and continue on a tapering course for up to 3 or 4 weeks. Breitbart et al.[63] recently described the psychiatric complications seen in cancer patients undergoing such treatment for epidural spinal cord compression. With the higher dosages of dexamethasone, 22% of patients with ESCC had a major depressive syndrome diagnosed, compared to 4% in the control group. Also, delirium was much more common in the dexamethasone-treated patients with ESCC, with 24% diagnosed with delirium during the course of treatment, compared to only 10% in the control group. Steifel et al.[64] described the spectrum of neuropsychiatric syndromes produced by corcicosteroids in cancer patients.

Cancer patients with advanced disease are a particularly vulnerable group. The incidence of pain, depression, and delirium increases with greater debilitation and advanced stages of illness.[65,66] Although the prevalence of depression in cancer patients varies across studies depending on which criteria are used to diagnose depression, it appears that the prevalence of depression increases over the course of the illness, with patients with advanced disease having a greater likelihood of depression than patients with less advanced disease. The prevalence of organic mental disorders (delirium) among cancer patients requiring psychiatric consultation has been found to range from 25% to 40% and to be as high as 85% during the terminal stages of illness.[66] Opioids such as meperidine, levorphanol, and morphine sulfate can cause confusional states, particularly in the elderly and the terminally ill.[67]

Rosenfeld et al.[58] described the psychological impact of pain in an ambulatory AIDS population. AIDS patients with pain reported significantly greater depression and functional impairment than those without pain. Psychiatric disorders, in particular the organic mental disorders such as AIDS dementia complex, can occasionally interfere with adequate pain management in the AIDS patients. Opioid analgesics, the mainstay of treatment for moderate to severe pain, may worsen dementia or cause treatment-limiting sedation, confusion, or hallucinations in patients with neurologic complications of AIDS.[68] The judicious use of psychostimulants to diminish sedation and neuroleptics to clear confusional states can be quite helpful. Other psychiatric disorders that have an impact on pain management in the AIDS population include substance abuse and personality disorders.

Pain and Suicide

Uncontrolled pain is a major factor in suicide and suicidal ideation in cancer and AIDS patients.[69–76] Cancer is perceived by the public as an extremely painful disease compared with other medical conditions. In Wisconsin, a study revealed that 69% of the public agreed that cancer pain could cause a person to consider suicide.[71] The majority of suicides observed among patients with cancer had severe pain, which was often inadequately controlled or tolerated poorly.[69] Although relatively few cancer patients commit suicide, they are at increased risk.[69,72,75] Patients with advanced illness are at highest risk and are the most likely to have the complications of pain, depression, delirium, and deficit symptoms. Psychiatric disorders are frequently present in hospitalized cancer patients who attempt suicide. A review of the psychiatric consultation data at Memorial Sloan-Kettering Cancer Center showed that one-third of cancer patients who were seen for evaluation of suicide risk received a diagnosis of major depression; approximately 20% met criteria for delirium, and more than 50% were diagnosed with adjustment disorder.[75]

Thoughts of suicide probably occur quite frequently, particularly in the setting of advanced illness,[69,75] and seem to act as a steam valve for feelings often expressed by patients as "If it gets too bad, I always have a way out." It has been our experience working with terminally ill pain patients that, once a trusting and safe relationship develops, patients almost universally reveal that they have had occasionally persistent thoughts of suicide as a means of escaping the threat of being overwhelmed by pain. Recent published reports, however, suggest that suicidal ideation is relatively infrequent in cancer and is limited to those who are significantly depressed.[69,75] Silberfarb et al.[77] found that only 3 of 146 ambulatory breast cancer patients with early-stage disease had suicidal thoughts, whereas none of the 100 ambulatory cancer patients interviewed in a Finnish study expressed suicidal thoughts.[76] A study conducted at St. Boniface Hospice in Winnipeg, Canada, demonstrated that only 10 of 44 terminally ill cancer patients were suicidal or desired an early death; all 10 were suffering from clinical depression.[78] In general, suicidal ideation is less common in early-stage disease and becomes more common as the disease advances. At Memorial Sloan-Kettering Cancer Center (MSKCC), suicide risk evaluation accounted for 8.6% of psychiatric consultations, usually requested by staff in response to patients' verbalizing suicidal wishes.[70] In the 71 cancer patients who had suicidal ideation with serious intent, significant pain was a factor in only 30% of cases. In striking contrast, virtually all 71 suicidal cancer patients had a psychiatric disorder (mood disturbance or organic mental disorder) at the time of evaluation.[75]

We recently examined the role of cancer pain in suicidal ideation by assessing 185 cancer-pain patients involved in ongoing research protocols of the MSKCC Pain and Psychiatry Services.[79] Suicidal ideation occurred in 17% of the study population, with the majority reporting suicidal ideation without intent to act. Interestingly, in this population of cancer patients, all of whom had significant pain, suicidal ideation was not directly related to pain intensity but was strongly related to degree of depression and mood disturbance. Pain was related to suicidal ideation indirectly in that patients' perception of poor pain relief was associated with suicidal ideation. Perceptions of pain relief may have more to do with aspects of hopelessness than pain itself. Pain plays an important role in vulnerability to suicide; however, associated psychological distress and mood disturbance seem to be essential cofactors in raising the risk of suicide in cancer patients. Pain has adverse effects on patients' quality of life and sense of control and impairs the family's abil-

ity to provide support. Factors other than pain, such as mood disturbance, delirium, loss of control, and hopelessness, contribute to cancer suicide risk.

A study of men with AIDS in New York City[80] demonstrated a relative risk of suicide 36 times greater than that of males in the general population. Many of these patients had advanced AIDS with Kaposi's sarcoma and other potentially painful conditions. However, the role of pain in contributing to increased risk of suicide was not specifically examined. Our group at MSKCC has also examined the prevalence of suicidal ideation in an ambulatory AIDS population and examined the relationship among suicidal ideation, depression, and pain.[70,58] Suicidal ideation in ambulatory AIDS patients was found to be highly correlated with the presence of pain, depressed mood (as measured by the Beck Depression Inventory), and low CD 4 lymphocyte counts. While 20% of ambulatory AIDS patients without pain reported suicidal thoughts, more than 40% of those with pain reported suicidal ideation. Only two subjects in the sample ($n = 110$) reported suicidal intent. Neither of these two men was in the pain group; however, both scored quite high on measures of depression. No correlations were observed between suicidal ideation and pain intensity or pain relief. The mean visual analogue scale measure of pain intensity for the group overall was 49 mm (range of 5 to 100 mm), thus falling predominantly in the moderate range. As in cancer-pain patients, suicidal ideation in AIDS patients with pain is more likely to be related to a concommitant mood disturbance than to the intensity of pain experienced. Although AIDS patients are frequently found to have suicidal ideation, these thoughts are more often context-specific, occurring almost exclusively during exacerbations of the illness, often accompanied by severe pain, or at times of bereavement.[80–82]

PHARMACOTHERAPIES FOR PAIN IN CANCER AND AIDS

Although the management of analgesic medications is more often undertaken by the oncologist or palliative-care specialist, it is essential that the psychooncologist have a thorough understanding of the analgesic medications most often used in the management of cancer or AIDS-related pain.

The World Health Organization has devised guidelines for analgesic management of cancer pain that the AHCPR has endorsed for the management of pain related to cancer or AIDS.[33] These guidelines, also known widely as the WHO Analgesic Ladder, have been well validated.[83] This approach advocates selection of analgesics on the basis of severity of pain. For mild to moderately severe pain, nonopioid analgesics such as NSAIDs (nonsteroidal anti-inflammatory drugs) and acetaminophen are recommended. For pain that is persistent and moderate to severe in intensity, opioid analgesics of increasing potency (such as morphine) should be utilized. Adjuvant agents, such as laxatives and psychostimulants, are useful in preventing as well as treating opioid side effects such as constipation or sedation, respectively. Adjuvant analgesic drugs, such as the antidepressant analgesics, are suggested for considered use, along with opioids and NSAIDs, in all stages of the analgesic ladder (mild, moderate, or severe pain).

This WHO approach, commonly used in the treatment of cancer pain, has also been recommended by the AHCPR and by clinical authorities in the field of pain management and AIDS.[23,33,84] Clinical reports describing the successful application of the principles of the WHO Analgesic Ladder to the management of pain in AIDS, with particular emphasis on the use of opioids, have also recently appeared in the literature.[84–86]

Foley and Portenoy[31,34,87] have described the indications for and the use of three classes of analgesic drugs that have applications in the management of cancer and AIDS patients with pain: nonopioid analgesics (such as acetaminophen, aspirin, and other nonsteroidal anti-inflammatory drugs [NSAIDs], opioid analgesics (of which morphine is the standard), and adjuvant analgesics (such as antidepressants and anticonvulsants).

Nonopioid Analgesics

The nonopioid analgesics (Table 9.3) are prescribed principally for mild to moderate pain or to augment the analgesic effects of opioid analgesics in the treatment of severe pain. The analgesic effects of the NSAIDs result from their inhibition of cyclooxygenase and the subsequent reduction of prostaglandins in the tissues.[88,89] The concurrent use of NSAIDs or acetaminophen and opioids provides more analgesia than does either of the drug classes alone.[33] In contrast to opioids, NSAIDs have a ceiling effect for analgesia, do not produce tolerance or dependence, have antipyretic effects, and have a different spectrum of adverse side effects.

The physiochemical properties of the NSAIDs' mechanisms of action, pharmacokinetics, and pharmacodynamics influence the analgesic response. The selection of the NSAID should take into account the etiology and sever-

Table 9.3   Oral Analgesics for Mild to Moderate Pain in Cancer and AIDS

Analgesic (by class)	Starting Dose (mg)	Duration (hours)	Plasma Half-Life (hrs)	Comments
NONSTEROIDAL				
Aspirin	650	4–6	4–6	The standard for comparison among nonopioid analgesics
Ibuprofen	400–600	——	——	Like aspirin, can inhibit platelet function
Choline magnesium trisalicylate	700–1500	——	——	Essentially no hematologic or gastrointestinal side effects
WEAKER OPIOIDS				
Codeine	32–65	3–4	——	Metabolized to morphine, often used to suppress cough in patients at risk of pulmonary bleed
Oxycodone	5–10	3–4	——	Available as a single agent and in combination with aspirin or acetaminophen
Proxyphene	65–13	4–6	——	Toxic metabolite norpropoxy accumulates with repeated dosing

ity of the pain, concurrent medical conditions that may be relative contraindications (e.g., bleeding diathesis), associated symptoms, and favorable experience by the patient as well as the physician. From a practical point of view, an NSAID should be titrated to effect as well as to side effects. There is also variability in patient response to both relief and adverse reactions; if the results are not favorable, an alternative NSAID should be tried.

The major adverse effects associated with NSAIDs include gastric ulceration, renal failure, hepatic dysfunction, and bleeding. The use of NSAIDs has been associated with a variety of gastrointestinal toxicities, including minor dyspepsia and heartburn, as well as major gastric erosion, peptic ulcer formation, and gastrointestinal hemorrhage. The nonacetylated salicylates, such as salsalate, sodium salicylate, and choline magnesium salicylate, theoretically have fewer gastrointestinal (GI) side effects and might be considered in cases where GI distress is an issue. Prophylaxis for NSAID-associated GI symptoms includes H2-antagonist drugs (cimetidine 300 mg tid.-qid. or ranitidine 150 mg bid); misoprostal 200 mg qid; omeprazole 20 mg qd; or an antacid. Patients should be informed of these symptoms, issued guaiac cards with reagent, and taught to check their stool weekly. NSAIDs affect kidney function and should be used with caution. Prostaglandins are involved in the autoregulation of renal blood flow, glomerular filtration, and the tubular transport of water and ions. NSAIDs can cause a decrease in glomerular filtration, acute and chronic renal failure, interstitial nephritis, papillary necrosis, and hyperkalemia.[90] In patients with renal impairment, NSAIDs should be used with caution, since many (i.e., ketoprofen, feroprofen, naproxen, and carpofen) are highly dependent on renal function for clearance. The risk of renal dysfunction is greatest in patients with advanced age, preexisting renal impairment, hypovolemia, concomitant therapy with nephrotoxic drugs, and heart failure. Prostaglandins modulate vascular tone, and their inhibition by the NSAIDs can cause hypertension as well as interference with the pharmacologic control of hypertension.[91] Caution should be used in patients receiving B-adrenergic antagonists, diuretics, or angiotensin-converting enzyme inhibitors. Several studies have suggested that there is substantial biliary excretion of several NSAIDs, in-

cluding indomethacin and sulindac. In patients with hepatic dysfunction, these drugs should be used with caution. NSAIDs, with the exception of the nonacetylated salicylates (e.g., sodium salicylate, choline magnesium trisalicylate), produce inhibition of platelet aggregation (usually reversible, but irreversible with aspirin). NSAIDs should be used with extreme caution or avoided in patients who are thrombocytopenic or who have clotting impairment.

The use of NSAIDs in patients with cancer and AIDS must be accompanied by heightened awareness of toxicity and adverse effects. NSAIDs are highly protein bound, and the free fraction of available drug is increased in cancer and AIDS patients who are cachectic, wasted, and hypoalbuminic, often resulting in toxicities and adverse effects. Patients with cancer and AIDS are frequently hypovolemic, on concurrent nephrotoxic drugs, and experiencing HIV nephropathy and so are at increased risk for renal toxicity related to NSAIDs. Finally, the antipyretic effects of the NSAIDs may interfere with early detection of infection in patients with cancer and AIDS.

Opioid Analgesics

Opioid analgesics are the mainstay of pharmacotherapy of moderate to severe intensity pain in the patient with cancer or HIV disease (Table 9.4). Principles that are useful in guiding the appropriate use of opioid analgesics for pain[33,34,87,92] include the following:

1. Choose an appropriate drug.
2. Start with lowest dose possible.
3. Titrate dose.
4. Use "as needed" doses selectively.
5. Use an appropriate route of administration.
6. Be aware of equivalent analgesic doses.
7. Use a combination of opioid, nonopioid, and adjuvant drugs.
8. Be aware of tolerance.
9. Understand physical and psychological dependence.

In choosing the appropriate opioid analgesic for cancer pain, Portenoy[34] highlights the following important considerations: opioid class, choice of "weak" versus "strong" opioids, pharmacokinetic characteristics, duration of analgesic effect, favorable prior response, and opioid side effects. Opioid analgesics are divided into two

Table 9.4 Opioid Analgesics for Moderate to Severe Pain in Cancer or AIDS Patients

Analgesic	Equi-analgesic Route	Dose (mg)	Analgesic Onset (hrs)	Duration (hrs)	Plasma Half-life (hrs)	Comments
Morphine	PO	30–60*	1–11/2	4–6	2–3	Standard of comparison for the narcotic analgesics. 30mg for repeat around-the-clock dosing; 60mg for single dose or intermittent dosing.
	IM, IV, SC	10	1/2–1	3–6		
Morphine	PO	90–120	1–11/2	8–12	——	Now available in long-acting sustained release forms.
Oxycodone	PO	20–30	1	3–6	2–3	In combination with aspirin or acetaminaphen it is considered a weaker opioid; as a single agent it is comparable to the strong opioids, like morphine. Available in immediate-release and sustained-release preparation.
	PO	20–40	1	8–12	2–3	
Hydromophone	PO	7.5	1/2–1	3–4	2–3	Short half-life; ideal for elderly patients. Comes in suppository and injectable forms.
	IM, IV	1.5	1/4–1/2	3–4	2–3	
Methadone	PO	20	1/2–1	4–8	15–30	Long half-life; tends to accumulate with initial dosing, requires careful titration. Good oral potency.
	IM, IV	10	1/2–1	——	15–30	
Levorphanol	PO	4	1/2–11/2	3–6	12–16	Long half-life; requires careful dose titration in first week. Note that analgesic duration is only 4 hours.
	IM	2	1/2–1		12–16	
Meperidine	PO	300	1/2–11/2	3–6	3–4	Active toxic metabolite, ormeperidine, tends to accumulate (plasma half-life is 12–16 hours), especially with renal impairment and in elderly patients, causing delirium, myoclonus, and seizures.
	IM	75	1/2–1	3–4	3–4	
Fentanyl Transdermal System	TD	0.1	12–18	48–72	20–22	Transdermal patch is convenient, bypassing GI analgesia until depot is formed. Not suitable for rapid titration.
	IV	.01		——	——	

PO = per oral; IM = intramuscular; IV = intravenous; SC = subcutaneous; TD = transdermal

classes, the agonists and the agonist-antagonists, on the basis of their affinity to opioid receptors. Pentazocine, butorphanol, and nalbuphine are examples of opioid analgesics with mixed agonist-antagonist properties. These drugs can reverse opioid effects and precipitate an opioid with-drawal syndrome in patients who are opioid tolerant or dependent. They are of limited use in the management of chronic pain in cancer and AIDS. Oxycodone (in combination with either aspirin or acetominophen), hydrocodone, and codeine are the so-called weaker opioid analgesics and are indicated for use in step 2 of the WHO ladder for mild to moderate pain. More severe pain is best managed with morphine or another of the stronger opioid analgesics, such as hydromorphone, methadone, levorphanol, or fentanyl. Oxycodone, as a single agent without aspirin or acetaminophen, is available in immediate and sustained-release forms and is considered a stronger opioid in these forms.

A basic understanding of the pharmacokinetics of the opioid analgesics[87] is important for the cancer and AIDS care provider. Opioid analgesics with long half-lives, such as methadone and levorphanol, require approximately five days to achieve a steady state. Despite their long half-lives, the duration of analgesia that they provide is considerably shorter (i.e., most patients require administration of the drug every 4 to 6 hours). As both methadone and levorphanol tend to accumulate with early initial dosing, delayed effects of toxicity can develop (primarily sedation and, more rarely, respiratory depression).

The duration of analgesic effects of opioid analgesics varies considerably. Immediate-release preparations of morphine or oxycodone often provide only three hours of relief and must be prescribed on an every-3-hour, around-the-clock basis (not as needed). Methadone and levorphanol may provide up to 6 hours of analgesia. There is individual variation in the metabolism of opioid analgesics, and there can be significant differences between individuals in drug absorption and disposition. These differences lead to a need for alterations in dosing, route of administration, and scheduling for maximum analgesia in individual patients. While parenteral administration (intravenous, intramuscular, subcutaneous) yields a faster onset of pain relief, the duration of analgesia is shorter unless a continuous infusion of opioid is instituted. The use of continuous subcutaneous or intravenous infusions of opioids, with or without patient-controlled analgesia (PCA) devices, has become commonplace in caring for cancer and AIDS patients with escalating pain and in hospice and home settings during late stages of disease.

The oral route is often the preferred route of administration of opioid analgesics from the perspectives of convenience and cost. Immediate-release oral morphine or hydromorphone preparations require that the drug be taken every 3 to 4 hours. Longer-acting, sustained-release oral morphine preparations (MS Contin, Oramorph SR) and oxycodone preparations (oxycontin) are now available that provide up to 8–12 hours of analgesia, minimizing the number of daily doses required for the control of persistent pain. Rescue doses of immediate-release, short-acting opioid are often necessary to supplement the use of sustained-release morphine or oxycodone, particularly during periods of titration or pain escalation. The transdermal fentanyl patch system (Duragesic) also has applications in the management of severe pain in cancer and AIDS.[86] Each transdermal fentanyl patch contains a 48- to 72-hour supply of fentanyl, which is absorbed from a depot in the skin. Levels in the plasma rise slowly over 12 to 18 hours after patch placement, so, with the initial placement of a patch, alternative opioid analgesia (oral, rectal, or parenteral) must be provided until adequate levels of fentanyl are attained. The elimination half-life of this dosage form of fentanyl is long (21 hours), so it must be noted that significant levels of fentanyl remain in the plasma for about 24 hours after the removal of a transdermal patch. The transdermal system is not optimal for rapid dose titration of acutely exacerbated pain; however, a variety of dosage forms are available. As with sustained-release morphine preparations, all patients should be provided with oral or parenteral rapidly acting short-duration opioids to manage breakthrough pain. The transdermal system is convenient and eliminates the reminders of pain associated with repeated oral dosing of analgesics. In cancer and AIDS patients, it should be noted that the absorption of transdermal fentanyl can be increased with fever, resulting in increased plasma levels and shorter duration of analgesia from the patch.

It is important to note that opioids can be administered through a variety of routes: oral, rectal, transdermal, intravenous, subcutaneous, intraspinal, and even intraventrularly.[86] There are advantages and disadvantages, as well as indications, for use of these various routes. Further discussion of such alternative delivery routes as the intraspinal route are beyond the scope of this chapter; however, interested readers are directed to the Agency for Health Care Policy and Research Clinical Practice Guideline: Management of Cancer Pain[33] available free of charge through 1-800-4cancer.

The adequate treatment of pain in cancer and AIDS also requires consideration of the equianalgesic doses of opioid drugs, which are generally calculated using morphine as a standard. Cross-tolerance is not complete among these drugs. Therefore, one-half to two-thirds of the equianalgesic dose of the new drug should be given as the starting dose when switching from one opioid to another.[87] For example, if a patient receiving 20 mg of parenteral morphine is to be switched to hydromorphone, the equianalgesic dose of parenteral hydromorphone would be 3.0 mg. Thus, the starting dose of parenteral hydromorphone should be approximately 1.5 to 2 mg. There is also considerable variability in the parenteral-to-oral ratios among the opioid analgesics. Both levorphanol and methadone have 1:2 intramuscular/oral ratios, whereas morphine has a 1:6 and hydromorphone a 1:5 intramuscular/oral ratio. Failure to appreciate these dosage differences in route of administration can lead to inadequate pain control.

Regular ("standing") scheduling of the opioid analgesics is the foundation of adequate pain control. It is preferable to prevent the return of pain as opposed to treating pain as it reoccurs. "As needed" orders for chronic cancer pain often create a struggle among patient, family, and staff that is easily avoided by regular administration of opioid analgesics. The typical prescribing of methadone is a notable exception. It is often initially prescribed on an as-needed basis to determine the patient's total daily requirement and to minimize toxicity (due to its long half-life).

Opioid Side Effects

While the opioids are extremely effective analgesics, their side effects are common and can be minimized if anticipated in advance. Sedation is a common CNS side effect, especially during the initiation of treatment. Sedation usually resolves after the patient has been maintained on a steady dosage. Persistent sedation can be alleviated with a psychostimulant, such as dextroamphetamine, pemoline, or methylphenidate. All are prescribed in divided doses in early morning and at noon. Additionally, psychostimulants can improve depressed mood and enhance analgesia.[93,94] Delirium, of either an agitated or a somnolent variety, can also occur while the patient is on opioid analgesics and is usually accompanied by attentional deficits, disorientation, and perceptual disturbances (visual hallucinations and, more com-

monly, illusions). Myoclonus and asterixis are often early signs of neurotoxicity that accompany the course of opioid-induced delirium. Meperidine (Demerol), when administered chronically in patients with renal impairment, can lead to a delirium resulting from accumulation of the neuroexcitatory metabolite normeperidine.[95] Opioid-induced delirium can be alleviated through the implementation of three possible strategies: lowering the dose of the opioid drug presently in use, changing to a different opioid, or treating the delirium with low doses of high-potency neuroleptics, such as haloperidol. The third strategy is especially useful for agitation and clears the sensorium.[96] For agitated states, intravenous haloperidol in doses starting at between 1 and 2 mg is useful, with rapid escalation of dose if no effect is noted. Gastrointestinal side effects of opioid analgesics are common. The most prevalent are nausea, vomiting, and constipation.[35] Concomitant therapy with prochlorperazine for nausea is sometimes effective. Since all opioid analgesics are not tolerated in the same manner, switching to another narcotic can be helpful if an antiemetic regimen fails to control nausea. Constipation caused by narcotic effects on gut receptors is a problem frequently encountered, and it tends to be responsive to the regular use of senna derivatives. A careful review of medications is imperative, since anticholinergic drugs such as the tricyclic antidepressants can worsen opioid-induced constipation and can cause bowel obstruction. Respiratory depression is a worrisome but rare side effect of the opioid analgesics. Respiratory difficulties can almost always be avoided if two general principles are adhered to: start opioid analgesics in low doses in opioid-naive patients; and be cognizant of relative potencies when switching opioid analgesics, routes of administration or, both.

Adjuvant Psychotropic Analgesics for Patients with AIDS and Cancer

Although opioid and nonopioid analgesics are the mainstay of management of pain associated with AIDS or cancer, adjuvant analgesics are another class of medications frequently prescribed for the treatment of chronic pain and have important applications in the management of pain in AIDS and cancer. Adjuvant analgesic drugs are used to enhance the analgesic efficacy of opioids, treat concurrent symptoms that exacerbate pain, and provide independent analgesia. They may be used in all stages of the analgesic ladder. Commonly used adjuvant drugs include antidepressants, anticonvulsants, psychostimulants, neuroleptics, corticosteroids, and oral anesthetics.[33,35,94]

Antidepressants

The current literature supports the use of antidepressants as adjuvant analgesic agents in the management of a wide variety of chronic pain syndromes, including cancer pain, postherpetic neuralgia, diabetic neuropathy, fibromyalgia, headache, and low back pain.[28,29, 97–102, 130] The antidepressants are analgesic through a number of mechanisms that include antidepressant activity,[98] potentiation or enhancement of opioid analgesia[103–105] and direct analgesic effects.[106] The leading hypothesis suggests that both serotonergic and noradrenergic properties of the antidepressants are probably important and that variations among individuals in pain (as to the status of their own neurotransmitter systems) is an important variable.[28] Other possible mechanisms of antidepressant analgesic activity that have been proposed include adrenergic and serotonin receptor effects,[107] adenosinergic effects,[108] antihistaminic effects,[107] and direct neuronal effects, such as inhibition of paroxysmal neuronal discharge and decreasing sensitivity of adrenergic receptors on injured nerve sprouts.[109] There is substantial evidence that the tricyclic antidepressants in particular are analgesic and useful in the management of chronic neuropathic and nonneuropathic pain syndromes.[130] Amitriptyline is the tricyclic antidepressant most studied and has been proved effective as an analgesic in a large number of clinical trials addressing a wide variety of chronic pain syndromes, including neuropathy, cancer pain, and fibromyalgia.[98,99,110–112,130] Other tricyclics that have been shown to have efficacy as analgesics include imipramine,[113,114] desipramine,[29,115] nortriptyline,[116] clomipramine,[117,118] and doxepin.[119]

The heterocyclic and noncyclic antidepressant drugs, such as trazadone, mianserin, and maprotiline, and the newer serotonin-specific reuptake inhibitors (SSRIs), fluoxetine and paroxetine, may also be useful as adjuvant analgesics for chronic pain syndromes.[28,94,99,106,115,120–125] Fluoxetine, a potent antidepressant with specific serotonin reuptake inhibition activity,[123] has been shown to have analgesic properties in experimental animal pain models[124] but failed to show analgesic effects in a clinical trial for neuropathy.[115] Several case reports suggest that fluoxetine may be a useful adjuvant analgesic in the management of headache[126] and fibrositis.[127] Paroxetine, a newer SSRI, is the first antidepressant of this class shown to be a highly effective analgesic in a controlled trial for the treatment of diabetic neuropathy.[125] Newer antidepressants such as sertraline, venlafaxine, and nefazodone may also eventually prove to be clinically useful as adjuvant analgesics. Nefazodone, for instance, has been demonstrated to potentiate opioid analgesics in an animal model.[128]

Given the diversity of clinical syndromes in which the antidepressants have been demonstrated to be analgesic, trials of these drugs can be justified in the treatment of virtually every type of chronic pain.[35,130] The established benefit of several of the antidepressants in patients with neuropathic pains,[111,115,125] however, suggests that these drugs may be particularly useful in populations, such as cancer and AIDS patients, where an underlying neuropathic component to the pain(s) often exists.[35] While studies of the analgesic efficacy of these drugs in HIV-related painful neuropathies have not yet been conducted, they are widely applied clinically using the model of diabetic and postherpetic neuropathies.

While antidepressant drugs are analgesic in both neuropathic and nonneuropathic pain models, their clinical use is most commonly in combination with opioid drugs, particularly for moderate to severe pain. Antidepressant adjuvant analgesics have their most broad application as "co-analgesics," potentiating the analgesic effects of opioid drugs.[33] The "opioid-sparing" effects of antidepressant analgesics has been demonstrated in a number of trials, especially in cancer populations with neuropathic as well as nonneuropathic pain syndromes.[99,102] In a placebo-controlled study, Walsh[102] demonstrated that imipramine was a potent co-analgesic when used along with morphine in the treatment of cancer-related pain, allowing for a reduction in morphine consumption of greater than 25%. Similar co-analgesic and opioid-sparing effects were demonstrated for amitriptyline and other antidepressants in two multicenter clinical trials for cancer pain.[99,101]

The dose and time course of onset of analgesia for antidepressants when used as analgesics appears to be similar to their use as antidepressants. There are those that have initially advocated a low-dose regimen of amitriptyline (10 to 30 mg) as being equally analgesic to a high-dose regimen (75 to 150 mg).[112] However, Zitman et al.[129] demonstrated only modest analgesic results from low-dose amitriptyline. Watson et al.[28] felt that there was a "therapeutic window" (20 to 100 mg) for the analgesic effects of amitriptyline. More recently, there is compelling evidence that the therapeutic analgesic effects of amitriptyline are correlated with serum levels, as are the antidepressant effects, and that analgesic treatment failure is due to low serum levels.[115] A high-dose regimen of up to 150 mg of amitriptyline or higher is suggested.[115] The proper analgesic dose for paroxetine is likely in the 40 to 60–mg range, with the major analgesic trial utilizing a fixed dose of 40 mg.[125] There is anecdotal evidence to suggest that the debilitated medically ill (e.g., cancer or AIDS patients) often respond (for both depression and pain) to lower doses of antidepressant than are usually required in the physically healthy, probably because of impaired metabolism of these drugs.[94] As to the time course of onset of analgesia, a biphasic process appears to occur. There are immediate or early analgesic effects that occur within hours or days, and these are probably mediated through inhibition of synaptic reuptake of catecholamines. In addition, there are later, longer analgesic effects that peak over a 2 to 4–week period that are probably a result of receptor effects of the antidepressants.[110,111]

Anticonvulsants

Selected anticonvulsant drugs appear to be analgesic for the lancinating dysesthesias that characterize diverse types of neuropathic pain.[130] Clinical experience also supports the use of these agents in patients with paroxysmal neuropathic pains that may not be lancinating and, to a far lesser extent, in those with neuropathic pains characterized solely by continuous dysesthesias. Although most practitioners prefer to begin with carbamazepine because of the extraordinarily good response rate observed in trigeminal neuralgia, this drug must be used cautiously in AIDS patients with thrombocytopenia, those at risk for marrow failure, and those whose blood counts must be monitored to determine disease status. If carbamazepine is used, a complete blood count should be obtained prior to the start of therapy, after two and four weeks, and then every 3 to 4 months thereafter. A leukocyte count below 4,000 is usually considered to be a contraindication to treatment, and a decline to less than 3,000 or an absolute neutrophil count of less than 1,500 during therapy should prompt discontinuation of the drug. Other anticonvulsant drugs may be useful for managing neuropathic pain in AIDS patients, including phenytoin, clonazepam, valproate, and gabapentin.[130]

Several newer anticonvulsants have been used in the treatment of neuropathic pain, particularly patients with reflect sympathetic dystrophy. These drugs include gabapentin, lamotrigine, and felbamate. Of these newer anticonvulsants, anecdotal experience has been most favorable with gabapentin, which is now being widely used by pain specialists to treat neuropathic pain of various types. Gabapentin has a relatively high degree of safety, including no known drug-drug interactions and a lack of hepatic metabolism.[130] Treatment with gabapentin is usually initiated at a dose of 300 mg per day and then gradually increased to a dose range of 900 to 3200 mg per day in three divided doses.

Psychostimulants

Psychostimulants, such as dextroamphetamine, methylphenidate, and pemoline, may be useful antidepressants in patients with cancer or AIDS who are cognitively impaired.[93,94,131] Psychostimulants also enhance the analgesic effects of the opioid drugs.[132] They are useful in diminishing sedation secondary to narcotic analgesics, and they are potent adjuvant analgesics. Bruera et al.[93] demonstrated that a regimen of 10 mg methylphenidate with breakfast and 5 mg with lunch significantly decreased sedation and potentiated the effect of narcotics in patients with cancer pain. Methylphenidate has also been demonstrated to improve functioning on a number of neuropsychological tests, including tests of memory, speed, and concentration, in patients receiving continuous infusions of opioids for cancer pain.[133] Dextroamphetamine has also been reported to have additive analgesic effects when used with morphine in postoperative pain.[134] In relatively low doses, psychostimulants stimulate appetite, promote a sense of well-being, and improve feelings of weakness and fatigue in cancer patients.

Pemoline is a unique alternative psychostimulant that is chemically unrelated to amphetamine but may have similar usefulness as an antidepressant and adjuvant analgesic in AIDS patients.[135] Advantages of pemoline as a psychostimulant in AIDS-pain patients include the lack of abuse potential, the lack of federal regulation through special triplicate prescriptions, the mild sympathomimetic effects, and the fact that it comes in a chewable tablet form that can be absorbed through the buccal mucosa and thus can be used by AIDS patients who have difficulty swallowing or who have intestinal obstruction. Clinically, pemoline is as effective as methyl-phenidate or dextroamphetamine in the treatment of depressive symptoms and in countering the sedating effects of opioid analgesics. There are no studies of pemoline's capacity to potentiate the analgesic properties of opioids. Pemoline should be used with caution in patients with liver impairment, and liver function tests should be monitored periodically with longer-term treatment.

Neuroleptics

Neuroleptic drugs, such as methotrimeprazine, fluphenazine, haloperidol and pimozide, may play a role as adjuvant analgesics[116,136–138] in AIDS or cancer patients with pain; however, their use must be weighed against what appears to be an increased sensitivity to the extrapyramidal side effects of these drugs in cancer patients or AIDS patients with neurological complications.[139] Anxiolytics, such as alprazolam and clonazepam, may also be useful as adjuvant analgesics, particularly in the management of neuropathic pains.[140–142]

Corticosteroids

Corticosteroid drugs have analgesic potential in a variety of chronic pain syndromes, including neuropathic pains and pain syndromes resulting from inflammatory processes.[35] Like other adjuvant analgesics, corticosteroids are usually added to an opioid regimen. In patients with advanced disease, these drugs may also improve appetite, nausea, malaise, and overall quality of life. Adverse effects include neuropsychiatric syndromes, gastrointestinal disturbances, and immunosuppression.

Oral Local Anesthetics

Local anesthetic drugs may be useful in the management of neuropathic pains characterized by either continuous or lancinating dysesthesias. Controlled trials have demonstrated the efficacy of tocainide and mexiletine, and there is clinical evidence that suggests similar effects from flecainide and subcutaneous lidocaine.[35] It is reasonable to undertake a trial with oral local anesthetic in patients with continuous dysesthesias who fail to respond adequately to, or who cannot tolerate, the tricyclic antidepressants and with patients with lancinating pains refractory to trials of anticonvulsant drugs and baclofen. Mexiletine is preferred in the United States.[55]

Placebo

A mention of the placebo response is important in order to highlight the misunderstandings and relative harm of this phenomenon. The placebo response is common, and analgesia is mediated through endogenous opioids. The deceptive use of placebo response to distinguish psychogenic pain from "real" pain should be avoided. Placebos are effective in a portion of patients for a short period of time only and are not indicated in the management of cancer pain.[2]

PSYCHIATRIC AND PSYCHOLOGIC MANAGEMENT OF PAIN IN CANCER AND AIDS

Optimal treatment of pain associated with advanced disease is multimodal and includes pharmacologic, psychotherapeutic, cognitive-behavioral, anesthetic, neurostimulatory, and rehabilitative approaches. Psychiatric participation in pain management involves the use of psychotherapeutic, cognitive-behavioral, and psychopharmacologic interventions, usually in combination. These are described in this section.

Psychotherapy and Pain

The goal of psychotherapy with medically ill patients with pain is to provide support, knowledge, and skills. Utilizing short-term supportive psychotherapy focused on the crisis created by the medical illness, the therapist provides emotional support, continuity, and information and assists in adaptation. The therapist has a role in emphasizing past strengths, supporting previously successful coping strategies, and teaching new coping skills such as relaxation, cognitive coping, use of analgesics, self-observation, documentation, assertiveness, and communication skills. Communication skills are of paramount importance for both patient and family, particularly around pain and analgesic issues. The patient and family are the unit of concern and need a more general, long-term, supportive relationship within the health-care system, in addition to specific psychological approaches for dealing with pain and dying that a psychiatrist, psychologist, social worker, chaplain, or nurse can provide.

Psychotherapy with the dying patient in pain consists of active listening with supportive verbal interventions and the occasional interpretation.[143] Despite the seriousness of the patient's plight, it is not necessary for the psychiatrist or psychologist to appear overly solemn or emotionally restrained. Often, it is only the psychotherapist, of all the patient's caregivers, who is comfortable enough to converse lightheartedly and to allow the patient to talk about his life and experiences, rather than focus solely on impending death. The dying patient who wishes to talk or ask questions about death and pain and suffering should be allowed to do so freely, with the therapist maintaining an interested, interactive stance. It is not uncommon for the dying patient to benefit from pastoral counseling. If a chaplaincy service is available, it should be offered to the patient and family. As the dying process progresses, psychotherapy with the individual patient may become limited by cognitive and speech deficits. It is at this point that the focus of supportive psychotherapeutic interventions shifts primarily to the family. In our experience, a very common issue for family members at this point is the level of alertness of the patient. Attempts to control pain are often accompanied by sedation that can limit communication between patient and family. This can sometimes become a source of conflict, with some family members disagreeing among themselves or with the patient about what constitutes an appropriate balance between comfort and alertness. It can be helpful for the physician to clarify the patient's preferences as they relate to these issues early so that conflict can be avoided and work related to bereavement can begin.

Group interventions with individual patients (even in advanced stages of disease), spouses, couples, and families are a powerful means of sharing experiences and identifying successful coping strategies. The limitations of using group interventions for patients with advanced disease are primarily pragmatic. The patient must be physically comfortable enough to participate and have the cognitive capacity to be aware of group discussion. It is often helpful for family members to attend support groups during the terminal phases of the patient's illness. Passik et al.[144] have worked with spouses of brain tumor patients in a psychoeducational group that has included spouses at all phases of the patient's illness. They have demonstrated how bereavement issues are often a focus of such interventions from the time of diagnosis on. The group members benefit from one another's support into widowhood. The leaders have been impressed by the increased quality of patient care that can be given at home by the spouse (including pain management and all forms of nursing care) when the spouse engages in such support.

Psychotherapeutic interventions that have multiple foci may be most useful. A prospective study of cancer pain has shown that cognitive-behavioral and psychoeducational techniques based on increasing support and self-efficacy and providing education may help patients deal with increased pain.[145] Results of an evaluation of patients with cancer pain indicate that psychological and social variables are significant predictors of pain. More specifically, distress specific to the illness, self-efficacy, and coping styles are predictors of increased pain.

Utilizing psychotherapy to diminish empirically symptoms of anxiety and depression, factors that can intensify pain, has beneficial effects on cancer-pain experience. Spiegel and Bloom[146] demonstrated, in a controlled randomized prospective study, the effect of both supportive group therapy for metastatic breast cancer patients in general and, in particular, the effect of hypnotic pain-control exercises. Their support group focused not on interpersonal processes or self-exploration but rather on a series of themes related to the practical and existential problems of living with cancer. Patients receiving group psychotherapy experienced significantly less psychological distress and pain than to patients who did not participate in group therapy.

While psychotherapy in the cancer-pain setting is primarily nonanalytical and focuses on current issues, exploration of reactions to cancer often involves insights into earlier, more pervasive life issues. Some patients choose to continue a more exploratory psychotherapy during extended illness-free periods or survivorship.

Cognitive-Behavioral Techniques

Cognitive-behavioral techniques can be useful as adjuncts to the management of pain in cancer and AIDS patients. Such techniques include passive relaxation with mental imagery, cognitive distraction or focusing, progressive muscle relaxation, biofeedback, hypnosis, and music therapy.[59] The goal of treatment is to guide the patient toward a sense of control over pain. Some techniques are primarily cognitive in nature, focusing on perceptual and thought processes, and others are directed at modifying patterns of behavior to help cancer patients cope with pain. Behavioral techniques for pain control seek to modify physiologic pain reactions, respondent pain behaviors, and operant pain behaviors.

Primarily cognitive techniques for coping with pain are aimed at reducing the intensity and distress that are part of the pain experience. This may be accomplished by the utilization of a number of techniques, including the modification of thoughts the patient has about pain or psychological distress, introduction of more adaptive coping strategies, and instruction in relaxation techniques. Cognitive modification (cognitive restructuring) is an approach derived from cognitive therapy for depression or anxiety and is based on how one interprets events and bodily sensation. It is assumed that patients have dysfunctional automatic thoughts that are consistent with their underlying assumptions and beliefs. In both cancer- and AIDS-pain populations, negative thoughts about pain have been shown to be significantly related to pain intensity, degree of psychological distress, and level of interference in functional activities.[51] By identifying and challenging dysfunctional automatic thoughts and underlying beliefs by restructuring or modifying thought processes, therapy allows a more rational response to pain to occur.[147] Examples of such automatic thoughts that have been shown to worsen pain experience are "The intensity of my pain will never diminish" or "Because my pain limits my activities, I am completely helpless." Patients can be taught to recognize and interrupt such thoughts and to develop a view of the pain experience as time limited and themselves as functional despite periods in which they are limited.

Although cognitive restructuring may be a useful technique in the earlier stages of cancer and AIDS, the goals change in the palliative-care context. In this setting, the goal is not necessarily to change the patient's maladaptive thoughts but to utilize techniques designed to diminish the patient's frustration, anxiety, and anger. Helping patients to employ more adaptive coping strategies, such as the avoidance of catastrophizing, and encouraging an increase in problem-solving skills may be helpful at this stage.[148-150]

Aside from modifying dysfunctional thoughts and attitudes, the most fundamental behavioral technique is self-monitoring. The development of the ability to monitor one's behaviors allows people to notice their dysfunctional reactions to the pain experience and to learn to control them. Systematic desensitization is useful in extinguishing anticipatory anxiety that leads to avoidance behaviors and in remobilizing inactive patients. Graded task assignment is essentially systematic desensitization as it is applied to patients who are encouraged to take small steps gradually so as to perform activities more readily. Contingency management is a method of reinforcing "well" behaviors only, thus modifying dysfunctional operant pain behaviors associated with secondary gain.[151,152]

Cognitive-behavioral interventions that are useful in the setting of advanced illness include a variety of techniques that range from preparatory information and self-monitoring to systematic desensitization and methods of distraction and relaxation.[153] Most often, techniques such as hypnosis, biofeedback, and systematic desensitization utilize both cognitive and behavioral elements, such as muscular relaxation and cognitive distraction.

Patient Selection for Cognitive-Behavioral Interventions for Pain

Many cancer and AIDS patients fear that focus on their pain will distract their physicians from treating the underlying causes of their disease and consequently are highly motivated to learn and practice cognitive-behavioral techniques. These techniques are often effective not only in pain control but in restoring a sense of self-control, personal efficacy, and active participation in one's care. It is important to note that these techniques must be used not as a substitute for appropriate analgesic management of pain but rather as part of a comprehensive, multimodal approach. The lack of side effects of these techniques make them attractive in the palliative-care setting as a supplement to already complicated medication regimens. The successful use of these techniques should never lead to the erroneous conclusion that the pain was of psychogenic origin and, as such, not "real." The mechanisms by which these cognitive and behavioral techniques relieve pain are not known; however, they all seem to share the elements of relaxation and distraction. Distraction or redirection of attention helps reduce awareness of pain, and relaxation reduces muscle tension and sympathetic arousal.[151]

Most patients with advanced illness and pain are appropriate candidates for useful application of these techniques; the clinician, however, should take into account the intensity of pain and the mental clarity of the patient. Ideal candidates have mild to moderate pain and can expect benefit, whereas patients with severe pain can expect limited benefit from psychological interventions unless somatic therapies can lower the level of pain to some degree. Confusional states interfere dramatically with a patient's ability to focus attention and thus limit the usefulness of these techniques.[152] Occasionally, these techniques can be modified to make them suitable even for mildly cognitive impaired patients. This often requires the therapist to take a more active role by orienting the patient, creating a safe and secure environment, and evoking a conditioned response to the therapist's voice or presence.

Barriers to engaging patients in cognitive-behavioral therapies can be divided into physician/nurse-based barriers and patient-based barriers. The health-care provider who works with patients with advanced illness may have particular difficulty in becoming comfortable with the use of behavioral therapies. Pharmacotherapy is highly effective in the management of pain, and to physicians it seems simpler and easier to use than labor-intensive and time-consuming nonpharmacologic interventions. Physicians and nurses have typical concerns about the practice of behavioral interventions, such as: "What if the

patient laughs, doesn't buy it?" or "It seems too theatrical, unscientific, nonmedical, too New Age!" The effort expended in overcoming such obstacles will be greatly rewarded. It is imperative that physicians working with patients with advanced illness be aware of the effective nonpharmacologic interventions for pain available and be able to make appropriate referrals to practitioners who can provide such interventions.

Patients themselves may be uncertain about the utility of behavioral therapies. Some may ask, "How can breathing take away my pain?" They may be frightened by the word "hypnosis" and its connotations. Hypnosis, as patients conceptualize it, is often associated with powerful and magical properties; some patients become frightened at the prospect of losing control or being under the influence of someone else. In our practice we generally attempt to introduce behavioral interventions only after we've been able to establish some rapport with the patient and engage him in an alliance with us. Occasionally, some patients may benefit from a discussion of the theoretical basis of these interventions; however, we stress that it is not important to understand why a technique works but rather to use the technique that works. Apprehensions must be affirmed and dealt with. Patients must also feel in control of the process at all times and be reassured that they can stop at any time.

General Instructions for Using Cognitive-Behavioral Therapy

A general approach to using cognitive-behavioral interventions with patients with advanced illness and pain involves the following: assessing the symptom, choosing a cognitive-behavioral strategy, and preparing the patient and the setting.

The main purpose of conducting a cognitive-behavioral assessment of pain is to determine what, if any, behavioral interventions are indicated.[152] One must initially engage the patient, establish a therapeutic alliance, and obtain a history of the pain symptom. One should review previous efforts to treat the patient's pain and collect data regarding the nature of the pain and its impact on the patient and his family.

The assessment process can lead to a variety of potential behavioral interventions. Choosing the appropriate behavioral strategy involves taking into consideration the patient's medical condition and physical and cognitive limitations, as well as such issues as time constraints and practical matters; for instance, patients with cognitive impairment or delirium will probably be unable to keep a pain diary or employ techniques that involve cognitive manipulation.

Relaxation Techniques   Several techniques can be used to achieve a mental and physical state of relaxation. Muscular tension, autonomic arousal, and mental distress exacerbate pain.[151,152] Some specific relaxation techniques include passive relaxation, focusing attention on sensations of warmth and decreased tension in various parts of the body; progressive muscle relaxation, involving active tensing and relaxing of muscles; and meditation. Other techniques that employ both relaxation and cognitive techniques include hypnosis, biofeedback, and music therapy and are discussed later in this chapter.

Passive relaxation, focused breathing, and passive muscle relaxation exercises involve the focusing of attention systematically on one's breathing, on sensations of warmth and relaxation, or on release of muscular tension in various body parts. Verbal suggestions and imagery are used to help promote relaxation. Muscle relaxation is an important component of the relaxation response and can augment the benefits of simple focused breathing exercises, leading to a deeper experience of relaxation and self-control.

Progressive or active muscle relaxation involves the active tensing and relaxing of various muscle groups in the body, focusing attention on the sensations of tension and relaxation. Clinically, in the hospital setting, relaxation is most commonly achieved through the use of a combination of focused breathing and progressive muscle relaxation exercises. Once patients are in a relaxed state, imagery techniques can then be used to induce deeper relaxation and facilitate distraction from or manipulation of a variety of cancer-related symptoms.

The following script is a generic relaxation exercise, utilizing passive relaxation or focused breathing. It is based on and integrates the work of Erickson,[150] Benson,[153] and others.[147]

Script for Passive Relaxation
(Focused Breathing)

"Why don't you begin by finding a comfortable position. It could be in a bed or in a chair. Slowly allow your body to unwind and just let it go. That's it. I wonder if you can allow your body to become as calm as possible . . . just let it go, just let your body sink into that bed (or chair) . . . feel free to move or shift around in any way that your body needs to, to find that comfortable position. You need not try very hard, simply and easily allow yourself to follow the sound of my voice as you allow your body to find itself a safe, comfortable position to relax in.

If you like, [patient's name here], you can gently allow your eyes to close, just let the lids cover your eyes . . . allow your eyes to sink back deeply into their sockets . . . that's it, just let them go, falling back gently and deeply into their sockets as your lids begin to feel heavier and heavier. As you allow your head to fall back deeply into the pillow, feeling the weight of your head sinking into the pillow as you breathe out, just breathe out, one big breath. Slowly, if you can begin to turn your attention to your breathing. Notice your breath for a few moments, how much air you take in, how much air you let out, and just breathe evenly and naturally, and with the sound of my voice I wonder if you can begin to take in more air, breathing in and out, in and out, that's it, gradually breathing in and out . . . in and out . . . breathing in calmness and quietness, breathing out tiredness and frustration, that's it . . . let it go, it's not important to you now . . . breathing in quietness and control, breathing out fear and tension . . . breathing in and out . . . in and out . . . you can enjoy breathing in this relaxed way for as long as you need to. You are peaceful now as you continue to observe your even and steady breathing that is allowing you to feel gentle and calm, breathing that is allowing you to feel a gentle calm, that's it, breathing relaxation in and tension out . . . in and out . . . breathing in quietness and control, breathing out tiredness and tension . . . that's it, [patient's name here]. Continue to notice the quietness and stillness of your body. Why don't you take a few quiet moments to experience this process more fully?"

It may be helpful for the clinician to mark the end of an exercise by increasing the pace, raising the volume of voice, and shifting position. Additionally, it is helpful for the clinician to both pace and model for the patient. This includes positioning yourself as similarly to the patient as possible (e.g., closing your eyes, assuming a position of relaxation, and breathing at the same rate). If the patient exhibits any visible anxiety or agitation, this can be briefly explored verbally, and then, if appropriate, the exercise can be continued.

Script for Active or Progressive Muscle Relaxation

This exercise involves having the patient actively tense and then relax specific body parts. Once again, it may be helpful if the clinician paces and models for the patient.

> "Now, I wonder if you can tense up every muscle in your body . . . that's it, squeeze in the muscles . . . hold it, and then just let it go . . . once more, tense up your muscles . . . make them very tight and tense, hold it, hold it . . . and then breathe out, and let your muscles relax, just let them go . . . Now, as your body begins to feel more and more relaxed, clench your jaw, squeeze it tight, clench it, and then let it go . . . now open your mouth wide, as wide as it will go, stick out your tongue, stick it way out, hold it and then let it go. Feel your head becoming more and more relaxed, as it sinks down into the pillow, allowing all the tension and tightness to drift out of it. . . . Now, I wonder if you can lift up your shoulders, lift them up, up to your ears, hold them there, squeezing them tightly, squeeze, and then let them drop down, just let them go . . . and then once more lift them up . . . hold it . . . then let them go . . . as you feel all the tightness and tension in your shoulders begin to drain away. . . . Now, I wonder if you can clench your hands into a fist, make a tight fist as your whole arm tightens, tense your arms as you squeeze in your fingers tighter and tighter . . . and now just let them go, once more now make a fist, a tight fist, hold it, and then let it go."

As with passive muscle relaxation, the clinician guides the patient through the exercise, requesting the patient to tense and release specific muscles in a progressive order.

Imagery/Distraction Techniques   Clinically, relaxation techniques are most helpful in managing pain when combined with some distracting or pleasant imagery. The use of distraction or focusing involves control over the focus of attention and can be used to make the patient less aware of the noxious stimuli.[154] One can employ imaginative inattention by picturing oneself on a beach. Mental distraction can be used and is similar to the practice of counting sheep to aid sleep. Keeping oneself busy is a form of behavioral distraction, Imagery—using one's imagination while in a relaxed state—can be used to transform pain into a warm or cold sensation. One can also imaginatively transform the context of pain, for example, imagining oneself in battle on the football field instead of the hospital bed. Disassociated somatization can be employed by some patients. In this technique they imagine that a painful body part is no longer part of their body.[152] It is important to note that not every patient finds these techniques acceptable, and the therapist must try out a number of approaches to determine which are consistent with the patient's style.

Imagery (often referred to as guided imagery) is most effective when the specific image is obtained from the patient. The clinician may ask the patient to close his or her eyes and think of a place, an activity, or an experience where the patient felt most safe and secure. The clinician may suggest that the patient visualize a favorite beach scene or a room in a house, or see himself riding a bicycle in a state park. Once the patient identifies the scene, the clinician may ask the patient to elaborate on the scene, asking for specific details, such as the temperature, season, time of day, type of ocean (calm, or with big waves), and so on. The clinician then utilizes this information and describes an image for the patient in detail. The skill is for the clinician to be as flexible and as creative as possible and to elaborate on the scene, utilizing all aspects of the senses and bodily sensations such as "feel the suns rays touching your skin, allow your skin to feel warm and tingly all over" or "breathe in the fresh, clear air, and allow it to fill your lungs with its freshness" or "feel the fresh dew of the grass under your feet." The clinician can focus on aromas in the garden or the sounds of birds singing, always reminding the patient to breathe evenly and steadily as he or she feels more and more relaxed and more and more in control. If possible, the clinician should avoid volunteering an image or scene for the patient because the clinician is unaware of the association or meaning the image may have for the patient. For example, a patient may have a fear of the water, and therefore a beach scene may evoke feelings of fear and loss of control.

Script for Pleasant Distracting Imagery

> "Once you are in a comfortable position, I wonder if you can continue lying there with your eyes closed, continuing to breathe in out . . . in and out

to the sound of my voice. Let your mind wander . . . just let it go . . . and if any unwanted thoughts come into your mind, you can allow then to pass out as easily as they came in. . . . You don't need them now . . . they are not important to you now. You have the ability to control your thoughts. You have the ability to be in control."

The clinician now begins to describe a specific image in detail as originally suggested by the patient.

"Slowly, I wonder if you can allow your mind to travel . . . to travel far away to your favorite beach. The beach that you have many fond memories of. I wonder if you can imagine that it's almost the end of the day and the beach is deserted . . . and the sun, while setting, is still warm, as it beats down . . . and makes your skin feel tingly and warm all over. As you begin to walk on the sand, you can feel the granules underneath your feet. Step evenly and steadily along the sand. As you look around, you can see the different colors in the sky. You can see for miles off into the distance, and you feel exhilarated and free because no one is around you. You are alone and in control. As you walk closer to the edge of the ocean, the sand is becoming a little damp, and you can feel the dampness underneath your feet—it feels refreshing. As you continue walking, you may notice a few odds and ends on the sand, maybe something that the ocean brought in . . . some shells perhaps. They may be broken from being knocked against the rocks . . . or there may be a few bits of seaweed or some jellyfish. You stop to notice them as you walk past . . . marveling at the wonders of nature. As you get to the edge of the ocean, you can feel the tiny little ripples of water washing over your feet . . . bouncing over your feet making you feel light and fresh. The water is warm—it soothes your feet. Washing back and forth . . . back and forth. As you keep walking, you see your rubber raft. This is your old, dependable rubber raft. You get to the raft, and you secure it in your hands and lie down on it, letting your whole body sink into the raft—just let it go . . . that's it. Slowly you kick off as the raft begins to take you away. The ocean is very calm and very gentle. Your whole body begins to unwind and sink deeper and deeper into the raft as you feel more and more relaxed. This raft allows you to drift off . . . and underneath you can feel the ripples of the ocean . . . rocking back and forth . . . back and forth as you continue to float away evenly and gently. You can become aware of the sun beating down in your skin. You are aware of the sounds around you—you can hear the ocean washing against the rocks as the waves rock back and forth . . . back and forth. You can hear the gulls crying in the distance. There is a very tiny protected bay that you are floating away in. It is a very calm and peaceful day, and you are feeling more and more relaxed. You are in control now . . . and as you continue to sail away, all your troubles and problems wash right out of you. They're not important to you now. You don't need them now. What's important is that your whole body, from the tip of your toes all the way up to the top of your head, is relaxed and calm in this very safe and private place that is your own. You can continue to lie here as you rock back and forth . . . back and forth for as long as you need to.

"When you are ready, you can slowly readjust yourself to the sound of my voice and I am going to count slowly backward from 10 and with each count backward, you can become more and more familiar with where you are. Perhaps when I get to number 5 you may want to open your eyes, or you can keep then closed for as long as you need to. Ten, 9 . . . become aware of the sounds around you . . . 8, 7 . . . become aware of the temperature of the room—how does it feel? how does your body feel? . . . 6, 5 . . . you can open your eyes now if you want to or you can keep them closed . . . 4, 3, 2, 1. You can stay in this relaxed position for as long as you need to. When you feel ready you may slowly prepare to sit up."

Hypnosis   Hypnosis can be a useful adjunct in the management of cancer pain.[146,155-158] In a controlled trial comparing hypnosis with cognitive behavioral therapy in relieving mucositis following a bone marrow transplant, patients utilizing hypnosis reported a significant reduction in pain compared to patients who used cognitive-behavioral techniques.[152] The hypnotic trance is essentially a state of heightened and focused concentration, and thus it can be used to manipulate the perception of pain. The depth of hypnotizability may determine the effectiveness as well as the strategies employed during hypnosis. One-third of cancer patients, as is the case with the general population, are not hypnotizable, and it is recommended that other techniques be employed for them. Of the two-thirds of patients who are identified as being less, moderately, and highly hypnotizable, three principles underlie the use of hypnosis in controlling pain:[155] use self-hypnosis; relax, do not fight the pain; and use a mental filter to ease the hurt in pain. Patients who are moderately and highly hypnotizable can often alter sensations in a painful area by changing temperature sensation or experiencing tingling. Less hypnotizable patients can often utilize an alternative focus by concentrating on a sensation in a nonaffected body part or on a mental image of a pleasant scene. The main disadvantage of hypnosis for cancer patients is that the technique frequently requires more attentional capacity than these patients have.

Biofeedback Fotopoulos et al.[159] noted significant pain relief in a group of cancer patients who were taught electromyographic (EMG) and electroencephalographic (EEG) biofeedback-assisted relaxation. Only 2 of 17 were able to maintain analgesia after the treatment ended. A lack of generalization of effect can be a problem with biofeedback techniques. Although physical condition may make a prolonged training period impossible, especially for the terminally ill, most cancer patients can often utilize EMG and temperature biofeedback techniques for learning relaxation-assisted pain control.[160]

Music, Aroma, and Art Therapies

Munro and Mount[161] have written extensively on the use of music therapy with cancer patients, documenting clinical examples and suggesting mechanisms of action. Music can often capture the attention like no other stimulus; it offers patients a new form of expression and helps patients distract themselves from their perception of pain, while expressing themselves in meaningful ways.[162]

Aromas have been shown to have innate relaxing and stimulating qualities. Our colleagues at Memorial Hospital have recently begun to explore the use of aroma therapy for the treatment of procedure-related anxiety (i.e., anxiety related to MRI scans). Utilizing the scent heliotropin, Manne et al.[163] reported that two-thirds of the patients in their study found the scent especially pleasant and reported feeling much less anxiety than those who were not exposed to the scent during MRI. As a general relaxation technique, aroma therapy may have an application for pain management, but this is as yet unstudied.

Art therapy allows less verbally skilled adults or children to express their fears and concerns in a more comfortable fashion. The creative experience can be used as both an important means of providing support and an avenue for providing patients with psychological insights into their experience.[164]

SUMMARY

The management of the pain associated with advanced disease such as AIDS or cancer represents a significant challenge for the palliative care practitioner, as well as the consultant psychiatrist, psychologist, or social worker. A thorough familiarity with both the pharmacological and nonpharmacological management of cancer and AIDS pain offers the mental health consultant the tools to help distinguish between the distress of unrelieved or poorly managed pain and the psychological distress that can accompany pain in advanced disease. Such knowledge also provides palliative care clinicians with the tools to decrease psychological distress for patients with pain and advanced disease, as well as improving overall quality of life.

References

1. Foley KM. Pain syndromes in patients with cancer. In: Bonica JJ, Ventafriddi V, Fink RB, Jones LE, Loeser JD, eds, *Advances in Pain Research and Therapy*. Vol 2. New York: Raven, 1975:59–75.
2. Foley KM. The treatment of cancer pain. *New England Journal of Medicine*, 1985; 313:84–95.
3. Breitbart W, Holland J. Psychiatric aspects of cancer pain. In: Foley KM et al, ed, *Advances in Pain Research and Therapy*. Vol. 16. New York: Raven Press, 1990:73–87.
4. Breitbart W. Psychiatric management of cancer pain. *Cancer*, 1989; 63:2336–2342.
5. Breitbart W. Psychiatric aspects of pain and HIV disease. *Focus: A Guide to AIDS Research and Counseling*, 1990; 5:1–2.
6. Massie MJ, Holland JC. The cancer patient with pain: psychiatric complications and their management. *Medical Clinics of North America*, 1987; 71:245–258.
7. Bonica JJ. Cancer pain. In: Bonica JJ, ed, *The Management of Pain*. 2nd ed. Vol 1. Philadelphia: Lea and Febiger, 400–460.
8. Twycross RG, Lack SA. *Symptom Control in Far Advanced Cancer: Pain Relief*. London: Pitman Brooks, 1983.
9. Marks RM, Sachar RJ. Undertreatment of med-

ical inpatients with narcotic analgesics. *Ann Intern Med*, 1983; 78:173–181.

10. Grond S, Zech D, Dienfenbach C, Bischoff A. Prevalence and pattern of symptoms inpatients with cancer pain: a prospective evaluation of 1635 cancer patients referred to a pain clinic. *Journal of Pain and Symptom Management*, 1994; 9:372–383.

11. Breitbart W, McDonald MV, Rosenfeld B, Passik SD, Hewitt D, Thaler H, Portenoy RK. Pain in ambulatory AIDS patients I: characteristics and medical correlates. *Pain*, 1996; 68:315–321.

12. Lebovits AK, Lefkowitz M, McCarthy D, et al. The prevalence and management of pain in patients with AIDS. A review of 134 cases. *Clinical Journal of Pain*, 1989; 5:245–248.

13. Schofferman J, Brody R. Pain in far advanced AIDS. In Foley KM et al, eds, *Advances in Pain Research and Therapy*. Vol. 16. New York: Raven, 1990:379–386.

14. Singer EJ, Zorilla C, Fahy-Chandon B, et al. Painful symptoms reported for ambulatory HIV-infected men in a longitudinal study. *Pain*, 1993; 54:15–19.

15. Kimball LR, McCormick WC. The pharmacologic management of pain and discomfort in persons with AIDS near the end of life: use of opioid analgesia in the hospice setting. *Journal of Pain and Symptom Management*, 1996; 11:88–94.

16. Larue F, Fontaine A, Colleau SN. Underestimation and undertreatment of pain in HIV disease: multicenter study. *British Medical Journal*, 1997; 314:223–228.

17. Larue L, Brasseur L, Massueault P, Demeulemeester R, Bonifassi L, Bez G. Pain and HIV infection: a French national survey. *Journal of Palliative Care*, 1994; 10:95. Abstract.

18. O'Neil WM, Sherrard JS. Pain in human immunodeficiency virus disease: A review. *Pain*, 1993; 54:3–14.

19. Penfold R, Clark AJM. Pain syndromes in HIV infection. *Canadian Journal of Anaesthesia*, 1992; 39:724–730.

20. Connolly GM, Hawkins D, Harcourt-Webster JN, Parsons PA, Husain OAN, Gazzard BG. Oesophageal symptoms, their causes, treatment and prognosis in patients with the acquired immunodeficiency syndrome. *Gut*, 1989; 30:1033–1039.

21. Eisner MS, Smith PD. Etiology of odynophagia and dysphagia in patients with the acquired immunodeficiency syndrome. *Arthritis and Rheumatism*, 1990; 31:A446.

22. Wexner SD, Smithy WB, Milsom JW, Dailey TH. The surgical management of anorectal dis-eases in AIDS and pre-AIDS patients. *Disease of the Colon and Rectum*, 1986; 29:719–723.

23. Breitbart W. Pain in AIDS: an overview. *Pain Reviews*, 1998; 5:247–272.

24. Steifel F. Psychosocial aspects of cancer pain. *Supportive Care in Cancer*, 1993; 1:130–134.

25. Saunders CM. *The Management of Terminal Illness*. New York: Hospital Medicine Publications, 1967.

26. Hanks GW. Opioid responsive and opioid non-responsive pain in cancer. *British Medical Bulletin*, 1991; 47:718–731.

27. Syrjala K, Chapko M. Evidence for a bio-physchosocial model of cancer treatment-related pain. *Pain*, 1995; 61:69–79.

28. Watson CP, Chipman M, Reed K, Evans RJ, Birkett N. Amitriptyline versus maprotiline in post herpetic neuralgia: A randomized double-blind, cross-over trial. *Pain*, 1992; 48:29–36.

29. Kishore-Kumar R, Max MB, Scafer SC, et al. Desipramine relieves post-herpetic neuralgia. *Clinical Pharmacological Therapy*, 1990; 47:305–312.

30. Portenoy RK, Foley KM. Management of cancer pain. In: Holland JC, Rowland JH, eds, *Handbook of Psychooncology*. New York: Oxford University Press, 1989:369–382.

31. Foley KM. The treatment of cancer pain. *New England Journal of Medicine*, 1985; 313:4–95.

32. World Health Organization. *Cancer Pain Relief*. Geneva: World Health Organization, 1986.

33. Jacox A, Carr D, Payne R, Berde CB, Breitbart W, et al. Clinical Practice Guideline Number 9: Management of Cancer Pain. U.S. Department of Health and Human Services, Public Health Service, Agency for Health Care Policy and Research, 1994; AHCPR Publication No. 94-0592: 139–41.

34. Portenoy RK. Pharmacologic approaches to the control of cancer pain. *Journal of Psychosocial Oncology*, 1990; 8:75–107.

35. Portenoy RK. Adjuvant analgesics in pain management. In: Doyle D, Hanks GWC, MacDonald N, eds, *Oxford Textbook of Palliative Medicine*. New York: Oxford University Press, 1993:187–203.

36. Elliot K, Foley KM. Pain Syndromes in the cancer patient. *Journal of Psychosocial Oncology*, 1990; 8:11–45.

37. Fishman B, Pasternack S, Wallenstein SL, et al. The Memorial Pain Assessment Card: a valid instrument for the evaluation of cancer pain. *Cancer*, 1987; 60:1151–1158.

38. Daut RL, Cleeland CS, Flanery RC. Development of the Wisconsin Brief Pain Questionnaire to Assess Pain in Cancer and Other Disease. *Pain*, 1983; 17:197–210.

39. Cleeland CS, Gonin R, Hatfield AK, et al. Pain and its treatment in outpatients with metastatic cancer: the Eastern Cooperative Oncology group's outpatient study. *New England Journal of Medicine*, 1994; 330:592–596.

40. McCormack JP, Li R, Zarowny D, Singer J. Inadequate treatment of pain in ambulatory HIV patients. *The Clinical Journal of Pain*, 1993; 9: 279–283.

41. Breitbart W, Rosenfeld B, Passik S, McDonald M, Thaler H, Portenoy RK. Undertreatment of pain in Ambulatory AIDS patients. *Pain*, 1996; 65:243–249.

42. Breitbart W, Passik S, McDonald MV, Rosenfeld B, Smith M, Kaim M, Furesh Esch J. Patient Related barriers to pain management in Ambulatory AIDS patients, *Pain*, 1998; 76:9–16.

43. Breitbart W, Rosenfeld B, Kaim M. Clinicians' perceptions of barriers to pain management in AIDS. *Journal of Pain and Symptom Management*, 1999; 18:203–212.

44. Charap AD. The knowledge, attitudes, and experience of medical personnel treating pain in the terminally ill. *Mt. Sinai Journal of Medicine*, 1978; 45:561–601.

45. Macaluso C, Weinberg D, Foley KM. Opiod abuse and misuse in a cancer pain population. (Abstract) Second International Congress on Cancer Pain.

46. Kanner RM, Foley KM. Patterns of narcotic use in a cancer pain clinic. *Annals of the New York Academy of Sciences*, 1981; 362:161–172.

47. Breitbart W, Rosenfeld B, Passik S, Kaim M, Furesh Esch J. A comparison of pain report and adequacy of analgesic therapy in ambulatory AIDS patients with and without a history of substance abuse. *Pain*, 1997; 72:235–243.

48. Bruera E, MacMillan K, Pither J, MacDonald RN. Effects of morphine on the dyspnea of terminal cancer patients. *Journal of Pain and Symptom Management*, 1990; 5:341–344.

49. Grossman SA, Sheidler VR, Sweden K, Mucenski J, Piantadosi S. Correlations of patient and caregiver ratings of cancer pain. *Journal of Pain and Symptom Management*, 1991; 6:53–57.

50. Daut RL, Cleeland CS. The prevalence and severity of pain in cancer. *Cancer*, 1982; 50:1913–1918.

51. Spiegel D, Bloom JR. Pain in metastatic breast cancer. *Cancer*, 1983; 52:341–345.

52. Padilla G, Ferrell B, Grant M, Rhiner M. Defining the content domain of quality of life for cancer patients with pain. *Cancer Nursing*, 1990; 13:108–115.

53. Payne D, Jacobsen P, Breitbart W, Passik S, Rosenfeld B, McDonald M. Negative thoughts related to pain are associated with greater pain, distress, and disability in AIDS pain. Presentation American Pain Society, Miami, Florida. 1994.

54. Payne D. *Cognition in Cancer Pain*. Unpublished dissertation. 1995.

55. McKegney FP, Bailey CR, Yates JW. Prediction and management of pain in patients with advanced cancer. *General Hospital Psychiatry*, 1981; 3:95–101.

56. Bond MR, Pearson IB. Psychological aspects of pain in women with advanced cancer of the cervix. *Journal of Psychosomatic Research*, 1969; 13:13–19.

57. Syrjala K, Chapko M. Evidence for a biopsychosocial model of cancer treatment-related pain. *Pain*, 1995; 61:69–79.

58. Rosenfeld B, Breitbart W, McDonald MV, Passik SD, Thaler H, Portenoy RK. Pain in Ambulatory AIDS patients II: impact of pain on physiological functioning and quality of life. *Pain*, 1996; 68:323–328.

59. Cleeland CS, Tearnan BH. Behavioral control of cancer pain. In: Holzman D, Turk D, eds, *Pain Management*. New York: Pergamon Press, 1986: 193–212.

60. Derogatis LR, Morrow GR, Fetting J, et al. The prevalence of psychiatric disorders among cancer patients. JAMA, 1983; 249:751–757.

61. Ahles TA, Blanchard EB, Ruckdeschel JC. The multidimensional nature of cancer related pain. *Pain*, 1983; 17:277–288.

62. Woodforde JM, Fielding JR. Pain and Cancer. *Journal of Psychosomatic Research*, 1970; 14:365–370.

63. Breitbart W, Stiefel F, Kornblith AB, Pannullo S. Neuropsychiatric disturbances in cancer patients with epidural spinal cord compression receiving high dose corticosteroids: A prospective comparison study. *Psycho-oncology*, 1993; 2:223–245.

64. Stiefel FC, Breitbart W, Holland J. Corticosteroids in cancer: Neuropsychiatric complications. *Cancer Investigation*, 1989; 7:479–491.

65. Bukberg J, Penman D, Holland J. Depression in hospitalized cancer patients. *Psychosomatic Medicine*, 1984; 43:199–222.

66. Massie MJ, Holland J, Glass E. Delirium in terminally ill cancer patients. *American Journal of Psychiatry*, 1983; 140:1048–1050.

67. Steifel F, Fainsinger R, Bruera E. Acute confusional states in patients with advanced cancer. *Journal of Pain and Symptom Management*. 1992; 7:94–98.

68. Breitbart W, Pharmacotherapy of pain in AIDS. In: Wormser GE, ed, *A Clinical Guide to AIDS and HIV*. Philadelphia: Lippincott-Raven Publishers, 1996:359–378.

69. Breitbart W. Cancer pain and suicide. In: Foley KM et al, eds, *Advances in Pain Research and Therapy*. Vol. 16. New York: Raven, 1990:399–412.

70. Sison A, Eller K, Segal J, Passik S, Breitbart W. Suicidal ideation in ambulatory HIV-infected patients: the roles of pain, mood, and disease status. (Abstract) *Current Concepts in Psycho-oncology IV*. New York. October 10–12, 1991.

71. Levin DN, Cleeland CS, Dan R. Public attitudes toward cancer pain. *Cancer*, 1985; 56:2337–2339.

72. Bolund C. Suicide and cancer: II. Medical and care factors in suicide by cancer patients in Sweden. 1973–1976. *Journal of Psychosocial Oncology*, 1985; 3:17–30.

73. Farberow NL, Schneidman ES, Leonard CV. Suicide among general medical and surgical hospital patients with malignant neoplasms. *Medical Bulletin 9*, Washington D.C., U.S. Veterans Administration. 1963.

74. Massie MJ, Gagnon P, Holland J. Depression and Suicide in Patients with Cancer. *Journal of Pain and Symptom Management* Vol. 9. 1994; 5:325–331.

75. Breitbart W. Suicide in cancer patients. *Oncology*, 1987; 1:49–53.

76. Achte KA, Vanhkonen ML. Cancer and the psych. Omega, 1971; 2:46–56.

77. Silberfarb PM, Manrer LH, Cronthamel CS. Psychological aspects of neoplastic disease, I: Functional status of breast cancer patients during different treatment regimens. *American Journal of Psychiatry*, 1980; 137:450–455.

78. Brown JH, Henteleff P, Barakat S, Rowe CJ: Is it normal for terminally ill patients to desire death. *American Journal of Psychiatry*, 1986; 143: 208–211.

79. Saltzburg D, Breitbart W, Fishman B, et al. The relationship of pain and depression to suicidal ideation in cancer patients. (Abstract) ASCO Annual Meeting. May 21–23, San Francisco, 1989.

80. Marzuk P, Tierney H, Tardiff K, Gross G, Morgan E, Hsu M, Mann J. Increased risk of suicide in persons with AIDS. *JAMA*, 1988; 259:1333–1337.

81. Abkin J, Remien R, Katoff L, Williams J. Suicidality in AIDS long-term survivors: what is the evidence? *AIDS-Care*, Vol 5, 1993; 4:401–411.

82. Belkin GS, Fleishman JA, Stein MD, Pieste J, Mor V: Physical symptoms and depressive symptoms among individuals with HIV infection. *Psychosomatics*, 1992; 33:416–427.

83. Ventafridda V, Caraceni A, Gamba A. Field testing of the WHO Guidelines for Cancer Pain Relief: summary report of demonstration projects. In: Foley KM, Bonica JJ, Ventafridda V, eds, *Proceedings of the Second International Congress on Pain. Vol 16, Advances in Pain Research and Therapy*. New York: Raven Press, Ltd., 1990a:155–165.

84. Anand A, Carmosino L, Glatt AE. Evaluation of recalcitrant pain in HIV-infected hospitalized patients. *Journal of Acquired Immune Deficiency Syndromes*, 1994; 7:52–56.

85. Kaplan R, Conant M, Curdiff D, et al. Sustained-release morphine sulfate in the management of pain associated with acquired immune deficiency syndrome. *Journal of Pain and Symptom Management* 1996; 12:150–160.

86. Lefkowitz M, Newshan G. An evaluation of the use of analgesics for chronic pain in patients with AIDS (Abstract) In: Proceedings of the 16th annual scientific meeting of the American Pain Society. 1997 Oct 23–26, p. 71, Abst # 684.

87. Foley KM, Intrussi CE. Analgesic drug therapy in cancer pain: principles and practice. In: Payne R, Foley KM, eds, *Cancer Pain Medical Clinics of North America*. Philadelphia: W.B. Saunders, 1987:207–232.

88. Kantor TG. Peripherally acting analgesics. In: Kuhar M, Pasternak C, eds, *Analgesics: Neurochemical, Behavioral and Clinical Perspectives*. New York: Raven Press, 1984:289–313.

89. Brooks MP, Day OR. Nonsteroidal anti-inflammatory drugs differences and similarities. *The New England Journal of Medicine*, 1991; 24:1716–1725.

90. Murray MD, Brater DC. Adverse effects of nonsteroidal anti-inflammatory drugs on renal function. *Annals of Internal Medicine*, 1990; 112:559–560.

91. Radeck K, Deck C. Do nonsteroidal anti-inflammatory drugs interfere with blood pressure control in hypertensive patients? *Journal of General Internal Medicine*, 1987; 2:108–112.

92. *American Pain Society: Principles of Analgesic Use in the Treatment of Acute Pain and Cancer Pain*, Third ed. Skokie, IL: American Pain Society, 1992.

93. Bruera E, Chadwick S, Brennels, Hanson J, MacDonald RN. Methylphenidate associated with narcotics for the treatment of cancer pain. *Cancer Treatment Report*, 1987; 71:67–70.

94. Breitbart W. Psychotrophic adjuvant analgesics pain in cancer and AIDS. *Psycho-Oncology*, 1998; 7:333–345.

95. Kaiko R, Foley K, Grabinski P, et al. Central nervous system excitation effects of meperidine in cancer patients. *Annals of Neurology*, 1983; 13: 180–183.

96. Breitbart W, Sparrow B. Management of delirium in the terminally ill. *Progress in Palliative Care*, 1998; 6:107–113.

97. Butler S. Present status of tricyclic antidepressants in chronic pain therapy. In: Benedetti, et al., eds, *Advances in Pain Research and Therapy and Therapy*. Vol. 7. New York: Raven, 1986:173–196.

98. France RD. The future of antidepressants: treatment of pain. *Psychopathology*, 1987; 20:99–113.

99. Ventafridda V, Bonezzi C, Caraceni A, et al. Antidepressants for cancer pain and other painful syndromes with deafferentation component: Comparison of amitriptyline and trazodone. *Italian Journal of Neurological Sciences*, 1987; 8:579–587.

100. Getto CJ, Sorkness CA, Howell T. Antidepressant and chronic malignant pain: a review. *Journal of Pain Symptom Control*, 1987; 2:9–18.

101. Magni G, Arsie D, Deleo D. Antidepressants in the treatment of cancer pain. A survey in Italy. *Pain*, 1987; 29:347–353.

102. Walsh TD. Controlled study of imipramine and morphine in chronic pain due to advanced cancer. In: Foley KM, et al., *Advances in Pain Research and Therapy*, vol. 16. New York: Raven Press, 1986:155–165.

103. Botney M, Fields HC. Amitriptyline potentiates morphine analgesia by direct action on the central nervous system. *Annals of Neurology*, 1983; 13:160–164.

104. Malseed RT, Goldstein FJ. Enhancement of morphine analgesics by tricyclic antidepressants. *Neuropharmacology*, 1979; 18:827–829.

105. Ventafridda V, Branchi M, Ripamonti C, et al. Studies on the effects of antidepressant drugs on the antinociceptive action of morphine and on plasma morphine in rat and man. *Pain*, 1990; 43:155–162.

106. Spiegel K, Kalb R, Pasternak GW. Analgesic activity of tricyclic antidepressants. *Annals of Neurology*, 1983; 13:462–465.

107. Gram LF. Receptors, pharmacokinetics and clinical effects. In: Burrows GD, et al., eds, *Antidepressants*. Amsterdam: Elsevier, Amsterdam, 1983: 81–95.

108. Mersky H, Hamilton JT. An open trial of possible analgesic effects of dipyridamole. *Journal of Symptom Management*, 1989; 4:34–37.

109. Devor M. Nerve pathophysiology and mechanisms of pain in causalgia. *Journal of the Autonomic Nervous System*, 1983; 7:371–384.

110. Pillowsky I, Hallet EC, Bassett EL, Thomas PG, Penhall RK. A controlled study of amitryptyline in the treatment of chronic pain. *Pain*, 1982; 14:169–179.

111. Max MB, Culnane M, Schafer SC, Gracely RH, et al. Amitryptyline relieves diabetic neuropathy pain in patients with normal and depressed mood. *Neurology*, 1987; 47:589–596.

112. Sharav Y, Singer E, Dione RA, Dubner R. The analgesic effect of amitriptyline on chronic facial pain. *Pain*, 1987; 31:199–209.

113. Young RJ, Clarke BF. Pain relief in diabetic neuropathy: the effectiveness of imipramine and related drugs. *Diabetic Medicine*, 1985; 2:363–366.

114. Sindrup SH, Ejlersten B, Froland A, et al. Imipiramine treatment in diabetic neuropathy: relief of subjective symptoms without changes in peripheral and autonomic nerve function. *European Journal of Clinical Pharmacology*, 1989; 37:151–153.

115. Max MB. Effects of desipramine, amitryptyline and fluoxetine on pain and diabetic neuropathy. *New England Journal of Medicine*, 1992; 326: 1250–1256.

116. Gomez-Perez FJ, Rull JA, Dies H, et al. Nortriptyline and fluphenazine in the symptomatic treatment of diabetic neuropathy: A double-blind cross-over study. *Pain*, 1985; 23:395–400.

117. Langohr HD, Stohr M, Petruch F. An open and double-blind crossover study on the efficacy of cloniramine (anafranil) in patients with painful mono- and polyneuropathies. *European Neurology*, 1982; 21:309–315.

118. Tiengo M, Pagnoni B, Calmi A, et al. Chlorimipramine compared to pentazocine as a unique treatment in post-operative pain. *International Journal of Clinical Pharmacology Research*, 1987; 7:141–143.

119. Hammeroff SR, Cork RC, Scherer K, et al. Doxepin effects on chronic pain, depression and plasma opioids. *Journal of Clinical Psychiatry*, 1982; 2:22–26.

120. Davidoff G, Guarracini M, Roth E, et al. Trazodone hydrochloride in the treatment of dysesthetic pain in traumatic myelopathy: a randomized, double-blind placebo-controlled study. *Pain*, 1987; 29:151–161.

121. Costa D, Mogos I, Toma T. Efficacy and safety of mainserin in the treatment of depression of woman with cancer. *Acta Psychiatrica Scandinavica*, 1985; 72:85–92.

122. Eberhard G, Von Khorring L, Nilsson HL, et al. A double-blind randomized study of clonimpramine versus maprotiline inpatients with idio-

pathic pain syndromes. *Neuropsychobiology*, 1988; 19:25–32.

123. Feighner JP. A comparative trial of fluoxetine and amitriptyline in patients with major depressive disorder. *Journal of Clinical Psychiatry*, 1985; 46:369–372.

124. Hynes MD, Lochner MA, Bemis K, et al. Fluoxetine, a selective inhibitor of serotonin uptake, potentiates morphine analgesia without altering its discriminitive stimulus properties or affinity for opioid receptors. *Life Sciences*, 1985; 36:2317–2323.

125. Sindrup SH, Gram LF, Brosen K, Eshoj O, Mogenson EF. The selective serotonin reuptake inhibitor paroxetine is effective in the treatment of diabetic neuropathy symptoms. *Pain*, 1990; 42:135–144.

126. Diamond S, Frietag FG. The use of fluoxetine in the treatment of headache. *Clinical Journal of Pain*, 1989; 5:200–201.

127. Geller SA. Treatment of fibrositis with fluoxetine hydrochloride (Prozac). *American Journal of Medicine*, 1989; 87:594–595.

128. Pick CG, Paul D, Eison MS, Pasternak G. Potentiation of opioid analegia by the antidepressant nefazodone. *European Journal of Pharmacology*, 1992; 2:375–381.

129. Zitman FG, Linssen ACG, Edelbroek PM, Stijnen T. Low dose amitriptyline in chronic pain: the gain is modest. *Pain*, 1990; 42:35–42.

130. Portenoy RK. Adjuvant analgesics in pain management. In: Doyle D, Hans GWC, MacDonald N, eds, *Oxford Textbook of Palliative Medicine*, 2nd Edition, Oxford: Oxford University Press, 1998: 361–390.

131. Fernandez F, Levy JK. Psychiatric diagnosis and pharmacotherapy of patients with HIV infection. In: Tasman A, Goldfinger SM, Kaufman, eds, *Review of Psychiatry*. Vol. 9. Washington, D.C. American Psychiatric Press, 1990:614.

132. Bruera E, Breuneis C, Patterson AH, MacDonald RN. Use of methyphenidate as an adjuvant to narcotic analgesics in patients with advanced cancer. *Journal of Pain and Symptom Management*, 1989; 4:3–6.

133. Bruera E, Fainsinger R, MacEachern T, Hanson J. The use of methylphenidate in patients with incident cancer pain receiving regular opiates: a preliminary report. *Pain*, 1992; 50:75–77.

134. Forrest WH, et al. Dextroamphetamine with morphine for the treatment of post-operative pain. *New England Journal of Medicine*, 1977;296:712–715.

135. Breitbart W, Mermelstein H. Pemoline: an alternative psychostimulant in the management of depressive disorders in cancer patients. *Psychosomatics*. 1992; 33:352–356.

136. Beaver WT, Wallerstein SL, Houde RW, et al. A comparison of the analgesic effect methotrimeprazine and morphine in patients with cancer. *Clinical Pharmacological Therapy*, 1966; 7:436–466.

137. Maltbie AA, Cavenar SO, Sullivan JL, et al. Analgesic and haloperidol: a hypothesis. *Journal of Canadian Psychiatry*, 1979; 40:323–326.

138. Lehin F, Vander Dijs B, Lechin ME, et al. Pimozide therapy for trigeminal neuralgia. *Archives of Neurology*, 1989; 9:960–964.

139. Breitbart W, Marotta RF, Call P. AIDS and neuroleptic malignant syndrome. *Lancet*, 1988; 2:1488.

140. Fernandez F, Adams F, Holmes VF. Analgesic effect of alprazolam in patients with chronic, organic pain of malignant origin. *Journal of Clinical Psychopharmacology*, 1987; 3:167–169.

141. Swerdlow M, Cundhill JG. Anticonvulsant drugs used in the treatment of lacerating pains: a comparison. *Anesthesia*, 1981; 36:1129–1134.

142. Caccia MR. Clonazepam in facial neuralgia and cluster headache: clinical and electrophysiological study. *European Neurology*, 1975; 13:560–563.

143. Syrajala K, Cummings C, Donaldson G. Hypnosis or cognitive behavioral training for the reduction of pain and nausea during cancer treatment: a controlled trial. *Pain*, 1992; 48:137–146.

144. Passik S, Horowitz S, Malkin M, Gargan R. A psychoeducational support program for spouses of brain tumor patients. (Abstract) *Symposium on New Trends in the Psychological Support of the Cancer Patient*. American Psychiatric Association Annual Meeting, New Orleans, LA, May 7–12, 1991.

145. Fishman B, Losalzo M. Cognitive-behavioral interventions in the management of cancer pain: principles and applications. *Medical Clinics of North America*, 1987; 71:271–287.

146. Speigel D, Bloom JR. Group therapy and hypnosis reduce metastatic breast carcinoma pain. *Psychosomatic Medicine*, 1983; 4:333–339.

147. Loscalzo M, Jacobsen PB. Practical behavioral approaches to the effective management of pain and distress. *Journal of Psychosocial Oncology*, 1990; 8:139–169.

148. Jensen M, Turner J, Romano J, Karoly. Coping with chronic pain: a critical review of the literature. *Pain*, 1991; 47:249–283.

149. Breitbart W, Holland JC. Psychiatric complications of cancer. In: Brain MC, Carbone PP, eds, *Current Therapy in Hematology Oncology-3*.

Toronto and Philadelphia: B.C. Decker Inc., 1988:268–274.

150. Erickson MH. Hypnosis in painful terminal illness. *American Journal of Clinical Hypnosis*, 1959; 1:1117–1121.

151. Turk D, Fernandez E. On the putative uniqueness of cancer pain: do psychological principles apply? *Behavior Research and Therapy*, 1990; 28, 1:1–13.

152. Fishman B. The treatment of suffering in patients with cancer pain. in: Foley K, Bonica J, Ventafridda V, eds, *Advances in Pain Research and Therapy*. Vol. 16, New York: Raven Press, 1990: 301–316.

153. Benson H. The relaxation response. New York: William Morrow, 1975.

154. Broome M, Lillis P, McGahhe T, Bates T. The use of distraction and imagery with children during painful procedures. *Oncology Nursing Forum*, 1992; 19:499–502.

155. Spiegel D. The use of Hypnosis in controlling cancer pain. *CA-A Cancer Journal for Clinicians*, 1985; 4:221–231.

156. Redd WB, Reeves JL, Storm RK, Minagawa RY. Hypnosis in the control of pain during hyperthermia treatment of cancer. In: Bonica JJ, et al., eds, *Advances in Pain Research and Theory*. New York: Raven Press, 1982:857–861.

157. Barber J, Gitelson J. Cancer Pain: psychological management using hypnosis. *CA-A Cancer Journal for Clinicians*, 1980; 3:130–136.

158. Levitan A. The use of hypnosis with cancer patients. *Psychiatry and Medicine*, 1992; 10:119–131.

159. Fotopoulos SS, Graham C, Cook MR. Psychophysiologic control of cancer pain. In: Bonica JJ, Ventafridda V, eds, *Advances in Pain Research and Therapy*. Vol. 2. New York: Raven Press, 1979:231–244.

160. Cleeland CS. Nonpharmacologic management of cancer pain. *Journal of Pain and Symptom Control*, 1987; 2:523–528.

161. Munro SM, Mount B. Music therapy in palliative care. *Canadian Medical Association Journal*, 1978; 119:1029–1034.

162. Schroeder-Sheker T. Music for the dying: a personal account of the new field of music thanatology-history, theories, and clinical narratives. *Advances*, 1993; 9:36–48.

163. Manne S, Redd W, Jacobsen P, Georgiades I. Aroma for treatment of anxiety during MRI scans. (Abstract) *Symposium on New Trends in the Psychological Support of the Cancer Patient*. American Psychiatric Association Annual Meeting, New Orleans, LA. May 7–12, 1991.

164. Connell C. Art therapy as part of a palliative cancer program. *Palliative Medicine*, 1992; 6:18–25.

10

Psychiatric Management of Eating Disorders in Palliative-Care Management of Cancer Patients

Lynna M. Lesko, M.D., Ph.D.

Cancer has often been associated with the symptoms of the disease and the side effects of its treatment. Common among these symptoms are cachexia (weight loss) and anorexia. Cachexia and subsequent failure to gain weight in children and adults with oncological diseases are most often attributed to altered metabolism and negative energy balance.[1,2] Changes in metabolism in such patients are usually manifested in altered carbohydrate and protein metabolism, whereas lipid metabolism is less affected. These metabolic changes usually lead to growth and maturation failure in pediatric patients and muscle wasting in adult patients. Negative energy balance in the cancer patient may be the result of decreased nutritional intake and/or increased nutritional expenditure. Much effort has gone into studying the effects of undernutrition on organ and cell function[3] and the effects of nutritional status on response to cancer therapy.[4] These mechanisms are much more prominent in the management of patients during their palliative-care treatment. Changes in appetite, anorexia (loss of appetite), and subsequent weight loss in such patients may result from the malignant disease itself, its treatment (e.g., radiation, surgery, chemotherapy), concomitant psychological syndromes, preexisting psychiatric syndromes, or behavioral issues. In this chapter, the physiological etiology of de-

creased or insufficient nutritional intake, the psychological mechanisms of cancer anorexia, and various currently used pharmacological, behavioral, and educational interventions are discussed. Other biologic aspects of negative energy balance, increased nutritional expenditure, and altered metabolism are summarized in other excellent review articles.[1]

GENERAL PATHOPHYSIOLOGY OF CANCER CACHEXIA/ANOREXIA

Cancer cachexia can be prevalent in patients with advanced or late-stage disease. Its main clinical manifestation, besides weight loss, is anorexia. Cachexia in cancer patients and in the animal models is common, complex, and, unfortunately, not well understood. Anorexia, reduction in caloric intake, and subsequent weight loss have a wide range of central and peripheral causes.[5,6] As Bernstein[7] states, the dilemma is that "the tumor-bearing organism fails to increased food intake (and more frequently decreases food intake) in the face of increased energy requirements imposed by tumor growth." In a simplistic model, cachexia in cancer patients, irrespective of the stage of their cancer treatment, may be the inability to maintain spontaneous food intake in order to keep up with necessary nutritional requirements. Peripheral causes of anorexia and subsequent cachexia include alterations in sensations of taste and smell, mechanical deficits secondary to surgery, altered physiology caused by surgery, radiation, and chemotherapy, and primary metabolic effects of tumor growth (inefficient or increased utilization of energy sources). The central nervous system regulatory mechanisms of normal food intake, appetite, and cancer anorexia are discussed later in this chapter.

Anatomically, it is well known from normal animal studies that "lesions" in or "ablation" of the lateral nucleus of the hypothalamus abolishes appetite and causes anorexia, whereas lesions in the ventromedial nucleus result in hyperphagia and weight gain. Unfortunately, lesion-ablation studies in tumor-bearing animals have revealed no direct and/or simple relationship between anorexia and food intake and the hypothalamic region.[7]

Researchers have also implicated the role of nonadrenergic, dopaminergic, serotonergic, and endorphinergic neurotransmitters in control and modulation of food intake. Elevations in tryptophan and 5-hydroxyindoleacetic acid (5-HIAA, a serotonin metabolite) and depletion of endorphin have been implicated in causing anorexia in tumor-bearing rats.[8,9] Bernstein[7] added that "the actual role of these transmitters in normal food intake regulation is as yet poorly understood and their role as mediators in cancer anorexia awaits further research."

Cancer-related cachexia may be explained by accelerated losses in skeletal protein. Some investigators feel that the rate of protein loss is greater in fed tumor-bearing animals than in fed control animals[10] and suggest that there is a "tumor-induced" acceleration of skeletal protecin loss independent of food intake. More recently, cachectin or tumor necrosis factor (TNF), a protein secreted by macrophages (which is disseminated via the circulation to interact with receptors on various end organs), has been implicated as an important central mediator in inducing toxic shock and wasting (cachexia) in animal models.[11–13] Cachectin produces a picture of weight loss, poor food intake, and apathy, as well as fever in animals. Elucidation of this important protein's mode of action may enhance our understanding of this problem in cancer.

Recently, several other factors have been suggested as mediators of cachexia associated with cancer. These include (1) other cytokines that alter the patient's metabolism indirectly, such as tumor necroses factors-alpha, gamma interferon, leukemia inhibitory factor, and interleukin-6, and (2) hormone-like compounds that result in a direct catabolism of host tissue, such as LMF or lipid mobilizing factor, which causes breakdown of adipose tissue.[14] The cytokines have several overlapping functions and activities, and the contribution of each one to cachexia in cancer patients still is uncertain.[15] Future physiological research will be important, particularly in sorting out causality of cachexia in both the newly diagnosed and the late-stage patient.

PHYSIOLOGICAL CAUSES OF ANOREXIA SECONDARY TO CANCER AND ITS TREATMENT

The anorexia and subsequent cachexia syndrome in patients with oncological disease has physiological and psychological causes. Table 10.1 includes a comprehensive list of the physiological (i.e., disease- and treatment-related) causes of cancer anorexia. The psychological aspects of cancer anorexia (e.g., depression, psychological distress, and behavioral paradigms such as learned food aversions) are discussed (for a concise background on the physiological causes of cancer anorexia, see review articles by Holland et al.,[16] Ohnuma and Holland,[17] Shils,[18] and Burish et al.[19]

DISEASE-RELATED ANOREXIA

Anorexia and secondary weight loss can occur either early or late in the course of certain gastrointestinal (GI) cancers, such as those of the stomach, colon, rectum, and pancreas, and in some cases can be the sole presenting symptom in early gastrointestinal disease. However, they may herald a late diagnosis of earlier quiescent disease. Occasionally, these symptoms are misinterpreted as depressive symptomatology, and the patient can mistakenly be referred to a psychiatrist. Metabolic abnormalities such as fever, anemia, uremia, hepatic dysfunction, protein-losing enteropathy, and other malabsorption difficulties can all produce transient anorexia in a patient at various stages of a malignant illness. These abnormalities may disrupt the feeding-satiety center of the hypothalamus, producing decreased hunger or early satiety. A growing area of interest concerning nutritional problems in lung cancer is the secretion of ectopic hormones, kinins, and various polypeptides. Such agents may affect peripheral or central systems to produce decreased appetite. Pain, discomfort, and GI obstruction and poor management of palliative care can lead to transient but profound anorexia in the later stages of disease.

TREATMENT-RELATED
CANCER ANOREXIA

Cancer anorexia can be a pervasive symptom secondary to a patient's cancer treatment and stage of illness. Loss of appetite can be caused by surgery, radiation, and/or chemotherapy (Table 10.1). Many of the chemotherapeutic drugs along or in combination with radiation may produce anorexia secondary to their effects on the hypothalamus or by their emetic potential.

The effects of ablative surgery for cancer treatment on taste and nutrition can often be profound, complicating the later chemotherapy- and radiation-induced anorexia. Ablative radical head and neck surgery can result in loss of normal oral architecture and/or decreased function (masticating and swallowing). The taste of food and the pleasure of eating can be altered by extensive and repetitive upper-GI surgery. Such surgery may require prolonged feedings via a nasogastric tube. Such indwelling tubes can produce throat irritation and psychological trauma that

Table 10.1   Early and Late Physiological Causes of Eating Disorders in Cancer Patients

Disease Related

- Early symptoms of pancreatic or gastrointestinal cancer
- Ectopic hormone production by tumors (lung)
- Fever
- Protein-losing enteropathy (gastric cancer)
- Tumor obstruction by advancing disease
- Chronic illness, anemia
- Cancer cachexia syndrome
- Metabolic changes (uremia and hepatic dysfunction)
- Pain or discomfort

Treatment Related

- Surgery
  Oropharyngeal resection: loss of dentition; chewing and swallowing difficulties
  Esophagectomy and reconstruction: gastric acid secondary to vagotomy, fibrosis
  Gastrectomy: gastric acid, malabsorption, "dumping" syndrome
  Pancreatectomy: diabetes, malabsorption
  Bowel resection: malabsorption, diarrhea secondary to bile salt loss, malnutrition
  Ileostomy or colostomy: fluid electrolyte imbalance
- Drug related
  Chemotherapeutic agents: fluid and electrolyte imbalance secondary to nausea and vomiting, stomatitis of alimentary canal, abdominal pain, constipation, intestinal ulceration, diarrhea, neuropathy, central nervous system complications
  Pain medication: somnolence, constipation
  Antifungal and antibacterial agents
- Radiation therapy
  Oropharyngeal area: decreased smell and taste, stomatitis
  Neck and mediastinal area: dysphagia, esophagitis, esophageal fibrosis/stenosis, fistulas
  Abdomen and pelvic area: nausea, vomiting, diarrhea, malabsorption, stenosis, fistulas
- Other
  Graft-versus-host disease (bone marrow transplantation): diarrhea, electrolyte imbalance, malabsorption

Source: Adapted from Lesko L, "Anorexia," In: Holland JC, Rowland, JH, eds, *Handbook of Psychooncology: Psychological Care of the Patient with Cancer*, New York: Oxford University Press, 1989:434–443.

interfere with appetite and the quality and sensation of taste and food intake. Gastrectomy and bowel resection can result in malabsorption and weight loss. Temporary or permanent colostomy in a small number of patients produces psychological trauma centered around food intake and excretion. Secondary anorexia and decreased oral intake can develop. Pancreatic resection and resultant loss of endocrine function can produce alterations in insulin control and subsequent nausea and decreased appetite.

Radiation therapy can cause transient and permanent sequelae that interfere with taste and oral consumption of nutrients. Radiation-induced anorexia often depends on the targeted area of such treatment, the amount of radiation, and the length of radiation treatments. Immediate effects of radiation treatment can often produce stomatitis of the oral areas, mucositis pharyngitis, esophagitis, nausea and/or vomiting, and diarrhea. Permanent and often more serious sequelae affecting appetite can develop. These involve a decreased sense of or change in taste,[20] change in saliva production, dysphagia secondary to esophageal fibrosis, and lower-GI obstruction secondary to stenosis or fistualization. Any time the oral canal, the senses involved in eating (i.e., smell and taste), or the secondary organ systems (i.e., saliva production) are affected by treatment, the experience of food intake is limited, and anorexia may develop.

Nausea, vomiting, decreased oral intake, fluid and electrolyte imbalance, and subsequent anorexia can be produced by almost all chemotherapeutic agents (e.g., cyclophosphamide [Cytoxan], nitrogen mustards, and cisplatin). Only a few agents, such as the alkylating agents (vincristine) and corticosteroids, are not associated with nausea, vomiting, and subsequent anorexia. Chemotherapy agents such as vincristine can, however, produce constipation and ileus, resulting in pain, discomfort, and subsequent anorexia. Stomatitis with oral ulcerations, glossitis, pharyngitis, and esophagitis are extremely common with methotrexate, fluorouracil, and high-dose doxorubicin (Adriamycin). Due to the rapid turnover of epithelial cells of the mucosal layer of the alimentary canal, the GI tract is extremely vulnerable to side effects of these agents, resulting in ulcerations, pain, and anorexia. Drugs other than chemotherapy agents (e.g., antibiotics and antifungal and pain medications) can produce transient anorexic syndromes. Analgesics may produce central nervous system somnolence, resulting in missed meals and poor nutrition.

A very serious long-term consequence of high-dose chemotherapy, radiation, and bone marrow transplantation is graft-versus-host disease (GVHD). Despite matching of donor and recipient at the major histocompatible antigen sites and adequate postgraft immunosuppression, 70% of patients can develop a GVHD syndrome.[21] Principal target organs of this syndrome include the skin, the GI tract, and the liver. Gastrointestinal dysfunction, usually manifest after the typical skin rash, is characterized by diarrhea, abdominal pain, ileus, anorexia, weight loss, malabsorption, and failure to thrive. Newer treatments of donor bone marrow with lectins and monoclonal antibodies can in most cases do away with GVHD and its sequelae.

PSYCHOLOGICAL ASPECTS
OF CANCER ANOREXIA

Even though anorexia is one of the most common symptoms of malignancy, it is the most difficult to treat because of its multiple etiologies. We often overlook the psychological causes and dynamics of anorexia in our haste to intervene (Table 10.2). In this section, loss of appetite is discussed in the context of psychiatric syndromes, learned food aversions, and behavioral issues. Case examples are included to illustrate the often complex nature of anorexia.

Psychiatric Causes of Appetite Loss

Often anorexia in patients with late-stage malignancies is seen in the context of an anxiety syndrome. We mistakenly make light of the complaint "I just don't feel like eating" and chalk it up to side effects of treatment or disease. It is well known in the psychiatric literature that patients without medical illness but with symptoms of anxiety or depression can experience a decreased interest in appetite and food intake. During the later stages of cancer, appetite can be exquisitely sensitive to anxiety. On learning that their cancer treatment may change or that treatment must change to take on a palliative nature, many patients note that, along with signs of distress such as insomnia and poor concentration, they lose

Table 10.2   Psychological Causes of Eating
Disorders in Cancer Patients During Palliative Care

Anxiety

Psychological fears related to meaning of weight loss,
assumed to be associated with tumor progression
Concerns about inability to eat
Issues about loss of normal appetite

Depression

Loss of appetite
Weight loss
Dysphoria
Hopelessness, helplessness
Withdrawal

Delirium

Altered mental status secondary to disease and its
treatment

Psychiatric Disorders

Affective disorders (e.g., depression)
Anorexia nervosa
Personality disorders
Schizophrenic disorders
Paranoia (suspiciousness of poisoning and refusal to
eat)

Food Aversions

Specific food aversions (e.g., decreased protein
tolerance, increased glucose tolerance)
Learned food aversions

Behavioral

Anticipatory nausea and vomiting

Source: Adapted from Lesko L, "Anorexia," in: Holland JC, Rowland,
JH, eds, *Handbook of Psychooncology: Psychological Care of the Patient
with Cancer*, New York: Oxford University Press, 1989:434–443.

their appetite. The loss of a few pounds is enough
to frighten such patients even more; their first assumption is that the now fulminent cancer is
causing the weight loss. Reassurance about the
emotional turmoil they are feeling may have an
impact on appetite and is often enough to reduce
the anxiety and encourage a return to whatever
the patient's normal food intake was. Occasionally, benzodiazepines are necessary to control levels of anxiety. The fear of relapse and recurrence
is greatest immediately after the end of treatment,
but it does not ever fully disappear. Concerned

and anxious family members, alarmed by signs of
poor eating, may attempt to force food on cancer
patients, making eating the source of family conflict. In some individuals, the fear of weight loss
and its potential significance as a sign of tumor
progression leads to compulsive overeating. Although less common, this is of equal concern.
Forced eating in the absence of hunger, as a compulsive habit, can result in obesity and appears
most often in women with breast cancer who are
undergoing chemotherapy. The following case
example illustrates the alarm that can be generated in patients and their families when eating
difficulties and weight loss complicate surgery for
a cancer of the gastrointestinal tract.

Case Example

Mrs. P, a 55-year-old grandmother, had a gastrectomy for a late-stage gastric carcinoma. She was previously anxious and had a history of several phobias. Her postoperative course was complicated by
anxiety attacks, chronic fears, and difficulty in eating and maintaining weight. Mrs. P and her family
were convinced that the problems with eating were
due to the immediate recurrence of cancer and unsuccessful surgery. A psychiatric consultation was
requested to help her deal with anxiety; however,
it soon became clear that some of her difficulty in
eating was related to uncontrolled anxiety. Intervention included psychotherapy, medication (antianxiety drugs), and repeated visits to the surgeon
to reassure Mrs. P and her daughter that the symptoms were not currently physical in origin but rather
an exacerbation of a previous psychiatric condition.
Regular periodic visits were suggested to monitor
the anxiety and its relationship to future stages of
advanced disease.

Anorexia can be a cardinal symptom of depression, but it is also a major symptom of advanced cancer. It is in the advanced states where
both are more common and the differential diagnosis between major depression and a physical
origin of anorexia becomes a difficult problem.
Anorexia may be a consequence of the medical
situation that results in secondary depression and
further inability to eat, or depression may be the
prime contributor. Patients may begin to feel helpless in the face of continuing anorexia and weight
loss, leading to despair and hopelessness. Such
painful emotional states require intervention. It is
important to make an accurate assessment of pos-

sible physical and psychological contributors to anorexia. Treatment of the psychological component includes counseling and pharmacological interventions aimed directly at appetite and at depressive symptoms. Often a therapeutic trial of an antidepressant medication is worth attempting, even when a diagnosis of major depression is not firm. The following case example illustrates how major psychiatric and intra-abdominal pathology can interact.

Case Example

Ms. C, a 60-year-old widow with pancreatic cancer, was treated with chemotherapy but experienced profound anorexia, weight loss, and abdominal pain. Subsequently, she developed severe depression and withdrawal, which her psychiatrist felt were due to a combination of functional (anticipatory mourning) and organic (pain medication) factors. She wished to be treated at her daughter's home and was kept comfortable by family and home-care nursing. Her treatment regime included analgesics, antidepressants (those with minimal sedating effects), and low-dose amphetamines. Frequent psychotherapeutic home visits with other children and grandchildren during the 3 months in which the disease progressed were useful in symptom control of depression, anorexia, and overall family anxiety.

Preexisting psychiatric disorders in individuals who develop late-stage cancer can complicate patient care and contribute to anorexia. In particular, affective and schizophrenic syndromes, personality disorders, and anorexia nervosa can result in altered intake and weight loss. Patients with such disorders present very complicated treatment issues. Anorexia nervosa, common among young women, has constituted a particularly difficult problem in anorexic individual who are later treated with extensive chemotherapy (with its concomitant nausea and vomiting). Weight loss, unusual difficulty with taste, and relentless preoccupation with food may be unrelated to the physical illness but evidence of a concurrent and complicating psychiatric disorder, as the following case examples illustrates.

Case Example

Ms. G was diagnosed at age 19 as having acute leukemia. The sixth of seven children, she had come to the United States with her parents from Sicily. Her leukemia treatment was uneventful until, during a second relapse, she began to "fake" taking drugs at home to avoid the nausea and vomiting, even injecting saline to fool her family. After the second relapse, she was hospitalized for an allogenic bone marrow transplantation. Her hospital course was complicated by a longer-than normal weaning period from total parenteral nutrition and disinterest in follow-up. She had developed mild chronic graft-vs-host disease posttransplant. Over 3 years, she had anorexia, difficulty swallowing, and an inability to take food except iced tea, and did not take oral medications regularly at home.

Ms. G was evaluated by several psychiatrists, who felt she had had early symptoms of anorexia nervosa (before leukemia), which were exacerbated by the transplantation procedure. She was hospitalized for infections, dehydration, failure to thrive, and weight loss. Her complaints of anorexia and difficulty swallowing continued; finally she refused to eat because it would "make me feel ugly." Her family, who were immigrants and could barely speak English, focused their attention on her cachexia, interpreting the symptoms as due to leukemia. Ms. G's noncompliance and passivity in the face of efforts to maintain her oral intake necessitated placement of a percutaneous feeding tube. She complained of bloating, abdominal pain, and diarrhea. Eventually she became immunologically compromised and died of generalized sepsis and failure to thrive.

Learned Food Aversions

Recently it has been suggested that appetite suppression in some cancer patients may be due to "learned food aversions."[7,22–27] According to Bernstein and colleagues,[25] who used animal models to study cancer anorexia, learned food aversions develop as a result of the association of certain foods with unpleasant internal symptoms (i.e., nausea and vomiting). Most of the research in this area has been in understanding food aversions in young children undergoing active cancer treatment. However, the findings have been applied to patients of all ages in late-stage disease.

This behavioral phenomenon of conditioned or learned taste aversion is similar to classical conditioning paradigms in which animals learn to associate a conditioned stimulus (taste) with an unconditioned response (symptom of the illness). In animal modes, (1) it is possible to introduce a delay of many hours between the conditioned stimulus and the subsequent discomfort (unconditioned response), and (2) the acquisition of such learning can occur rapidly, with only one trial.

In an attempt to examine this response in humans, Bernstein[22] examined learned food aversions in children receiving chemotherapy for cancer. These elegant studies are of particular importance because this phenomenon had not been previously demonstrated in humans. Children receiving chemotherapy (producing moderate to severe nausea and vomiting) were randomized to control or experimental groups. Patients in the experimental group were offered a novel food (maple toffee ice cream) shortly before their scheduled chemotherapy treatment. Patients in one control group received no novel food but were occupied with a toy. Other control groups consisted of patients receiving chemotherapy with little emetic potency or patients receiving no chemotherapy at all. All patients were tested for food aversions to the ice cream at 1 to 4 weeks. Patients exposed to the novel food stimulus were three times more likely to develop a significant food aversion than patients in the control groups ($P < .01$). These studies were expanded to determine whether patients receiving chemotherapy regimens developed food aversions to common, preferred, or familiar foods. The researchers concluded that food aversions are fairly specific to food eaten before therapy that produces GI distress and that they may occur not only with novel foods presented before chemotherapy but also with regular foods in the patient's diet, which may have been eaten up to several hours before treatment. Other studies by Bernstein and colleagues[24] in animal models have indicated that learned food aversions can occur in animals that are anorexic secondary to tumor growth. However, they demonstrated that it is possible to increase caloric intake by presenting a novel diet.

In summary, both clinical and laboratory studies have indicated that learned food aversions in cancer patients result from both treatment and tumor growth and suggest an interesting but causal role in the development of tumor anorexia. Such a food aversion model has been used to test various interventions for eliminating or reducing these problems. In these studies (e.g., Broberg and Bernstein),[28] the only intervention that significantly lowered the magnitude of drug-induced

food aversion was the presentation of a novel food or diet on the days of treatment. These preliminary studies using animal models are useful in identifying potential interventions that may be effective in clinical practice.

Occasionally, eating itself may result in biochemical changes and altered metabolism, which in turn may precipitate a learned food aversion. De Wys[1] noted that patients with cancer produce elevated levels of lactate, a metabolite known to cause nausea if infused into control subjects. De Wys suggested that for cancer patients, irrespective of the stage of their disease, eating even a normal-size meal or a high-carbohydrate diet may induce nausea, which then in turn becomes a learned response.

The final case example presents the interplay between the psychological (anxiety and conflict around weaning from total parenteral nutrition and subsequent discharge), physiological (liver damage and change in taste secondary to radiation and chemotherapy), and behavioral (learned food aversions) etiologies of anorexia. The psychological intervention for this patient was multimodal and included behavioral and pharmacological management. The patient's liver dysfunction slowly resolved without any physiological treatment.

Case Example

Mr. P, a 55-year-old man with acute leukemia, was treated with a chemotherapy regimen of induction and consolidation that resulted in acute but transient episodes of nausea, vomiting, anorexia, and change in taste. He was then rapidly admitted to a sterile room for an allogenic bone marrow transplantation. Over 3 months he received hyperalimentation, which was necessary secondary to stomatitis. Weaning from parenteral nutrition was stormy: Despite the absence of any physical problem, he had severe anorexia. However, after struggles with his physician, who wanted him to eat more, he was discharged with continued anorexia and nausea. After weeks at home on a bland diet, Mr. P became dehydrated and was started on parenteral nutrition. He subsequently relapsed and underwent a second transplant. During a very stormy convalescent period, he became depressed and developed nausea, first to solids and then to semisolids. Finally, the smell of food or sight of his menu resulted in anxiety and nausea. Antiemetics in adequate doses produced side effects, and he was finally successfully treated by desensitization and relaxation.

CLINICAL MANAGEMENT OF ANOREXIA AND EATING DISORDERS

Although cancer anorexia may for the most part be physiological and metabolic in nature, psychological interventions may be extremely useful in its treatment. Current and promising interventions such as psychopharmacological agents and psychoeducational-behavioral techniques are highlighted in this discussion. The goals of supportive nutritional interventions should include a proactive nutritional assessment, early and aggressive intervention that is cost-efficient, somewhat standardized, and supports nutritional status of the late-stage cancer patient so that functional status and quality of life are maintained.[29]

In caring for the patient with cancer-related anorexia, a full assessment of the patient's stage of cancer and its physiological causes of altered metabolism, appetite change, and decreased food intake metabolism is required. The reassurance gained by the patient from an understanding of the cause of the anorexia is of the utmost importance. Involving both the patient and family members is critical. Weekly supportive sessions often begin with a review of appetite changes and general changes in medical/physical condition and discussion of emotions and concerns about the illness. Assessment and treatment of underlying anxiety or depression or potential personal problems contributing to anorexia must be part of each evaluation. Referral for diet education or behavioral interventions is always helpful and often critical for patient management. Books and information on high-caloric foods, how to serve tasteful meals, new recipes, and other techniques for increasing food intake, such as frequent meals, are useful.

Pharmacological Intervention

Several pharmacological agents are known to be useful in promoting weight gain in patients with oncological disease.[16] They include antihistamines (cyproheptadine), steroids (dexamethasone and prednisone), amphetamine-like agents (dexamphetamine and methylphenidate), antidepressants with anticholinergic effects (tricyclic antidepressants), cannabinoids (tetrahydrocannabinols (Δ9-THC]), and progestational agents (megestrol) (Table 10.3).

It is often difficult to separate out whether appetite loss in cancer patients undergoing palliative care is due to the tumor or cancer therapy or represents an early symptom of depression. As mentioned, above, appetite loss may be the first symptom of depression in cancer patients. In particular, elderly patients may exhibit only one or two of the cardinal symptoms of depression, which include weight loss, anorexia, and difficulty sleeping. Consequently, a trial of an antidepressant (in low doses) can be extremely helpful to patients in regaining their appropriate food intake. Steroids can produce a mild euphoria and an enhanced sense of well-being that initially improves appetite. Over time, however, increased appetite can result in obesity and severe problems in controlling weight.

Table 10.3   Possible Pharmacological Interventions in the Management of Cancer-Related Eating Disorders

Pharmacological Drug (Trade Name)	Class	Dose
Cyproheptadine (Periactin)	Antihistamine	4 mg po tid (tablet or elixir)
Dexamethasone (Decadron); prednisone	Steroids	Variable
Dextroamphetamine[a] (Dexedrine)	Amphetamine	5–10 mg bid
Methylphenidate (Ritalin)[a]	Stimulant	2.5–5 mg bid
Tricyclic antidepressants	Antidepressant	25–100 mg/day
Tetrahydrocannabinols [Δ^9-THC]	Cannabinoids	15 mg/day po or inhalation
Megestrol acetate (Megace)[b]	Progestional	160–800 mg/day
Hydrazine sulfate		60 mg po tid

[a]Should be taken in morning or early afternoon to prevent insomnia.

[b]800 mg/day may be the optimal daily dose (Loprinzi, 1994).

Source. Adapted in part from Lesko L, "Anorexia," in: Holland JC, Rowland, JH, eds, *Handbook of Psychooncology: Psychological Care of the Patient with Cancer*, New York: Oxford University Press, 1989:434–443.

Megestrol acetate, used in breast cancer regimens, may promote increased appetite and subsequent weight gain and may prove an important pharmacological intervention for anorexia and cachexia in terminal illness and acquired immunodeficiency syndrome (AIDS).[30–33] Early studies employing megestrol acetate have proven successful. Cruz et al.[34] studied approximately 200 women with advanced breast cancer, comparing a standard regimen of 160 mg per day with one of 800 mg per day; weight gain was directly correlated to the dose and length of megestrol acetate treatment. Megestrol acetate, at a dose of 160 mg per day, resulted in a 5-lb. weight gain in a significant portion of cancer patients.[31] In a large randomized, double-blind, placebo-controlled trial of megestrol acetate in patients with cancer-associated anorexia and cachexia,[30] patients receiving 800 mg per day of megestrol experienced significant appetite stimulation and weight gain (16% gained 15 lb. or more) with little associated toxicity. Tchekmedyian et al.[35] have also studied high-dose regimens of megestrol acetate (e.g., 480 to 1600 mg per day) and found that such a regimen could be helpful in cancer anorexia.

More recent studies have continued to demonstrate the positive effect of megestrol acetate on weight gain and appetite stimulation. In one study of patients with external pelvic radiation, patients taking 120 mg daily megestrol acetate or 30 mg daily prenisolone for 21 days demonstrated improvement in body weight, appetite, performance status, and sense of well-being. However, only appetite improvement was statistically significant ($P = .024$) in the megestrol patient group.[36] Again, oral megestrol acetate at 320 mg daily stimulated appetite and nonfluid weight gain in 24 patients with advanced bladder or colorectal cancer.[37] In a large, 342-patient study evaluating four doses of megestrol acetate (160, 480, 800, and 1280 mg daily), Loprinzi et al.[38] elegantly demonstrated a dose-response effect on appetite stimulation ($P = .02$), with the optimal dose being 800 mg per day. The experience with doses of megestrol acetate in excess of 800 mg per day is limited, however, and care should be exercised with any use of this drug above such a dose.[39]

Amphetamine and amphetamine-like agents also stimulate appetite. Small doses of dextroamphetamine or methylphenidate in the morning reduce the withdrawal and apathy experienced by patients with advanced disease and also reduce somnolence caused by analgesics. Excessive doses, however, reduce appetite and if given toward evening can inhibit sleep. Dizziness, somnolence, depersonalization, and dysphoria can occur with cannabinoids at doses sufficient to improve appetite, which limits their usefulness.

Hydrazine sulfate, a drug originally studied in cancer patients 70 years ago, is currently under study as a potentially useful agent in the treatment of cancer anorexia and cachexia. In a study of 101 patients,[40] 83% maintained or increased their weight on hydrazine sulfate 60 mg tid, compared to 58% in the placebo group. In contrast, in another randomized, placebo-controlled study of 127 patients with advanced colorectal cancer, there were no significant differences between the groups for anorexia or weight loss.[41]

Delta-9 THC in one study proved to be an effective appetite stimulant in patients with advanced cancer from various malignancies when efficacy, satisfaction, and acceptability were evaluated at 2 and 4 weeks. It appeared to be well tolerated at low doses of 2.5 mg po tid taken 1 hour before meals.[5,6]

As mentioned earlier, cancer-related cachexia associated with abnormalities of energy balance and metabolism may be related to the macrophage-reduced cytokine TNF. Several agents such as hydrazinesulfate, corticosteroids, and pentoxifylline have been proported to diminish TNF production in animals. Pentoxifylline, a derivative of methyxanthine, has been reported to decrease TNF mRNA levels in cancer patients and also decreases replication of the AIDS virus. In one randomized, double-blind, placebo-controlled trial, 35 patients received 400 mg of pentoxifylline tid with follow-up for 2 months. Pentoxifylline did not cause any toxicity or side effects but unfortunately did not spur improvement in appetite or induce weight gain.[42]

In summary, despite small, positive pilot studies, large randomized trials with hydrazine sulfate, cyroheptadine, and pentoxifylline have been unable to prove the efficacy of these agents in inducing weight gain and appetite improvement.

Behavioral and Educational Techniques

Quite often, simple behavioral and educational techniques are overlooked by distraught patients and their families. Some very basic behavioral techniques can be used by hospital staff and families to improve oral intake and possibly reverse symptoms of appetite loss (Table 10.4). These may not be available in every hospital but often can be found in hospice and palliative-care treatment centers. A dietary consultation can be helpful in educating patients and families on the nutritional content of certain foods, especially those high in calories and protein; the necessity for small and frequent meals; novel ways of preparing favorite foods; and new recipes with tempting visual presentations. Often such a consultation is mandatory when a patient has undergone head and neck surgery and required special pureed foods or prosthetic devices. Patients receiving chemotherapy or radiation often avoid strongly flavored foods like barbecued meats and fish and may prefer canned fruits, cottage cheese, and milk supplements. Stomatitis secondary to radiation or chemotherapy and oral candidal infections involve not only the oral mucosa but also the esophagus, and patients with such conditions may require pureed or liquid foods because of pain.

Radiation and mucosal GVHD may change the characteristics of the patient's saliva or decrease its volume, necessitating more liquid with meals or saliva-like additives to moisten the oral cavity. In these situations, saliva becomes thick and difficult to cough up; patients do not toler-

ate milk products that appear to aggravate this problem. In addition, candidal infections treated with oral medications (nystatin) often make food taste undesirable. If anorexia and decreased caloric intake become profound, nutritional consultation may be necessary for artificial feeding (either enteral through a nasogastric tube or feeding gastrostomy or parenteral via a Hickman-Broviac catheter).

The ambiance at meal time can be very important for improving caloric intake. Having a family member share a meal with the hospitalized patient, serving a favorite wine or beer, or using candles and special table settings can add many of the social aspects that physically well individuals associate with a pleasant meal. If possible, a gathering of two or three patients who can eat communally creates an ambiance more conducive to joyful and pleasurable eating.

A variety of more sophisticated behavioral techniques have been applied to eating disorders in cancer, especially among children. Because anorexia may be accompanied by anxiety, worry concerning food intake, and anticipatory anxiety or nausea before a meal, the fear, anxiety, worry, and anorexia may become behaviorally linked. In such situations, several behavioral techniques, such as relaxation or self-hypnosis, can lower anxiety and anticipatory phenomena around eating and improve fluid and caloric intake. Conflicts about eating often necessitate meetings with staff and family members. Attention to situations that create problems and are associated with refusal to eat are important and should be recognized early in the course of the illness. If anxiety is the center of the problem, relaxation exercises before meals in an effort to reduce the focus on eating and diminish anticipatory distress symptoms, coupled with use of anxiolytic medication, can improve the anorexia. Sometimes patients complain of nausea at the thought or sight of food, and relaxation with an antiemetic may be appropriate. Symptoms may be experienced more in socially embarrassing situations, such as in a restaurant, in which the inability to eat or the onset of nausea increases patients' self-consciousness and may become a reason to remain at home and not eat with others.

Contingency management, in which rewards such as family visits, exercise, permission to watch television, or tokens are dependent on

Table 10.4   Psychoeducational-Supportive and Behavioral Interventions in the Management of Cancer-related Eating Disorder

---

Psychoeducational-Supportive

  Supportive psychotherapy for psychiatric issues and psychological fears related to weight loss

  Advice about meals with caloric and protein content, appetizing recipes, visually appealing presentations, relaxing ambiance at mealtime, novel ways of preparing favorite foods

  Special consultation for medically related problems of head and neck tumors (e.g., stomatitis, artificial feeding, pain control)

Behavioral

  Relaxation techniques to reduce anxiety and anticipatory phenomena before meals

  Techniques to reduce learned food aversions

  Operant conditioning methods for weight gain

weight gain or caloric intake, have been successful in patients with primary anorexia nervosa. There has been no research in the literature to investigate whether this behavioral method can be applied to cancer patients with anorexia. However, a few cancer patients may develop secondary anorexia nervosa indistinguishable from that seen in the psychiatric population. The etiology of this syndrome is unknown; one theory is that anorexic-like features or characteristics that have been dormant in some individuals are triggered by the cancer diagnosis and its treatment. An operant conditioning-based treatment may be of help in such cases (W.H. Redd, personal communications, 1992).

SUMMARY

Cancer anorexia, with its associated decreased food intake and weight loss, is a common and profoundly important symptom in late-stage malignancy, and one that has at times a psychological as well as a physical component. Most poorly understood is the anorexia-cachexia syndrome of advanced disease. When physical in origin, it may be caused directly or indirectly by the disease process or treatment. Psychological causes often reflect anxiety about cancer, its progression, depression, anticipatory phenomena, and learned food aversions. Preexisting psychiatric disorders, especially anorexia nervosa or paranoid states, can substantially complicate cancer treatment. Recent research indicates that learned food aversions may play a role in cancer anorexia and can occur as a result of the pairing or association of foods with tumor growth or with the side effects of chemotherapy. The management of nutrition in the oncological setting can be enhanced by the use of various types of artificial feeding (i.e., parenteral or enteral administration) and by judicious use of various pharmacological drugs that control nausea and vomiting or stimulate appetite. Regardless of the etiology of the psychological management of the problem is often helpful. Optimal management often involves the use of a combination of modalities—psychotherapeutic, behavioral, and/or pharmacological treatment, supplemented by education, counseling, and support. Many of these are available in palliative-care treatment centers. Behavioral techniques such as relaxation exercises are useful tools to alter this response as well as to relieve the anxiety precipitated by patient concerns about anorexia and weight loss. Environmental interventions and nutritional advice can also be of considerable value in reversing the negative effects of this distressing symptom in cancer. Artificial feeding, used for poor intake,[43] poses a special set of psychological problems for patient and family depending on whether it is accomplished by tubes (enteral) or catheters (parenteral). Mental health professionals can play an important role in the management of the cancer anorexia/cachexia syndrome, particularly if they have a fundamental knowledge of the pathophysiology of anorexia/cachexia, as well as familiarity with the pharmacologic and nonpharmacologic interventions that can be effective.

References

1. De Wys WD. Pathophysiology of cancer cachexia: Current understanding and areas for future research. *Cancer Research*, 1982; 42(suppl):721S–726S.

2. Kisner DL, De Wys WD. Anorexia and cachexia in malignant disease. In: Newell GR, Ellison NM, eds. *Nutrition and Cancer: Etiology and Treatment*. New York: Raven, 1981:355–365.

3. Good RA, West A, Day NK, et al. Effects of undernutrition on host cell and organ function. *Cancer Research*, 1982; 42(suppl):737S–746S.

4. Van Eys J. Effects of Nutritional status on response to therapy. *Cancer Research*, 1982; 42(suppl): 747S–753S.

5. Nelson K, Walsh D, Sheehan F. A phase II study 8 delta-9-tetrahydrocannabinol for appetite stimulation in cancer-associated anorexia. *Journal of Palliative Care*, 1994; 10(1):14–18.

6. Nelson KA, Walsh D, Sheehan FA. The cancer-anorexia-cachexia syndrome. *Journal of Clinical Oncology*, 1994; 12(1):213–224.

7. Bernstein IL. Physiological and psychological mechanisms of cancer anorexia. *Cancer Research*, 1982; 42(suppl):S715–S720.

8. Krause R, James JH, Ziparo V, et al. Brain tryptophan and the neoplastic anorexia-cachexia syndrome. *Cancer*, 1979; 44:1003–1008.

9. Lowry MT, Yim GKW. Similar feeding profiles in tumor-bearing and dexamethasone-treated rats suggest endorphin depletion in cancer cachexia. *Neuroscience Abstracts*, 1980; 6:518.

10. Norton JA, Shamberger R, Stein TP, et al. The influence of tumor-bearing on protein metabolism in the rat. *J Surg Res* 1981; 30:456–462.

11. Beutler B. Cachexia: a fundamental mechanism. *Nutrition Review,* 1988; 46:369–373.

12. Beutler B, Cerami T. Cachectin: more than a tumor necrosis factor. *New England Journal of Medicine,* 1981; 305:375–381.

13. Olds LJ. Tumor necrosis factor (TNF). *Science,* 1985; 230:630–632.

14. Tisdale MJ. Cancer-cachexia. *Anti-Cancer Drugs,* 1993; 4(2):115–125.

15. Keller U. Pathophysiology of cancer-cachexia. *Supportive Care in Cancer,* 1993; 1(6):290–294.

16. Holland JC, Rowland JH, Plumb M. Psychological aspects of anorexia in cancer patients. *Cancer Research,* 1977; 37:2425–2428.

17. Ohnuma T, Holland JF. Nutritional consequences of cancer chemotherapy and immunotherapy. *Cancer Research,* 1977; 37:2395–2406.

18. Shils ME. Nutritional problems induced by cancer. *Med Clin North Am* 1979; 63:1009–1025.

19. Burish TG, Levy SM, Meyerowitz BE. *Cancer, Nutrition and Eating Behavior.* Hillsdale, NJ: Lawrence Earlbaum, 1985.

20. Huldij A, Giesberg A, Klein Poelhuis EH, et al. Alterations in taste appreciation in cancer patients during treatment. *Cancer Nurs* 1986; 9:38–42.

21. Deeg HJ, Storb R. Acute and chronic graft versus host disease. *Journal of the National Cancer Institute,* 1986; 76(6):1325–1328.

22. Bernstein IL. Learned taste aversion in children receiving chemotherapy. *Science,* 1978; 200:1302–1303.

23. Bernstein IL. Etiology of anorexia in cancer. *Cancer,* 1986; 581:1881–1886.

24. Bernstein IL, Sigundi RA. Tumor anorexia: a learned food aversion. *Science,* 1980; 209:414–418.

25. Bernstein IL, Webster MM. Learned food aversions: a consequence of cancer chemotherapy. In: Burish TG, Levy SM, Meyerowitz BE, eds, *Cancer, Nutrition and Eating Behavior.* Hillsdale, NJ: Lawrence Earlbaum, 1985:103–116.

26. Bernstein IL, Wallace MI, Bernstein ID, et al. Learned food aversions as a consequence of cancer treatment. In: Van Eys J, Seelig MS, Nichols BL, eds. *Nutrition and Cancer.* New York: SP Medical & Scientific Books, 1979:159–164.

27. Mattes RD, Arnold C, Borass M. Learned food aversions among cancer chemotherapy patients: incidence, nature and clinical implications. *Cancer,* 1987; 60:2576–2580.

28. Broberg DJ, Bernstein IL. Candy as a scapegoat in the prevention of food aversions in children receiving chemotherapy. *Cancer,* 1987; 60:2344–2347.

29. Ottery FD. Supportive nutrition to prevent cachexia and improve quality of life. *Seminars in Oncology,* 1995; 22(2 suppl 3):98–111.

30. Loprinzi CL, Ellison NM, Schaid DJ, et al. Controlled trials of megestrol acetate for the treatment of cancer anorexia and cachexia. *Journal of the National Cancer Institute,* 1990; 82:1127–1132.

31. Tchekmedyian NS, Tait N, Moody M, et al. Appetite stimulation with megestrol acetate in cachectic cancer patients. *Semin Oncol* 1986; 13:37–43.

32. Tchekmedyian NS, Hichman M, Sian J, et al. Megestrol acetate in cancer anorexia and weight loss. *Cancer,* 1992; 69:1268–1274.

33. Von Roenn JH, Armstrong O, Kotler DP, Cohn DL, Klimas NG, Tchekmedyian NS, Cone L, Brennan PJ, Weitzman SA. Megestriol acetate in patients with AIDS related cachexia. *Annals of Internal Medicine,* 1994; 121:393–399.

34. Cruz JM, Mus HB, Brockschmidt JK, et al. Weight changes in women with metastatic breast cancer treated with megestrol acetate: a comparison of standard versus high-dose therapy. *Seminars in Oncology,* 1990; 17(suppl 9):S63–S67.

35. Tchekmedyian NS, Tait N, Moody M, et al. High dose megestrol acetate: a possible treatment for cachexia. *Journal of the American Medical Association,* 1987; 257:1195–1199.

36. Lai YL, Fang FM, Yeh CY. Management of anorexia patients in radiology: a prospective randomized comparison of megestrol and prednesone. *Journal of Pain and Symptom Management,* 1994; 9(4):265–268.

37. Neri B, Gemelli MT, Tarantini P, Benvenuti F, Khader A, Ludovici M, Michelotti R, Fabbroni S. The role of megestrol acetate in neoplastic anorexia and cachexia. *Current Therapeutic Research, Clinical and Experimental,* 1995; 56(2):183–189.

38. Loprinzi CL, Bernath AM, Schaid DJ, Malliard JA, Athmann LM, Michalak JC, Tschetter LK, Hatfield AK, Morton RF. Phase III evaluation of 4 doses of megestrol acetate as therapy of patients with cancer anorexia and/or cachexia. *Oncology,* 1994; 51(suppl 1):2–7.

39. Bruera E. Current pharmacological management of anorexia in cancer patients. *Oncology,* 1992; 6:125–137.

40. Chlebowski RT, Bulcavage L, Grosvenor M, et al. Hydrazine sulfate in cancer patients with weight loss: a placebo-controlled clinical experience. *Cancer,* 1987; 59:406–410.

41. Loprinzi CL, Kuross SA, O'Fallin JR, Gesme DH, Gerstner JB, Rospons RM, Cobau CD, Goldberg

RM. Randomized placebo-controlled evaluation of hydrazine sulfate in patients with advanced colorectal cancer. *Journal of Clinical Oncology*, 1994; 12(6):1121–1125.

42. Goldberg RM, Loprinzi CL, Maillard JA, O'Fallon JR, Krook JE, Ghosh C, Hestorff RD, Chong SF, Reuter NF, Shanahan TG. Pentoxifylline for treatment of cancer anorexia and cachexia? A randomized, double-blind, placebo-controlled trial. *Journal of Clinical Oncology*, 1995; 12(11):2856–2859.

43. Brennan MF. Total parenteral nutrition in the cancer patient. *New England Journal of Medicine*, 1981; 305:375–381.

44. Lesko L. Anorexia. In: Holland JC, Rowland JH, eds. *Handbook of Psychooncology: Psychological Care of the Patient With Cancer*. New York: Oxford University Press, 1989:434–443.

11

Psychiatric Aspects of Fatigue in the Terminally Ill

Susan Abbey, M.D., FRCPC

Fatigue complicates a variety of terminal illnesses, compromises quality of life, produces significant suffering, and in cancer and AIDS patients is associated with suicidal intent and wish for early death.[1,2] Yet it has received remarkably little attention. Therapeutic nihilism has predominated. Psychiatric professionals have an important role with the fatigued terminally ill patient, given their medical background and their expertise in a range of psychotherapeutic and psychopharmacological interventions that may improve fatigue or assist the patient in coping with fatigue that cannot be treated. Familiarity with medical causes of fatigue is important, given that they are the predominant source of fatigue in the terminally ill. The psychiatrist or psychiatric nurse often sorts out medical and psychiatric contributors to fatigue and frequently needs to encourage the medical team to optimize medical status. Psychiatric factors are often inappropriately invoked by exasperated physicians whose treatments have failed.[1]

This chapter focuses primarily on fatigue in patients with advanced cancer as a model for understanding the psychiatric dimensions of fatigue and the potential role of mental health professionals in the management of fatigue in the palliative setting. While fatigue in the terminally ill has received the most attention to date in the cancer literature, it is still remarkably underresearched. Fatigue is regularly associated with terminal illness secondary to acquired immune deficiency syndrome, end-stage respiratory diseases, end-stage cardiac diseases, and neurological diseases and yet has received little formal study. While the mechanisms underlying the physical causes of fatigue differ across these groups, they share possible common psychiatric causes of fatigue. The treatment of fatigue shares many similarities across these disparate diagnoses. Given the polysymptomatic nature of terminal illness, it is important to improve treatable symptoms. Fatigue is increasingly seen as one symptom that can be improved in some patients.

DEFINING FATIGUE

Fatigue is a word with a wide range of different meanings whose definition has bedeviled researchers for the past 100 years.[3] It is used to describe experiences such as tiredness, weariness, lassitude, inertia, lethargy, exhaustion, weakness, lack of energy, and lack of vitality. Unfortunately, most studies of fatigue in the medically ill do not specifically define their conceptualization or operationalization of fatigue. Fatigue is used in the cancer literature to refer to feelings of tiredness, weariness, weakness, exhaustion, and lack of energy.[4] Fatigue is commonly distinguished from somnolence. The boundary between fatigue and weakness is more controversial. Most researchers agree that fatigue is a multidimensional concept that includes physical, cognitive, affective, and motivational components and temporal descriptors (i.e., acute versus chronic). The Fatigue Coalition, in studying fatigue in cancer patients, has described fatigue as a general feeling of debilitating tiredness or loss of energy significant enough to impact how patients go about their daily routine.[5] While there has long been the hope of "objectively" measuring fatigue, clearly the situation is analogous to pain, that is, fatigue is experiential and defined by the patient. Self-report measures designed to evaluate fatigue are often not validated in palliative-care patients. Cella[6] notes the importance of measuring fatigue in the context of other dimensions of quality of life or well-being such as physical, functional, emotional, and social well-being.

LIMITATIONS IN RESEARCHING FATIGUE

While the largest limitation is that fatigue in terminal illness has been vastly understudied, the literature that does exist is problematic. Richardson[7] reviews limitations in the cancer literature regarding fatigue and finds that they are similar to those for other terminal diseases: problems of sample size; lack of control groups; design and measurement problems, including significant difficulties in measuring and characterizing fatigue; the paucity of well-validated, reliable questionnaires; and lack of information about other aspects of individual's lives that would make it possible to accurately assess the impact of the disease and other etiological factors. Future studies of fatigue in palliative-care patients need to operationalize their definition of fatigue and to characterize it carefully.

THE ROLE OF PSYCHIATRIC FACTORS IN FATIGUE

Fatigue is closely associated with psychological and psychosocial morbidity in studies of healthy community samples,[8,9] in primary care,[10] and in a variety of medical illnesses.[11] The mechanisms by which psychological distress is transduced into fatigue are complex and remain poorly understood. The relationship between fatigue and medical illnesses is complex and may be the result of cause, effect, or covariate.[11] Weisman,[12] in his classic monograph *Coping with Cancer*, emphasized that fatigue in the cancer patient is both a symptom of and a cause for emotional distress. Disentangling the relationship between fatigue and psychiatric and psychosocial distress in an individual patient may be complex and may require considerable experience and skill.

Psychiatric disorders most commonly associated with fatigue have psychophysiological concomitants, including fatigue, and are associated with somatic amplification in which bodily symptoms or perceptions are experienced as intense, noxious, or disturbing.[13] Depressive disorders are characterized by decreased energy, easy fatigability, and sleep disturbances. Anxiety disorders such as acute stress disorder and generalized anxiety disorder are associated with sleep disturbance and the latter with easy fatigability. Panic attacks, with their intense, episodic, and intensely somatic nature, are often followed by fatigue. Substance abuse must be considered in the psychiatric differential diagnosis of fatigue. A small subset of fatigued terminally ill patients may be abusing analgesics, sedative-hypnotics, or marijuana to deal with intolerable effects of disease or medications. Terminally ill patients are particularly vulnerable to depression, anxiety, and bodily preoccupation.

FATIGUE IN TERMINAL CANCER

Fatigue is the most commonly reported symptom of cancer and cancer therapies[14] and a major source of distress for patients with advanced cancer. The systematic study of fatigue and potential interventions directed toward it have become a topic of growing interest in clinical oncology, reflecting an increasing awareness of the impact of fatigue on a wide variety of life domains and an appreciation of the unique distress that it causes patients.[4,7,15–17]. According to Winningham et al., "Fatigue has important implications for cancer care. Patients discontinue treatment because of fatigue; doses of various forms of treatment are limited by fatigue; patients attribute impairment in quality of life to fatigue."[17] The Fatigue Coalition was developed in 1996 to advocate for greater attention to fatigue in cancer patients and research into its management.[5] Experts have emphasized the importance of both prevalence and intervention studies related to fatigue in advanced cancer.[18]

The Importance of Fatigue in Cancer Patients

Patients' ($n = 419$), caregivers' ($n = 200$), and oncologists' ($n = 197$) perceptions of cancer-related fatigue have been studied.[5] Fatigue was reported by 78% of patients who had undergone chemotherapy or radiotherapy and were recruited through a survey of 100,000 randomly selected households. Fatigue was described in their patients by 86% of caregivers. Fatigue was seen as more adversely affecting daily life than cancer pain by 61% of cancer patients, and 12% reported that fatigue made them want to die. The treatment of fatigue was seen by 16% of patients to be as important as treating their cancer, and 41% felt its treatment was more important than the treatment of pain. Only 27% of patient reported that their oncologists suggested a treatment for fatigue.

Epidemiology

Most studies have focused on earlier disease and have documented rates of fatigue between 60% and 90% during chemotherapy and between 31% and 100% in the radiotherapy literature.[17] Rates vary with the type of tumor and treatment. Fatigue persists following completion of treatment in many chemotherapy and radiotherapy patients.[17] One large study of symptoms in advanced cancer patients found that easy fatigability was the second most prevalent and second most severe problem reported by 1,000 patients. It was clinically important in 48% of the total sample and in 77% of those affected.[19] Of patients reporting fatigue, approximately 56% described moderate severity, with the remainder split equally between mild and severe. Lack of energy was the most prevalent or second most prevalent symptom in four tumor types, ranging from 68% of ovarian cancer patients to 80% of breast cancer patients.[14]

Etiological Mechanisms for Fatigue in Advanced Cancer

Mechanisms postulated to explain fatigue in cancer patients can be broadly grouped by patho-physiology to include direct effects of the tumor, effects of treatment, outcome of other symptoms of cancer (e.g., pain), and emotional distress. Terminally ill cancer patients vary with respect to which mechanism(s) are most responsible for their symptomatology. Prudent health care professionals must consider the relative contributions of each of these factors in a given patient. A variety of theoretical models have been proposed to integrate these diverse etiological mechanisms and to structure patient assessment.[17] While a detailed discussion of nonpsychiatric factors is beyond the scope of this chapter, they are summarized here to highlight their complexity. Direct effects of tumor include a variety of fatigue-producing metabolic and biochemical changes. Cancer may be associated with alterations in the Krebs cycle, increased futile cycle pathways, and increased glucose uptake.[20] Muscle changes in cancer patients may contribute to reduced capacity for physical exertion,[20] although it is unclear whether this is specific to cancer or an epiphenomenon secondary to inactivity, which produces muscle atrophy. Treatments for cancer, including surgery, chemotherapy, radiotherapy, and immune therapies, may produce or exacerbate fatigue through a wide variety of mechanisms.[7,15] Chemotherapy and radiotherapy result in cellular lysis and necrosis of tumor mass, with the liberation of intracellular products and metabolites. They have important emotional side effects, including anxiety and sleep disturbance, which may produce fatigue. Anemia is associated with fatigue, although the relationship is not consistent and may be most relevant at extremely low levels of hemoglobin. Studies of fatigue with biological response modifiers (e.g., interferon, interleukin-2) were among the first to demonstrate the role of cytokines in the genesis of fatigue states. Fatigue and malaise associated with their use is a key dose-limiting side effect.[17] Fatigue continues past treatment cessation, although the mechanism remains poorly understood. Cancer symptoms may produce fatigue. Gastrointestinal disturbances (e.g., vomiting, diarrhea) alter electrolyte and metabolic parameters, inducing fatigue, pain, and abnormal muscle metabolism. Pain acts through a variety of mechanisms, including interfering with sleep and increasing emotional distress. Sleep disruption significantly contributes to fatigue, although it has received little systematic study in cancer.[21–23] Sleep disturbances were reported by 5% to 29% of advanced cancer patients[19,24] and were a clinically important problem for 68% of those with sleep problems.[19] Sleep problems may be a symptom of the cancer, a side effect of treatment, a sequelae of cancer symptoms such as pain or nausea, or a reaction to the stress of having cancer[21] or to environmental disruptions related to care.[23] Multiple factors may contribute to sleep disturbance, including perturbations in the immune system, pain, gastrointestinal distress, dyspnea, fever, anxiety, and depression. Patients in inpatient settings contend with environmental conditions that impact on sleep. Cachexia and weight loss are anecdotally implicated in the genesis of fatigue and may act through impaired energy synthesis, alterations in muscle function, and loss of muscle mass.[17] Research is now focusing on the role of altered cytokine metabolism in impaired energy metabolism and weight loss.[20] Physical deconditioning related to periods in bed of even as little as several weeks has been implicated in fatigue. Psychosocial, psychological, and psychiatric factors are important in the genesis of fatigue in some patients. The relationship between depression and fatigue in cancer patients is complicated, as there is the dilemma of sorting out "which cancer patients are merely tired and which are tired and depressed."[25] In advanced disease, higher levels of fatigue are reported by depressed patients than nondepressed patients.[26]

FATIGUE IN AIDS

More than 50% of AIDS (CDC IV) patients have problematic fatigue that interferes with daily functioning,[27] only one-third describe feeling alert during the morning hours, and more than one-third have significant sleep problems.[27] Fatigue in AIDS patients is related to both immunological and psychological factors. Organic mental disorders and mood and anxiety disorders are common in terminally ill AIDS patients.[1,28]

FATIGUE IN END-STAGE HEART AND LUNG DISEASES

Little has been written about fatigue in end-stage heart and lung diseases, although studies are now under way. Physical factors appear paramount in fatigue in both groups, but preliminary research is suggesting that psychiatric disorders associated with fatigue are relatively common and may contribute to fatigue in some terminally ill patients. End-stage lung disease is commonly accompanied by depression[29] and panic disorder.[30]

FATIGUE IN END-STAGE NEUROLOGICAL DISEASE

Fatigue is a common and often profoundly debilitating symptom of end-stage neurological disease that requires multidisciplinary approaches to assessment and treatment.[31] Studies in amyotrophic lateral sclerosis show that perceived fatigue is a complex phenomenon including both central and peripheral factors, although psychiatric distress has not been adequately evaluated.[32]

FATIGUE IN CARE PROVIDERS

No discussion of fatigue in palliative medicine is complete without addressing caregiver fatigue. Caregivers face significant psychosocial stresses, including bearing the practical burden of assisting patients with tasks they cannot do, providing physical care, fulfilling their own social roles, and at times dealing with added financial stresses.[33–35] A minority of caregivers develop depressive or anxiety disorders that warrant treatment. Holistic care for the palliative-care patient includes attention to the needs of caregivers, including helping caregivers set priorities with respect to competing demands on their time, optimizing coping and stress management, encouraging rest and relaxation, assisting in organizing respite care, and reinforcing the importance of leisure activities for the caregiver.

TREATMENT APPROACHES TO FATIGUE IN THE PALLIATIVE PATIENT

Interventions for fatigue in terminally ill patients have not been systematically studied. From a practical standpoint, it is important to address any factor that is potentially modifiable. Psychiatric professionals have an important role to play in assessing and managing fatigue from a biopsychosocial perspective. Familiarity with medical issues is required for optimal effectiveness, given that they may need to encourage optimization of medical interventions and educate patients and families. Even small improvements in fatigue or the ability to cope with it may be associated with decreased suffering and improved quality of life. Analogies that present fatigue as a depletion of a "bank account" of energy may be helpful to both patients and caregivers as they attempt to "increase deposits" and "minimize withdrawals."

Optimizing Medical Status

The psychiatrist must ensure that a comprehensive assessment, including physical examination and laboratory investigations, has been done to identify potentially remediable medical factors that contribute to fatigue. Adequate hydration and optimal electrolyte and metabolic balance are important. Thyroid function should be assessed. Anemia may be treated. Recombinant human erythropoietin is being used for the anemia of advanced cancer, although clinically significant effects may take 2 to 6 weeks.[36] Red blood cell transfusions may be improve quality of life in the severely fatigued anemic patient.[37] Dyspnea should be treated aggressively, given its multiple mediating effects on fatigue.[38] The diagnosis of hypoactive delirium may have been missed and should initiate the search for reversible causes and symptomatic treatment (see chapter 5). Steroids have been prescribed to fatigued and weak patients with transient improvement at times but on balance do not seem helpful.[1]

Reviewing Medications and Optimizing Analgesia

Each medication should be reviewed for its sedative potential. Drug interactions that might increase sedation should be considered. Analgesic medications require particular attention in terms of (1) their potential role in producing sedation and fatigue, and (2) achieving optimal pain control, as inadequately treated pain is emotionally distressing and fatiguing. Drowsiness and fatigue are well-recognized complications of opioid therapy. Optimizing the use of nonopioid analgesics and adjuvant medications may reduce fatigue.[39]

Psychostimulants used to counteract opioid-induced drowsiness and sedation include both dextroamphetamine[40] and methylphenidate.[41]

Optimizing Nutritional Status

Nutritional strategies for ameliorating fatigue in terminally ill patients are in development. Nutritional assessment in terms of dietary intake is important, as it is clear that the terminally ill patient may have difficulty taking in adequate calories and fluids. Commonsense advice includes eating small amounts throughout the day in addition to conventional meals, sipping fluids to ensure adequate intake, and consuming foods that are both high in calories and enjoyable to the patient. Recent data in healthy volunteers suggests that n-3 polyunsaturated fatty acids (e.g., flax seed oil, fish oil) may decrease cytokines such as tumor necrosis factor alpha and interleukin 1 beta and be helpful in increasing weight and appetite and decreasing fatigue in patients with advanced cancer.[20] Compounds such as thalidomide and megestrol acetate may stimulate appetite.[20,42]

Beginning Physical Reactivation and Exercise

Physical reactivation in the terminally ill patient may counteract the multiple effects of physical deconditioning, including alterations in muscle functioning, sleep-wake cycle, and social isolation. However, it may be difficult to convince patients of the value of reactivation and physical exercise, as it is counterintuitive to patients who are advised to "rest up," "take it easy," and "look after themselves". Exercise may be beneficial if it can be physically tolerated. In women with less advanced breast cancer, there is preliminary evidence that it improves physiological and psychological well-being and decreases symptoms such as anorexia, asthenia, and cachexia.[43] Studies in chronic congestive heart failure have focused on nonhospitalized patients and have demonstrated improvements in aerobic and ventilatory capacity and fatigue with short-term exercise training using interval exercise methods.[44] Exercise may reduce symptoms in patients with end-stage lung disease.[45] Exercise may be integrated into daily life by beginning slowly, keeping within what is tolerated, slowly increasing duration, setting a regular exercise time, and involving a buddy or partner.

Introducing Energy Conservation Techniques

Occupational therapists are very helpful in modifying the home to maximize conservation of patient energy (e.g., installing grab rails in the shower, raising toilet seats, positioning chairs to allow for a rest along long hallways or near stairs). Motorized scooters may be helpful for some patients. Patient education materials outline a large number of techniques and strategies for coping with the challenges of dressing, meal preparation, and housekeeping.[46,47] Techniques, including planning, prioritizing, and pacing, are designed to conserve energy so that it can be spent on those activities of most value to the patient. Regular rest and relaxation periods are essential, should be routinely scheduled into the day, and may be added prior to periods of activity or visitors. Relaxation techniques may contribute to rest periods. Psychological factors may be obstacles to effectively incorporating rest into daily schedules, and an exploration of patient's reluctance to schedule rest periods may lead to discussions of core beliefs related to the importance of activity for self-worth, which in the context of terminal illness are maladaptive and limiting. A diary may be a useful tool in helping the patient, family, and health care professionals to fully appreciate the various dimensions of and the factors involved in the patient's fatigue. An explicit discussion needs to be held around help seeking. Many individuals are reluctant to ask family and friends for help. At times, this reluctance reaches maladaptive levels and requires intervention, such as exploring the meaning of help seeking and reframing help seeking as an adaptive strategy. Helping individuals to make lists of activities that they could ask others to do and helping them decide whom they could ask for help may be important. While involving community agencies is important for most terminally ill patients, it is essential for those without adequate social supports and as a respite for those with caregivers who have little support. Prioritizing activities is a hallmark of energy conservation and yet often one of the most difficult to do. Maladaptive core beliefs may intrude, and mental health professionals may help in exploring beliefs and value systems and sorting out what patients' priorities are at this point in their life. Individuals can be encouraged to cultivate interests that are less strenuous but nonetheless rewarding. These may be easier or shorter versions of highly valued activities or substitutes that maintain interest and offer pleasure but require less physical exertion. For example, an outdoorsman might find some pleasure in fishing shows or reading about the outdoors. Encouraging interests in reading, music, and videos may be helpful. Assisting the patient in coping with continuing decrements in function is important; for example, the avid reader may need to make peace with shorter articles and eventually looking at pictures as his energy and concentration decrease.

Developing Strategies to Overcome the Negative Effects of Fatigue

Many patients note problems with memory and concentration related to their fatigue. Simple techniques such as making notes, keeping lists, and involving caregivers may be helpful. Relaxation techniques such as mindfulness meditation, yoga, and visual imagery may be beneficial.

Treating Sleep Disturbances

Sleep disturbance contributes to fatigue and must be addressed. Attention should first be directed to remediable factors in the environment (e.g., timing of treatments, decreasing nocturnal awakenings for care) and the identification of specific cause(s) of sleeplessness. The potential role of medications in daytime sedation and rebound insomnia should be considered.[21] Assessment for and treatment of concomitant psychiatric disorders, particularly major depression and delirium, are essential. Management should then focus on principles of sleep hygiene and move on to behavioral interventions and pharmacotherapy if necessary. Sleep hygiene includes having regular times for going to bed and getting up; limiting daytime napping; relaxing before bed; decreasing sources of stimulation in the evening hours (e.g., exercise, caffeine and alcohol consumption, smoking); adjusting ambient temperature and humidity; ensuring support and comfortable body positioning by using pillows or rolled blankets; getting up from bed if unsuccessful in falling asleep. Ensuring adequate analgesia through the period of sleep is essential. Complementary therapies, including aromatherapy, guided meditations and imagery, and herbal treatments and teas may help. Behavioral interventions of value include progressive muscle relaxation training[48] and relaxation and imagery techniques.[49] Sedative-hypnotic medications may be indicated when sleep problems are related to medication side effects or other physical factors. The use of sedative-hypnotic medications requires an assessment of the balance between risk (e.g., daytime sedation, impaired cognition) and benefit. The goal of pharmacotherapy is a good night's sleep with minimal daytime sedation or "hangover." The choice of specific agent will depend on other medications that the patient is taking and concern about side effects or interactions with these drugs. The most commonly prescribed sedative medications in the medically ill include the cyclopyrrolones (e.g., zopiclone, zopilidem), benzodiazepines (e.g., lorazepam, clonazepam), and low doses of sedating heterocyclic antidepressants (e.g., trazodone, doxepin, amitriptyline). Dosing should start low and be increased as needed. Caution must be employed, as sedative-hypnotics may impair cognition in the palliative-care patient, and arguments have been made for discontinuing their use. In a sample of 120 palliative-care cancer patients, rapid discontinuation of hypnotics resulted in no significant change in the intensity of insomnia but an improvement in cognition.[50]

Identifying and Treating Psychiatric Disorders and Reducing Emotional Distress

Fatigued patients should be assessed for depressive disorders, anxiety disorders, and delirium and provided with aggressive treatment if indicated (see chapters 2, 4, 5). Supportive attention to emotional distress that does not meet diagnostic criteria may assist the patient in coping better with irreversible fatigue or decreasing fatigue that has a psychosocial component. While psychosocial, psychological, and psychiatric factors are transduced through the central and autonomic nervous systems, there unfortunately remains a common perception that when such factors are involved in fatigue, the fatigue is somehow less "real" or disabling. This leads to difficulties in engaging many patients in psychiatric treatment they see as stigmatizing. Nonetheless, it is essen-

tial that psychiatric disorders and psychosocial correlates of fatigue be identified, as they are common and often remediable.

Psychoeducation

Providing information about fatigue and the role of physical and emotional factors in its origin and perpetuation may encourage patients to accept help. Even when fatigue is entirely based in physical factors, the psychiatrist's clear explanation of these factors may do much to allay the patient's and the family's anxiety and may decrease the suffering associated with the fatigue. Education can address faulty attributions made about fatigue and distortions in understanding its prognostic implications. For example, a patient who is experiencing fatigue secondary to palliative chemotherapy or radiotherapy may mistakenly interpret the fatigue as evidence that they are near death. Learning that fatigue in response to such treatments is normative relieves emotional distress.

Social Interventions

Enhancing social support may be beneficial for patients whose fatigue has resulted in significant isolation.[25] Community supports may be invaluable for both patients and caregivers. Encouraging participation in support groups where feasible may be helpful. Telephone contact and the Internet offer support for the housebound patient.

Relaxation Techniques

Professionals should be aware of and comfortable instructing patients and caregivers in a variety of relaxation techniques or refer them for such instruction. Commonly used techniques include stretching,[51] yoga,[52] progressive muscle relaxation,[53] the relaxation response,[54] mindfulness meditation,[55] guided visual imagery,[56] and self-hypnosis.[57] All of these techniques may diminish anxiety, aid in sleep induction, improve the quality of rest periods, and decrease pain.

Psychotherapy

Psychotherapeutic interventions to reduce emotional distress in terminally ill patients include a wide range of modalities and techniques, as discussed later in this book (see chapters 12–16).

There has been no systematic attention to the use of psychotherapy in managing fatigue in the terminally ill. A positive impact on fatigue has been reported by investigators using tailored counseling in patients with less advanced cancer,[58–60] although these studies did not specifically select patients complaining of fatigue; other studies have found no effect. Cognitive therapy techniques related to energy conservation techniques are described earlier. They may assist in dealing with bodily preoccupation.[61] Chapter 15 describes cognitive therapy in the palliative setting in detail. A cognitive model has been used with success in patients with end-stage pulmonary disease.[62,63]

Pharmacotherapy

Patients with major depressive disorders, panic disorder, and generalized anxiety disorder warrant pharmacotherapy (see chapters 2, 4). The role of pharmacotherapy in patients with fatigue who do not have a psychiatric disorder is less clear. Many clinicians give a trial of a psychostimulant to fatigued patients. Psychostimulants act on the central nervous system to produce wakefulness, alertness, elevation of mood, and increased initiative and motivation, and their use in the medically ill has recently been reviewed.[64] Although they have been used primarily to treat major depression, adjustment disorders, and cognitive disturbance, clinically it appears that fatigue, apathy, and "giving up" are the symptoms most responsive to psychostimulants. Psychostimulants may increase a patient's energy and break an established cycle of hopelessness and inactivity. Methylphenidate and dextroamphetamine are the most commonly prescribed stimulants and are relatively free of side effects. Discontinuation due to treatment emergent side effects is typically less than 10%.[64] Pulse and blood pressure may be checked prior to and 1 hour after the first dose to monitor for sinus tachycardia or hypertension. Debilitated patients may be started on low doses (e.g., methylphenidate 2.5 mg or 5 mg at 8 A.M., dextroamphetamine 2.5 mg at 8 A.M.) and increased until there is a response or side effects emerge. Methylphenidate requires dosing at 8 A.M. and noon, while dextroamphetamine requires only a single 8 A.M. dose. Despite their efficacy, there remain a number of barriers to their use, including myths regarding addiction, abuse, toler-

ance, and anorexiant effects.[64] While amphetamines suppress normal appetite, they tend to normalize poor appetite.[1,64] There is a case report of methylphenidate's value in the management of psychological distress and somatization in a terminal cancer patient.[65] Dextroamphetamine increases energy and mood in depressed AIDS patients with debilitating low energy.[66] In patients who refuse pharmacotherapy, it is important to explore the meaning of pharmacotherapy to the patient. Patients who are already taking a number of drugs may be reluctant to add an additional medication and may perceive pharmacotherapy as evidence of loss of control, personal weakness, or moral failure.

FUTURE DIRECTIONS

We are beginning to shed the therapeutic nihilism toward fatigue that has impeded research to date. Recently, several new, brief, and well-validated fatigue assessment tools appeared in the literature, including the Brief Fatigue Inventory,[67] the Revised Piper Fatigue Scale,[68] and the Fatigue Severity Index.[69] With better assessment tools, newer, hopefully effective interventions for fatigue can be tested in diverse palliative care populations. When we also accept the seriousness of fatigue in terms of its prevalence and its negative impact on quality of life in the terminally ill, we are poised for significant developments in the field akin to the explosion in knowledge about cancer pain in the 1980s and 1990s. In the interim, we have a number of strategies that can benefit fatigued, terminally ill patients today.

References

1. Breitbart W, Passik SD. Psychiatric aspects of palliative care. In: Doyle D, Hanks G, MacDonald N, eds, *Oxford Textbook of Palliative Medicine*. New York: Oxford University Press, 1993; 609–626.
2. Coyle N, Adelhardt J, Foley KM, Portenoy RK. Character of terminal illness in the advanced cancer patient: pain and other symptoms during the last four weeks of life. *Journal of Pain and Symptom Management*, 1990; 5:83–93.
3. Berrios GE. Feelings of fatigue and psychopathology: a conceptual history. *Comprehensive Psychiatry*, 1990; 31:140–151.
4. Aistars J. Fatigue in the cancer patient: a concep-

tual approach to a clinical problem. *Oncology Nursing Forum*, 1987; 14:25–30.

5. Vogelzang NJ, Breitbart W, Cella C, Curt GA, Groopman JE, Horning SJ, Itri LM, Johnson DH, Scherr SL, Portenoy RK. Patient, caregiver, and oncologist perceptions of cancer-related fatigue: results of a tripart assessment survey. *Seminars in Hematology*, 1997; 13(3 Suppl 2):4–12.

6. Cella D. The functional assessment of cancer therapy—anemia (FACT-An) scale: a new tool for the assessment of outcomes in cancer anemia and fatigue. *Seminars in Hematology*, 1997; 34(3 Suppl 2):13–19.

7. Richardson A. Fatigue in cancer patients: a review of the literature. *European Journal of Cancer Care*, 1995; 4:20–32.

8. Walker EA, Katon WJ, Jemelka RP. Psychiatric disorders and medical care utilization among people in the general population who report fatigue. *Journal of General Internal Medicine*, 1993; 8:436–440.

9. Pawlikowska T, Chalder T, Hirsch SR, Wallace P, Wright DJ, Wessely SC. Population-based study of fatigue and psychological distress. *British Medical Journal*, 1994; 308:763–766.

10. Bates DW, Schmitt W, Buchwald D, Ware NC, Lee J, Thoyer E, Kornish RJ, Komaroff AL. Prevalence of fatigue and chronic fatigue syndrome in a primary-care practice. *Archives of Internal Medicine*, 1993; 153:2759–2765.

11. Abbey SE, Garfinkel PE. Chronic fatigue and depression: cause, effect or covariate. *Reviews of Infectious Disease*, 1991; 13(Suppl 1):S73–83.

12. Weisman A. *Coping with Cancer*. New York: McGraw-Hill, 1979.

13. Abbey SE. Somatization and somatoform disorders. In: Rundell JR, Wise MG, eds, *The American Psychiatric Press Textbook of Consultation-Liaison Psychiatry*. Washington, DC: American Psychiatric Press, 1996:369–401.

14. Portenoy RK, Thaler HT, Kornblith AB, Lepore JM, Friedlander-Klar H, Coyle N, Smart-Curley T, Kemeny N, Norton L, Hoskins W, Sher H. Problems, characteristics, and distress in a cancer population. *Quality of Life Research*, 1994; 3:183–189.

15. Glaus A. Assessment of fatigue in cancer and non-cancer patients and in health individuals. *Supportive Care in Cancer*, 1993; 1:305–315.

16. Smets EMA, Garssen B, Schuster-Uitterhoeve ALJ, deHaes JCJM. Fatigue in cancer patients. *British Journal of Cancer*, 1993; 68:220–224.

17. Winningham ML, Nail LM, Barton Burke M, Brophy L, Cimprich B, Jones LS, Pickard-Holley S, Rhodes V, St. Pierre B, Beck S, Glass EC, Mock VL, Mooney KH, Piper B. Fatigue and the cancer experience: the state of the knowledge. *Oncology Nursing Forum*, 1994; 21:23–36.

18. Breitbart W, Bruera E, Chochinov H, Lynch M. Neuropsychiatric syndromes and psychological symptoms in patients with advanced cancer. *Journal of Pain and Symptom Management*, 1995; 10:131–141.

19. Donnelly S, Walsh D. The symptoms of advanced cancer: identification of clinical and research priorities by assessment of prevalence and severity. *Journal of Palliative Care*, 1995; 11:27–32.

20. Kalman D, Villani LJ. Nutritional aspects of cancer-related fatigue. *Journal of the American Dietetic Association*, 1997; 97:650–654.

21. Hu DS, Silberfarb PM. Management of sleep problems in cancer patients. *Oncology*, 1991; 5:23–27.

22. Malone M, Harris AL, Luscombe DK. Assessment of the impact of cancer on work, recreation, home management and sleep using a general health status measure. *Journal of the Royal Society of Medicine*, 1994; 87:386–389.

23. Sheeley LC. Sleep disturbances in hospitalized patients with cancer. *Oncology Nursing Forum*, 1996; 23:109–111.

24. Vainio A, Auvinen A, Members of the Symptom Prevalence Group. Prevalence of symptoms among patients with advanced cancer: an international collaborative study. *Journal of Pain and Symptom Management*, 1996; 12:3–10.

25. Hayes JR. Depression and chronic fatigue in cancer patients. *Primary Care: Clinics in Office Practice*, 1991; 18:327–339.

26. Grassi L, Indelli M, Marzola M, Maestri A, Santini A, Piva E, Boccalon M. Depressive symptoms and quality of life in home-care-assisted cancer patients. *Journal of Pain and Symptom Management*, 1996; 12:300–307.

27. Darko DF, McCutchan JA, Kripke DF, Gillin JC, Golshan S. Fatigue, sleep disturbance, disability, and indices of progression in HIV infection. *American Journal of Psychiatry*, 1992; 149:514–520.

28. Worth HL, Halman MH. HIV Disease/AIDS. In: Rundell JR, Wise MG, eds., *The American Psychiatric Press Textbook of Consultation-Liaison Psychiatry*, Washington, DC: American Psychiatric Press, 1996:832–877.

29. Gift AG, McCrone SH. Depression in patients with COPD. *Heart & Lung*, 1993; 22:289–297.

30. Smoller JW, Pollack MH, Ottow MW, Rosenbaum JF, Kradin RL. Panic anxiety, dyspnea, and respiratory disease. Theoretical and clinical considerations. *American Journal of Respiratory and Critical Care Medicine*, 1996, 154:6–17.

31. Krupp LB, Pollina DA. Mechanisms and management of fatigue in progressive neurological disorders. *Current Opinion in Neurology*, 1996; 9:456–460.

32. Sharma KR, Kent-Braun JA, Majumdar S, Huang Y, Mynhier M, Weiner MW, Miller RG. Physiology of fatigue in amyotrophic lateral sclerosis. *Neurology*, 1995; 45:733–740.

33. Hinds C. The needs of families who care for patients with cancer at home: are we meeting them? *Journal of Advanced Nursing*, 1985; 10:575–581.

34. Stetz KM. Caregiving demands during advanced cancer: the spouse's needs. *Cancer Nursing*, 1987; 10:260–268.

35. Folkman S, Chesney MA, Christopher-Richards A. Stress and coping in caregiving partners of men with AIDS. *Psychiatric Clinics of North America*, 1994; 7:35–53.

36. Henry DH, Abels RI. Recombinant human erythropoietin in the treatment of cancer and chemotherapy-induced anemia: results of double-blind and open-label follow-up studies. *Seminars in Oncology*, 1994; 21(2 Suppl 3):1–28.

37. Monti M, Castellani L, Berlusconi A, Cunietti E. Use of red blood cell transfusions in terminally ill cancer patients admitted to a palliative-care unit. *Journal of Pain and Symptom Management*, 1996; 12:18–22.

38. Ziment I. Use of medication in end-stage disease. *Seminars in Respiratory and Critical Care Medicine*, 1996; 17:491–502.

39. Gron S, Zech D, Schug SA, Lynch J, Lehmann KA. Validation of World Health Organization guidelines for cancer pain relief during the last days and hours of life. *Journal of Pain and Symptom Management*, 1991; 6:411–422.

40. Kreeger L, Duncan A, Cowap J. Psychostimulants used for opioid-induced drowsiness. *Journal of Pain and Symptom Management*, 1996; 11:1–2. Letter.

41. Bruera E, Miller MJ, Macmillan K, Kuehn N. Neuropsychological effects of methylphenidate in patients receiving a continuous infusion of narcotics for cancer pain. *Pain*, 1992; 48:163–166.

42. Strang P. The effect of megestrol acetate on anorexia, weight loss and cachexia in cancer and AIDS patients. *Anticancer Research*, 1997; 18:657–662.

43. Friedenreich CM, Courneya KS. Exercise as rehabilitation for cancer patients. *Clinical Journal of Sports Medicine*, 1996; 6:237–244.

44. Meyer K, Schwaibold M, Westbrook S, Beneke R, Hajric R, Gornandt L, Lehmann M, Roskamm H. Effects of short-term exercise training and activity restriction on functional capacity in patients with severe chronic congestive heart failure. *American Journal of Cardiology*, 1996; 78:1017–1022.

45. Ries AL. Rehabilitation for the patient with advanced lung disease: designing an appropriate program, establishing realistic goals, meeting the goals. *Seminars in Respiratory and Critical Care Medicine*, 1996; 17:451–463.

46. Rosenbarum EH, Dollinger M, Piper BF, Rosenbaum I. Coping with treatment side effects. In: Dollinger M, Rosenbaum EH, Cable G, eds, *Everyone's Guide to Cancer Therapy*. 2nd ed., Kansas City: Somerville House, 1994:25–128.

47. Di Lima DM, ed. *Completing Daily Tasks When Coping with Cancer. Oncology Patient Education Manual*. Gaithersburg, MD: Aspen Publishers, 1994:638–641.

48. Cannici J, Malcolm R, Peck LA. Treatment of insomnia in cancer patients using muscle relaxant training. *Journal of Behaviour Therapy and Experimental Psychiatry*, 1983; 14:251–256.

49. Stamm H, Bultz B, Pittman C. Psychosocial problems and interventions in a referred sample of cancer patients. *Psychosomatic Medicine*, 1986; 48:539–548.

50. Bruera E, Fainsinger RL, Schoeller T, Ripamonti C. Rapid discontinuation of hypnotics in terminal cancer patients: a prospective study. *Annals of Oncology*, 1996; 7:855–856.

51. Anderson B. *Stretching*. Bolinas, CA: Shelter Publications, 1980.

52. Christensen A, Rankin D. *Easy Does It: Yoga for Older People*. New York: Harper and Row, 1979.

53. Jacobson E. *Progressive Relaxation*. Chicago: University of Chicago Press, 1974.

54. Benson H, Beary JF, Carol MP. The relaxation response. *Psychiatry*, 1974; 37:37–46.

55. Kabat-Zinn J. *Full Catastrophe Living: Using the Wisdom of Your Body and Mind to Face Stress, Pain and Illness*. New York: Dell, 1990.

56. Epstein G. *Healing Visualization: Creating Health Through Imagery*. New York: Bantam, 1989.

57. Alman BM, Lambrou P. *Self-Hypnosis: The Complete Manual for Health and Self-Change*. New York: Brunner/Mazel, 1992.

58. Spiegel D, Bloom JR, Yalom I. Group support for patients with metastatic cancer: a randomized prospective outcome study. *Archives of General Psychiatry*, 1981; 38:527–533.

59. Worden JW, Weisman AD. Preventive psychosocial intervention with newly diagnosed cancer patients. *General Hospital Psychiatry*, 1984; 6:243–249.

60. Forester B, Kornfeld DS, Fleis JL. Psychotherapy during radiotherapy: effects on emotional and

physical distress. *American Journal of Psychiatry*, 1985; 142:22–27.

61. Salkovskis P. Somatic problems. In: Hawton K, Salkovskis PM, Kirk J, Clark DM eds, *Cognitive Behaviour Therapy for Psychiatric Problems, A Practical Guide*. New York: Oxford University Press, 1989:235–276.

62. Littlefield C. Psychological treatment of patients with end-stage pulmonary disease. *Monaldi Archives of Chest Disease*, 1995; 50:58–61.

63. Abbey SE, Littlefield C, Bright J. Assisting the patient and family to cope with advanced disease: the psychosocial aspects of end-stage disease. *Seminars in Respiratory Critical Care Medicine*, 1996; 17:533–542.

64. Masand PS, Tesar GE. Use of stimulants in the medically ill. *Psychiatric Clinics of North America*, 1996; 19:515–547.

65. Vigano A, Watanabe S, Bruera E. Methyphenidate for the management of somatization in terminal cancer patients. *Journal of Pain and Symptom Management*, 1995; 10:167–170.

66. Wagner GJ, Rabkin JG, Rabkin R. Dextroamphetamine as a treatment for depression and low energy in AIDS patients: a pilot study. *Journal of Psychosomatic Research*, 1997; 42:407–411.

67. Mendoza TR, Wang XS, Cleeland CS, Morrisey M, Johnson BA, Wendt JK, Haber SC. The rapid assessment of fatigue severity in cancer patients: use of the Brief Fatigue Inventory. *Cancer*, 1999; 85:1186–1196.

68. Piper BF, Dibble SL, Dodd MJ, Weiss MC, Slaughter RE, Paul SM. The revised Piper Fatigue Scale: psychometric evaluation in women with breast cancer. *Oncology Nursing Forum*, 1998; 25:677–684.

69. Hann DM, Jacobson PB, Azzarello LM, Martin SC, Curran SL, Fields K, Greenberg H, Lyman G. Measurement of fatigue in cancer patients: development and validation of the Fatigue Symptom Inventory. *Quality of Life Research*, 1998; 7:301–310.

PART III

Psychotherapeutic Intervention
and Palliative Care

12

Individual Psychotherapy for the Patient with Advanced Disease

Gary Rodin, M.D., FRCPC
Laurie A. Gillies, Ph.D., Cpsych

Psychological response to chronic or serious medical disease is determined by a complex interaction of factors related to the illness, the individual, and the social milieu. Those who have been previously well adjusted may experience unfamiliar and severe emotional distress in the wake of serious or terminal illness. With children who are ill, coping may be impaired by limitations in their ability to comprehend the nature of the disease or the reasons for their suffering. For adolescents and young adults who are struggling to be independent, the inevitable loss of independence or autonomy as a result of illness can be particularly distressing. The terminally ill adolescent, in particular, must accept the loss of innumerable unfulfilled possibilities. Those in their middle years face disappointments in terms of anticipated accomplishments. In the elderly, distress may be compounded when there is little support from peers, many of whom may also be frail or ill. Serious or terminal illness highlights the sense that life is finite and that there are not endless possibilities for achieving one's aspirations. Indeed, awareness of a shortened life span is often an unspoken backdrop to all thoughts and feelings that emerge after the illness is diagnosed.

AIDS deserves special consideration as one of the more common causes of serious illness and death in young adults. Indeed, most young adults in urban centers have known someone who has died of AIDS. Those in the gay community have often witnessed the literal decimation of their network of friends, confidants, and peers. The multiple and progressive complications of AIDS, the stigma and, in many cases, the elimination of available support, add considerably to the burden of this disease.

Signs of successful adaptation to a chronic or serious disease include the maintenance of self-esteem, the relative preservation of self-concept, acceptance of the illness such that treatment recommendations can be followed, engagement in occupational, family, and social activities to the extent that physical ability permits, and the ability to experience feelings related to the illness without persistent anxiety or depression.[1] Initial grief reactions and a subsequent mourning process are common following the onset of a serious or terminal illness. The term "grief" refers to the initial response to the perception of loss. It may include feelings of shock, disbelief, emotional numbness, and denial of the objective reality of the illness. These symptoms resemble those observed in posttraumatic stress disorder. The term *anticipatory grief* has been used to describe the perceived damage to one's life trajectory, hopes, and aspirations following the onset or diagnosis of a serious or terminal illness. After the immediate grief response, a broader range of feelings may emerge. These are based on the personal meaning of the illness experience. Feelings of sadness, loss, defectiveness, isolation, and helplessness are common at this stage. In addition, damage to an individual's sense of identity and value may arise due to bodily alterations related to the illness or its treatment, loss of the ability to work or to engage in pleasurable activities, and alterations in family relationships.

There are marked individual differences in the way in which illness-related feelings are experienced, articulated, and understood. Such differences are influenced by the emotional awareness and coping style of the individual, the number and quality of available confidants, and sociocultural attitudes regarding the expression of feelings. For some, the working through of feelings related to the illness is an important and necessary aspect of adjustment. Others may place personal value on stoicism or quiet suffering and/or may belong to cultures or societies in which there are proscriptions against overt expression of personal distress.

Although serious or terminal illness is most often a psychologically damaging experience, it sometimes facilitates a process of psychological reorganization and growth. This may include a review of one's life history, with a renewed attempt to find meaning in it. The imminence of death can be a stimulus to engage in life with conviction, pleasure, and growth and to accomplish and enjoy what can be done in the time that remains. For such individuals, the thought of dying actually enables them to live more effectively in the present. Active coping mechanisms in such cases help to maintain physical activity and overcome or adjust to the complications of the illness. For such individuals, the process of dying continues in the context of a life lived. Unfortunately, for others, the onslaught of disease results in demoralization, unresolved grief and mourning, and the premature relinquishment of possibilities that might still be available. In these individuals, the illness may trigger passivity and intense feelings of disappointment, injury, or victimization. In contrast to many textbook descriptions of death and dying, relief may not occur until the late stages of the disease, when neurological impairment or pharmacological analgesia alters the level of consciousness. The placid acceptance of illness and the calm review of one's life accomplishments is a goal that many terminally ill patients never achieve.

INDICATIONS FOR PSYCHOTHERAPY

The relationship with a primary medical caregiver is potentially the most important psychotherapeutic tool for many patients with serious illness.[2,3] Patient groups and self-help and other support groups may also be extremely helpful in providing information and support in reducing feelings of ineffectiveness. However, the detection of distress by medical caregivers is extremely variable.[4] Those who notice depression in their patients sometimes ignore it because they consider it to be a "normal" or unavoidable response to catastrophic illness rather than an indication for assistance. This is unfortunate, because many patients are unwilling or unable to communicate their distress unless invited to do so by a caregiver. Other health-care providers are so uncomfortable with emotional distress that they refer patients directly to mental health professionals before attempting to provide any support. A referral for a specific psychotherapeutic intervention should take into account the severity of the patient's distress, the need for support, the available support network, the patient's motivation for psychological assistance, and the capacity to learn new coping strategies and/or to engage in a process that involves introspection and the expression of feelings. Patients who are referred for psychotherapy are most often those with unexpected disability or distress, those with persistent symptoms of anxiety, depression, or demoralization, or those who wish to understand and communicate feelings that have been activated by the illness.

TYPES OF PSYCHOTHERAPY

Individual psychotherapeutic treatment for patients with terminal illness should be considered together with other psychosocial approaches. These may include social network interventions, including family, friends, community agencies, and treatment teams, and self-help groups. The latter may be particularly valuable in diminishing feelings of stigma and social isolation generated by the illness. The individual's cultural, ethnic, and religious support should also be routinely considered in terms of the possibilities for adjunctive support and for the provision of meaning for the suffering.

The most common psychotherapeutic approaches in those with advanced disease are (1) the promotion of active coping strategies to maintain the level of functioning, and (2) assistance with understanding, managing, and working through feelings related to the disease. These approaches can often be successfully integrated for optimal care.

Promotion of Active Coping Strategies

An individual's sense of competency and mastery can be severely challenged by a chronic or terminal illness, triggering feelings of helplessness, ineffectiveness, and uncertainty. A number of active therapeutic approaches can help patients to regain a sense of mastery.[5] Some cancer patients prefer receiving all available information, while others prefer to know less. Group therapy, particularly self help groups, may assist with practical concerns and information sharing and can reinforce active coping strategies. Sharing of the experience of illness or treatment with others who have been in similar circumstances can help to combat the emotional isolation that may accompany illness.

Behavioral strategies, including relaxation, biofeedback, guided imagery, and hypnosis, may be helpful in pain management and in preventing demoralization and despair. Cognitive-behavioral therapy directed toward identifying cognitive distortions related to the illness and replacing dysfunctional thoughts with more adaptive ones may also diminish feelings of helplessness and promote a sense of mastery. Education of families about the medical condition can also be helpful if it is based on the identified wishes and needs of the family. These approaches may be used separately or in combination with anxiolytic and analgesic medication to reduce symptoms and to increase feelings of control over the illness.

Psychodynamic Therapy

Supportive Therapy

The usual goal of supportive psychotherapy is to bolster established adaptive coping mechanisms, to minimize maladaptive ones, and to decrease adverse psychological reactions such as fear, shame, and self-loathing. Such treatment can often be provided by the primary-care practitioner or by interested nursing or social work staff. It may lessen the need for analgesic or psychotropic medication and may improve compliance with medical treatment. With any seriously ill patient, a consistent, reliable, and supportive relationship with a medical practitioner is likely to be a key factor in maintaining morale and a sense of well-being. The primary physician's role is most important in this regard because his authority, expertise, and prior knowledge of the patient places him in a special position of trust. The importance of listening to the concerns of the seriously or terminally ill patient may be underestimated by physicians who feel pressured to act in response to their patients' emotional distress by prescribing unnecessary medication, offering unsolicited advice, or ordering investigations or treatments that are not needed.

There is no clear boundary between supportive and expressive therapies. The goal of both approaches in the medically ill is to provide support and assistance in adapting to and understanding the illness. Supportive psychotherapy tends to be more focused on symptomatic relief and maintaining or restoring psychological equilibrium. This is generally accomplished by providing an empathic posture, a stable therapeutic relationship, and a way for individuals to understand their experience. Reassurance is helpful when it is based on a specific understanding of the individual's needs. Premature or unrealistic reassurance may be experienced as distancing or unsupportive. Therapists who are knowledgeable about the medical condition may be best able to provide the patient with a cognitive framework to understand the illness and to distinguish trivial symptoms from those that are serious or that require further medical interventions. This approach, which may include exploration of treatment options, helps to diminish feelings of helplessness, ineffectiveness, and despair.

Case Example

A 47-year-old married woman developed a serious neurological demylinating condition, accompanied by a variety of symptoms, including an inability to walk, loss of hearing, and a painful neuropathy in her feet. She was subsequently referred for psychiatric consultation because of extreme health-related anxiety, which persisted after her physical symptoms remitted. Because of her underlying fears about the recurrence of her medical condition, current minor medical symptoms generated profound health-related anxiety, which, in a circular fashion, amplified her pain. Clarifying and explaining the origin of her symptoms and helping her distinguish the symptoms of irritable bowel syndrome and muscular tension from those of her neurological disease provided enormous relief. This clarification and cognitive restructuring, together with the support of a therapeutic relationship, allowed the patient to resume many of her former activities and to be relatively free of anxiety.

Insight-Oriented Psychotherapy

Insight-oriented psychotherapy is intended to promote self-understanding and the development of new means to cope with a broad range of emotional experience. It should be conducted by specifically trained mental health professionals and is appropriate for only a minority of medical patients. It is most suitable for those with significant psychological distress or interpersonal difficulties who are motivated to explore their feelings. The ability to form an alliance with a therapist is critical to this treatment. Expressive psychotherapy can be especially helpful to patients who fear that discussing their feelings with family members or others in their support network would alienate, antagonize, or overwhelm them.

There are a number of contraindications for expressive psychotherapy in the medically ill.[1] These include medical conditions in which emotional arousal may be medically hazardous, e.g., recent myocardial infarction; medical crises or other stresses that have already overloaded the patient's capacity to tolerate anxiety or further emotional disruption; and organic brain syndromes, due to cardiovascular, neurological, metabolic, or other disorders. Cognitive impairment may limit the patient's ability to make use of verbally based treatments, and associated emotional lability can increase the tendency of the patient to experience distress or disorganization in response to emotional stimuli.

Interpersonal Therapy

Interpersonal Therapy (IPT) is an effective psychotherapeutic treatment in which the focus is on discrete, manageable psychological and inter-

personal issues. IPT is often suitable for patients with serious medical illness because the resolution of conflicts or difficulties in important personal relationships is critical for many individuals in coming to terms with a serious illness or the possibility of death. Current research with HIV-seropositive patients[6] and breast cancer shows promise for the use of IPT. The availability of a treatment and research manual[7] is an additional advantage of this method, which permits standardized training and evaluation.

Case Example

A 28-year-old single woman was referred for therapy following mastectomy, radiation, and chemotherapy for breast cancer. She was profoundly depressed and was convinced that her cancer would return. She felt devastated by the physical changes resulting from the treatment and mourned the loss of her long, beautiful hair. She had had a number of suitors previously and had twice been engaged prior to her cancer diagnosis. Her most recent relationship ended during her cancer treatment, and she had not dated since. She struggled in therapy to sustain a sense of identity, which included not only being a cancer patient but other aspects of her healthy self. She was able to grieve her losses and to accept reasonable new role expectations. She began dating near the end of therapy and then could foresee a life for herself that included marriage and adopting children, plans that had always been important to her.

THE INITIATION OF TREATMENT

Most patients who seek or are referred for psychotherapy want relief from distress. Once such relief occurs, a wide range of other issues may need to be addressed. These include fears of abandonment, threats to the sense of identify, feelings of helplessness, and relationships with family, friends, and caregivers. There may be pressing decisions regarding treatment options or life supports that need to be explored. It is sometimes necessary to explore whether a decision to refuse further treatment represents a rational choice to end unbearable suffering or is a manifestation of clinical depression. In some cases, the fear of being burdensome to caregivers affects treatment decisions. Therapists need to explore the range of feelings and be prepared to accept patients' decisions, which may differ from their own personal preferences or opinions. The psychotherapeutic situation allows patients' feelings to be explored, apart from the reactions or concerns of family or caregivers.

Case Example

A 35-year-old woman recently diagnosed with cancer accepted limited surgical resection but adamantly refused recommended chemotherapy. An academic herself, she was aware of the statistics regarding improved survival with chemotherapy. Nevertheless, she regarded the chemotherapeutic drugs as "poison" that would kill her, and she persistently refused even to consider them. The potential loss of her hair following chemotherapy represented for her an unbearable threat to her sense of femininity and identity. At the same time, she expressed a desperate wish to live, both for herself and for her children. Exploration of her feelings in psychotherapy allowed her to consider the range of feelings that she experienced in relation to acceptance or refusal of this treatment option. She eventually became more confident about being able to preserve her sense of self, even with hair loss, and eventually decided to accept chemotherapy. This final decision was made with a sense of empowerment, although the previous delay decreased her chances for a successful outcome.

Some patients seek psychotherapy with an acknowledged or unconscious wish to prolong life or even to cure the illness through this treatment. This can range from a realistic hope that life may be extended by reducing emotional distress to unrealistic beliefs that psychotherapy will cure the illness. Some of these beliefs may have been reinforced by the recent attention in the media to the role of psychological factors in illness. Although there is some scientific evidence[8,9] that links psychological treatment with increased survival rates, improved quality of life is a more realistic treatment goal. Grossly unrealistic expectations should be addressed early in the therapy, with care not to undermine patients' need for hope.

A common dilemma for therapists is whether and when to challenge or explore patients' denial of illness. Such denial may be manifest in a delay in initial help seeking or in the apparent lack of awareness of the severity of the illness or of the imminence of death. One patient who arrived for a psychotherapy session had to be taken directly to the emergency department because of obvious respiratory distress related to a metastatic pleural effusion. The adaptive function of denial must be respected, except when it interferes with appropriate treatment or necessary personal tasks, such as arranging a will or settling personal financial matters. In some cases, the gradual assumption of the many necessary tasks of dying gradually allows patients to face the reality of their situation.

Case Example

A 23-year-old man presented with symptoms of anxiety and depression. He had been diagnosed with AIDS and was recovering from a bout of pneumonia. The treatment sessions initially focused on his anxiety about telling others about his illness. This led to exploration of his feelings about his homosexuality and his fear that disclosure to his family would lead to rejection by them. As a result of the therapy, he was able to discuss the AIDS diagnosis with them and to initiate the painful but important process of saying goodbye. He had previously felt dominated by his parents and responded to this feeling with rebelliousness and oppositionality. He was now able to be frank with them about his illness and his homosexuality but ceded to their wishes that others not be told he had AIDS. He felt satisfied with this because he no longer wished to maintain an oppositional stance with them. The therapy began twice weekly in the therapist's office and continued in the patient's hospital room and, later still, in his home as he was dying. During this period, he felt able to accept his condition, to focus on such tasks as arranging 24-hour home nursing care, and to maintain the quality of life to the extent possible.

THE PROCESS OF TREATMENT

Although therapy with patients who are seriously ill resembles that with other patients, there are some important differences. When patients are incapacitated, the treatment must sometimes continue at a hospital bedside, by telephone, or with briefer or less frequent visits. The length of a treatment session may need to be adjusted according to the stamina of the patient, with briefer sessions arranged when patients are ill or fatigued. Rescheduling of appointments is often necessary to coordinate sessions with medical treatments or appointments. Fluctuations in the medical condition may require a shift in the focus of treatment. Emotional exploration generally requires that the patient not be experiencing severe pain or anxiety or be in the midst of a medical crisis. At those times, the treatment usually shifts to bolster short-term coping strategies and to maintain psychological equilibrium. Patients and therapists must be prepared to allow the treatment to proceed as circumstances permit or require. Sometimes therapy must be conducted at the bedside on a busy ward, with frequent interruptions by hospital personal. Some patients request that a significant other participates in the treatment, while others request that another member of the treatment team attend one or more sessions.

Countertransference

Terminally ill patients may provoke a variety of emotional responses and reactions, referred to broadly as countertransference, in the therapist. Such responses include concern or overconcern about the patient's dilemma, feelings of helplessness and frustration at being unable to alter the course of events, anxiety or even repulsion in response to the patient's debilitation or disfiguration, and a tendency to offer unrealistic reassurance. Therapists need to explore their own feelings about illness and mortality in order to understand their patients' feelings more deeply and to disentangle their feelings from those of their patients.

A patient's condition may evoke illness-related anxieties or irrational fears in the therapist that need to be addressed. Some therapists become overly directive in order to counterbalance feelings of frustration and impotence evoked by their patient's dilemma. Such approaches, however well intended, may diminish the patient's sense of autonomy and self-sufficiency. The overly solicitous therapist may also make it difficult for a patient to express frustration and anger. Alternatively, therapists may become detached in order to avoid feeling overwhelmed. Such detachment may be overt or may be evident in subtle objectification of patients who are emaciated or disfigured. "Finding the person" in the ill and physically wasted patient is critical to preserve the patient's sense of humanity. Super-

vision or peer support is helpful for therapists who have not previously worked with dying patients or for those whose workload is predominantly focused on this population.

Collaboration with the Primary-Care Physician

Psychotherapy with patients suffering from serious medical illnesses usually benefits from communication among caregivers. Sometimes patients' negotiations with specialists and medical caregivers become a primary focus of psychotherapy. This may be the case with patients who react to their illness or to caregivers in a way that antagonizes caregivers or adversely affects their care. The therapist must be prepared to listen empathically to the patient's experience, while supporting the alliance with the treatment team. Some patients tend to establish special relationships with some caregivers while denigrating others, thereby creating tensions in the treatment team. The therapist must try to maintain a balanced perspective but also be prepared to act as an advocate or mediator between the patient and other caregivers. The benefits of collaboration and communication among caregivers must always be weighed against the patient's need and wish for confidentiality. Decisions regarding the boundaries of privacy must be made on a case-by-case basis in consultation with the patient. At the beginning of the treatment, a review with the patient about what should remain confidential can be useful. Even when there is permission, therapists should avoid unnecessary communications of personal information about the patient to other caregivers.

Case Example

A 29-year-old woman with a history of sexual abuse and an unhappy early home life was referred for psychiatric assessment and treatment after the diagnosis of ovarian cancer. She was mistrustful of those in positions of authority but responded well to clear and direct explanations and recommendations. Her anger when caregivers communicated incorrect or inconsistent information and her tendency to be suspicious caused the treatment team to be rejecting of her. The therapist played an important mediating role in helping the patient understand how her reactions affected her caregivers and in helping the treatment team develop a more sympathetic understanding of her. This approach was valuable to the patient, who came to appreciate the importance for her of the relationships with the caregivers on whom she depended so much.

Grief and Mourning

Grief and mourning are common responses to the perceived losses associated with a serious medical illness. These include the loss of a sense of well-being, of bodily integrity, of future life possibilities, and of the ability to work, engage in personal relationships, and experience pleasure. Exploration of feelings related to these losses with patients with advanced disease may allow the process of mourning to proceed. In the initial phase of treatment, the goal is to establish an atmosphere in which the patient can speak openly about such difficult feelings. Gradually, the patient may come to trust that the therapist is able to listen and to act as a witness to his experience. This includes developing an understanding of the patient prior to the onset of illness as well as the patient's own unique response to illness. This longitudinal perspective helps to counteract the tendency of some patients to lose the sense of their prior identity and to think of themselves only in terms of their illness.

Therapists who explore patients' feelings about their illness must be prepared to help them modulate the intensity of affective expression so that it remains within a tolerable range. This may include providing structure sufficient to prevent the patient from feeling overwhelmed but that permits greater depth and breadth of the patient's experience to emerge. When there have been multiple medical complications or a rapidly deteriorating course, patients may enter a state of unresolved grief and mourning in which they may feel too detached or numb to access feelings. In some of these cases, psychotherapy facilitates resolution of the mourning process. In other cases, however, such factors as the progression of the illness and of medical complications, ongoing psychological stress, or fluctuations in the patient's level of consciousness interfere with such resolution.

Case Example

A 29-year-old woman who had been previously well was referred for assessment because of symptoms of depression that developed one year after the diag-

nosis and successful treatment of Hodgkin's disease. She had previously been an energetic and ambitious individual who was successful in her career and who tried to view herself and life events in positive terms. Although she was able to suppress her emotions during the diagnosis and treatment of her disease, profound feelings of sadness and loss emerged after the disease remitted. She then became clinically depressed, with symptoms that met criteria for major depression. Her vegetative symptoms responded to antidepressant medication, but psychotherapy was also needed to address profound and persistent feelings of sadness and loss. She came to understand how her need to "think positive" had limited her ability to process her response to the illness and contributed to her subsequent depression. Ongoing exploration of her feelings over the course of one year allowed her to understand her response to the illness and to be able to tolerate a wider range of emotions. It was anticipated that these changes would not only allow her to resume her former activities but protect her from becoming depressed in response to further episodes of illness or other life stress.

The Sense of Mastery

Serious medical illness may be damaging to an individual's sense of competence and mastery. Disability caused by the illness and the greater need to depend on others often evokes feelings of helplessness. Although a new repertoire of behaviors and coping strategies is often needed, such a change may further threaten an individual's sense of stability. A sense of competence and mastery can be enhanced in several ways with psychotherapeutic treatment. It may be facilitated when individuals learn to master moment-to-moment waves of affective experience or develop new coping strategies. These changes should be distinguished from less adaptive responses, such as social withdrawal, which provide only a veneer of self-sufficiency. For individuals who regard the expression of emotions as a sign of weakness, it can be empowering to reframe the dilemma and to point to the courage required to face and express feelings.

THE END OF THERAPY

Many patients with terminal illness die while still in active treatment. Indeed, sessions that are productive and engaging may occur very near to a patient's death. Therapy at such times may reflect denial of an imminent reality or, alternatively, may reflect living fully in the moment. Some therapists recommend that treatment be structured to include time for therapist and patient to say farewell. Such an approach ought to arise from the patient's wishes and should be conducted with the understanding that saying goodbye does not signify that the therapist is "giving up." Some therapists decide to attend memorial services or funerals, but this must also be based on the expressed wishes of patients and their families.

SUMMARY

The potential value of psychotherapy is often underestimated for medically ill patients, including those who are terminally ill. Psychotherapy may help to provide relief from emotional distress, to develop new coping strategies, to explore and work through emotions related to the illness, and to regain a sense of competence and mastery. Unresolved grief and mourning are common problems that may be responsive to treatment in this population. Supportive psychotherapy can often be provided by primary medical caregivers. Suitability for insight-oriented psychotherapy must be carefully assessed and should be conducted by a trained mental health professional. Patients with cognitive impairment, marked anxiety, or severe physical distress may not benefit from such an approach. The focus of dynamic therapy with the terminally ill may be on the meaning of the illness, the sense of loss, the disruption in personal relationships, or the damage to an individual's sense of competence and mastery. Psychotherapy can enable terminally ill patients to process feelings and to alleviate unresolved or blocked states of grief and mourning.

A variety of technical modifications may be necessary in the conduct of psychotherapy with patients who suffer from serious medical illness. These include modifications regarding the timing, circumstance, and depth of therapy and collaboration with caregivers. Further, there are a variety of difficult countertransference feelings that therapists who treat the medically ill often need to address. Although the challenges for therapists and patients are great when there is a terminal illness, the rewards can also be significant. Patients who suffer from dire illness may be capable of dramatic insight or behavioral change that improve their quality of life. Therapists have an opportunity to participate in a process with terminally ill patients that can be a rich and rewarding experience.

References

1. Rodin G. Psychiatric care for the chronically ill and dying patient. In: Goldman H, ed, *Review of General Psychiatry*, 4th ed. Norfolk, CT, Appleton and Lange, 1995.
2. Rodin G. Expressive psychotherapy in the medically ill: resistances and possibilities. *International Journal of Psychiatry in Medicine*, 1984; 14:99–108.
3. Suchman AL, Matthews DA. What makes the patient-doctor relationship therapeutic? exploring the connexional dimension of medical care. *Annals of Internal Medicine*, 1988; 108:125–130.
4. Rodin G, Craven J, Littlefield C. *Depression in the Medically Ill: An Integrated Approach.* New York: Brunner/Mazel, 1991.
5. Trijsburg RW, Van Knippenberg FC, Rijpma SE. Effects of psychological treatment on cancer patients: a critical review. *Psychosomatic Medicine*, 1992; 54:489–517.
6. Markowitz JC, Klerman GL, Perry SW. Interpersonal psychotherapy of depressed HIV-positive patients. *Hospital and Community Psychiatry*, 1992; 43:885–890.
7. Klerman GL, Weissman MM, Rounsaville BJ, Chevron ES. *Interpersonal Psychotherapy of Depression.* New York: Basic Books, 1984.
8. Spiegel D, Bloom JR, Kraemer HC, Gottheil E. Effect of psychosocial treatment on survival of patients with metastatic breast cancer. *Lancet*, 1989; 2(8668):888–901.
9. Spiegel D. Can psychotherapy prolong cancer survival? *Psychosomatics*, 1990; 31:361–366.

13

Existential Psychotherapy in Palliative Care

James L. Spira, Ph.D., M.P.H.

Existentialism can be thought of as the philosophical study of the experience of living. It includes recognizing and enhancing meaning, purpose, and value in one's everyday life. Existential psychotherapy, then, has traditionally offered both an evaluation and a reevaluation of one's relationship to life, with the goal of helping patients live more fully in each moment.

While commonly considered an approach for those who are highly motivated and who have the "luxury" of considering how to improve their quality of life, existential psychotherapy is in fact nowhere more appropriate than in helping people facing a terminal illness. This is so because such people are highly motivated, are confronted daily with choices affecting their quality of life, and have lives filled with challenges to meaning, purpose, and values that have been built up over a lifetime.

This chapter discusses the theoretical foundations of existential group psychotherapy, the process of facilitating this approach for persons with advanced-stage illness, such as advanced cancer, incurable cardiac illness, and AIDS, and the benefits to the patient that might be expected on the basis of research that has examined principles found in existential psychotherapy. Specifically, existential psychotherapy for patients with advanced illness is intended to assist these persons to better cope with diagnosis, adjust to living with the illness, and live more fully in the time they have left. Because existential psychotherapy is more of an orientation than a technique per se, this chapter provides a framework that can serve to guide any therapist who works with this population, no matter what therapeutic orientation is adopted.

RESEARCH

Briefly, existentialism is the study of living life to its fullest. Almost all people have experienced times in their lives when they were able to derive maximum meaning, purpose, and value from each moment of their day. The experience of love and that of helping another person to live more fully are two examples commonly associated with this experience. At such times, people report that they feel open and honest in relationship to themselves, others, and the world and are able to feel comfortable and focused in the moment. This experience leads them to feel that they are living as fully as possible, able to go to sleep knowing that their lives are complete. The converse occurs when a person feels isolated or hopeless or is distracted by worries about the future, or when one suppresses one's feelings and thoughts, or tries to be in complete control over uncontrollable events and is unable to accept what is happening to them. These experiences have been identified as contributing to disease incidence, progression, and survival.

Only a few studies have been conducted utilizing existential principles and methods. However, there is sufficient indication from the literature of the need for this approach to warrant its widespread use. Such support comes from studies that identify existential principles as contributing to health outcomes and interventions utilizing existential methods as associated with increased psychological and physical health of patients.

Not surprisingly, persons diagnosed with cancer undergo substantial changes in mood and psychophysical functioning and in the existential aspects of their lives. The way that patients cope with their illness influences their emotional state and their ability to adjust to living with the illness.[1,2] Moreover, it is also possible that psychosocial factors may influence the course of the disease itself.[3] Specifically noteworthy is research emphasizing the importance of social support in survival rather than isolation,[4,5] open expression of affect rather than inhibition of expression[6] or uncontrolled hostility,[7] honest expression of cognitive concerns rather than denial/avoidance,[8] and active coping rather than passive compliance.[9] In brief, avoidance of feelings, denial of concerns, feelings of helplessness or passive compliance with other's demands, and social isolation are bound to result in poor quality of life, if not increased risk of disease incidence, progression, or mortality. On the other hand, open, honest expression of affective and cognitive concerns to another person in an effort to actively improve one's condition clearly corresponds to higher quality of life and also appear to be related to one's physical health.[10,11]

Fortunately, all these psychosocial factors can be improved through the existential group psychotherapy format. Many descriptions of group therapy for medically ill patients that have some features of existential psychotherapy exist in the literature.[12–15] While they provide helpful descriptions of group therapy formats, relatively few of the reports have been grounded in prospective randomized designs that attempt to demonstrate specific benefits of specific interventional styles.

Although in-depth reviews of group intervention studies can be found elsewhere,[16–19] it is valuable at least to note here that empirical studies of group intervention with an existential orientation have illustrated the benefit of group therapy for cancer, HIV, and cardiac patients.

Since the late 1970s, research has consistently demonstrated the benefits of group therapy for improving cancer patients' quality of life (such as improving mood and coping skills, relieving psychophysical distress, and improving physical functioning). With one exception, all reported studies of group therapy have been short term (fewer than 12 meetings); for the most part they follow a cognitive-behavioral format emphasizing educational information, coping skills, and emotional/social support.[20–24] The exception is a research group based on the existentially oriented work of Irvin Yalom.[25] The group met weekly for an entire year and emphasized a more traditional interactive, emotionally supportive therapeutic style.[26] Another existentially oriented intervention was conducted by Mulder and associates[27] with HIV patients. In a 16-session intervention, they found improved quality of life for patients compared to control groups. This study is important as it shows that, at least for medically ill patients, briefer, existentially oriented therapy can be effective in improving quality of life.

Four studies indicate that group therapy that addresses existential issues to varying extents may also be effective for improving physical health.

Supportive evidence for the benefits of group therapy with some existential focus in reducing the rate of disease recurrence and improving survival comes from a study of patients with malignant melanoma conducted by Fawzy et al.[28,29] and a study of patients with HIV by Antoni and associates.[30,31] In these studies, brief, structured interventions urged patients to confront their maladaptive coping strategies and encouraged open discussion of their concerns, as well as the active pursuit of meaningful activities in their lives. Investigators found not only improved mood and coping but also buffered immunity in treatment patients for up to 1 year following treatment. These studies also found improved survival rates for treatment patients at later follow-ups.

Friedman and associates took a large cohort of Type-A post-myocardial infarction patients, and randomized half to long-term therapy, meeting weekly for the first year and then monthly thereafter.[32] In the best existential tradition, they attempted to uncover habitual personality patterns that had been socially and developmentally shaped (e.g., Type-A patterns of hostility and competitiveness[33]) and addressed issues of living more fully and authentically in relationship with others. Investigators found not only decreases in Type-A behaviors but a concomitant reduction in recurrent cardiac events.[34]

The year-long group therapy based on Yalom's existential approach to group psychotherapy found in a retrospective follow-up analysis that patients with recurrent breast cancer who had been randomly assigned to receive group therapy lived an average of 18 months longer from study entry than did control patients.[35] However, Fox[36] has pointed out that the treatment group lived only as long as the national and local average, whereas the control group died at a faster than expected rate, suggesting that statistical sampling error accounted for the survival effect. Whether or not the intervention had any effect on patients' quantity of life, its effect on their quality of life is notable. After meeting in groups weekly for 1 year, intervention patients had less mood disturbance and psychophysical distress. In a replication of the earlier study, we found that, in an environment of group support and therapeutic facilitation, patients were able to both raise and address existential issues in an open and honest fashion.[37]

It must also be noted that initial blunting of feelings and avoidance of what the diagnosis entails may be helpful initially to buffer extreme distress.[38–40] However, studies that suggest the beneficial effects of covering up distress were interested in assessment only, not in intervention. It is reasonable to assume that persons who need to avoid such distress may have lacked the external social support or internal resources to deal with the event.[41] Persons without such support may indeed benefit from temporary initial blunting but may be at greater risk for subsequent posttraumatic stress disorder, especially at a point of disease progression.[42,43] While the intervention studies described earlier that offered group therapeutic support to such persons indicate that those who are offered interventive support do better than those who do not, the type of intervention is important. Should the supportive intervention encourage expression of distress or further covering up of one's fears?

A study based on the work of Bernie Siegel failed to find survival benefits for treatment subjects.[44] One major distinction between this study and the others that show positive survival outcomes is the style of therapy. The Siegel groups emphasized considering a more positive future without dwelling on the negative, whereas the Yalom-style and coping-skills groups directly addressed negative feelings and thoughts and encouraged expression of distress, as well as considered active coping strategies.[45] This difference parallels the literature, which suggests that confronting distress in an open and honest manner, rather than avoiding feelings and thoughts, may contribute to improved health outcomes.[46,47] Perhaps future research will demonstrate that optimism is healthy as long as it does not entail avoidance of important behaviors. "Positive thinking" could then be considered openly and actively dealing with ways to improve one's life.

The concepts of openness of thoughts, expression of honest emotions, and active coping with one's current situation require a maturity that comes from confronting death and the life that remains. With loss of function comes loss of self-image and of the meaning and values patients have carried with them for a lifetime. With their lifetime assumptions challenged on a daily basis, patients face the choice, possibly for the first time in their lives, whether to cling to images and values that seemed to serve them well in the past or instead to challenge these old assumptions in order to live as fully and meaningfully an existence as is possible in the days remaining to them.

Thus, while their physical health may be benefited by their addressing the existential aspects of their lives, even more important are the daily quality-of-life issues that confront terminally ill patients. Coping with pain serves to demonstrate the existential psychotherapeutic approach to quality of life. Existentially, pain can be distinguished from suffering. With psychosocial intervention, intensity of and suffering due to pain can be reduced, even though frequency and duration of pain are unchanged. This can occur since suffering can be seen in large measure as a reaction to the physical cause of pain. Similarly, existential psychotherapy can reduce suffering in life, even though the pain of loss exists. Here, suffering can be seen as a reaction to loss of function, hopes, and relationships. If the experience of living is attending to one's self-image, then abandoning this self-image is tantamount to the experience of death. And the inability to release one's prior self-image out of fear of death corresponds to the extent to which one will suffer. In this regard, pain can be seen as a gift, in that when a self-image can no longer be maintained, one must abandon it and examine what one's life is truly about. Pain can therefore lead to an awakening of the spirit and an ultimate reduction in suffering.

Drawing on the traditions of philosophical existentialism and existential psychotherapy and the adaptation of existential psychotherapy for the terminally ill, the rest of this chapter offers suggestions on how therapists can facilitate the patients' ability to move beyond the way they were and to adjust to their current circumstances in order to live as fully as possible in each moment of each day remaining to them. Since existential psychotherapy is more of a set of guiding principles than a collection of specific techniques, the philosophical and therapeutic basis of these principles is outlined.

BACKGROUND

To better appreciate the thrust of existential psychotherapy for terminally ill patients, it is useful to review the tenets of existentialism, as well as the way these have been utilized in existential psychotherapy for psychosocial concerns in general.

Existentialism

Existentialism is the study of the experience of living life to its fullest. This includes attempting to understand one's self, one's relationship to others and the world, and the meaning, purpose, and commitment in one's life. Existential writers have described the ways one's relationship to life has been conditioned and automatically/habitually conducted, diminishing one's experience, and the ways it is possible to live a more fully conscious, authentic, and valued existence. Different existential writers have emphasized various aspects of

human experience. A brief summary of existential principles will help readers appreciate the applications of these philosophical ideals to psychotherapy for persons with advanced illness.

Early Influences

Several important philosophical and social science traditions influenced the formation of existentialism and existential psychotherapy. *German Idealism*[48-50] emphasized the constructivist nature of our experience. Rather than having direct access to the nature of existence, we create our experiences out of social conditioning, past experience, and current desires and expectations.

The study of *hermeneutics*[51-53] extends idealist thought into the realm of interpretations of an individual's expression. Understanding a person's meaning can be achieved only by considering both the individual expressor and the social-historical context within which the expression occurred.

Phenomenology[54-56] is the study of how we impose our interpretations on the world we perceive[54-56] and of what our world is like once we suspend interpretation. Interpretations are revealed when there is a "breakdown" of normal functioning. When some aspect of our world suddenly ceases to function in the intended fashion, our assumptions about that object is revealed, and we may gain a brief glimpse into that object as it is, distinct from our intentions for it.

Zen Buddhism[57,58] shares characteristics with each of the traditions already mentioned. Major tenets relevant to existential psychotherapy are that (1) suffering stems from considering one's constructed image of self or other as if it were real; (2) freedom from suffering entails the suspension of one's illusory interpretive foreground (fixed image) in order to return to one's natural foundation of interpretationless unity with existence (Spirit, or *Geist*, in Hegel's terms); (3) only by experiencing this foundation can one emerge in full authentic relationship with and commitment to life; (4) meditation is the most direct method of accomplishing this authentic relationship.[59] From the Zen Buddhist tradition, modern existentialism derives the notion of being more fully present in each moment, without the need to worry about the future or to regret the past, along with the release from self-made suffering and the richness of life that comes from living more fully in the moment.

Existential Philosophy

The study of existentialism arose out of a need to appreciate individual experience, rather than a more metaphysical (and less personal) philosophical tradition. Existential writers have ranged from those interested in describing life as it is lived to those concerned with living more authentically and richly in everyday life.

Schopenhauer,[60] who wrote in the early nineteenth century, was the first Western philosopher to study Buddhism. He felt that there is a strong drive on the part of Spirit to return the individual back to its source—that is, the will to "de-evolve," or to release ego back to its unified oneness. Only an acceptance of death allows one's spirit to shine forth in its fullest potential.

Søren Kierkegaard is generally considered the first Existentialist. Kierkegaard argued that social conventions led individuals to develop an inauthentic relationship to Spirit (God). In fact, Kierkegaard[61] believed that it was only when we can entirely remove societies' influences that our authentic nature can manifest itself with pure freedom. Yet the rejection of social convention leaves one with anxiety that stems from being responsible for forming one's own opinions and choosing one's own actions.[62] By accepting one's anxiety over separation from society and entering into self-responsibility, one also can enter into an authentic relationship with life. The old, socially conditioned self "dies" so that the pure self can emerge,[63] free to choose and free to love with all of one's being.

Friedrich Nietzsche[64] not only advocated distancing oneself from social institutions but also advised separating from one's own thoughts, which are formed by social convention. He argued that meaning, purpose, and value in our lives are not our own but rather given to us by society. Our self-image is formed in large measure by society; therefore, only self-death can free one from oneself. Like a phoenix rising out of the ashes, one can then manifest fully, creating a self-generated life authentically rich in meaning, purpose, and value.[65] Nietzsche reasoned that it is only through suffering that one is ready to abandon social convention and to one's full potential.

Martin Heidegger was influenced by Nietzsche and by Zen Buddhism.[66–68] He believed that inauthentic thought and action can be noticed only from a standpoint of nonthought. Only from this background of nothingness (*Nichte*) can the thoughts and meanings that form one's consciousness be noticed. Only from this perspective can one choose actions authentically, in a way that will bring the most meaning, purpose, and value to one's life. The release of social convention usually follows a breakdown of normal assumptions (e.g., diagnosis of cancer). One can try to cover up these breakdowns, fleeing into social convention once again (becoming a "patient," expecting the doctor to effect a cure). But when the breakdown is sufficiently severe (diagnosis of recurrent cancer), covering up may become impossible, and one is left watching one's assumptions about life crumble. Only once one can accept this perishing of the self and accept that all prior assumptions about one's life have no real basis—only then can one manifest authentically, living fully in each moment.

Other existentialists, especially those who have written plays, novels, and poems (e.g., Eliot, Rilke, Camus, Sartre, Ionesco, and Dostoyevsky), have contributed to the dissemination of existential ideas. From the standpoint of defining the tradition that has had such an impact on existential psychotherapy, however, the traditions described are the most central to the existential thesis. This thesis can be summarized by these five major components:

1. *Hermeneutic basis of the self*. Since we are interpretive beings, we are fundamentally unified through the social interpretations given to us by society. An individual's expression of his own meaningful existence can be understood only by appreciating the person's personal experience and the historical-social context within which the expression of meaning is made.

2. *Inauthentic assumptions of our world and our self*. We do not realize that our self-image and our images of the world are merely mental constructions that are provided to us by society by a lifetime of unconscious conditioning, we form habits that in turn limit our perceptions and our freedom of actions. Instead, we believe that our impression of life (ourselves and our world) directly matches the "world as it is." We tend to take ourselves as fixed entities that exist in stable form and similarly view our world as fixed and regular. Failing

to appreciate that the way we think of self, others, and the world is dictated by social rules that we learn, we do not appreciate that what we think of as free choice in our lives is nothing more than the inauthentic constraints of society that in large measure dictate what we consider to be our options. Such unconscious assumptions form the basis of suffering and limit our freedom to choose meaningful activity.

3. *Breakdown of inauthentic assumptions.* Since one's ego exists to safeguard itself and to perpetuate its stability, an external crisis is required to shatter one's assumptions. There are small, everyday breakdowns, such as a mechanism's (e.g., door knob) not working, which leads to temporary recognition of our assumptions (we assumed that turning the knob would open the door), until we can find an alternative mechanism to work for us (a lock). Whenever possible, we "cover up" such breakdowns of our habitual assumptions, fleeing into conveniently provided social conventions. Yet there are more serious breakdowns, such as the loss of a loved one or the diagnosis of terminal illness, where the usual alternative habitual mechanism just simply does not work. When the breakdown is so severe that we cannot simply flee into social convention, we instead experience anxiety (*Angst*); our usual, everyday activity appears to be absurd, and we feel a sense of dissociated depersonalization (*Unheimlicheit*). Such a state occurs because there is no longer the usual conditioned basis for understanding what is occurring, and we recognize that what we took for granted has been in fact artificial, inauthentically derived and maintained.

4. *Moment of vision.* When an external crisis facilitates a breakdown and thus our recognition of assumptions, we experience a kind of emptiness. An awareness of the emptiness of an a priori order to and meaning of life (*nicht*) for the first time affords an authentic look at our inauthentically derived and maintained foregrounded assumptions about our life. The extent to which our breakdown cannot be covered up corresponds to the depth of authentic understanding about our life activities. For instance, if a person assumes his health to be adequate, he will probably give issues of health or longevity little consideration. Yet, after a diagnosis of coronary artery disease followed by a coronary artery bypass graft (CABG), he must consciously and seriously address the actual state of his health and the extent to which he can influence it. If a woman breaks up with a man she had dated for several months, she can justify the breakup by blaming him or circumstance. However, if her husband of 40 years dies suddenly of acute myocardial infarction, any amount of rationale or social convention will provide little comfort. And, occasionally, one is thrust into examining not only the specific assumption that has been disrupted (about, e.g., health or relationships) but further may be compelled to reconsider one's attitude toward life itself. Once one recognizes that one has been primarily "fooled by oneself," then the potential for authentic consideration of one's unconsciously derived assumptions becomes possible. The more those assumptions break down, the more one is able to recognize one's prior assumptions. Tolstoy[69] tells the story of Ivan Illych, who only on his deathbed realized that his misery resulted from the fact that he had done none of the things that *he* trully found rewarding but only those things others expected of him.

5. *Authentic commitment.* The more one is able to recognize one's prior assumptions, the more one is able to enter into authentic action. If the "moment of vision" is limited to one element (e.g., one's heart), one's freedom to choose authentically will be limited to that realm (e.g., cardiac rehabilitation). If one's "vision" extends to recognizing a more general concept (life at risk), then one has the opportunity to reevaluate one's life in light of the potential of dying soon, and may therefore reevaluate how one wants to live more fully in the time remaining. Finally, if one's vision encompasses the general notion that all of one's prior assumptions about one's self and one's life have all been unconsciously and largely other-derived and -maintained, then one has the potential to begin anew to reevaluate one's life activities and to select those that will bring greatest meaning, purpose, and value to one's life.

Existential psychotherapy for seriously ill patients can help to facilitate the breakdown of assumptions (to whatever extent the patient is able to tolerate it), avoid the need to cover up their distress, and facilitate exploration of authentic activities to which they can commit themselves in order to live life to its fullest extent (see Table 13.1).

EXISTENTIAL PSYCHOTHERAPY

Existential psychotherapy stands in contrast to other approaches, which tend to cover up the ex-

Table 13.1 Aspects of Existential Maturity

1. **Hermeneutic basis** (the *"self"* arises from and is part of a sociohistorical context)
2. **Inauthentic self** (even though self is formed from a lifetime of social conditioning, one has the illusion of freedom and takes one's self to be a free and independent agent). This inevitably leads to a:
3. → **Breakdown of inauthentic self** (external circumstance lead to the breakdown of unconscious assumptions), leads to either:
4. → **Covering up this breakdown** (fleeing into alternative social convention, returning to (2), or else leading to
   → **Moment of Vision** (becoming aware of the assumptions one has unconsciously been making in one's life)
5. **Authentic Commitment** (choosing actions that will bring the greatest meaning, purpose, and value to one's life)

NOTE: The severity of the external disruption (e.g., a life-threatening diagnosis) corresponds to the extent to which assumptions break down (life as it has been lived), corresponds to the extent to which one will recognize prior assumptions (habitual, nonchosen activities), which in turn corresponds to the extent to which new activities can be authentically chosen for greatest meaning, purpose, and value in one's life.

istential cause of distress and facilitate "fleeing into social convention." These approaches quickly assist with finding specific solutions to specific problems, without regard to patients' existential concerns about the extent to which they authentically live each moment of their lives. Moreover, many approaches to psychotherapy for medically ill patients too often support the inauthentic existence of patients. It is not a particular psychotherapeutic technique that operates in contrast to existential considerations but rather the paradigm of individual practitioners who wish to dull patients' pain, yet, while doing so, dull the opportunity for patients to get the most out of the days remaining to them. Ideally, approaches can be found that reduce suffering while at the same time enhancing the extent to which patients can live as fully as possible. This is the intent of existential psychotherapy for patients in palliative care.

Three approaches to existential psychotherapy have emerged over the past century, influenced by hermeneutics, phenomenology, and Buddhism. Existential psychotherapy for the medically ill uses aspects found throughout the history of this approach. A brief review will provide a useful context for applications to the terminally ill.

Hermeneutic Influence

The earliest forms of existential psychotherapy put into practice the hermeneutic principles of allowing meaningful expression to be understood from patients and their context. Thus, existential psychotherapy opposes the imposition of a deductive theoretical framework on patients by testing them with standard assessment tools, categorizing them

into preexisting categories, and treating them according to standards appropriate to that category. In reaction to the deductive approach, Karl Jaspers[70] and Ludwig Binswanger[71] felt that therapists could best serve their patients by understanding their existence through a thorough study of the patients' direct experience and the context within which their experience had arisen. The hermeneutic orientation is constructivist. As Viktor Frankl[72] pointed out, patients create their own unique sense of order and meaning in the world. Yet our construct of the world may not keep up with the constant changes that occur in the world or in ourselves. This gap between patients' constructs of their lives and the challenges constantly provided by a changing world is the basis of neurosis.

The task of the existential psychotherapist, therefore, is to find the gaps in a patient's world order, providing a link to help patients relate to world events. According to Medard Boss,[73] the role of the therapist is to point out the inconsistencies in the way the world has been created by the patient, and to do so as much as possible from within the patient's perspective. Through first understanding and then questioning the patient's created world, the existential psychotherapist provides a setting where a "lateral perspective" can be gained, viewing life from various points of view. Moreno[74] helped bring background beliefs and assumptions into the foreground by having patients act out various archetypal aspects of their meaningful life, thus making their unconscious patterns conscious. The way that cognitive therapists challenge patient's belief systems[75,76] can be seen as operating within this hermeneutically influenced existential tradition.

Phenomenologic Influence

The phenomenologically oriented existential psychotherapist attempts to help patients notice their foregrounded activities from the background of *nicht* (nothingness). This is usually achieved by having patients consider their living in the face of loss or even death. The old adage "You don't appreciate something until it is gone" applies here. From this perspective, the existential psychotherapist can serve to (1) facilitate the breakdown of a patient's inauthentic assumptions, (2) help avoid covering up so that a "moment of vision" can be obtained, and (3) facilitate authentic commitment to chosen activities that will bring the greatest meaning, value, and purpose to the patient's life.

A breakdown of normal assumptions may begin with the diagnosis. The therapist can facilitate this process. It is only when such breakdowns occur that authentic growth can occur, along with easier adjustment to one's new situation. Adjustment is difficult when we hold onto a fixed image of the way we consider ourselves and the world to be. By forming an authentic relationship with the patient and providing the skills to ease the excess anxiety, the therapist frees the patient to allow the breakdown to occur and to resist the tendency to flee immediately into a comfortable convention. Once the patient is able to tolerate discussion of his situation, the therapist can assist in the release of such habitual fixed images by first making them conscious and then helping the patient accept that this life is now past and it is best to look to the future. In this way, one can begin to consider how one wants to live, rather than the way one was living out of habit.

Yalom[77,78] has applied existential psychotherapy of this sort to patients facing incurable cancer, as well as to their families. Patients are encouraged to accept the fact of their illness and eventual death so that they can also fully accept their lives. No effort is made to deny or reject the negative aspects of the patient's life in favor of concentrating on the positive or the hopeful. Bugental[79] has developed a series of exercises to help both therapists and patients appreciate what it means to face one's death honestly, enabling one to live more authentically and fully in each moment. For example, he might ask, "If you had six months to live, what would you do that would bring greatest meaning into your life, that would allow you to live your fullest in that last year of life?" For medical patients, this type of exercise helps facilitate authentic exploration of issues that are current and relevant. For therapists, family members of medically ill patients, or patients with psychosocial dysfunction, it helps explore existential issues that have been largely ignored. Exercises of this sort are likely to stimulate a great deal of authentic discussion in therapy. Similar exercises are presented later in this chapter.

Zen Buddhist Influence

Buddhist-influenced approaches to existential psychotherapy stem from a different sort of fundamental assumption than do hermeneutically or phenomenology-oriented approaches. Hermeneutics concerns itself with expression as having meaning only within a social context. Phenomenology recognizes foregrounded meaning in contrast to a background of nothingness (*nicht*, empty of a priori interpretation and meaning, purpose, value). In contrast, Buddhism examines life in light of a ground of nondiscriminative unity with all existence. The main tenet of Buddhism is that once interpretation has been suspended, one experiences a sense of oneness and well-being. It is from this greater sense of fullness with life (which comes from suspending interpretation) that one is able to confront one's life as it is, and as it could be.

Existential psychotherapists who are influenced by Buddhism maintain that once a person suspends thinking (interpreting, reflecting), he also suspends cognitive distortion, affective distress, physiological disturbance, and behavioral habits. Letting go of interpretation even for an instant has long-term ramifications. This suspension of interpretation leaves one with a fuller awareness of the moment, greater affective fluidity and physiological equilibrium, and increased control over one's actions.[80] Most cognitive or affective distress stems from worry about the future and an inability to let go of the past. When one is able to focus more fully on the present moment, one is usually able to feel a greater sense of well-being.[81,82] The feeling of the breath and warmth of the body, simple patterns of light and sounds, tastes and smells, all combine to afford one the same sense of presence that a young baby experiences after it has had its fill of milk and when it is bundled in its mothers arms, or a cat or dog feels resting by the fireplace. Even pain is better handled when the patient addresses it directly, rather than dissociate from it.[83]

The practice of meditation is intended to facilitate the ability of a person to be more fully present in the moment, free of socially influenced interpretation and thus in a fuller and freer relationship with life. Maslow[84] describes this way of being as a "peak experience," after which one's sense of joy at being in the world increases tremendously. Fritz Perls[85] knew the value of being totally "in the moment" and "in one's body," and he used this fundamental state as an opportunity to examine how patients tended to flee into their anxieties (clinging to what they are afraid to let go of). Gendlin[86] described this presence in the moment as a "felt sense," and, like Perls, used it as a basis for exploring existential issues. In a technique Gendlin calls "focusing," a therapist serves as an active mirror for the patient, being in this "felt sense," as well as asking the patient questions that help him notice how he is fleeing from this "felt sense," and finally lead the patient to feel "integrated" when he allows himself to operate from this "felt sense." Modern-day followers of Reich[87] use deep breathing and rapid movement (rather than free association) in an extension of Freud's efforts to break down resistance to unconscious fears. By releasing somatic stress, patients allow past fears and their present manifestations to surface. By discussing these fears while remaining calm, they are able to work through this neurosis and manifest more freely in their lives. Reynolds[88] describes what he calls "the quiet therapies," methods of psychotherapy that incorporate silence into their methodology. Used by the Japanese, this approach combines Zen meditation with Western psychotherapy. In one of these applications, developed by Shomno Morita,[89] patients are kept in social and sensory isolation for some time, often in a quiet room or even in bed, for 1 week. Here, habitual thoughts, emotions, and impulses become more evident and can begin to subside; at the least, they can be the topic of later discussion. Even without formal psychotherapy, persons who are confined to their house or a bed will find that forced "silence" is sure to surface their habitual "noise."

Experiential activities such as Zen meditation, yoga, and tai chi can be especially useful for persons with advanced-stage illness.[90] By focusing on the breath or on simple comfortable movements, patients are able to reduce attention to distressful thoughts or feelings over which they have no control and that serve only to accentuate suffering. Instead, they begin to attend more fully to each moment, where they find a great deal with which they can participate. It is important to note that these methods are not used to "cover up" or avoid existential issues. Rather, they are used to help the patient become more open to such considerations.

METHODS OF EXISTENTIAL PSYCHOTHERAPY IN PALLIATIVE CARE

There are numerous ways in which the existentially oriented therapist can facilitate patients' existential development during the final period of their lives.

Establish an Authentic Counseling Relationship

First and foremost among the methods utilized by the existential psychotherapist is the establishment of an authentic relationship. Rather than maintain a role as the doctor, the therapist enters into an honest interaction with the patient. While therapists should not use the interaction as an opportunity for their own psychotherapy, they should be able to treat the encounter as a learning experience for both therapist and patient. Each moment is precious, and each patient's experience and potential is to be respected. Thus, all patients are to be taken on their own terms, from the perspective of their own lives as well as in the context within which they have lived. Acknowledging and exploring patients' cognitive and emotional lives, along with their potential for existential maturity, models for the patient an appreciation of entering into fuller relationship with others and with life. This acceptance of the patient entails not covering up distress but rather an awareness at all times of the patient's full potential.

The therapist can employ specific methods to encourage authentic expression on the part of the patient. Focusing on existential content as well as process is useful. Active listening, which summarizes the patient's feeling and topics of concern, helps develop rapport. In addition, ther-

Table 13.2   Establishing an Authentic Therapist-Patient Relationship

Establish rapport—Practice active listening, acknowledging patient statements of existential concern and emotional tone.

Explore existential Issues—Ask questions that force patients to consider what is important to them in the time they have left.

Lead to existential process—Ask questions that facilitate the process of open intimacy with self-and others and active participation in meaningful activities.

Cognitive openness:	Acceptance (personal and specific statements) vs. denial (external or general statements)
	(Can you give me a specific example of how that affects you personally?)
Explore affect:	Integrated feeling vs. repression and intellectualization
	(How does that make you feel? Or That must make you angry.)
Interpersonal:	Intimate, open, and honest expression to another person (therapist, family, friend) vs. remaining isolated
	(Can you tell your children your fears about losing control?)
Active coping:	Exploring ways to active participate in what one can control, while letting go of what one cannot control
	(What can you do to reduce your pain? Or Can you tell the med tech when it gets too painful?)

apists can ask questions that encourage exploration of existential issues and development of existential maturity. Therapists can encourage cognitive openness by asking questions that require a personal and specific answer, that inquire about current unexpressed affect, that encourage intimate interaction with the therapist or family members, and that assist in consideration of active coping strategies (see Table 13.2).

Facilitate the Breakdown

Perhaps what most distinguishes existential psychotherapy from other approaches for seriously ill patients is that, rather than helping cover up patients' distress, it directly acknowledges their suffering and explores more fully the basis of such suffering. Thus, illness is considered an opportunity for growth.

First establishing rapport and then using appropriate questioning, the therapist can help the patient let go of old assumptions that simply serve to increase suffering and are minimally beneficial to the patient, since they were for the most part other-determined. Patients whose lives are disrupted due to illness and disability are ripe for understanding that the way they thought about themselves and their world no longer applies to the current circumstances. In order to cope with their current circumstances, they must be willing to let go of prior assumptions about their lives. Most such assumptions are maintained unconsciously, so the therapist must assist the patient

in making such unconscious assumptions conscious.

There are several ways in which the existential psychotherapist can assist in making unconscious assumptions conscious. One approach is to facilitate the development of a "lateral perspective," where a patient explores alternative ways of viewing a situation: How do others (family, doctors, friends, other patients) view what is going on? From such exploration, it becomes quickly apparent that no single way is correct, that different views are merely convenient from various perspectives. A patient, although possibly initially confused by such an approach, can come to appreciate the idea that any view is personally created over a lifetime, rather than mirroring a "realistic" view of the world. Following such a realization, patients find it easier to suspend their fixed view of self and life in order to explore ways of being that facilitate adjustment to current circumstances.

Another way of facilitating the breakdown of inauthentic assumptions is to contrast one's views against a background of nothingness. When patients consider dying, activities they habitually engage in become somewhat absurd, especially those activities that are done out of habit, with no real value or meaning to the patient. Openly discussing dying, and how one wants to live in the time one has left, goes far in helping to reprioritize what is important and what is not.

Offering alternative perspectives as well as examining one's life in the face of dying can be accomplished through dialogue or special exercises. Interactive conversation allows therapists to gently yet directly encourage patients to examine their assumptions that limit their ability to live more fully in the time they have left. Especially useful are cognitive methods of confronting absolutes (e.g., all, should, never), while challenging patients to imagine alternative ways of being.[91,92] First in conversation, then in imagination, and finally in practice, patients can experiment with recognizing their own fixed way of seeing things and then wondering what it would be like to see things from a different perspective, or possibly no way at all! For example, if a man recently diagnosed with cardiomyopathy has believed that hard work is the measure of success, security, and ultimate happiness, he will find forced semi- or full retirement to be very difficult. It will be necessary to discuss with him alternative ways of living that others have found to be of value and that he might be able to find to be of value as well. If the patient is especially fixed in his views, he will no doubt find it difficult to even consider alternative ways of looking at life, let alone to adjust his lifestyle to accommodate his new situation. Therefore, some direct challenge of the "absolute nature" of his prior beliefs can be helpful.

Numerous structured exercises can be utilized to help patients explore existential issues that help break down restrictive assumptions and examine alternative ways to live more fully in the time one has left. These are especially useful:

1. *Living in the face of dying.* Considering an (existentially) optimal future in the time one has left can be conducted in discussion or as a paper and pencil exercise.

Exercise 1. Considering an Optimal Future

"If you had one year (month, week) to live and you wanted to make it the most meaningful year of your life:

- What personal characteristics (self-image, personality, assumptions about life) would you want to let go of?
- What activities would you let go of that you find more of a burden than a joy?
- What personal characteristics would you want to have to help you make this year a valuable one for you?
- What activities would you want to engage in

that would bring greatest meaning and value to your life?
- What is stopping you from having these qualities and doing these activities now?
- What can you do to overcome these barriers live more fully?"

2. *Restrictive beliefs.* In this exercise, the therapist helps a patient identify beliefs, attitudes, and assumptions about life or the world that appear to limit the patient's ability to adjust to current circumstances and live as fully as possible. These may include the need to help others rather than let others help one, the tendency to find a specific reason for the illness, a need to minimize the seriousness of the illness or one's own suffering, or difficulty trusting others. The following questions help to put such beliefs in perspective:

Exercise 2. Beliefs Exercise

"When was this belief developed? Under what circumstances did you form this belief?

- How did this belief help you at that time? How does this belief still help you now?
- How has this belief limited you in the past? How does this belief limit you at this time?
- What is an alternative belief that would help you at this time, and would keep the habit belief in check?
- In what situations will the old belief influence you, and what will help you recall the alternative belief?"

3. *Being in the moment.* The following exercise helps patients live more fully in each moment they have left in their lives and also serves to reveal what thoughts and feelings take them "out of the moment." When working with very distressed patients, a therapist can notice how difficult it is for them to consciously "remain in the room." They may talk excitedly about the past or the future but rarely say anything about what is occurring in the moment. Frequently, patients experiencing pain have an increased sense of suffering because they are attending as much to the way they were and what the pain means for the future as they are to the somatic sensation itself. It can be useful to ask such patients to describe their present state but not to "leave the room" in doing so. For many of these patients, it soon becomes apparent that the problem is that they are unable to focus on the present and are con-

tinually pulled away by thoughts of an uncomfortable past and future. Patients can be asked to discuss what they feel in their bodies, what they see in the room, what sounds come to their ears, or how they feel in the relationship with the therapist. Once a highly distressed patient is able to simply describe the present moment, most of their discomfort soon extinguishes, and they are able to consider more calmly and maturely how they wish to address their concerns. These patients can be told to practice this each day for one minute and then to use this "presencing" method to become calm whenever they start "thinking too much."

Support a "Moment of Vision"

From a hermeneutic standpoint, a moment of vision occurs when patients realize they are more than their limited view of themselves. They also come to appreciate that they contain all the resources they have from their entire lives, releasing their full potential for acting. Ways to elicit these resources include group therapy, where others can discuss ways of coping with a problem and finding meaningful activities to engage in. Asking about times in the past when a patient was able to cope with difficult situations or find meaning and value in some purposeful activity can also be a valuable means of awakening talents and attitudes that have been forgotten.

Phenomenologically, a moment of vision occurs when one's habitual assumptions are revealed through the breakdown of normal daily events. It is important that, following a catastrophic illness and the subsequent breakdown of normal life assumptions, therapists offer support for this phase of a patient's development. Following such a breakdown, patients usually experience what would be coded as an adjustment disorder with depressed or anxious mood. However, this can be considered a normal and healthy result of recognizing that one's assumptions about oneself and one's life were merely transient phenomena and not the state of the world one assumed it to be. Relinquishing deeply held beliefs requires a period of mourning, and this mourning may manifest as internalized or externalized anger or blame, sadness, or even a sense of despair. Positive commitment to life only can progress after one fully accepts the release of inauthentic assumptions. Thus, the grieving phase must be fully and authentically experienced. Existential matu-

rity can be said to correspond to the extent to which one can accept one's suffering without covering up and fleeing into another inauthentic image. Therefore, the existential psychotherapist must allow full grieving to occur, supporting this state of despair, until such time as the patient can fully accept his condition without attempting to flee it. From this point the patient can begin anew, determining what is of maximum value and purpose in his lives.

From a Buddhist perspective, a moment of vision occurs when all interpretations of one's life and the nature of the world are abandoned, allowing one to be more fully present in the moment. Once one has let go of images of self and other and has therefore recognized one's images as conditioned mental creations, one can for the first time experience true freedom of perception and action. Freedom of perception comes from being able to take each moment on its own terms, rather than continually viewing every event in terms of an imagined context ("How will this affect me in the future, or Why bother with this since I have no future?"). The existential psychotherapist can support the suspension of contextual vigilance (a state that occurs more frequently as patients become cognitively and physically weaker) by allowing patients to be more fully present in the moment (rather than needing to discuss the future or the past), or by simply permitting periods of silence and simple physical contact.

By teaching meditation, the therapist can encourage the patient to spend more time letting go of thought and attending to simple visual, auditory, and somatic sensation, sensations that are for the most part soothing and effortless. In fact, the less one tries to think about the future or the past, the more one can attend to the natural sensations that occur effortlessly in the moment and have the time to consider what is important for one's life at that moment.

Hypnotherapy[93] can also be used to explore existential dimensions. By using simple controlled dissociation, one is able to consider difficult issues in a relaxed state and in a way that bypasses old habitual ways of interpreting the situation. However, hypnosis that merely focuses on comfort and wishful thinking can be used to cover up rather than uncover one's existential concerns.

Excess distress can limit the patient's ability to examine existential issues. Miller et al.[94] have demonstrated that cancer patients manifest cognitive-affective avoidance when they become overwhelmed by thoughts and feelings about events over which they have little control. For this reason, assisting patients to achieve a moment of calm clarity is a useful starting place for existential psychotherapy. Living more frequently in this state is also a goal of existential psychotherapy. Therefore, concomitant with establishing rapport, entering into an authentic relationship, and facilitating a breakdown of inauthentic assumptions, therapists should support a patient's "moment of vision."

It must be kept in mind that different patients will have different capacities for existential development in their lives. Thus, therapists must be sufficiently flexible to support patients in the way that works best for them. In general, the depth of insight that is revealed to patients corresponds to the depth of breakdown that has occurred in their lives, and this level of insight in turn is related to the level of authentic commitment they are able to make. Coming to a new level of comfort (through hypnosis or meditation) reveals the tendency to cling to worry or fear. Being able to attend more fully to the moment reveals the tendency to flee to the past and the future, which perpetuates one's suffering. And the experience of unity (between patient and therapist or spouse or simple sensation) reveals the tendency to separate self from other. To the extent the therapist can facilitate the patient's acceptance of his current situation, that is the extent to which a "moment of vision" will propel the patient into finding greater meaning, purpose, and value in his remaining life.

Encourage the Pragmatic Development of Commitment

No matter how much time remains to the patient, the existential psychotherapist should promote active strategies to develop meaningful actions in the patient's life. This could entail reprioritizing the patient's activities so that he spends more time on relationships that are of special value while minimizing those of less import and does those activities that he has been waiting to do his whole life or that now have the greatest value. As in other approaches to existential psychotherapy, a combination of structured exercises and Socratic dialogue is highly ef-

fective in helping patients to find ways to engage in committed activity.

A typical exercise to help patients reprioritize life activities follows.

Exercise 3. Reprioritizing Life Activities

1. Make a list of activities you spend your time doing during a typical week.
2. Prioritize this list, with the activities you spend most time with at the top and those you spend less time on toward the bottom.
3. Prioritize these activities again, but this time list at the top the activities that bring more meaning and personal value to your life, with progressively less meaningful activities toward the bottom. To this list can also be added any activities that you wish you were doing, even though you have not gotten around to them.
4. Examine the last two columns. If the lists are ordered differently, then it is important to ask what you can do to spend more time engaged in those activities that bring more meaning and value to your life and less in activities that you do out of habit.

Simply asking what would bring most value and meaning to their lives in the time they have left can be of great importance to patients. Finally, behavioral counseling, which includes setting goals, developing a reasonable action plan, and trying out the activity, can be instrumental in assisting the patient to begin active commitment and provide the confidence boost required to take bold new action.

In order for one's commitment to stay "freshly authentic," it is important that the patient be able to reflect about it from time to time (or "take it all back," as Heidegger puts it).[95] In this way, one can continue to derive full value from whatever one commits to, whether it be spending more time with family, taking a trip, delving into religion, or doing volunteer work, and avoid having it become just another unconsciously performed habit.

Summary of Principles

Highlights of existential psychotherapy for medically ill patients are presented in Table 13.3.

It should be kept in mind that the facilitation of existential maturity, as presented in this chapter, is not a unidirectional process. Rather, it re-

Table 13.3   Principles of Existential Psychotherapy

Existential Psychotherapy emphasizes:
  Development of an authentic relationship between therapist and patient, and between patient and others
  The value of patient experience, resources, and capacity for development at any point in life
  The importance of facilitating the breakdown of conditioned habitual assumptions about life
  Assisting patients to accept their suffering and potential for death without attempting to cover up
  Helping patients to trust in the present moment as the fullest experience possible in life
  Engaging in activities that bring greatest meaning, purpose, and value to one's life

quires a continuous recycling through the various stages. While patients may begin to explore how to live more fully once they have received a diagnosis of a terminal illness, it is equally the case that once patients have experienced living more fully in each moment, they are then better able to notice the habitual assumptions that have kept them from examining their options sooner.

"Living in the moment" does not mean ignoring responsibilities or giving into impulses—quite the opposite. Rather than acting unconsciously from habitual and neurotically based impulses, and who lives more fully in the moment can become more fully conscious of habits and impulses, along with optimal actions, so that one is free to make informed choices. This is true responsibility.

FORMATS OF DELIVERY

Existential psychotherapy can be performed in an individual format, in a group setting, or in combination with other approaches. This approach works well in the psychotherapy office or by the patient's bedside (hospital or home). The more time one has to meet, the deeper the progress that can be made. However, with a population in crisis, and therefore highly motivated, even one session can prove useful. Simply hearing that it is all right to feel as one does and to have such thoughts can be a relief and a revelation to a patient. And letting the family know that showing its suffering is all right can bring everyone closer.

Whenever possible, group existential psychotherapy is especially useful in facilitating existential maturity in the patient.[96] Hearing about others experience can provide a "lateral experience" that allows alternative ways of understanding and action to be considered. Relating to a group also demands that one to some extent suspend one's own perspective in order to appreciate another's. Both factors aid in facilitating a

breakdown of fixed assumptions about life, aiding in adjustment to current circumstances, and selecting actions that are truly meaningful for one's life. The group experience can serve to "normalize" patients' experiences so that they are less likely to cover up their concerns. However, the therapist must take care that the group does not foster a culture in which one way of perceiving or acting predominates. Rather, each patients' experience and process must be respected as valuable. At its best the group has the potential to help reveal experience, while at its worst it has the power to aid in covering up.

Existential psychotherapy uses techniques developed in other approaches to psychotherapy, as well as heuristically guiding other psychotherapeutic modalities, which are all too often devoid of underlying principles when serving critically ill populations. For instance, the Socratic method of questioning assumptions found in cognitive therapy are of value in confronting inauthentic assumptions and stimulating consideration of meaningful activities for medically ill patients. Cognitive therapists, on the other hand, may find the stages of existential psychotherapy presented here useful for guiding patients' development. Behavioral methods can help patients reduce distress in order to consider their current situation or develop an effective action plan for engaging in new meaningful activities. Behavioral therapists may find existential principles useful to ensure that they are helping patients to be more fully present in the moment and in their relationship with others, rather than merely covering up distress and consequently any potential for personal development.

CONCLUSION

Existential psychotherapy provides a framework for treating persons with serious medical illness.

It offers an understanding of the difficulties facing persons whose usual approach to life is in major transition. It also offers the therapist guidance in how to facilitate the transitional period of life and elicit the maximum meaning, purpose, and value possible in the time the patient has left.

Persons with a terminal illness naturally fear losing control at some point and becoming a burden to others. However, most patients with cancer and cardiac disease are very functional until a few weeks before death, and very few are actually a burden on their loved ones. If you were to ask a man, "If your wife were sick, and you were caring for her, would you want your wife to end her life so that she would no longer be a burden to you?" the answer would usually be, "Absolutely not!" Rather than being a burden, this relationship can build a deep and mature caring beyond what the partners have previously experienced. In part, this happens because in this novel situation, all involved must release their prior experiences of each other and their world and enter into a new relationship, based on the authentic present moment that is currently unfolding. Frankly, in such circumstances, there is really very little choice. Thus, relationships at the end of one's physical life offer an excellent opportunity for authentic intimacy and maturity. By entering into such a relationship with patients, existentially oriented psychotherapists can facilitate such maturity in their patients, as well as in themselves.

Many persons who are diagnosed with a terminal illness consider suicide as a viable option. From an existential standpoint, it is useful to consider death, even the possibility of taking one's life, since choosing to live will then have that much greater meaning and value to it. However, from a Buddhist standpoint, the ego that decides to live or die is a small part of one's entire being. One should be careful about making a conscious choice from the standpoint of the inauthentic self. If considered from the standpoint of an authentic moment of vision, one's commitment to life would be such that one would never consider taking one's life.[97] Ending one's life prematurely simply robs one of the potential for living as fully as one ever has. The example of Lynn might help to demonstrate this point.

Case Example

Lynn was a widow who moved to a new state to enjoy her retirement years. Soon after arriving she was diagnosed with inoperable metastatic ovarian cancer. Lynn was a very social person, optimistic by nature, and full of energy. She presented for therapy because she heard "psychotherapy was useful in prolonging survival." She was confident she "was going to beat this thing" and was determined "not to let it get me down." Her "positive energy," however, served to cover up important considerations, such as choice of treatment, arranging for nursing care in the months ahead, and preparing her family and her friends for the likelihood of her dying in the upcoming year. She was continually pulling for reassurance that "everything would be all right," and incessantly talked about her past life. One time, early in treatment, Lynn called to say that she had just been told by the oncologist that there was no point in continuing chemotherapy, since the tumors were continuing to grow and spread, despite rigorous treatment. She said that she needed to cancer our session for that afternoon, and I responded that while I understood that she was distressed by the news, I thought that this would be an important session to keep. She agreed about the need for the session but said that the reason she was canceling was not because of the bad news but because the O.J. Simpson trial was on, and she just "couldn't" miss it! It turned out that this trial was her only real interest at this time. Needless to say, this provided fertile material for subsequent sessions.

Over the course of the year, Lynn was gradually able to tolerate consideration of the fact that she was going to die (although we could not be sure when this would be). As we worked to tolerate being in the moment through meditation and personal interaction, she reduced her tendency to flee into the past and became calmer and more reflective. She was able to reject an experimental treatment that had a small chance of temporarily reducing tumor size but a high probability of debilitating side effects. She made arrangements for home nursing care, began saying goodbye to her family and friends, and even choreographed her own funeral. As she weakened, she let go of irrelevant activities (that she eventually realized were mostly distractions) and began to focus on important relationships in her life. She found herself capable of more intimate relationships than she had ever been capable of. In our final session at her bedside, Lynn told me she was dying well, able to get from each moment whatever it had to offer. Indeed, during her last breath, Lynn let go of her idea of time and space, of self and other. Her last breath never stopped for her. And as she drew her friends into that final breath, we all experienced a moment of intimate unity with Lynn, and with one another.

References

1. Dunkel-Schetter C, Feinstein LG, Taylor SE. Patterns of coping with cancer. *Health Psychology*, 1992; 11(2):79–87.
2. Goldstein DA, Antoni MH. The distribution of repressive coping styles among non-metastatic and metastatic breast cancer patients as compared to non-cancer patients. *Psychology and Health*, 1989; 3:245–258.
3. Greer S. Psychological response to cancer and survival. *Psychological Medicine*, 1991; 21:43–49.
4. Helgeson VS, Cohen S, Fritz HL. Social ties and cancer. In: Holland J, ed, *Psycho-Oncology*. New York: Oxford University Press, 1998:99–109.
5. Reifman A. Social relationships, recovery from illness, and survival: a literature review. *Annals of Behavioral Medicine*, 1995; 17(2):124–131.
6. Temoshok L. Biopsychosocial studies on cutaneous malignant melanoma: Psychosocial factors associated with prognostic indicators, progression, psychophysiology, and tumor-host response. *Social Science and Medicine*, 1985; 20:833–840.
7. Shekelle RB, Gale M, Ostfeld AM, Paul O. Hostility, risk of coronary heart disease, and mortality. *Psychosomatic Medicine*, 1983; 45(2):109–14.
8. Dunkel-Schetter C, Feinstein LG, Taylor SE. Patterns of coping with cancer. *Health Psychology*, 1992; 11(2):79–87.
9. Fawzy FI, Kemeny ME, Fawzy N, Elashoff R, Morton D, Cousins N, Fahey JL. A structured psychiatric intervention for cancer patients, II: changes over time in immunological measures. *Archives of General Psychiatry*, 1990; 47:729–735.
10. Fox B. Psychosocial factors in cancer incidence and prognosis. In: Holland J, ed, *Psycho-Oncology*. New York: Oxford University Press, 1998:110–124.
11. Williams R, Haney T, Lee K, et al. Type A behavior, hostility, and coronary heart disease. *Psychosomatic Medicine*, 1980; 42:539–549.
12. Winick L, Robbins GF. Physical and psychologic readjustment after mastectomy: an evaluation of Memorial Hospitals' PMRG program. *Cancer*, 1977; 39(2):478–486.
13. Wood PE, Milligan M, Christ D, Liff D. Group counseling for cancer patients in a community hospital. *Psychosomatics*, 1978; 19:555–561.
14. Frenkel EM, Torem M. Management of a dying patient in group therapy. Group, *Journal of the Eastern Group Psychotherapy Society*, 1981; 5(1): 54–61.
15. Cella D, Sarafian B, Snider P, Yellen S, Winicour P. Evaluation of a community-based cancer support group. *Psycho-oncology*, 1993; 2:123–132.
16. Trijsburg RW, van Knippenberg FCI, Rijpma SE. Effects of psychological treatment on cancer patients: a critical review. *Psychosomatic Medicine*, 1992; 54:489–517.
17. Spira J, Spiegel D. Group Psychotherapy of the Medically Ill. In: Stoudemire A, Fogel B, eds, *Psychiatric Care of the Medical Patient*. 2nd ed, New York: Oxford University Press, 1993:31–50.
18. Fawzy FI, Fawzy NW, Arndt LA, Pasnau RO. Critical review of psychosocial interventions in cancer care. *Archives of General Psychiatry*, 1995; 52:100–113.
19. Forester B, Kornfelf DS, Fleiss JL, Thompson S. Group psychotherapy during radiotherapy: effects on emotional and physical distress. *American Journal of Psychiatry*, 1993; 150(11):1700–1706.
20. Weisman A, Worden J, Sobel H. Psychosocial Screening and Intervention With Cancer Patients: *Research Report*. Cambridge, Mass: Shea Bros., 1980.
21. Vachon ML, Lyall WA, Rogers J, Cochrane J, Freeman S. The effectiveness of psychosocial support during post-surgical treatment of breast cancer. *International Journal of Psychiatry Medicine*, 1982; 11:365–372.
22. Heinrich R, Schag C. Stress and activity management: group treatment for cancer patients and spouses. *Journal of Consulting and Clinical Psychology*, 1985; 33:439–446.
23. Berglund G, Bolund C, Gustafsson U, Sjoden P. A randomized study of a rehabilitation program for cancer patients: the "starting again" group. *Psycho-oncology*, 1994; 3:109–120.
24. Fawzy FI, Fawzy NW, Hyun CS. Short-term psychiatric intervention for patients with malignant melanoma: effects on psychological state, coping, and the immune system. *The Psychoimmunology of Cancer*. New York: Oxford University Press, 1994:292–319.
25. Yalom I. *Theory and Practice of Group Psychotherapy*. 3rd ed. New York: Basic Books, 1985.
26. Spiegel D, Bloom J, Yalom I. Group support for patients with metastatic cancer. *Archives of General Psychiatry*, 1981; 38:527–533.
27. Mulder CI, Antoni MH, Emmelkamp PM, Veugelers PJ, Sanfort TP, Vijver FA, deVries MJ. Psychosocial group intervention and the rate of decline of immunological parameters in asymptomatic HIV infected gay men. *Psychotherapy and Psychosomatics*, 1994; 63:185–192.

28. Fawzy FI, Kemeny ME, Fawzy N, Elashoff R, Morton D, Cousins N, Fahey JL. A structured psychiatric intervention for cancer patients, II: changes over time in immunological measures. *Archives of General Psychiatry*, 1990; 47:729–735.

29. Fawzy FI, Fawzy NW, Hyun CS, Elashoff R, Guthrie D, Fahey JL, Morton D. Malignant melanoma: effects of an early structured psychiatric intervention, coping, and affective state on recurrence and survival 6 years later. *Archives of General Psychiatry*, 1993; 50:681–689.

30. Antoni MH, Schnneiderman N, Fletcher MA, Goldstein DA, Ironson G, Laperrier A. Psychoneuroimmunology and HIV-1. *Journal of Consulting and Clinical Psychology*, 1990; 58(1):38–49.

31. Antoni M. Cognitive behavioral intervention for persons with HIV. In: Spira J, ed, *Group Therapy for Medically Ill Patients*. New York: The Guilford Press, 1997.

32. Friedman M, Thoresen CE, Gill JJ, et al. Alteration of type A behavior and its effect on cardiac recurrences in post-myocardial infarction patients: Summary results of the current coronary prevention project. *American Heart Journal*, 1986; 112:653–665.

33. Friedman M, Rosenman R. *Type-A Behavior and Your Heart*. New York: Alfred A. Knopf, 1974.

34. Thoresen C, Bracke P. In: Spira J, ed, *Group Therapy For The Medically Ill*. New York: Guilford Press, 1996.

35. Spiegel D, Bloom JR, Kraemer HC, Gottheil E. Effect of psychosocial treatment on survival of patients with metastatic breast cancer. *The Lancet*, 1989; November:889–891.

36. Fox B. A critique of psychosocial factors and cancer incidence and mortality. In: Holland J, ed, *Textbook of Psycho-Oncology*. (in press) Oxford University Press.

37. Spiegel D, Spira JL. *Supportive Expressive Group Therapy: A Treatment Manual of Psychosocial Intervention for Treating Women With Recurrent Breast Cancer*. Department of Psychiatry, Stanford University, Palo Alto, CA, 1991.

38. Miller S, Brody D, Summerton J. Styles of coping with threat: implications for health. *Journal of Personality and Social Psychology*, 1988; 54:345–353.

39. Reed GM, Kemeny ME, Taylor SE, Wang H-YW, Visscher BR. Realistic acceptance as a predictor of reduced survival time in gay men with AIDS. *Health Psychology*, 1994; 13:299–307.

40. Taylor S. Attributions, beliefs about control, and adjustment to breast cancer. *Journal of Personality and Social Psychology*, 1984; 46(3):489–502.

41. Spira J. Existential group psychotherapy for advanced breast cancer and other life-threatening illnesses. In: Spira J, ed, *Group Therapy for Medically Ill Patients*. New York: The Guilford Press, 1997.

42. Spira J. *Dissociation and PTSD in the Medically Ill*. (ABSTRACT) Academy of Psychosomatic Medicine, New Orleans, LA, November, 1993.

43. Passik S, Grummon K. PTSD and dissociative disorders. In Holland J, ed, *Psycho-Oncology*. New York: Oxford Press, 1998:595–607.

44. Gellert GA, Maxwell RM, Siegel BS. Survival of breast cancer patients receiving adjunctive psychosocial support therapy: a 10-year follow-up study. *Journal of Clinical Oncology*, 1993; 11(1):66–69.

45. Siegel B, Spira J, and Ulmer D. Panel discussion: The effects of group therapy on medically ill patients. *Fourth Mind, Body, and Immunity Conference*, sponsored by the Institute for the Clinical Application of Behavioral Medicine; Hilton Head, SC, December, 1992.

46. Watson M, Greer S. Personality and Coping. In: Holland J, ed, *Psycho-Oncology*. New York: Oxford University Press, 1998:91–98.

47. Pennebaker JW, Kiecolt-Glaser JK, Glaser R. Disclosure of traumas and immune function: health implications for psychotherapy. *Journal of Consulting and Clinical Psychology*, 1988; 56:239–245.

48. Fichte JG. *The Science of Knowledge* (P. Heath & J. Lachs, Trans.). London: Cambridge University Press. (Original work published 1794), 1982.

49. Jacobi FH. Open Letter to Fichte 1799. In: Behler E, ed, *Philosophy of German Idealism*, (pp. 126–7). New York: Continuum, 1987.

50. Behler E. *Philosophy of German Idealism: Fichte, Jacobi, and Schelling*. New York: Continuum, 1987.

51. Schleiermacher F. *Hermenetik*. Kemmerle H, ed, Heidelberg: Carl Winter, Universtatsverlag, 1959.

52. Dilthey W. *Selected Writings*. Ed. Rickman, HP, ed, Cambridge University Press.

53. Heidegger M. (1927). *Being and Time*. (Macquarrie & Robinson, Trans.). New York: Harper and Row, 1962.

54. Zimmerman M. *Eclipse of the Self: The Development of Heidegger's Concept of Authenticity*. Athens, Ohio: University of Ohio Press, 1986.

55. Husserl E. *Logical Investigations*. Vols. 1 and 2. (J.N. Findlay), Boston: Routledge and Kegan Paul, 1900.

56. Merleau-Ponty M. *Phenomenology of Perception*. (Colin Smith, Trans.). London: Routledge and Kegan Paul, 1962.

57. Bodhidharma. *The Zen Teachings of Bodhidharma*, (R. Pine, Trans.). Port Townsend, WA: Empty Bowl, 1987.

58. Suzuki DT. *Introduction to Zen Buddhism*. New York: Causeway Books, 1974.

59. Rahula W. *What The Buddha Taught*, New York: Grove Press, 1959.

60. Schopenhauer A. *The World As Will And Representation*. Vol II. (EF Payne, trans), New York: Doubleday, 1958.

61. Kierkegaard S. (1847) Works of Love. In: Bretall R, ed, *A Kierkegaard Anthology*, New Jersey: Princeton University Press, 1946.

62. Kierkegaard S. *Fear and Trembling* (orig. 1841) and *Sickness Unto Death* (orig. 1848), Lowrie, W (trans). New Jersey: Princeton University Press, Fifth edition, 1974.

63. Kierkegaard S. *Fear and Trembling* (orig. 1841) and *Sickness Unto Death* (orig. 1848), Lowrie, W (trans), Princeton University Press, Fifth edition, 1974.

64. Nietzsche F. *The Will To Power*. (original notes completed in 1888), W. Kaufmann (trans.) New York: Vintage, 1967.

65. Nietzsche F. *Thus Spoke Zarathustra* (orig. 1883). Hollingsdale (trans), New York: Penguine, 1961.

66. Heidegger M. Conversations on a country path about thinking. In: *Discourse On Thinking* (orig. 1944–45). New York: Haper Torchbooks, 1966.

67. Nishitani K. *Religion and Nothingness*. Berkeley: University of California Press, 1982.

68. Zimmerman M. *Eclipse of the Self: The Development of Heidegger's Concept of Authenticity*. Athens, Ohio: Ohio University Press, 1986.

69. Tolstoy L. The death of Ivan Ilych. In: *The Death of Ivan Ilych and Other Stories*. New York: Signet, 1966/1960.

70. Jaspers K. *Allgemeine Psychopathologie* Berlin: Springer, 1913.

71. Binswanger L. Selected Papers of Ludwig Binswanger. Translated and with a critical introduction to his existential psychoanalysis by Jacob Needleman. New York: Harper and Row, 1968.

72. Frankl V. *The Unheard Cry for Meaning*. New York: Simon and Schuster, 1978.

73. Boss M. *The Analysis of Dreams*, (A. Pomerans, trans.). New York: Philosophical Library, 1958.

74. Moreno J. *Psychodrama: Volume I*. New York: Beacon House, 1946.

75. Ellis A. *Reason and Emotion in Psychotherapy*. New York: Lyle Stuart and Citadel Press, 1962.

76. Glasser W. *Reality Therapy*. New York: Harper & Row, 1965.

77. Yalom ID. *Existential Psychotherapy*. New York, NY: Basic Books, 1980.

78. Yalom ID, Greaves C. Group therapy with the terminally ill. *American Journal of Psychiatry*, 1977; 134:396–400.

79. Bugental J. Confronting the existential meaning of "my death" through group exercises. *Interpersonal Development*, 1973–74; 4:148–163.

80. Zimmerman M. *Eclipse of the Self: The Development of Heidegger's Concept of Authenticity*. Athens, Ohio University Press, 1986.

81. Miller I., et al. Applying cognitive-social theory to health-protective behavior: breast self-examination in cancer screening. *Psychological Bulletin*, 1996; 119:1–24.

82. Spira, in preparation.

83. Spiegel D, Spira J. The use of hypnosis in managing medical symptoms. *Psychiatr Med* 1991; 9: 521–533.

84. Maslow A. *Toward a Psychology of Being*. 2nd ed. Princeton, NJ: Insight Books, 1968.

85. Perls FS. *Gestalt Therapy Verbatim*. Moab, Utah: Real People Press, 1969.

86. Gendlin E. Experiential Psychotherapy. In: Corsini R, ed, *Current Psychotherapies*. 2nd ed. Itasca, IL: F.E. Peacock Publishers, 1979:340–373.

87. Reich W. *The Function of the Orgasm*. T. Wolfe (trans), New York: Noonday Press, 1942.

88. Reynolds DK. *The Quiet Therapies: Japanese Pathways To Personal Growth*. University Press of Honolulu, Hawaii, 1980.

89. Reynolds D. *Morita Psychotherapy*. Berkeley: University of California Press, 1976.

90. Spira J. *Tai Chi Chuan and Zen Meditation For Medically Ill Patients*: Videotape and Manual. Durham, NC: Duke University Center For Living, 1994.

91. Ellis A. *Reason and Emotion in Psychotherapy*. New York: Lyle Stuart and Citadel Press, 1962.

92. Glasser W. *Reality Therapy*. New York: Harper & Row, 1965.

93. Spira J, Spiegel D. Hypnosis and related techniques in pain management. *Hospice Journal*, 1992; 8 (1,2):89–119.

94. Miller et al. Applying cognitive-social theory to health-protective behavior: breast self-examination in cancer screening. *Psychological Bulletin*, 1996; 119:1–24.

95. Heidegger M. *Being and Time*. (orig. 1927, Macquarrie & Robinson, Trans.). New York: Harper and Row, 1962.

96. Spira J. Existential group psychotherapy for persons with advanced stage illness. In: Spira J ed, *Group Therapy For the Medically Ill*. New York: Guilford Press, 1997:55–64.

97. Levine S. *A Gradual Awakening*. New York: Bantam, Doubleday & Dell, 1989.

14

The Supportive Relationship, the Psychodynamic Life Narrative, and the Dying Patient

Milton Viederman, M.D.

This chapter explores the fundamentals of a particular supportive therapy in patients with cancer and in those confronted with death. The treatment is to be viewed as a specific treatment, requiring skill and based on a psychodynamic theory of the mind. It is distinguished from long-term, expressive, insight-oriented therapies by its goals and techniques. In general, the supportive therapist utilizes rather than interprets the transference, does not encourage regressive behavior, and is less bound to a neutral, anonymous, and nongratifying stance. The aim of the therapy is not to effect profound personality change (although this may be possible in situations of crisis[1–3] but rather to help the patient to reestablish a previous homeostasis rooted in greater comfort, to ameliorate dysphoric symptoms such as anxiety or depression, and to facilitate the establishment of a sense of hope about what is possible in the context of severe illness. This treatment presumes that a previous homeostasis has been disturbed by a new danger situation. This situation reflects a new reality that inevitably evokes unconscious phantoms, and amalgams of past and present unconscious fantasies. Appropriate clarification of aspects of these fears and a view of them as residues of the past can help to mute and soften them. This is a reparative therapy that resides in the view that appropriate knowledge of irrational fears dimin-ishes them. Of no less importance is the emphasis on the relationship with the therapist. If the therapist is sensitive to what the patient needs and will tolerate and to the need to support self-esteem and the expressed valuation of what the patient admires in himself, the protective soothing of a supportive human relationship, that is, positive transference, will be evoked. Central to the establishment of this relationship is the concept of appropriate communicated understanding.

Supportive psychotherapy is commonly misunderstood as handholding or being nice to the patient or simply caring for the patient. In fact, it requires the development of skill in elucidating the personal and idiosyncratic responses of the patient that reflect his unique life experience. It is a therapy based on a search for meaning, for specific understanding of the patient's dilemma as he experiences it. It involves the translation of this meaning into terms that the patient can hear, accept, and integrate. It is this *appropriate communicated understanding* that solidifies the powerful bond with the therapist. This bond decreases the isolation and the loneliness of a patient confronted with a new and fearful reality.

The physician confronted with an ill patient has multiple tasks. One is to use his or her expertise and knowledge to diagnose and positively affect the pathophysiological state we call *disease*.

A second, equally important goal is to relieve or at least alleviate the patient's distress, a component of the complex phenomenon we call *illness*, namely the patient's subjective experience. In many cases, this relief may be the only positive good that the doctor can offer. in order to offer this relief, the physician must establish a particular type of trusting relationship with the patient, one that will be therapeutic, both in facilitating the patient's collaboration with the doctor in the treatment and in affording relief from concern, anxiety, and depression. It is unlikely that any physician would argue with this as a reasonable goal, although physicians vary considerably in the attention they pay to this aspect of their role.

The particular ways of conceptualizing the predicament of the patient and the particular skills needed to implement this goal are the subject of this chapter. Being nice to the patient and reassuring him or her is not an adequate substitute for the application of knowledge with skill. Reassurance, in particular, is helpful only if directed toward the real source of the patient's concern and not to what the physician infers is a reasonable concern for such a patient with such a disease. Reassurance about something not of primary concern to the patient is alienating.

An important principle underlies the approach to be outlined in this chapter. This has to do with meaning as an intervening variable between the disease and the patient's distress. Individuals have highly varied emotional reactions to illness. The assumption, for example, that depression is a usual and expected response to the diagnosis of cancer is clearly incorrect, since some patients become depressed and others do not. Simple illnesses without apparent serious implications from the physician's point of view may still lead to profound anxiety and depression. Conversely, serious and life-threatening illnesses may be met with remarkable courage, optimism, the will to live, and a desire to experience maximum pleasure and satisfaction. These varied reactions do not reside simply in personality characteristics and attitudes of patients but reflect the special meanings of the experience in the context of the patient's life, present and past. Does the cancer or its treatment imply necessary dependence, loss of control, disfigurement, unrelenting pain, or abandonment?

Appropriate communicated understanding of the meaning of the diagnosis for the patient is of prime importance and powerfully influences the patient's attitude toward his or her physician. One may understand much more than one should appropriately communicate at a particular moment. Part of how one communicates and what one decides to communicate is influenced by one's understanding of the personality of the patient, an area described by Kahana and Bibring.[4] Much depends on the state of the patient at a given moment. The task of physicians is to convey to the patient that they understand the implications of what the illness means for the patient in the context of his or her life and to thereby offer a "presence," establishing a bond that patients typically do not expect to have with their physicians. It is in this type of interaction that the patient feels "noticed" and reciprocally notices the physician, not simply in the role of physician but as a person in the life of the patient. This is of special importance when an individual is confronted by the crisis of physical illness.

THE PREDICAMENT OF THE PATIENT

The experience of illness isolates patients, who are confronted with a bewildering new reality that demands that they change their perceptions of themselves in the multiple roles in which they have functioned—spouse, parent, worker, employer, and so on. The patient's anticipated life trajectories and perceptions of themselves in the world must be altered. If the disease has potentially fatal consequences, they may feel categorically set apart from others—"the healthy people"—whose perspective on life they can no longer share. The illness, the limitations that it imposes, the treatment demands—these evoke threatening and fearful fantasies on varying levels of consciousness that have echoes in childhood conflicts, fantasies, and concerns. Anxiety is generated by the breakdown of coherence, order, and predictability. Moreover, patients must develop new modes of behaving in the world. The dramatic change in their experience of reality becomes a crisis when the psychological demands cannot be handled adequately by the usual repertoire of coping devices. Hence, crisis in this regard may involve the following three components: (1) the disruption of the usual psychic equilibrium that depends on a stable, familiar, and predictable world, now no longer present; (2) regressive tendencies, with the evocation of childhood fears and wishes, accompanied by the wish and need to be protected by the parental figures of the past, often defended against; and (3) an inclination to examine the trajectory of one's life in an effort to integrate the new experience and to give it meaning that will permit its integration in the previous life experience.

THE PSYCHODYNAMIC LIFE NARRATIVE

A psychotherapeutic intervention, the psychodynamic life narrative,[5,6] has evolved from work with the physically ill. It has implications for use with individuals confronted by other crises, as well. It is to be understood not only as a therapeutic maneuver but as a way of conceptualizing responses to physical illness and the meaning of illness to a particular patient. This intervention is particularly useful for those individuals whose relatively successful adaptation or homeostasis has been disrupted by a crisis, specific life event, or such as a physical illness that has led to anxiety, depression, or demoralization.

The psychodynamic life narrative is a therapeutic intervention designed to address these components of crisis. It is a construct offered to patients to give their current experience meaning in the context of their life histories and to reveal their current reactions as logical products of previous life experience, rather than as an inevitable response to illness that is therefore unmodifiable. It offers coherence, order, and logic in a situation where patients experience chaos. Moreover, it gratifies the need for a protective figure. By presenting a narrative that spans the patient's life, the physician conveys a sense of having known the patient over time. Like the good parent who has a perspective on the child— where he has been and what he is becoming— the physician captures in the life narrative the quality of a shared experience over time and becomes, in the crisis situation, a reassuring figure reminiscent of the good parent. A powerful bond is generated by this intervention, which gives the physician a special status in the patient's experience that remains useful in their continued relationship.

The narrative may be constructed on different levels and may be striking in its simplicity if the proper questions are asked. Following are two examples of narratives—one only partially formulated, used in the context of a dying patient, the other used with a seriously ill AIDS patient to facilitate her acceptance of support.

Case Example

The patient, a lawyer, was a 77-year-old married father of three, hospitalized with severe pulmonary disease secondary to bronchiectasis, who now required constant use of prednisone. This led to multiple cervical and lumbar fractures. The patient requested consultation for depression.

Mr. D was an engaging, intelligent, coherent, and interesting man who spoke spontaneously and appropriately. He described his life history easily and with great self-awareness. His engagement, his general interest in life, his sense of humor, and his general optimism belied significant depression. It was pointed out to the patient that he was not depressed but appeared to be experiencing grief about his impending death. He had been aware of the seriousness of his illness and the fact that he was confronted with an extremely truncated life span.

The patient was one of two children born to a family that included many generations of lawyers. He expressed considerable anger at his father, who had insisted that he go into law and give up a promising career as an English professor. He was an amateur poet and highly valued his poetry writing, noting that he had not completed his last poem. His mother was a strong and appealing woman.

The patient had led a vigorous life with many close relationships. His second marriage was good, although not without conflict. Most important to him was his very special relationship with his three daughters. He became tearful as he spoke of his impending death and the fact that he would be leaving these daughters behind and bereft. It was at this point that I presented a narrative to him.

"You are very fearful of what your daughters will experience when you die. It is clear that your relationship with them has been central to your life and a source of great gratification to both yourself and to them. Clearly you have been able to offer them something that you had never received from your father, who was unable to recognize your poetic potential and to resonate with your needs. It is clear that they will be very pained by your death, but it is certain that the very positive relationship that you have had with them over the years will remain as a very important part of their life experience." The patient responded with tears and indicated that he felt very relieved. He had been aware of the special importance of his relationship with his daughters and recognized the truth of his continuing influence on them and the special importance that this had for him in light of his own experience with his father. He stated that it was a curious thing but that he had extremely warm feelings toward me and likened them to those one would have for a mentor, an experience he had had in a psychoanalysis many years before with his analyst. "It is curious," he said, "that, although you are many years younger than I, I can experience you as a good father."

When I visited him shortly thereafter, he expressed great appreciation for our encounter, indicating that the discussion had been "like lancing an abscess." He had felt much freer to talk to his daughters and his wife since then and indicated that he had not been able to cry before and now felt that he had gotten a great deal out of his system. Moreover, he had even felt some desire to eat.

One month later I noted an obituary in the newspaper that indicated the patient had died. I wrote a letter of condolence to his family, commenting on how important they had been to him. His wife wrote a letter in response.

Your letter was an enormous gift to us. For us to hear about D from someone who knew him only during his illness and for you to give us the landscape of the D you saw touches me deeply. He told me about his first visit with you and how wise and sensitive you were.

So look what you have done: You helped D during his terrible and difficult time, and now you have helped us. With my thanks.

The intervention described is not a complete life narrative, but it does make an important link between the patient's early life experience and the value he placed on his relationship with his daughters. In this regard, he was helped to understand that there was permanence in his relationship with his daughters. Through this relationship he had achieved what Lifton[7] has described as "symbolic immortality," the experience of immortality that resides in one's progeny. He felt relieved of some of the pain of his approaching death, particularly as he anticipated how it would affect his daughters. Moreover, he spontaneously indicated that a powerful positive paternal transference had been evoked in which I played a role for him like that he had played for his daughters. This brief intervention demonstrated that the patient's distress was not related directly to the fear of death itself but had its own special meaning in the context of his life. Work with such a patient can be extremely gratifying.

Case Example

The patient was a 40-year-old woman who had been diagnosed with AIDS one year earlier and who was now admitted with pneumocystis, lymphoma, and a bacterial infection. Consultation was requested because she appeared to be depressed.

The patient was an attractive, intelligent, articulate, and spontaneous woman who had had family therapy in the past. Although she did not appear profoundly depressed, she became tearful when certain important themes were touched.

Information provided by the resident who had begun an evaluation revealed that the patient had lived with a boyfriend for $5^1/_2$ years. In the context of her illness, she felt removed from him and feared abandonment. His dissatisfaction in the relationship related to the difficulty that he had in being with her and a sense that she was depressed and unresponsive. A separate discussion with him had revealed, however, that he had no intention of leaving her.

The following is a description of the evolution of the interview to give a sense of how the information was obtained and utilized with the patient.

The interview began with the patient's musing about why she had not actively confronted her boyfriend about her fear of abandonment, even though she had been in family therapy and had learned that this was the best way of dealing with such problems. I asked whether she was fearful of alienating him, and she remarked that she was afraid that he would abandon her. In response to the question about whether the fear of abandonment was an important theme in her life, the patient responded in the affirmative. I asked about this sense of vulnerability and asked what thoughts she had about this as it related to her earlier life, suggesting that she tell me whatever thoughts came to mind without attempting to explain them. The patient responded by saying that she had been abandoned by her beloved father when she was 13. Apparently they had had a very close relationship, which the mother resented. There had been much conflict in the family, and the father began to drink more and more and to leave the family for long periods of time. The patient felt very hurt about the father's departures. She was asked whether the father was abusive. "Yes, he was physically abusive and he attempted to abuse me sexually when he was in an alcoholic state and I was 16. It was then that I took flight. I always take flight from things that bother me." I commented, "This is exactly what you did in relationship to your boyfriend, as well, by not speaking to him." "That is certainly the case," she said. "Moreover, my mother had said, 'What do you expect when you walk around dressed as you are?' I had always felt guilty and felt that I was responsible for my father's seductiveness and his having left. This certainly has a lot to do with what is going on with my boyfriend. I am amazed that this has come out so easily." I asked, "But tell me how this developed. How did he react when you got AIDS?" The patient initially told a somewhat confused story about being depressed immediately and not recognizing it. However, with careful examination she revealed that, although she was very shocked at the beginning, her boyfriend took a semester off from college and she had felt quite cared for. I asked when this had changed, and she revealed that it was only the summer before. "What had happened, then, in August or September?" "Oh," she said, "I suddenly remember, he returned to school and I felt that he was betraying me, that he was leaving me and moreover began to imagine that he might be having an affair with someone else." "So once again you expected to be abandoned and betrayed, and you couldn't talk to him about it." "I was always afraid of being abandoned, and in fact at that point I ceased to have sex with him, believing that he would be at risk. I stayed in bed and had no motivation to do anything. I must have been depressed but didn't realize that I was." I commented, "And so in a way you left him before he left you." "Yes, that is certainly true, and I was afraid to talk to him about it. This is really amazing, it is so clear."

I then presented a narrative to the patient. "Look, it seems so clear how you got into this difficulty. You were always the beloved daughter of your father. You had a special relationship, and your mother may even have been competitive and moved closer to your older sister because of this. It must have been a terrible shock to you when your father betrayed you and could leave for such long periods of time. The betrayal led to you. You also felt responsible. You went off and started to drink and take drugs at this time."

The patient became very tearful as she remembered all of this. She indicated that it was painful to think about it. I continued, "You stopped taking drugs 7 years ago and stopped drinking 3 years ago. You were really pulling your life together and establishing this wonderful relationship with your boyfriend, and then the roof fell in. You found that you had AIDS." The patient interrupted and said, "I was so bitter and angry. I had done everything right and looked what happened to me." I continued, "But nonetheless your boyfriend was very responsive for these first 6 months and took care of you and reassured you. Yet it was when he returned to college that you felt that he was going to abandon you, just as your father had done. This was so distressing, and yet you were afraid to talk to him about it. As was characteristic of you, you pulled out before he could do it." The patient said, "I even thought of moving out of the apartment at that point. It is so remarkable. It all seems so simple. I feel very grateful to you."

In this somewhat lengthy case description, the evolution of the interview is described with a focus on very active interventions, inferences made from the material, and decisions made about the accuracy of the interventions as reflected in the patient's responses. The patient felt more and more relieved as the interview progressed and the narrative was presented. At times she became tearful, having been touched by the material, and at the end she felt relieved. In this case, the psychodynamic life narrative was a summary statement of material that had been covered before but organized and placed in context.

Although the primary goal in the use of the narrative is to provide symptom relief and to effect a return to an earlier homeostasis, both of these patients experienced change in the context of the encounter. How might one conceptualize such change?[1,2]

As we think about human behavior, it is readily apparent that we are motivated to achieve ideals. The discrepancy between the way we experience ourselves and the ideal way that we would choose to behave or be acts as a motivational system throughout life, directed toward change to attain the ideal. Especially in time of crisis, individuals may be motivated to test new versions of themselves through action in the world, or the crisis itself may precipitate such a test. If these actions take place in the presence of important individuals who support them, a change can occur in the patient's self-perception. Part of this change may involve an identification with the supportive person. The physician may be the catalyst for such change, even in a relatively brief contact. The model I propose involves four elements:

1. A defective sense of self and a lifelong motivation to modify this self-perception to achieve an ideal
2. A decision to test a new sense of self through an action in the world
3. The presence of an important individual in the person's life who helps to consolidate a new perception of self
4. An identification with this individual

We are motivated to change, and we consolidate that change through action in the world. Positive and negative aspects of our sense of self are developed in the context of these actions. Actions can be taken to facilitate the crystallization of a new sense of self. This is more likely to occur in the presence of a supportive person who may be viewed in a somewhat idealized way and may in the process become the object of identification. A person who is revealed as being understanding and supportive at such a moment, even if previously a stranger, may take on special status in the patient's eyes and thereby become an important person in the patient's life.

Transference

The conceptualization of the change process can be broadened to include the concept of transference and the psychotherapeutic stance of enactment. Stated most simply and nontechnically, it implies that present relationships resonate with unconscious echoes of earlier important ones and that this resonance, to a greater or lesser extent, affects the current relationships. This is of special importance in the states of regression that have been alluded to. Much depends on the quality of early relationships, particularly parental ones. If these relationships were more benevolent than malevolent, the substrate for positive influence is present. As physicians, our greatest external difficulty in establishing trusting relationships with certain patients resides in their early negative experiences with caretaking figures. In the face of distrust, if the physician uncovers a story of early deprivation and communicates to the patient how this early experience may affect the present relationship, the patient may well be able to respond.

For those patients who were favored by early positive experiences, the generous and supportive presence of a responsive physician will be experienced as supportive even though the roots of this relationship may never become manifest.

Listening and understanding should be the basis for the therapeutic intervention but not its sole components. The passive approach tends to create, not a neutral field but rather one of a special nature. Passivity and inactivity have as powerful an effect on the interaction between two people as does activity. The model limited to receptive listening is inadequate as a mode of dealing with terminally ill patients.

Special Considerations When Dealing with the Dying Patient

The management of denial represents a special problem for those who treat the physically ill, and in particular the dying patient.[8,9] Denial is defined as a type of "scotoma" directed toward external reality, in contrast to the defense of repression, which is directed toward internal impulses, wishes, and fantasies. In general, the extensive use of denial in physically healthy people is considered maladaptive since a relatively accurate perception of reality is likely to permit a more effective adaptation to it. The situation changes significantly with physical illness, where denial serves a very useful function in protecting against distress and anxiety. Intense denial directed against the cognitive appreciation that one has a disease may be highly maladaptive if it interferes with the individual's willingness to seek appropriate treatment. However, often patients who accept treatment continue to deny the implications of their disease, if not the fact of it. Breznitz[10] points out that there is a sequence in denial that involves denial of information, denial of threatening information, denial of personal relevance, denial of urgency, denial of vulnerability or responsibility, denial of affect, and denial of affect relevance. This conceptualization is useful, although one might argue with some of the terminology. It implies that one can be quite aware of a presence of a disease cognitively but deny its implications or that one may attribute affects generated by the awareness of the disease to other sources, all in the service of defense. Of importance, however, is the fact that denial is extremely variable in the same patient from moment to moment, and the patient's acknowledgement of a serious condition in the morning may be followed by considerable denial in the afternoon. The psychotherapist works at the limits of the patient's denial, neither intruding on it as a defense and evoking anxiety nor avoiding threatening subjects that the patient is able to acknowledge.

It is important to distinguish denial from suppression, the conscious pushing away of feelings and thoughts of which the patient is aware. Often patients who are fearful of their own predicament and of what the future may bring suppress their thoughts and feelings in order to "protect" those around them. In so doing, these individuals become isolated and, often, depressed because of the loneliness that follows their inability to communicate. It is the physician's task to test the patient's ability to describe his current predicament by testing the limits of the patient's awareness with questions such as "Are there things that you fear talking about?" "How do you see the future?" "What is the most disturbing aspect of your current predicament?"

The issue of denial is closely related to recent research on the question of illusion. Taylor and Brown[11] suggest that unrealistically positive views of self are extremely helpful in adaptation to various forms of cancer. Moreover, illusions of control or unrealistic optimism clearly promote better states of mental equilibrium and should not be disturbed. The cognitive concept of "reframing" may be helpful in this regard. This technique was used to support a patient who had a brain tumor. Although the first round of treatment seemed not to be effective, this fact was reframed as a suggestion that the tumor had not progressed, a statement that relieved the patient.

The broad principles that underlie any dynamic therapy apply to the treatment of the dying patient, as well. The particular experience of the patient is what determines the therapeutic approach. It is to be emphasized that there is no single way to die. The views of Kübler-Ross et al.[8] on the sequential stages that precede death—denial, rage, bargaining, depression, and acceptance—is a useful organizing model but it is to be emphasized that the sequential transition through these stages is rare, and individuals may experience none or all of the elements in this progression. Indeed, there are individuals who appear to maintain their denial to the very end of life without excessive suffering.

Clearly, most dying patients do not require psychotherapy. In general, psychotherapy may be of help if there are major disturbances in communication between the sick and dying patient and the family. The role of the psychiatrist may be to facilitate communication between members of the family and to overcome anxieties about meaningful discussion at a level tolerable for the patient and for other members of the family.[9] In particular, a dying patient requires a psychotherapist who is "present"—one who is authentically involved with the patient. A therapist who undertakes such treatment may be obliged to work with the patient until his or her death, perhaps including making visits to the patient's home.

The concept of meaning as a variable in deciding on a therapeutic intervention has as much applicability to work with the dying patient as to work with any other patient. The presumption that there is a primary fear of death (questioned by Freud)[13] may or may not be valid, but the specter of death evoke fears that are unique to each patient and reflective of his life experience. These may include the fear of helplessness, dependency, pain, separation, abandonment, lack of fulfillment, body disintegration, loss of control, change of self-image, loss of function, and danger of regression. The use of the narrative may be helpful in clarifying special meanings to the patient and in demonstrating their origin in the patient's life history. Although regression may not be encouraged in the treatment of the dying patient, it often occurs, and it may be the therapist's task to tolerate the regression and to respond to regressive wishes as the patient approaches death. Often anticipatory grief is manifest and is to be distinguished from depression.

CONCLUSION

Patients have certain expectations of doctors, and they tell their stories in particular ways. The presence of a physician who actively engages patients may come as an unexpected surprise and may lead to a personal dialogue hardly anticipated. The idea that this type of engagement should be reserved for the experienced physician or, in the more extreme case, only for the psychiatrist is in error. Although there may be lapses in sensitivity and awareness, physicians who have been grounded early in the principles of psychological medicine often return to such interests later in their careers, particularly as they anticipate long-term relationships with patients and feel the need for establishing a therapeutic alliance. Learning about this kind of treatment is a lifelong task that is fraught with difficulty, yet graced with the rewards of achievement.

References

1. Viederman M. Personality change through life experience (I): a model. *Psychiatry*, 1986; 49(3):204–217.
2. Viederman M. Personality change through life experience (II): the role of ego ideal, personality and events. 111–132. In: Cooper, ed, *Psychoanalysis: Toward the Second Century*. New Haven: Yale University Press, 1989:111–132.
3. Viederman M. Personality change through life experience (III): two creative types of response to object loss. In: Dietrich D and Shabad P, eds, *The Problem of Loss and Mourning: Psychoanalytic Perspectives*. New York: International Universities Press, 1989:187–212.
4. Kahana RJ, Bibring GL. Personality types in medical management. In: Zinberg N, ed, *Psychiatry and Medical Practice in a General Hospital*. New York: International Universities Press, 1964.
5. Viederman M. Psychodynamic life narrative in a psychotherapeutic intervention useful in crisis situations. *Psychiatry*, 1983; 46:236–246.
6. Viederman M, Perry S. Use of the psychodynamic life narrative in the treatment of depression in the physically ill. *General Hospital Psychiatry*, 1980; 2:177–185.
7. Lifton RJ. Twentieth annual Karen Harvey lecture: the sense of immortality—on death and the continuity of life. *American Journal of Psychoanalysis*, 1973; 33:3–15.
8. Kübler-Ross E, Wessler S, Arcoli LV. On death and dying. *Journal of the American Medical Association*, 1972; 221:174–179.
9. Norton J. Treatment of a dying patient. *Psychoanalytic Study of the Child*, 1963; 18:541–561.
10. Breznitz S. *The Denial of Stress*. New York: International University Press, 1983.
11. Taylor SE, Brown JD. Illusion and well-being: a social psychological perspective on mental health. *Psychological Bulletin*, 1988; 103:193–210.
12. Freud S. *The Ego and the Id*. London: Hogarth Press, 1961. Originally published 1923.

15

A Cognitive-Behavioral Approach to Symptom Management in Palliative Care

Augmenting Somatic Interventions

Dennis C. Turk, Ph.D.
Caryn S. Feldman, Ph.D.

Although medicine has made tremendous strides in the prevention, detection, and treatment of diseases, inevitably we all die. For a significant majority of people, death is not unexpected, more likely, there is a steady decline following a downward course. At some point during this progression, palliation of symptoms is unfortunately the best that can be offered. Despite the significant advances medicine has made in the development of sophisticated pharmacological and surgical interventions, the range of noxious symptoms that accompany the process of dying (e.g., fatigue, disturbances of appetite and sleep, nausea, dyspnea, and pain) may not be totally eliminated, and there is a need to provide palliative care.[1-3]

Pain, in particular, is dreaded more than anything else about dying. This should not be surprising, since pain has the capacity to negatively affect every aspect of a person's life. It can and does affect a patient's mood, will to live, family relations, social life, sleep, appetite, spirituality, and ability to participate in physical activity for self-care or enjoyment. When left untreated, pain can cause a patient's emotional and spiritual death long before that the actual end of life.

Sadly, a significant minority of patients report that their symptoms are not adequately relieved. Some have argued that the reason symptoms such as pain are not ameliorated is that the knowledge we do have about drugs is not adequately applied or that physicians have not treated pain in a sufficiently aggressive manner.[4] Others have speculated that the problem is the patient's failure to comply with the recommended drug regimen.[4] Although these explanations are plausible, it is also possible that some of the reported pain is associated with a host of psychological factors that may exacerbate the perception of and subsequent reports of pain.[5] If psychological factors play a role in pain perception, then a host of noninvasive interventions may be of use in assisting these patients.

Before we proceed, an important caveat needs to be stated. Although we will suggest that psychological factors may modify the perception of pain and other symptoms and augment their experience, this is not to suggest that psychological factors cause the symptom. Nor is it to suggest that the reported symptom is imaginary. Rather, it is the intention of this chapter to sensitize readers to the importance of considering the role of psychological factors in pain and other symptoms and to alert them to a set of strategies that may be useful to complement the usual pharmaco-logical and surgical modalities already in their armamentarium.[6-8] A broader perspective is needed, one in which psychological concepts, variables, and treatment modalities receive greater consideration in keeping with their recognized contributions to symptom management and the promise they hold for alleviating suffering.[9]

Psychological techniques have been developed and used in conjunction with more traditional medical interventions to alleviate symptoms, disturbed thoughts, mood, and behavior commonly associated with dying.[10] For example, fears that typically accompany a diagnosis of terminal disease include loss of bodily function, disfiguring treatments, loss of autonomy and independence, abandonment and isolation, becoming a burden, financial strain, the end of known existence, and uncontrollable pain. These fears, along with the diagnosis of terminal status, contribute to feelings of anger, anxiety, and depression. Family members' responses run a similar gauntlet of fears and emotions (see Chapter 19 in this volume).

In this chapter we review the central role that psychological factors play in the perception of symptoms, with emphasis on pain as an example. We describe how these psychological factors may impact on the quality of life and symptom severity of patients with advanced disease. Finally, we describe a set of cognitive and behavioral methods that can be used with patients during the terminal phase. We give particular attention to practical suggestions regarding the selection of treatments and the matching of treatments to patients' characteristics and disease status.

DIVERGING PERSPECTIVES ON PAIN IN TERMINAL ILLNESS

A common assumption that is pervasive in palliative care is that pain is directly linked to tissue pathology and less subject to the psychological variables that are implicated in other classes of clinical pain.[11] The assumption seems to be that if terminal patients report pain, these subjective reports are veridical reflection of an objective state of their anatomy and physiology. The palliative-care literature has tended to ignore research on chronic pain and continues to be guided by sensory models that have been shown to be inadequate.[12] Unfortunately, this sensory-physiological model is incomplete. It cannot explain why many individuals with the same extent of tissue pathology differ so widely in their report

of pain intensity; do not report any pain despite objective radiographic evidence of bony degenerative changes; complain of severe pain in the absence of significant physical pathology; and, with the same physical diagnosis and identified tissue pathology treated with the same intervention, respond in distinctly different ways.

Psychological factors such as anxiety, expectancy, cognitive appraisal, self-efficacy, and perceived control, along with principles of operant conditioning and observational learning, have been shown to influence reports and experience of physiological processes, fatigue, appetite and sleep disturbance, nausea, and pain not associated with advanced disease. These factors have been largely disregarded in the palliative-care literature. The influential gate control model of pain,[12,13] postulating motivational-affective and cognitive-evaluative as well as sensory-discriminative contributions to the perception of pain, appears to have had relatively little impact in cancer pain. In short, the fund of knowledge about pain in general seems to be underutilized in the cancer pain arena.

PSYCHOLOGY OF TERMINAL ILLNESS AND PHYSICAL SYMPTOMS

Symptom Preoccupation

A physical symptom is the awareness of some aspect of an internal state. Note that this definition does not mean that there necessarily is any physiological concomitant of the symptom. The symptom is a perception. A stomachache may signal indigestion, food poisoning, intestinal flu, appendicitis, or anxiety.

The very act of monitoring sensations for signs of change increases the probability that expected changes (ipso facto exacerbation of pain) will be perceived. The cancer patient may become increasingly preoccupied with his or her body in order to monitor any changes related to disease progression. Constant monitoring of the body will likely lead to identification of bodily signs that in other situations might be ignored or never even perceived. Thus, there may be anticipation of noxious stimulation and reports of such sensations even in their absence.

Much of the diversity of people's responses to threatening events or ambiguous sensations is attributable to variations in the appraisal process.

An individual's appraisals influence emotional arousal and the behavioral response to a situation. The more ambiguous the event, the greater the reliance on subjective interpretations and appraisals and subsequent responding. Cancer is, by its very nature, an ambiguous disease. It is often of unknown origin, its course is unpredictable and erratic, the likelihood of arresting the disease progression is uncertain, and the physical sensations created by the disease, treatment, and physiological arousal in response to the diagnosis are often vague and diffuse. When an individual has cancer, he or she may become sensitized to, continually monitor, and become preoccupied with bodily sensations. Physical sensations serve as a constant reminder of the disease, with all that it connotes, and are capable of being interpreted or misinterpreted.[14,15] They may also lead to overreaction and outright panic.[16] Continual vigilance and monitoring of noxious stimulation and the belief that physical changes signify disease progression may render even low-intensity nociception less bearable. Nonphysical factors can influence behavioral communications of distress and suffering. Overt communications of suffering elicit responses from health-care providers, as well as from family and friends. A terminal illness presents a particular dilemma. When symptoms are associated with a nonterminal disease, complaints of symptoms can result from a range of possible reinforcers. In these instances, where continuous reporting of symptoms contributes little information that is diagnostically or therapeutically useful, treatment efforts are often directed toward discouraging patients from reporting symptoms. In the case of patients with advanced disease, however, report of symptoms may signal change in disease status and may be necessary for proper titration of treatment for both the disease and pain. Thus, terminal patients are encouraged to focus on symptoms and to report exacerbations of symptoms to family members and medical staff. This attention, however, may lead to increased reporting. This difference between symptoms in terminal and those in nonterminal patients is an important one and needs to be considered in assessing reports of symptoms. However, it does not remove the probability that reinforcement factors can influence the report. The dilemma is how to differentiate appropriate reports of symptoms from maladaptive illness behaviors. The health-care provider must acknowledge the symptoms but provide reassurance and attention for "healthy behaviors" (e.g., activity) and support, even in the absence of symptom reporting, so that complaints are not consciously used as means for gaining attention and support.

A range of psychological variables have been identified that influence patients' perceptions and reports of symptoms, especially pain.[5,17] We highlight only some findings that carry implications for symptoms associated with advanced disease.

Fear and Anxiety

Anxiety has been demonstrated to be both a cause and a correlate of symptom reports. Anxiety can initiate a sequence of physiological changes, instigating nociception through heightened sympathetic nervous system activity that provokes muscle spasm, vasoconstriction, visceral disturbances, and release of pain-producing substances (e.g., substance P, Bradykinin). Furthermore, in an anxious state, patients may not be able to differentiate signs of sympathetic arousal from aversive stimulation. Thus, anxiety may exacerbate symptoms by altering the discriminability of physical sensations so that a lower threshold is used for labeling sensory events as noxious.[18] Barber[19] concluded:

> It appears that some procedures that are said to reduce pain actually reduce anxiety, fear, worry, and other emotions that are usually intermingled with pain. For instance, the pain relief that follows the administration of morphine and other opiates may be closely related to the reduction of anxiety or fear. Although the patient who has received the opiate may still experience pain sensations, the reduction in anxiety, fear or other emotions apparently leads him to report that pain is reduced (p. 453)

Symptoms that accompany terminal diseases may be exacerbated by emotional distress. For example, Spiegel and Bloom[20] found that mood disturbance and the meaning of pain to a patient predicted patients' reported pain intensity in a sample of 86 women with metastatic breast cancer. They reported that greater mood disturbance and the belief that pain signaled a worsening of their disease were significantly correlated with reported pain intensity. The authors concluded that since the patient sample was homogeneous with regard to medical status, the differential pain experiences reported were due in large part to the patients' emotional status.

The influence of the situation in which the symptom occurs is particularly important in patients with advanced disease, because of the fear and anxiety often evoked by their health status. This is demonstrated by a study of 667 cancer patients in which pain was perceived as interfering with activity and enjoyment of life (as reported by patients) to a greater degree when pain was perceived to be caused by cancer than when it was thought to have another cause.[21] Ahles, Blanchard, and Ruckdeschel[14] noted that 61% of patients studied were afraid that pain signified a progression of their disease. These patients had significantly higher scores on several measures of anxiety and depression than did the group that did not consider pain as indicative of worsening or progressive disease.

Perceived Controllability

Attribution of control is another factor implicated in symptom reporting.[15] Several clinical studies indicate that perceived control (i.e., the belief that one has control), whether veridical or not, is sufficient to produce significant pain relief.[22] Hill, Saeger, and Chapman[23] used patient-controlled analgesia (a patient-controlled drug infusion pump) for cancer patients undergoing painful bone marrow transplantation. The pain produced by this procedure is very severe and persists for up to 4 weeks. The authors found that those with the pump used approximately one-third as much morphine to achieve *equivalent* levels of pain control as those whose narcotics were administered by nurses. Thus, perception as well as actual ability to control pain appears to be capable of alleviating the intensity of the pain experienced.

COGNITIVE-BEHAVIORAL PERSPECTIVE ON TERMINAL ILLNESSES

The role of cognitive factors has been emphasized in perception and behavioral response to noxious symptoms.[24] The cognitive-behavioral perspective has two basic assumptions. First, individuals are active processors of information, rather than passive recipients of environmental stimuli. People attempt to make sense of, understand, predict, and control their lives. The amount of threat, arousal, or stress they experience is a joint function of the idiosyncratic appraisals of the novel stimuli and their adaptive resources. Second, cognitions, emotions, behaviors, and the social environment are to some extent causally related. Cognitions can elicit feelings, potentiate emotions, reduce arousal, and serve as an impetus for behavior. Conversely, feelings and behaviors can facilitate or inhibit the production of cognitions, and behaviors and emotions can influence the type of response from the environment. Thus, behavior is reciprocally determined by both the individual and his or her environment. As Turk and Rudy[25] suggest, the cognitive-behavioral perspective that focuses on individual appraisals, interpretations, and expectancies, as well as physiology and environmental influences, may be more essential to achieve successful results than any specific technique.

Cognitive-behavioral intervention for adverse symptoms has three foci: alteration of maladaptive behaviors; alteration of ongoing self-statements, images, and feelings that interfere with adaptive functioning; and alteration of cognitive schema (tacit assumptions and beliefs) that give rise to habitual ways of construing the self (i.e., as helpless) and cancer (as uncontrollable, inevitably causing pain). The objective of the intervention is not necessarily to abolish the symptom altogether but to promote well behaviors that facilitate health, as well as help patients cope with varying degrees of discomfort in order to maximize their quality of life for whatever period of time remains.

The specifics of treatment as outlined by Turk and Holzman[26] include:

- Reconceptualize the cause of the patient's symptom so that it is consistent with the rationale underlying the treatment.
- Foster a sense of optimism.
- Individualize the treatment to match the needs of each patient.
- Emphasize active patient participation and responsibility to the extent possible.
- Provide skills acquisition.

Central to the cognitive-behavioral approach is the collaborative therapeutic relationship. Failure of this relationship will doom any psychological intervention, no matter how potent. The therapist is an ally who is primarily the disseminator of options and a facilitator of the treatment process. Treatment is designed to assist patients to relinquish the passive, helpless victim role and to accept an active, self-management role whenever possible, given their physical status.

Therapists should anticipate that patients hold sensory views of their symptom. Without challenging or expanding on this view, it may be futile to encourage the use of certain techniques (e.g., relaxation). A brief explanation of the multidimensional nature of pain and other symptoms will usually satisfy most patient's questions and provide a rationale for the involvement of the therapist. Some patients may feel as if they are "crazy" (i.e., it's all in their head) for complaining about the symptom, especially if medication has failed to eradicate the problem. Patients may thus be exquisitely sensitive to the suggestion that they meet with a mental health professional (MHP).

Although they may not ask, many patients will wonder why such a referral was made. When suggesting the possibility of involvement with an MHP, the health care provider might say something like the following: "I know you are suffering quite a bit with your [adverse symptom], despite your doctor's best efforts at controlling it. I wanted to make you aware of some additional forms of symptom management, with which you may be less familiar. These techniques have been found to be helpful with many patients, and we expect that they will be helpful with you, too."

Psychological interventions should be described as short term, skills oriented and focused on the present. In our experience, terminally ill patients are usually not only receptive to involvement with an MHP but often very appreciative of the opportunity to talk with someone about whatever problems they might be having.

COGNITIVE-BEHAVIORAL THERAPY IN PALLIATIVE-CARE PATIENTS

Stage 1: Assessment

The assessment and reconceptualization phases of cognitive-behavioral treatment are interdependent. The assessment phase serves several distinct functions, namely:

- To provide a baseline against which the progress and success of treatment can be compared

- To provide the therapist with detailed information about the nature of the patient's medical condition, previous treatments, perceptions of his or her medical condition, expectations about treatment, resources, competencies, difficulties in coping with the symptom, and view of various aspects of his or her life (e.g., family relationships)
- To assist in the establishment of appropriate treatment goals
- To foster the reconceptualization process by assisting patients and significant others in becoming aware of the situational variability and psychosocial factors that influence the nature and degree of adverse symptom(s)
- To examine the important role of significant others in the maintenance of maladaptive behaviors and as resources in the change process

For patients with advanced disease, the assessment process may need to be abbreviated, depending on the unique circumstances of the patient. For example, asking the patient to imagine the last time that he or she experienced moderate to severe intensity of the symptom and to recall the thoughts and feelings experienced at that time will likely reveal how cognitive and affective factors contribute to their perception of the symptom. The patient is then encouraged to use negative cognitions and feelings as cues to instigate more adaptive strategies. For example, patients who report thoughts that they are overwhelmed by their symptoms and have no control over them are encouraged to become aware of the times they engage in such thinking and to appreciate how such thoughts may exacerbate their overall level of distress and become self-fulfilling prophecies. Alternative thoughts such as realistic appraisal of the situation can instead be taught.

Stage 2: Reconceptualization

A central goal of cognitive-behavioral treatment is to facilitate the emergence of a new conceptualization of the symptom(s). Reconceptualization permits problems to be translated into difficulties that can be pinpointed and viewed as circumscribed and addressable, rather than as vague, overwhelming experiences. The reconceptualization process is also designed to help the patient become more receptive to psychological approaches to symptom management.

People are constantly thinking, evaluating, and appraising information and their situation. It has been suggested that the thoughts that people have can greatly influence their mood, their behavior, and some of their physiological processes. Conversely, people's mood, behaviors, and physiological activity can influence their thoughts. Thus, it is important for patients with advanced disease to become aware of the thoughts and feelings that are associated with their symptoms. *Cognitive restructuring* is a method that encourages people to identify and change stress-inducing thoughts and feelings that are associated with the noxious sensations they experience.

It is hard for some patients to accept that their thoughts and emotions can affect their bodies. In these instances, it is useful to have the patient self-monitor the thoughts and feelings that precede, accompany, and follow symptom exacerbation. When patients monitor their thoughts, a number of beliefs that might lead to increased muscle tension and increased emotional distress are frequently identified. For example, patients may find that they have some of the following thoughts:

I feel as if I can't take it any more.

I can't do anything when my pain is bad.

It is terrible to feel so helpless. I feel useless.

These types of thoughts are maladaptive in that they can increase the individual's perceptions of symptoms through increased autonomic arousal and prevent efforts to cope with the situation.

Once specific associations of thoughts, emotions, and symptoms are identified, the patient can consider alternative thoughts and strategies that might be used in similar circumstances. He or she can try substituting these alternative thoughts and observe the effects.

Helping patients to alter maladaptive thoughts requires a delicate blend of empathy and reason. It is helpful to convey that their thoughts are quite understandable and that most other patients in similar circumstances have them as well. It is equally important, however, to have patients examine the consequences of having these thoughts. Given their understanding of their symptom and its relationship to stress, how do they view their thoughts? Patients are usually able to see that their responses are not adaptive and have an interest in modifying them. The crucial

element in successful treatment is bringing about a shift in the patient's repertoire from habitual and automatic but ineffective responses to systematic problem solving and planning, control of affect, behavioral persistence, or disengagement when appropriate.

Treatment is a collaborative process by which the therapist carefully elicits the troublesome thoughts and concerns of patients, acknowledges their bothersome nature, and then constructs an atmosphere in which the patient can critically challenge the validity and utility of those beliefs. Rather than suggest alternate thoughts, the therapist attempts to elicit competing thoughts from the patient and then reinforces the adaptive nature of these alternatives where appropriate. Patients have well-learned and frequently rehearsed thoughts about their condition. Only after repetition and practice in cuing competent interpretations and evaluations will patients come to change their conceptualizations.

A constructive assignment might be to have patients create adaptive self-statements about their symptoms. Examples include:

Relax. Focus on your breathing.

Stay calm. Getting upset will only make me feel worse.

I have coped with the [symptom] before and I can do it again.

I am getting better at handling this [symptom].

I will not let this [symptom] get the better of me.

The [symptom] comes and goes. Hold on.

We encourage patients to write these statements down, perhaps along with other inspiring quotes or passages (e.g., the Serenity Prayer) in a notebook to use when needed. The patient's family members might read these statements out loud during difficult times, or they may be tape recorded. The therapist will also encourage patients in their efforts and suggest that they positively reinforce themselves for the effort and not necessarily for the result, as changing habitual ways of thinking can take time.

A distinct subset of patients may require cognitive restructuring prior to learning other self-management skills. These patients have historically been caretakers themselves, either formally in the type of work they have done or informally as homemakers, spouses, or children caring for an ill parent. It is not uncommon for these patients to make comments reflecting their difficulty being in the patient (i.e., dependent) role, no less in a self-management role. These are the patients who say they have spent their lives taking care of someone else and feel uncomfortable or "selfish" receiving help.

In order to self-manage adverse symptoms, patients must be motivated (usually inherent in the discomfort from the symptom) and value themselves and their needs enough that they want to do something about it. A surprising number of otherwise motivated patients are initially unresponsive to a self-management approach. We are not speaking here of patients who are greatly debilitated and simply do not have the capacity for a self-management approach. Instead, we are speaking of patients who have the physical and psychological stamina but who are uncomfortable with the approach. We have found it helpful in these cases to explore the etiology of their caretaker role and their belief that caring for their own needs is "selfish." Many patients will readily recognize that these beliefs stem from childhood roles and experiences.

For example, we had one patient who was very interested in learning nonpharmacologic approaches to her pain problem but was dismayed with herself for not practicing the relaxation on her own. We reviewed her understanding of how to practice the relaxation, and it was clear that her lack of information was not the problem. We then explored what it was like for her to engage in self-nurturing behavior, and things became clearer. She described how she had been taught as a child that her role in life was to take care of others and that she was "bad" or "selfish" to do things for herself. The patient was amazed at how such beliefs were still affecting her so many years later, especially as she very much wanted to help herself. Fortunately, this awareness led to insights about her failure to take care of herself, and she was able to make a conscious effort to change her behavior.

Regardless of the etiology, however, recognizing that an old belief is not what the patient would choose to believe at present may be the turning point toward self-care. Once patients acknowledge that they want more self-control and that self-management is central to that goal, they are often amenable to change.

Spirituality should not be overlooked as an important source of coping. In an excellent over-

view of religion and spirituality as resources for coping with cancer, Jenkins and Pargament[27] discuss the fact that most clinicians come from secular backgrounds and may dismiss religion. The authors explore the multiple reasons that clinicians might reject religion and wisely frame religion and spirituality within the context of belief systems. In this way, the therapist can then assess the patient's spiritual beliefs as varying along a continuum of adaptive (active coping with a higher power as an ally) or maladaptive (passively deferring to a higher power). It is also important that, regardless of a clinician's religious or spiritual beliefs, he or she not let personal views interfere with an assessment of the patient's spiritual needs and that the clinician make referrals to clergy where appropriate. This is an extremely important issue, as, given a limited period of time to live, most patients reflect on existential issues (see Chapter 13 in this volume). We have had a surprising number of patients who view their religious and spiritual beliefs as separate from their distressing symptom and have not yet made the connection that spirituality can be an important source of solace for them. It certainly behooves the clinician to raise these issues for discussion and exploration.

In sum, cognitive restructuring is a technique designed to make patients aware of the role cognitions and emotions play in potentiating and maintaining stress. The process involves eliciting the patient's thoughts, feelings, and interpretations of events, gathering evidence for or against such interpretations, identifying habitual self-statements and images that occur, and testing the validity of these interpretations. The therapist helps the patient identify automatic thoughts that may set up an escalating stream of negative, catastrophizing ideation and learn how such habitual thoughts may exacerbate stress and interfere with performance of adaptive coping responses.

Stage 3: Skills Acquisition

The skills acquisition phase begins once the basic goals of treatment have been established. During this phase, the therapist provides education, guidance, and practice in the use of a range of specific cognitive coping skills. Coping can occur prior to a stressful event (i.e., anticipatory coping) or in response to a direct stress. In cancer, some teaching about coping has to be reactive, rather than anticipatory. In other instances, such as the patient who anticipates nausea at meal time or painful dressing changes, anticipatory coping is appropriate. Anticipatory coping concerns the way individuals engage in the regulation of emotional reactions, planning, choosing, tolerating, and avoiding maladaptive thoughts.

Relaxation Techniques

It is helpful to begin relaxation exercises early in treatment because they can be readily learned by almost all patients, and most view them as credible techniques. There are a range of relaxation strategies that can be used, and there is little evidence to recommend one method over another. More important is the message to the patient that relaxation is a skill that can be learned and that there are a wide range of techniques available. The therapist can help the patient find one or more techniques that are most helpful for that particular individual.

Instruction in the use of relaxation is designed to teach an incompatible response and to help patients develop a set of coping skills that can be employed in any situation in which adaptive coping is required. The therapist can discuss with patients how to identify bodily signs of physical tension, the stress-tension cycle, how occupying one's attention can short-circuit stress, how relaxation can reduce anxiety because it presents something they can do to exert control, how relaxation and tension are incompatible states, and how unwinding while living with chronic stress can be therapeutic. Patients are asked to practice relaxation on a regular basis and in situations where they perceive themselves as becoming tense, anxious, or distressed (e.g., when the adverse symptom occurs).

Throughout the practice of relaxation, the therapist continues to take the collaborator's role. This is very important for developing the conceptualization of relaxation as a self-management skill, thereby facilitating self-control of stress, affective distress, and, at times, physical symptoms. The therapist also should assume a role that fosters the patient's perception of success. All possible indications and reports of success by the patient should be reinforced.

All too often, we have found therapists focused more on the patient's technical proficiency than on the patient's thoughts with respect to the relaxation experience. The patient's thoughts regarding the relaxation process far outweigh the importance of technical proficiency. It does little good for patients to practice diaphragmatic breathing "correctly" while simultaneously worrying that their nausea has not subsided.

When we teach relaxation, we initially downplay the importance of technique and emphasize the importance of the patient's thoughts. Most commonly, patients are relieved to hear that they will not be expected to "perform" (i.e., have technical proficiency) when they are already feeling depressed, anxious, or fatigued.

When speaking of emphasizing thoughts regarding relaxation, we refer to patients' expectations, the tone of inner voice they take, and the process by which they learn a new skill. Common problems we encounter are patients with perfectionistic, impatient, self-critical, pessimistic, and distractible tendencies. Rather than wait for these tendencies perhaps to interfere with treatment, we take a proactive approach. One primary therapist goal is to help patients focus on thoughts that give themselves permission to relax. It is this permission that is often central in letting tensions go. We might say something like the following:

> In our experience, the way that a patient talks to him- or herself about the relaxation experience is sometimes even more important than the relaxation technique itself. I know that you have a lot on your mind right now, and we certainly don't want to add to your stress level by having you worry about doing the relaxation "perfectly." Instead, all I'm going to ask that you do is set aside your troubles for the 15-minute period during which time we'll practice the relaxation.

It's funny, but the way we're wired means that we can't just simply tell our bodies to relax and have them fully cooperate! Instead, we almost have to "trick" our bodies into relaxing. In other words, if we relax our mind, then the rest of our body typically relaxes, too. For example, if you take a very critical or demanding tone with yourself, even if it is with the instruction to relax, your mind is not going to relax, because no one likes to be criticized. Instead, if you take a tone that is supportive and encouraging, like you might take toward a young child learning a new skill, your body will, in all likelihood, respond in a relaxed manner.

We also emphasize that patients have learned other skills (e.g., driving a car, acquiring proficiency with a hobby) through patience, persistence, and faith in their ability to learn. We remind patients that we know of no reason why they cannot be successful with the relaxation as well.

For highly self-critical, impatient patients, we often use the analogy of teaching a young child how to ride a bicycle. By asking patients how they could best help that child learn to ride the bike, we encourage them to see how impatience and criticism would inhibit the child's learning. Asking patients what kind of comments they might make that would be encouraging to the child typically results in supportive, patient, encouraging comments that are exactly the kinds of statements they can make to themselves. In other words, thoughts that interfere with a patient's ability to benefit from relaxation are typically amenable to cognitive restructuring.

Controlled Breathing   Deep breathing is probably the most versatile of all the relaxation techniques. It is the simplest to learn, can be used in almost any situation, is palatable to most patients, can be helpful for controlling all aversive symptoms, and is helpful even with patients with some cognitive limitations. As simple as the technique may be, it can be one of the most effective methods for patients to release tension and focus on nonsymptom somatic functioning. Deep breathing can be used in conjunction with other techniques, either as a prelude or conjointly.

Certainly, for patients with breathing difficulties this technique may be contraindicated. Depending on the patient's level of cognitive functioning, breathing techniques may be either quite simple or extremely complex. Table 15.1 contains a sample of a controlled-breathing exercise.

Progressive Muscle Relaxation   Progressive muscle relaxation (PMR) is useful because it has face validity, it is a concrete procedure and thus easy to recall and practice, and it is less prone than passive relaxation techniques to failure because of distraction by symptoms or cognitive intrusions. Slight symptomatic exacerbations that often accompany muscle tensing clearly demonstrate to the patient the role of muscle activity in symptom perception and possibly exacerbation. If muscle tension results in increased symptoms, it can be reasoned that the converse, muscle relaxation, leads to symptom reduction. Also, the results of even the first relaxation training session are often inherently reinforcing because they reduce generalized arousal. Table 15.2 describes a progressive muscle relaxation exercise.

In our experience, PMR is more helpful with symptoms such as insomnia or a mood disturbance than with pain. Although we certainly find the technique helpful with many pain patients, we advise caution in using it. Given that tight muscles can aggravate pain, the tension phase of PMR runs with it the risk of increasing pain. We have tried having patients tense only nonpainful areas or gently tense all muscle groups, but we have not had good results. As a result, we tend to use this approach most with pain patients who are unusually tense and have a high need for control.

In general, we find PMR most helpful with patients who have trouble "letting go" or who need to relax by "doing" and for unusually hesitant or skeptical patients. By using such a concrete physical activity, even the most cynical of patients can usually be convinced of the technique's efficacy.

Autogenic Training   Autogenic training is a technique based on cognitive exercises that involve

---

Table 15.1   A Controlled Breathing Exercise

1. Have patient sit or lie down in a comfortable, relaxed position.
2. Instruct the patient to inhale slowly and deeply through their nose.
3. Instruct the patient to count up to five at one-second intervals and then to slowly exhale.
4. Instruct the patient to think of a single word such as "calm" or "peace" between each count to help free the mind of distracting or stressful thoughts.
5. Instruct the patient to hold his or her breath for 5 seconds and then to exhale slowly through the mouth, counting backward from 5 to 1, and to think of the chosen word. While exhaling, instruct the patient to let his or her chest and stomach muscles relax and, if the person is seated, to let the shoulders sag.)
6. Repeat this cycle at least 3 times, but continue for 3 to 5 minutes.
7. If patient reports feeling light-headed, suggest alternation of a few shallow breaths and the deep breaths.
8. After the exercise is over, ask patient about the experience and whether he or she experienced any difficulties.

Table 15.2   Sample Progressive Relaxation Exercises

You can ask the patient to perform these exercises either seated or lying down, with their eyes closed or focusing on a picture of a pleasant scene. As the patient becomes more proficient in the techniques, the exercises can be performed in different settings. The exercise may be audiotaped and a copy provided to the patient for home practice.

About 30 seconds should be devoted to each task, 10 seconds for tensing each group of muscles, 20 seconds for relaxing them. Note that the order of the exercise is not important, and some may be deleted, depending on the nature of the patient's pain. For example, you might not have headache patients tense the muscles of the scalp and neck. Repeat each exercise twice.

1. Curl the toes of your left foot toward the bottom of your foot or the floor. Hold this tense position. Feel the cramped tightness in your ankle and the sole of your foot that you have created. Pay attention to how this feels.
2. Now, relax your foot by moving your toes away from the bottom of your foot or the floor. Let your toes relax. Let the tension drain from your toes. Feel the warm comfortable sensations of relaxation that you have been able to produce. Pay attention to these feelings, and notice how they differ from the cramped tight feeling you experienced when you tensed your muscles.
3. Repeat 1 and 2.

The therapist can then proceed, using the same methods with muscles throughout the body:

- "Pull the toes of your left foot up toward your face."
- "Tense the muscles in your left thigh by pressing hard against your other leg."
- "Tighten the muscles of your buttocks by pulling them toward each other."
- "Tighten the muscles of your stomach as if you were trying to protect yourself from being punched."
- "Pull your shoulder blades toward each other."
- "Hunch your shoulders toward your ears."
- "Press the upper part of your left arm against your left side."
- "Make a tight fist with your left hand."
- "Push the back of your head hard against the floor or chair to tighten your neck muscles."
- "Clench your teeth together, push your tongue against the roof of your mouth, and smile to expose as many teeth as you can."
- "Squint your eyes tightly shut, and wrinkle your nose."
- "Raise your eyebrows as high as you can to wrinkle your forehead."

focusing on limb heaviness and warmth, breathing, and coolness in the forehead. Patients can decrease tension and fatigue and improve their blood flow by generating heaviness and warmth in their extremities. Patients are given a set of self-statements dealing with warmth, heaviness, and mental calm to say to themselves several times over. Despite its simplicity, this technique has a powerful ability to produce deep relaxation. Some autogenic suggestions are as follows:

- My left hand feels heavy.
- My left hand feels heavy and warm.
- My left hand feels loose and relaxed.
- I feel quite quiet.

- My left arm feels heavy.
- My left arm feels heavy and warm.
- My left arm feels loose and relaxed.

Autogenics can be helpful even with those patients who are distractible, since it involves simple and concrete statements that a patient could make repeatedly even when distracted. We have otherwise found the technique less helpful with patients who have cognitive limitations.

Meditation   Many of the elements of meditation are similar to those of other relaxation techniques: a quiet environment, an object (word, sound, symbol) to focus on, a passive attitude, and a comfortable position. In meditation, however, thoughts, feelings, and images drift in the mind but are not concentrated on and are allowed to pass.

We have often found that patients naturally gravitate toward this technique when given a variety from which to choose. Although in many ways it is very simple, we have found that many patients have difficulty with it. These patients tend to be self-critical, goal oriented, and with higher control needs. Many of these patients can be successfully guided through discussion of their frustration-engendering cognitions, but there remain those patients for whom the technique is not appropriate.

Attentional Training

The role of attention is a major factor in perceptual activity, and therefore it is of primary concern in efforts to change behavior. The act of attending has both a selective and an amplifying function. The therapist may note that people can focus their attention on only one thing at a time and that, although people can, to some extent, control what they attend to, at times this maybe more difficult than others. The therapist may wish to draw an analogy to television; despite the simultaneous availability of numerous channels, a viewer can attend fully to only one channel at any one time. The therapist might state: "Attention is like the TV or searchlight; we can control what we attend to and what we avoid. With instruction and practice, you can learn how to more effectively control your attention."

Guided imagery may be used in order to enhance patients' ability to use all their sensory modalities (i.e., vision, audition, olfaction, gustatory, and kinesthetic) and thereby increase their absorption of what is around them. The therapist may ask the patient to imagine such scenes as a pleasant day at the beach. Such practice can be of assistance to patients by providing them with opportunities to try out a range of different scenes so that they can learn to use all their senses and to generate a set of images that is of particular use for them. It is important that the therapist assist the patient to discover personally relevant attention diverting scenes rather than impose a specific and predetermined one.

Attempts should be made to involve patients actively in their own treatment. As with relaxation, the data on attentional training do not unequivocally support the effectiveness of any one strategy over any other.[28] What appears to be more important is the extent to which patients can become actively absorbed in any imaginary scene.

Distraction   Some research has suggested that preoccupation with one's own body can lead to increased awareness and overestimation of sensory information. Because it is possible to attend fully to only one thing at a time, taking one's mind off pain by attending to something else may lead to reduced perceptions of pain and reduce levels of stress arousal. People who have persistent pain or other aversive symptoms often try to distract themselves by reading books, watching television, engaging in hobbies, or listening to music. Using thoughts and imagination can also help people distract themselves from their bodies and symptoms.

Cognitive techniques consist of several different types of procedures, including cognitive distraction or attention diversion. Terminally ill patients are often preoccupied with their bodily symptoms. Every new sensation is seen as an indication of deterioration or a potential new problem. *Cognitive distraction techniques* are best used during episodes where the patient experiences an exacerbation of symptoms.

A great deal of research on attentional focus has been conducted on the relative efficacy of various cognitive distraction techniques. Fernandez and Turk[28] reviewed the literature on the range of different cognitive coping strategies that have been studied. They classified these into five groups: (1) those that focus on the environment rather than on the body; (2) neutral images; (3) dramatized images where the painful part is included in the image (for example, imaging that one is a spy who has been wounded but is trying to escape); (4) pleasant images; and (5) rhythmic activity (for example, singing a song). Each strategy has been shown to be effective for mild to moderate pain. Fernandez and Turk[28] concluded that no one coping strategy is consistently more effective than any other.

The therapist might ask patients to close their eyes and to focus attention on some part of their body. The therapist then notes some ambient sound such as the ventilation system and suggests that while, attending to their body, the patients were not aware of the sound of the air conditioning. The therapist may call attention to the sound of ventilation but then remind patients that they have stopped focusing on their body. The therapist also might call attention to some part of the body that the patients were not attending to, such as the gentle pressure of their watches on their wrists. The point is that there is environmental (internal and external) input that remains out of conscious attention until one focuses directly on it. The objective is to communicate to patients that people commonly employ various methods to get some degree of control over the focus of their attention.

Providing patients with education and practice in the use of many different types of strategies may be the best approach. A variety of cognitive coping images and attention-diverting tasks may be reviewed in an attempt to find those that are most appealing to individual patients.

Distraction is one technique that is particularly amenable to family involvement. Not only can the family members be helpful with describing relaxing scenes to the patient, but they may also be distracting in other ways. Playing cars, word games, or board games, even if only for brief periods of time, may be useful in breaking the symptom focus. Listening to music, singing, or reading the Bible or another book out loud for a few minutes can also be helpful. One of the authors had a patient who spent her time writing jokes. She knew that her "material" was not exactly worthy of a standup comedian, but she so enjoyed herself and thereby kept her frame of mind positive. Selective use of positive reminiscence through stories and/or looking at pictures may not only distract but also help the patient and family with their grief process.

Imagery   Imagery has a long history of successful use with patients having advanced disease for a variety of symptom complaints. Indeed, the technique looked so promising that some advocated its use as a possible method of eradicating cancer itself.[29] Although it is still used by some in this capacity, it is now used primarily for symptom relief.

Imagery techniques are limited only by the creative imagination of patient and therapist and may be used with such diverse symptoms as nausea, breathing problems, sleep difficulties, pain, appetite disturbance, and fatigue. Relief may also come in surprising packages. One of our patients

who was particularly troubled by fatigue found that by putting on music and imagining herself dancing as she loved to do for many years, she became exhilarated and felt afterward as if she had a long nap. Another patient with metastatic lung cancer had trouble accepting relaxation as a legitimate way to spend her time. Together we found another method that she deemed more acceptable. The patient had always been a "doer" and could not find sitting still relaxing. Instead, we agreed that she would take a slow walk through her apartment and imagine how she would redecorate if money were not an object. The patient found this to be a very effective distraction and was able to stay focused and calm for progressively longer periods of time. Imagery may be used to transform the adverse sensation (as with hypnosis) or for distraction purposes (as with attentional training).

We encourage patients who are alert and who have reasonably good cognitive functioning to practice on their own. For those who have lower energy levels or who are more distractible or concrete, we might do a guided imagery, using images that the patient or family member previously described as a particularly positive memory or fantasy. Taping the guided imagery or having the family member observe and learn how to relax by describing the image(s) would also be appropriate in this situation. We might introduce a guided imagery session this way:

> Guided imagery is very much like having a pleasant daydream or fantasy . . . something we are all familiar with. The only real difference between the two is that in this situation I will be helping you to improve your skills at imagining by directing you through the fantasy. Of course, you are always free to focus on whatever you choose . . . I am here only as a guide. My guiding you through this procedure is similar to your listening to a radio program; it allows you to create in your mind the action and images related to the story to which you're listening.
>
> Allowing yourself to become relaxed and highly focused on an image is a skill that can be learned by anyone. And, just like other skills, it requires active participation and practice. In many ways you already have skill in this area. What's different about today's procedure is that we're actively and consciously letting go and focusing on an image so that you have the ability to focus less on [the adverse symptom]. While you will become very relaxed, you will not fall asleep. Although your eyes

will close just as they do when you go to sleep, you will be aware of what is happening throughout the entire procedure. If at any time you choose to tune my voice out and make it like the background hum of the air conditioning, that is fine, as long as you are instead allowing yourself to focus on something pleasant or relaxing. Do you have any questions before we begin?

Hypnosis Hypnosis has been used successfully with cancer patients with different types and stages of the disease, as well as for various symptom complaints. It has been found to reduce anxiety, pain, insomnia, nausea and vomiting with chemotherapy,[30,31] alter moods,[32] produce local anesthesia for venipuncture, spinal taps, bone marrow aspirations, biopsies and injections, and develop rigidity or flaccidity of the body to allow for care of wounds during radiology.[33]

Although it is always good practice to explain to patients what types of sensations they might experience with relaxation, we have found this to be more important when using hypnosis. Perhaps because of factors such as media exposure to hypnosis for entertainment purposes (e.g., stage hypnotists), patients tend to have a number of misconceptions about the procedure. Several researchers, when examining the use of hypnosis to alleviate cancer chemotherapy side effects, have found that not all patients agree to be hypnotized.[30] Explanations for rejection typically involve misperceptions about the process of hypnosis and potential posthypnotic effects. Whereas Redd and his colleagues now refer to their hypnotic procedure as "passive relaxation training with guided imagery" and meet with greater patient acceptance, we handle the situation in a different manner. We might say the following:

> The aim of using this procedure is to enable you to become as calm and relaxed as possible. It is expected that by becoming relaxed you will find the experience of [adverse symptom] to be less unpleasant. Have you every been hypnotized?
>
> Yes . . . what was the experience like? *or* No . . . what have you heard about hypnosis? What do you expect hypnosis to be like?
>
> Hypnosis is a state of enhanced concentration that can be reached by anyone who is willing to be receptive and responsive to suggestions. Allowing yourself to be hypnotized is very much like learning any other skill. It requires active participation and practice. While some people believe that hyp-

notic "sleep" and ordinary sleep are one and the same, this is not the case. The hypnotic state is qualitatively different from both sleep and the normal waking state. Although your eyes will close, you will be aware of what is happening throughout the entire procedure. If at some point you experience unusual feelings like tingling or a floating sensation, there is no need for alarm. Nothing bad is happening. On the contrary, such different sensations seem to be signposts that your muscles are beginning to loosen and that you are responding appropriately.

> One proven characteristic of people who are hypnotized is that they tend to be more responsive to suggestion than if they were in the normal waking state. However, it is clear from research that when people are hypnotized they cannot be made to do anything that they wouldn't normally do in the waking state. You will be undergoing a normal, standard hypnotic induction procedure, and then I will make various suggestions to you that you will likely find to be pleasant. I expect that you will benefit from this experience. Most people who undergo hypnosis describe it as an enjoyable and interesting experience, and I see no reason why you should be different from them.
>
> Do you have any questions? If for any reason you want to stop the procedure, you are always free to do so. The procedure is really quite simple. All you do is listen and just let things happen.

More often than not, we find that with such explanations and reassurance patients are receptive. If a patient is not receptive, there is a wide range of other techniques worth using.

The primary purpose of the induction is to focus the patient's attention. It sets the stage for the patient to view the hypnosis as a unique time and carries a mystique that can be very useful. Although this mystique may bring misconceptions with it, as previously indicated, many patients view hypnosis as a potentially powerful technique that may fit with their conception of what is needed to treat their problem.

Before using hypnosis for symptom management, the therapist is well served by eliciting from the patient what images, in their eyes, would ease the problem. Asking questions such as "What, in your wildest imagination, might ease your nausea?" or "What color might you imagine as soothing to your discomfort?" is typically useful. Gather as many different ideas as possible from the patient, as the most meaningful soothing images will come from the patients themselves. A question like "What do you think is causing your lack of appetite?" might reveal thoughts that reflect great misconceptions about a patient's physical status and for which soothing imagery easily follows. Asking patients to describe vivid examples of when they did not suffer with the symptom is also potentially helpful.

For example, we had some success with a man who was losing weight secondary to chronic nausea and anxiety. We learned that he longingly recalled memories of having a healthy appetite, looking forward to meals and to his wife's cherry pie. On the basis of his symptoms and imagery, we agreed to work on suggestions of enjoyable anticipation of the smell and taste of cherry pie, stomach distension, and enjoyable digestion of food. We worked on developing his self-hypnosis skills, and then he regularly applied them before meals. His hypnotic suggestions went something like the following:

> Now that you are feeling calm and relaxed and peaceful, you might begin to notice some additionally enjoyable sensations. Perhaps you do not recognize these sensations at first, as if they are awakening after a long and pleasant slumber. You may begin to notice, however, that your mouth is more moist then usual. At first this may seem a little surprising to you, but you'll probably find that if you scan your body you're nevertheless continuing to feel at ease, secure, and calm. And as you notice this calm, you may find that your mouth is becoming, more moist . . . almost salivating. And you may slowly begin to recognize this familiar feeling as your mouth wanting something . . . and as you continue to feel calm and relaxed you may be able to smell a familiar smell. The aroma of crust and fruit blended together that almost reflexively intensifies your salivating. I don't know if you can recall what it would taste like . . . anticipating the sensation of hot pie on your tongue, activating your taste buds. And again almost reflexively you might begin to notice your stomach wanting to participate in the enjoyment of your favorite food. Your stomach may want to be soothed as it distends and waits to be sated. Can you anticipate the calming feeling of sitting down at your kitchen table as you have so many times before? And once you begin to taste that first bite, savoring each mouthful in an unhurried manner, letting your taste buds relish the sweet and tart and hot and flaky as you chew and enjoy . . . allowing yourself to swallow and let your stomach, which has grown large in anticipation of this delight, finally begin to be quenched . . . letting your-

self enjoy the feeling of your stomach becoming more and more comfortably full as you delight in each bite. . . .

Another strategy for symptom management with hypnosis includes changing the adverse sensation to a different one. This is most often done with pain, where a sensation of cramping, for example, might be replaced by a sensation such as tingling. The alternate sensation should not necessarily be a pleasant one, as this may be too great a leap. For example, we might say:

> You may begin to notice that your discomfort is almost imperceptibly starting to change . . . a feeling akin to a slow leak in a tire . . . the unpleasantness slightly decreasing and in its place a slow spread of icy cold numbing . . . and as you notice the icy cold numbing you may begin to experience a sense of relief as any sensation other then your initial discomfort is probably much more tolerable.

Strategies that involve maintaining a certain degree of discomfort, such as that just described, should not be used as a first line of attack in the treatment of adverse symptoms, however. First efforts should invariably involve distracting the patient from the adverse sensation if at all possible. However, should the discomfort be diagnostically useful or if it cannot be overcome with distraction, the strategy described is appropriate. The strategies available are varied, and the choice of one will depend on the patient's adverse symptom, cognitive functioning, physical status, various personality characteristics, and level of susceptibility to hypnosis.

In our experience, the most simple and likely successful scenario involves a patient with low symptom levels, no cognitive limitations, and high susceptibility to hypnosis. We also find this technique most helpful with patients who have a relatively lower need for control. Patients who can "let go" and trust their experience and their creative imagination seem to respond more favorably than patients who have a higher need for control. For these latter patients, we recommend a technique like progressive muscle relaxation, where the patient may feel more control.

The most challenging scenario is a patient with higher symptom severity, some cognitive limitations (due either to brain metastases or the obtunding effects of opiate analgesics or other medications), and poor hypnotic susceptibility. In this case, we recommend using tape recordings of inductions or teaching the patient and a family member a less demanding skill, such as deep breathing.

SUMMARY AND CONCLUSIONS

Psychological principles and variables have been found to be important in the perception of and behavioral response to adverse symptoms. However, these approaches and principles have seldom been systematically and consistently incorporated into treatments of patients with advanced disease. We have argued that this is primarily a result of some misconceptions regarding terminal diseases as unique by virtue of its organicity and association with impending death.[9] Noxious symptoms, however, as discussed throughout this chapter, involve perceptions that are subject to modulation by numerous psychological variables, prominent among which are controllability, expectancy, anxiety, appraisal

processes, perceived self-efficacy, and contingencies of reinforcement. The manipulation of such variables can help patients to reinterpret noxious sensations as less intense, to relabel physical perturbations in other terms, and to engage in coping and other well behaviors. The successful use of such techniques also adds to a sense of control over what many view as an uncontrollable disease and thus can further alleviate suffering.

Although some patients may initially be hesitant to pursue psychological intervention for fear that it suggests that their symptoms are "all in their head," it must be emphasized that all symptoms are multidimensional, with sensory, cognitive, and affective components. These components are affected by environmental contingencies, and each of these needs to be addressed by a multifaceted approach that gives broader consideration to both biomedical and psychosocial contributors. It is important to acknowledge that the association between symptoms and psychological distress in patients with advanced dis-

Table 15.3   Factors to Consider in Selecting Psychological Techniques

	Symptom Severity	Patient Control Needs	Cognitive Functioning
Progressive muscle relaxation (PMR)	+ Mild pain − Moderate to severe pain + All other symptoms	+ High control	− Poor concentration + Limited, concrete patients
Breathing exercises	+ All symptoms + All severity levels	+ Most patients	+ Most patients
Autogenics	+ Mild to moderate pain − Severe pain + All other symptoms	+ High control needs + Low control	± Limited, concrete + Low enegy
Imagery	+ Mild to moderate pain + All other symptoms	+ Low control needs ± High control needs	− Low energy, distractable ± Concrete patients
Meditation	+ Mild to moderate pain + All other symptoms	+ Low control	+ Low energy + Distractability
Hypnosis	+ Mild to moderate pain + All other symptoms	+ Low control needs ± High control needs	− Low energy − Distractability + Moderate to high hypnotizability

+ = most useful

− = least useful

ease may be one of reciprocal causality.[34] The occurrence of aversive symptoms may contribute to patients' psychological distress; conversely, the occurrence of psychological distress may amplify patients' perceptions of the symptoms. When patients report exacerbation of symptoms, the worsening symptoms often have several indistinguishable causes, including progression of the disease and an increase in the level of psychological distress. Both of these contributors need to be addressed. In the palliative-care literature, the former has been addressed repeatedly, but the latter is rarely given sufficient emphasis.

We have described a set of techniques that has been shown to have promise in alleviating symptoms. MHPs need to decide which techniques to use, depending upon the patient disease status, capabilities, and preferences. Table 15.3 summarizes some of the factors that need to be considered in selecting a specific psychological technique.

We believe that the most appropriate treatment of patients with advanced diseases is by an interdisciplinary team that includes MHPs, along with the usual range of other health-care professionals (e.g., physicians, nurses, physical therapists, social workers, and pharmacologists). MHPs can play an important role simultaneous with the use of somatic modalities, as well as assist patients in understanding the role of appraisal processes, body preoccupation, and environmental contingencies and how such factors can contribute to symptom perception and suffering. Therapists can also teach patients a range of cognitive and behavioral techniques to increase their sense of control over the symptoms they experience, if not the disease, and thereby reduce the demoralization frequently encountered in patients with advanced disease. Furthermore, MHPs may serve as consultants to other members of the palliative-care team by alerting them to the role of cognitive and behavioral factors in the report, maintenance, and exacerbation of suffering.

References

1. Breitbart W, Passik SD. Psychiatric aspects of palliative care. In: Doyle D, Hanks WEC, MacDonald N, eds, *Oxford Textbook of Palliative Medicine*. London: Oxford University Press, 1993:609–626.
2. Ferrell B, Grant M, Rhiner M, Cohen J. Pain as a metaphor for illness: Part I: Impact of cancer caregivers' pain on family. *Oncology Nursing Forum*,
3. Padilla GV, Ferrell B, Grant MM, Rhiner M. Defining the content domain of quality of life for cancer patients with pain. *Cancer Nursing*, 1990; 13:108–115.
4. Rimer BK, Kedziera P, Levy MH. The role of patient education in cancer pain control. In: Turk DC, Feldman CS, eds, *Noninvasive Approaches to Pain Management in the Terminally Ill*. New York: Haworth, 1992:171–192.
5. Turk DC, Feldman CS. Noninvasive approaches to pain control in terminal illness: the contribution of psychological variables. In: Turk DC, Feldman CS, eds, *Noninvasive Approaches to Pain Management in the Terminally Ill*. New York: Haworth, 1992:1–24.
6. Foley KM, Inturrisi CE. Analgesic drug therapy in cancer pain: principles and practice. *Medical Clinics of North America*, 1987; 71:207–232.
7. Portenoy RK. Practical aspects of pain control in the patient with cancer. *CA: A Cancer Journal for Clinicians*, 1988; 38:327–352.
8. World Health Organization. *Cancer Pain Relief*. Geneva: WHO, 1986.
9. Turk DC, Fernandez E. On the putative uniqueness of cancer pain: do psychological principles apply? *Behavior Research and Therapy*, 1990; 28:1–13.
10. Meyer TJ, Mark MM. Effects of psychosocial interventions with adult cancer patients: a meta-analysis of randomized experiments. *Health Psychology*, 1995; 14:101–108.
11. McGuire DB. Cancer pain. Pathophysiology of pain in cancer. *Cancer Nursing*, 1989; 12:310–315.
12. Melzack R, Wall PD. Pain mechanisms: a new theory. *Science*, 1965; 50:971–979.
13. Melzack R, Casey KL. Sensory, motivational and central control determinants of pain: A new conceptual model. In: Kenshalo D, ed, *The Skin Senses*. Springfield, Ill: Charles C Thomas, 1968:423–443.
14. Ahles TA, Blanchard EB, Ruckdeschel JC. The multidimensional nature of cancer-related pain. *Pain*, 1983; 17:277–288.
15. Pennebaker JW. *The Psychology of Physical Symptoms*. New York: Springer, 1982.
16. Rachman S, Levitt K, Lopatka C. Panic: the links between cognitions and bodily symptoms. *Behaviour Research and Therapy*, 1987; 25:411–423.
17. Turk DC, Rudy TE. Cognitive factors and persistent pain: a glimpse into Pandora's box. *Cognitive Therapy and Research*, 1992; 16:99–122.
18. Yang JC, Wagner JN, Clark WC. Psychological distress and mood in chronic pain and surgical patients: a sensory decision analysis. In: Bonica JJ, Lindblom U, Iggo A, eds, *Advances in Pain Research and Therapy*. New York: Raven, 1983:901–906.

19. Barber TX. Toward a theory of pain: relief of chronic pain by prefrontal leucotomy, opiates, placebos, and hypnosis. *Psychological Bulletin*, 1959; 56:430–460.

20. Spiegel D, Bloom JR. Group therapy and hypnosis reduce metastatic breast carcinoma pain. *Psychosomatic Medicine*, 1983; 45:333–339.

21. Daut RL, Cleeland CS. The prevalence and severity of pain in cancer. *Cancer*, 1913–1918.

22. Holroyd KA, Holm JE, Hursey KG, Penzien DB, Cordingley GE, Theofanous AG, Richardson, SC, Tobin DL. Recurrent vascular headache: Home-based behavioral treatment versus abortive pharmacological treatment. *Journal of Consulting and Clinical Psychology*, 1984; 56:218–223.

23. Hill HF, Saeger LC, Chapman CR. Patient controlled analgesia after bone marrow transplantation for cancer. *Postgraduate Medicine*, 1986; August, 33–40.

24. Turk DC, Meichenbaum D, Genest M. Pain and behavioral medicine: a cognitive-behavioral perspective. New York: Guilford Press, 1983.

25. Turk DC, Rudy TE. An integrated approach to pain treatment: beyond the scalpel and syringe. In: Tollison CD, ed, *Handbook of Chronic Pain Management*. Baltimore, MD: Williams & Wilkins, 1989:223–237.

26. Turk DC, Holzman AD. Commonalities among psychological approaches in the treatment of chronic pain: specifying the meta-constructs. In: Holzman AD, Turk DC, eds, *Pain Management: A Handbook of Psychological Approaches*. New York: Pergamon Press, 1986:269–275.

27. Jenkins RA, Pargament KI. Religion and spirituality as resources for coping with cancer. *Journal of Psychosocial Oncology*, 1995; 13:51–74.

28. Fernandez E, Turk DC. The utility of cognitive coping strategies for altering pain perception: a meta-analysis. *Pain*, 1989; 38:123–135.

29. Simonton OC, Matthews-Simonton SM, Creighton JL. *Getting Well Again*. New York: Basic Books, 1978.

30. Hendler CS, Redd WH. Fear of hypnosis: the role of labeling in patients' acceptance of behavioral interventions. *Behavior Therapy*, 1986; 17:2–13.

31. Spiegel D. The use of hypnosis in controlling cancer pain. *CA: A Cancer Journal for Clinicians*, 1985; 35:221–231.

32. Newton BW. The use of hypnosis in the treatment of cancer patients. *American Journal of Clinical Hypnosis*, 1983; 25:104–113.

33. Rosenberg SW. Hypnosis in cancer care: imagery to enhance the control of psychological "side effects" of cancer therapy. *American Journal of Clinical Hypnosis*, 1983; 25:122–127.

34. Davis M, Vasterling J, Bransfield D, Burish TG. Behavioral interventions in coping with cancer-related pain. *British Journal of Guidance and Counseling*, 1987; 15:17–28.

16

Group Psychotherapy and the Terminally Ill

David Spiegel, M.D.
Sara L. Stein, M.D.
Tamara Z. Earhart, B.A.
Susan Diamond, L.C.S.W.

The emergence of support groups in the care and treatment of the terminally ill is a twentieth-century phenomenon. Chronic and terminal illnesses were at one time associated with considerable stigmatization, which in turn reinforced social isolation and loneliness.[1] Diseases were discussed using vague euphemisms such as "female trouble" or "stomach problems," rather than the correct name (i.e., breast cancer or prostate cancer). Families and caregivers often made paternalistic assumptions that open discussion of illness and death would worsen the patient's psychological state rather than provide relief, support, and enlightenment.[2,3] Support and self-help groups were originally created to inform patients with cancer and their families about prognosis and treatment and have evolved into one of the most important sources of social support outside the family.[1]

In recent years, patients have become active participants in their own illnesses and treatments, and even in their own deaths. This disease-related consumer activism has been stimulated, in part, by the findings that quality of life, psychosocial distress, and even disease progression may be modulated by interventions such as group support.

Followers of illness-related psychosocial research find that it is often difficult to distinguish between "psychosocial adjustment" and "quality of life." These two interrelated constructs are often used synonymously, but they exist independently. Generally, quality-of-life instruments contain considerably more physical symptoms and activities of daily living measures than measures of psychological distress. In a small but illustrative study of 32 women following radical gynecological surgery, Roberts and colleagues demonstrated that psychosocial adjustment and quality of life are not synonymous.[4] The majority of patients rated quality of life as high, while simultaneously reporting significant levels of psychological distress on the Symptom Checklist-90-Revised (SCL-90-R). This finding is significant in assessing the impact of support groups. even though anxiety can be increased when a patient meets with others who are confronting similar problems, such as disease progression and death, such experiences can have stress inoculation effects, helping members to face what they fear head on, cope more actively, and reorder their life priorities. Thus, quality of life can improve even though distress is higher.

We assume that terminally ill patients suffer from a wide range of disease-related sequelae, both physical and psychological. In discussing terminal illness, we refer to the overall process of a progressive, incurable illness, rather than the remaining duration of life or level of physical vitality.

This chapter is designed to familiarize the clinician with the use of group therapies with the terminally ill. The first section is an examination of the essential components of group intervention for the terminally ill: social support, emotional expression, coping, education, and relaxation. In the second section, we review the growing body of literature that suggests that stress-reducing group interventions can improve quality of life and may even prolong survival time in the terminally ill. The third section explores the specific issues that should be addressed during group therapy and related techniques that may assist the clinician.

THE COMPONENTS OF
GROUP INTERVENTION

Support groups combine a variety of principles: social support, emotional ventilation, education, and cognitive restructuring. Some combine all of these approaches, while others emphasize 1 or 2 of them.

Social Support

Human beings are naturally social animals, and a number of large epidemiological studies have found that social isolation increases morbidity and mortality.[5,6] Social support has been estimated in terms of quality, quantity, and degree of relatedness. The well-known Alameda County Study examined social networks of thousands of people in relationship to their odds of dying. Lack of community was associated with elevated mortality from all causes.[7] In a reanalysis of the Alameda County data, Reynolds and Kaplan[8] showed that poor social support in the form of fewer social contacts was related to higher cancer incidence in women and more rapid disease progression in men. Similarly, Goodwin and colleagues[9] reported that being married strongly predicted better outcome among several thousand cancer patients. Other studies have confirmed the relationship between the presence of social support and improved survival in patients with myocardial infarction and end-stage renal disease as well.[7,10,11]

These conditions may be replicated in support groups for cancer patients. Support groups have been shown to (1) reduce feelings of isolation by providing a sense of universality among the members;[12,13] (2) decrease psychological distress symptoms in both trauma victims and cancer patients;[12,14] and (3) buffer the effects of the stressful conditions.[15]

The beneficial effects of group support for terminally ill patients can be offset by unsatisfactory or inadequate relationships within the family. These may be preexisting conflicts, or they may be brought on by the demands and side effects of serious illness. The accessibility of social support, the quality of relationships, and the ability of the patient to interact with others may be affected. For example, Strang[16] found that cancer-related pain led to decreased physical and social activity. Although patients reported feeling supported by friends and family, 85% of patients in the sample reported less self-initiated contact with friends, and 65% reported that they isolated themselves due to the intensity of their pain. Lewis and Hammond[17] found that breast cancer patients who were depressed suffered impaired marital and family relationships when the depression became chronic.

Unfortunately, a good relationship with another individual did not compensate for a difficult or inadequate relationship with one's partner.[18] A 1992 study by Ward and colleagues demonstrated a peculiar thing: For some cancer patients, increased communication about the cancer with "supportive" others led to lower self-esteem.[19] This relationship disappeared if the supportive other was appropriately sensitized to the emotional and physical needs of the cancer patient.

This raises three points. First, not all social relationships are supportive, nor are all supportive relationships consistent in the level of support provided at all times. Second, relationships may change after one member is diagnosed with cancer. Third, brief interventions within the family system can often produce large positive effects on the quality of support received. Thus, constructing new social networks for cancer patients via support groups and other means is doubly important: This intervention comes at a time when natural social support may erode and when more is needed.[20]

Psychotherapy, especially in groups, can provide a new social network with the common bond of facing similar problems.[21] Just at a time when the illness makes a person feel removed from the flow of life, when many others withdraw out of awkwardness or fear, psychotherapeutic support provides a new and important social connection. This is particularly true among dying patients, for whom illness is transformed into an admission ticket to such groups, providing a surprising intensity of caring among members right from the beginning.

Emotional Expression

Emotional expression in a supportive, empathic environment is a key component in the reduction of psychological distress in ill patients.[21–23] Depression is a common underlying cause of the desire for death and requests for physician-assisted suicide among the terminally ill, with major depression affecting as many as 60% of such patients.[25] The expression of emotion is important in reducing social isolation and improving coping. Yet it is often an aspect of patient adjustment that is overlooked or suppressed. The supportive/expressive model of group support encourages therapists to facilitate open ventilation of fears of dying and death, anxiety about the future, and sadness regarding life losses.[21] Even grieving the deaths of other members can be reassuring by helping those who are dying experience the depth of feeling others will have for them when they die. Some also feel fortunate, reappraising their situation as more fortunate than that of someone else in the group who has died of the same illness.[26] Emotional suppression and avoidance inhibit active coping and are associated with reduced intimacy among family members. Those who are able to ventilate strong feelings directly cope better with illness, perhaps through improved support.[21,27–31]

The act of disclosure as a component of expression also appears to be "good for one's health." Subjects who disclosed personal trauma in journal form as part of a study design had both fewer doctor visits and improved immune function.[32] Recent studies have begun to explore the relationship between nonexpression of strong emotion and cancer progression. Women with more advanced breast tumors at the time of diagnosis demonstrated a tendency to suppress emotion, to trivialize, and to display self-pity.[33] In a study of 2,000 women seen in a breast cancer screening clinic, the correlation between ma-

lignancy and a recent single acute life stressor was strongest in those women who were unable to express their emotions.[34]

There is much that can be done in both group and individual psychotherapies to facilitate the expression of emotion appropriate to the illness.[35] Disease-related dysphoria may be amplified by the patient's perception of isolation or alienation. The psychotherapeutic setting provides an organizing context for the individual's experience of illness or dying. This benefit can extent to social and family interactions and communications with health-care providers, as well as to management of intrusive or distressing thoughts. Many patients are able to "shelve" painful affect when there is a specified time and place reserved for exploration. Being in a group where many others express similar distress normalizes their reactions, making them less overwhelming.

Education

Some groups emphasize imparting medical and psychosocial information about a disease and its treatment. They are structured as a series of lectures, with health-care professionals discussing the nature of the illness, its course and prognosis, and the varieties of available treatments. Meetings tend to be highly structured, with a schedule similar to a class syllabus. They are usually time limited, with a series of 5 to 10 weekly or monthly meetings. Educational forums gather larger audiences and are often the first group contact for newly diagnosed persons. Psychoeducational groups combine education with psychotherapy in brief, time-limited series directed at improving coping and quality of life.[36]

Cognitive Restructuring

Many treatment approaches involve teaching cognitive techniques for managing disease-related psychological distress. These include learning to identify developing emotions, understanding sources of emotional response, and shifting from emotion-focused to problem-focused coping. These approaches help the patient take a more active stance toward the illness. Rather than feeling overwhelmed by an insoluble problem, they learn to divide problems into smaller and more manageable ones. If I don't have much time left, how do I want to spend it? What effect will further chemotherapy have on my quality of life?

Following a diagnosis of cancer, patients can invoke a variety of coping strategies, including positive reappraisal and cognitive avoidance.[37] However, denial and avoidance have their costs, including an increase in anxiety and isolation. Facing even life-threatening issues directly can help patients shift from emotion-focused to problem-focused coping.[38,39] When worked through, life-threatening problems can come to seem real but not overwhelming.[21] For example, most terminally ill patients are more afraid of the process of dying than they are of death itself. Discussion of these issues can lead to further specification of sources of anxiety: being in pain, losing control of treatment decisions, being isolated from loved ones. Identification of these specific concerns in group therapy can lead to more active strategies to cope with them, ameliorating the situation if not eliminating the problem.

Many group and individual psychotherapy programs teach specific coping skills designed to help patients reduce cancer-related symptoms such as anxiety, anticipatory nausea and vomiting, and pain. Techniques used include specific self-regulation skills such as self-hypnosis, meditation, biofeedback, and progressive muscle relaxation.[38,40–46]

PSYCHOSOCIAL INTERVENTIONS: IMPACT ON DISEASE PROGRESSION AND SURVIVAL

There is now clear evidence that various psychotherapies for cancer patients are effective in reducing anxiety and depression,[9,12,20,40,47–49] improving coping skills,[22,50] and reducing symptoms such as pain and nausea and vomiting.[43,51,52]

There is provocative evidence that psychotherapy may affect not only adjustment to medical illness but survival time as well. Three of six published studies have demonstrated that both the psychosocial and the physical sequelae of progressing malignant disease can be modulated by psychosocial interventions. The three studies that demonstrated improvement in both disease progression and overall survival all had strikingly similar interventions. In these studies, patients were provided with social support, an arena for emotional expression, and direction in facing and coping with life-threatening illness.

Spiegel and colleagues randomly assigned 86 women with metastatic breast cancer, all receiving standard medical care, to conditions of either treatment (weekly group therapy) or control (nonintervention).[24] The intervention technique, supportive-expressive group psychotherapy, consisted of a weekly support group designed to encourage expression of strong emotion, deal with fears of death and dying, intensify mutual support, improve relationships and doctor-patient communication, and manage pain through self-hypnosis. Women assigned to the intervention group showed reduced mood disturbance and pain over the initial intervention year and lived an average of 18 months longer than those in the control group. By 48 months after the study had begun, all of the control patients had died, whereas one-third of the intervention subjects was still alive.

Richardson and colleagues randomly assigned lymphoma and leukemia patients to one of two conditions: (1) an active intervention consisting of home visiting by a professional trained to deliver both education and empathic support or (2) a control group that received routine care.[53,54] Not surprisingly, the intervention group demonstrated significant improvement in adherence to medical treatment. However, independent of that effect, the intervention group had significantly longer survival time. This suggests that an enriching patient-caregiver relationship that included support, coping, and empathy extended the educational benefits. Neither the duration of intervention nor the method of delivery (individual versus group) appears to negatively influence the beneficial effect on both psychological outcome and prolonged survival.

Fawzy and colleagues[22] randomly assigned 80 malignant melanoma patients either to routine care or to 6 weeks in intensive group psychotherapy that included expressive and supportive components, cognitive restructuring, and education. They found that at the 6-month follow-up, the intervention patients had significantly better alpha-interferon-augmented natural-killer-cell activity.[23] This effect was not evident at the 1-year follow-up. However, at the 6-year follow-up, the intervention group had fewer recurrences and significantly fewer deaths.[55] In this study, intervention status correlated with medical outcome, while baseline natural-killer-cell activity predicted rates of recurrence. This raises the question whether the timing of intervention (i.e., the time from diagnosis or treatment) may influence outcome years later.

Three published studies of psychosocial intervention in cancer patients demonstrated no survival benefit in the intervention groups.[56–58] In an early study by Linn and colleagues,[56] terminally ill patients (primarily with lung and gastrointestinal cancers) were randomized to counseling that focused on quality-of-life issues. Despite an improvement in quality of life, there was no difference in either functional status or survival between the 2 groups: Most of the patients died within a year. One possible explanation is that psychosocial intervention cannot alter cancer progression in the setting of overwhelming tumor burden.

In the two other studies, however, the psychological intervention was problematic. Gellert and colleagues followed up on the Exceptional Cancer Patient Program developed by Dr. Bernie Siegel by matching participants with breast cancer in the Exceptional Cancer Patient Program to others receiving routine care at 10-year follow-up.[57,59] There was no difference observed in subsequent survival time. In the three previously cited studies with survival advantage,[22,24,53] the expressive components of the interventions consisted of open patient expression of "negative thoughts" (such as fear of dying, anger, hopelessness). In the Gellert study, the intervention, which centers around the use of "positive" thoughts, places much of the "work" of fighting cancer in the patient's own internal psyche. This may potentially increase rather than relieve the individual's stress response by making the patient feel responsible for the occurrence or progression of her cancer.

The third study without survival advantage was a randomized trial in which breast cancer patients received a poorly defined assortment of group therapies led by a mixture of trained and untrained therapists.[58] The patients received no psychological benefit; thus, it is not surprising that there was also no survival advantage. These results suggest that the skill and training of the therapists in conducting the psychotherapy also play a role in outcome.

There are currently two major randomized trials under way with metastatic breast cancer patients to examine whether longer survival time is associated with participation in supportive/expressive group therapy, one in our laboratory at Stanford,[21,60] the other in Canada.[61] Trials in Australia and Europe are also being developed.

Mechanisms for Prolonged Survival

There are four classes of possible mechanisms that may account for the relationship between social support and expressiveness and prolonged longevity as illustrated in the studies discussed in the first section. The mechanisms underlying such an effect may involve influence on daily activities such as diet, exercise, and sleep or on adherence to medical treatment, or they may involve changes in endocrine and immune function.[62] Various psychotherapeutic stress management techniques have effects on the endocrine[63,64] and immune systems.[65–67]

Diet, Sleep, and Exercise

For the patient who feels isolated, depressed, or withdrawn as a result of a terminal illness, group support may provide emotional nurturing. As a result of improved psychological well-being and active coping and improved symptom management, patients may eat better, sleep better, and exercise more than those with similar disease who feel demoralized and unsupported. While studies of dietary manipulation do not demonstrate enormous differences in the survival of all cancer patients,[68] it is certainly possible that these variables, taken as a whole, play a role in mediating the effect of psychosocial support on illness.

Medical Treatment Utilization

Another possibility is that patients who have the benefit of better support seek, adhere to, or receive more vigorous treatment.[54] They may be more assertive in getting their doctors to detect disease progression earlier and respond to it more quickly. They may comply better with administered treatments because they feel more like partners and more in control of their health care. It is also possible that they elicit more vigorous intervention from their doctors. Patients who appear vigorous and determined to live their life fully may seem more capable of sustaining continuing arduous treatment.

Psychoneuroendocrinology

It is well known that stress has complex effects on the body, ranging from elevations in heart rate and blood pressure to excess secretion of stress hormones such as cortisol and prolactin. These hormones in turn have many effects on body function, including metabolism, immune function, and the control of mood, including depression and anxiety. Depression has in fact been found to be associated with high levels of cortisol that are not easily regulated and appear to lose their reactivity.[63,69] Medical illness is in and of itself stressful. One theory holds that a cycle of stress response is set up that in turn damages the body's ability to fight the illness.

A secure social environment may reduce an individual's full neuroendocrine response to stressors such as loneliness and isolation. In order to achieve a beneficial effect, the social support must be adequate in quantity and nonconfrontational in quality and must add the elements of commonality and stability within the group. For example, squirrel monkeys subjected to an aversive conditioned stimulus had a reduced cortisol stress response when accompanied by another animal during administration of the stressor.[64] The cortisol increase disappeared entirely when 5 such "friends" surrounded the monkey.

Psychoneuroimmunology

It is now recognized that there is a complex and important relationship between the two memory systems of the body, the brain and the immune system.[67] There is a growing body of research that demonstrates the transduction of psychosocial stress and/or support into altered immune function and therefore disease vulnerability and progression.[70] The effect of psychosocial stress on immune function appears to be modulated by social support and emotional expression.[15,32,71–73] In studies of heterogeneous cancer patients, increased mood disturbance, decreased life expectancy, and decreased natural-killer-cell activity all correlated with a lack of social support.[70,74–77] These findings are corroborated by Fawzy and colleagues in their study of group intervention in pa-

tients with malignant melanoma. Improvement in mood disturbance on the Profile of Mood States in the intervention patients was related to increases in alpha-interferon-induced natural-killer-cell activity, suggesting that the psychosocial intervention positively influenced immune function.[22,23,78]

SUPPORTIVE-EXPRESSIVE GROUP PSYCHOTHERAPY FOR THE TERMINALLY ILL

Supportive/expressive group therapy for metastatic breast cancer patients has been shown to result in better mood, fewer maladaptive coping responses, fewer phobic symptoms,[12] and reduced pain.[40] This treatment model[12,24] has been compared in a randomized prospective trial to cognitive/behavioral treatment in a sample of HIV-infected patients[79] and was found to be more effective in reducing mood disturbance. Two trained facilitators emphasize seven themes in weekly 90-minute sessions.

1. *Encourage mutual support.* The first goal involved in group psychotherapy is to help patients establish a new social-support network. Most patients experience some degree of bidirectional isolation: As a result of their illness, they may feel removed from the flow of life and may also be avoided by friends and family.[38,80] In the group setting, the illness that sequesters them from one social network serves to unite them in the new one. Group members come quickly to care deeply about one another, visit one another in the hospital, make phone calls, accompany one another to physicians' offices. They are no longer helpless; they gain in self-esteem by providing concrete help to others.

2. *Detoxifying dying.* Death anxiety and depression are common among cancer patients, even those with a good prognosis.[25,81] There is understandable concern that confrontation with disease progression and death in the group might demoralize patients. In our study, 27% of the sample died during the initial year, and yet mood disturbance decreased in the treated group.[12] For many terminally ill patients, however, it is the process of dying that is threatening, rather than death itself. Direct discussion of death anxiety can help to divide the fear of death into a series of problems: loss of control over treatment deci-

sions, fear of separation from loved ones, anxiety about pain. Discussion of these concerns can lead to means of addressing if not completely resolving each of these issues. Thus, even facing death can result in positive life changes. When they can observe someone coping with the process of dying, they can identify not simply with their dying but with their adaptive abilities in coping with the fear of death.

3. *Reordering life priorities.* The acceptance of a progressive terminal illness carries with it an opportunity for reevaluating life priorities, which can be usefully discussed in groups. Exercises are conducted in which patients imagine giving up attributes they value (e.g., teacher, hiker, skier) and ponder what remains of importance to their identity.[82] Patients who are able to face their future death and reprioritize realistically may gain precious time for accomplishing life projects, communicating openly with family and friends, and setting affairs in order. Facing the threat of death can aid in making the most of life.[12] This can help patients take control of those aspects of their lives they can influence, while grieving and relinquishing those they cannot.

4. *Realign social networks.* Serious illness changes most relationships, including friends and family. They either improve or get worse. Social relationships require a great deal of energy from the individual, and troubled relationships may be particularly draining to the very ill. The group is a protected arena for examining the rewards and demands of current relationships, talking through how to improve some and dispense with others. Group members become adept at conserving information sharing, obtaining needed social support, and also insisting on privacy when desired. They learned greater empathy for the sense of helplessness that often afflicts their friends and family. They learn to identify and assign tasks to those who want to help but may not know what to do. One husband suggested using voice mail to spare his wife the constant reporting of her condition: "Press 1 if you want to know how Martha slept; press 2 if you want to know the results of her bone scan. . . . " While tongue-in-cheek, this example points out that information sharing can be burdensome, and selecting those who should know is important.

5. *Communication with physicians.* Support groups can be quite useful in facilitating better communication with physicians and other health-care providers. Patients often leave doctors' offices with more of their questions unanswered than answered. Treatment adherence can be enhanced when patients feel like partners in their care and understand and agree with treatment protocols. Groups provide mutual encouragement to get questions answered, to participate actively in treatment decisions, and to consider alternatives carefully. Among patients who have treatment alternatives, those who are involved in the decision-making process are more satisfied with the results.[83] Such groups must be careful not to interfere with medical treatment and decisions but rather to encourage clarification and the development of a cooperative relationship between doctor and patient.

6. *Enhancing family support.* Psychotherapeutic interventions can be helpful in improving communication among family members by identifying needs, increasing role flexibility, and aiding in adjustment to new medical, social, vocational, and financial realities. There is evidence that an atmosphere of open and shared problem solving in families results in reduced anxiety and depression among the terminally ill.[84] Thus, facilitating the development of open discussion of common problems is a useful therapeutic goal. The group format is especially useful for such a task; members can use the group as rehearsal for clarifying how they can best communicate their needs and wishes within the family.

Cancer afflicts families as well as patients. Group participants are encouraged to develop role flexibility within the family, a capacity to exchange roles or to develop new ones as the pressures of the illness demand. One woman, for example, who became unable to carry out her usual household chores wrote an "owner's manual" for the care of the house so that her husband could better help her and carry on after her death.

Direct and open communication with important family and friends reduces the strain that comes with maintaining secrets, increases intimacy and empathic understanding of what the ill person is going through, and increases cooperative problem solving. The natural desire to protect one another from bad news becomes impossible in the setting of progressive, terminal illness. Sharing information enhances mutual caring and coping.

For children, feeling included may be more important than actively caregiving. Younger children who are isolated or excluded from the patient's illness may believe they have contributed to the illness in some way. Providing clear explanations and allowing them to help in some way can reduce their anxiety and guilt and enable them to anticipate each step as it occurs.

Family members often suffer separately rather than together. In addition to patient therapy groups, monthly group meetings can be held for family members. In these groups, husbands, children, and parents of cancer patients may express their sadness and fear about the effects of the illness, their anxiety about managing family responsibilities, anticipated losses, and their frustration at the burdens imposed upon them. Many family members of terminally ill patients have a natural reticence to express such feelings. Some believe that taking time to examine their own pain is selfish or a sign of weakness or may unleash uncontrollable anger. By bringing family members together, group therapy can help normalize unwanted or threatening feelings. Group interventions for family members can be very helpful, teaching them to be flexible about family roles and giving family members a place to work through their own anticipatory or postloss grief. As one husband of a breast cancer patient put it, "This is a place where I come to feel better about feeling bad."

7. *Symptom control.* Physical complaints related to either disease progression or treatment are common problems among up to 90% of terminally ill patients and may markedly alter quality of life.[85] Pain afflicts more than two-thirds of advanced cancer patients and often coexists with depression and anxiety.[16,86–90] The presence of pain may cause the individual to become isolated and withdraw from social contacts.[16] Fifty-seven percent of our sample of metastatic breast cancer patients reported significant pain, which was not associated with site of metastasis.[91] The pain was associated with two factors: their mood disturbance scores and their belief that worsening pain directly reflected worsening disease. This underscores findings that cognitive and affective factors are major determinants of pain intensity.[92,93] Pain can be both exacerbated by and reinforced by depression, anxiety, and fears of worsening disease.

At the end of each of our support groups, we teach patients to use a simple self-hypnosis exercise, inducing physical relaxation and analgesia. Hypnosis is a simple form of focused concentration with a relative suspension of peripheral awareness, something like the experience of being so caught up in a good novel or a movie that one enters the imagined world.[94] Patients in pain can learn to direct their attention away from pain stimuli by focusing on pleasant sensations such as a feeling of floating, a sense of warmth or coolness or lightness or heaviness, or sensations in a nonpainful part of the body.

Limitations of Support Groups

Many of the psychotherapies that have shown promise in improving emotional adjustment and influencing survival time involve encouraging open expression of emotion and assertiveness in assuming control over the course of treatment, life decisions, and relationships.[12,22,24,80] Recent research has shown that belief that one has control over the *course* of the disease leads to better outcome, whereas belief that one had control over the *cause* of the disease leads to poorer outcome.[95]

One limitation of some support groups is their desire to maintain an optimistic atmosphere by avoiding confrontation with the risks and problems associated with many medical illnesses. In some support groups, a member who suffers progression of disease can be made to feel unwelcome, as if the member were "bad example" to the others.[96] This is doubly unfortunate: It makes the member who is not well feel excluded at a time when he or she needs extra help,[21] and it conveys to the other members an uncomfortable message—recurrence of disease is too terrible to be faced and will lead to the individual's being isolated and rejected by the group.

Other support groups emphasize having the "right mental attitude" about illness, instructing members to visualize their white blood cells killing cancer cells or convincing them that illness can be cured only when one believes that it will be cured. For example, one popular book on the relationship between mental attitude and cancer recommends that each person with cancer be asked: "Why did you need the illness?," implying that the cancer occurred or progressed to fulfill an emotional need for it.[59] While having a positive outlook and believing in one's medical treatment is helpful, it is not a cure for disease. Thus, what may seem initially to be harmless, if unsupported, optimism may have the adverse consequence of making medically ill patients, especially those with terminal illness, feel even worse by blaming them for a disease that they do not control.

CONCLUSION

Support groups are an effective means of helping the terminally ill and their families confront and work through issues related to dying and death. The very aspect that might seem most frightening about such groups, witnessing others die of the same illness, can be the most reassuring. Patients in well-run groups learn that others can resolutely face their deaths and die with dignity. They learn through firsthand experience the sense of grief that others will feel for them and understand more deeply the responsibilities they have to their loved ones up to the moment of their death. They also learn skills to help with pain and anxiety control, to better manage and participate in medical decision making, and to get the most help from their support networks. Such groups provide much-needed social support at a time when our social denial of death often leads to increased isolation of patients. Support groups can improve the quality of both living and dying.

References

1. Muzzin LJ, Anderson NJ, Figueredo AT, et al. The experience of cancer. *Social Science and Medicine,* 1994; 38:1201–1208.
2. Davis DB, Cowley SA, Ryland RK. The effects of terminal illness on patients and their carers. *Journal of Advanced Nursing,* 1996; 23:512–520.
3. Super A, Plutko LA. Danger signs: coalition points to causes and consequences of inadequate care of the dying. *Health Progress,* 1996; 77:50–54.
4. Roberts CS, Rossetti K, Cone D, et al. Psychosocial impact of gynecologic cancer: a descriptive study. *J Psychosoc Oncol,* 1992; 10:99–109.
5. House JS, Robbins C, Metzner HL. The association of social relationships and activities with mortality: prospective evidence from the Tecumseh Community Health Study. *American Journal of Epidemiology,* 1982; 116:123–140.
6. House JS, Landis KR, Umberson D. Social relationships and health. *Science,* 1988; 241:540–544.
7. Berkman LF, Syme SL. Social networks, host re-sistance, and mortality: a nine-year follow-up study of Alameda County residents. *American Journal of Epidemiology,* 1979; 109:186–204.
8. Reynolds P, Kaplan G. Social connections and risk for cancer: prospective evidence from the Alameda County Study. *Behavioral Medicine,* 1990; Fall:101–110.
9. Goodwin JS, Hunt WC, Key CR, et al. The effect of marital status on stage, treatment and survival of cancer patients. *JAMA,* 1987; 158:3125–3130.
10. McClellan WM, Stanwyck DJ, Anson CA. Social support and subsequent mortality among patients with end-stage renal disease. *Journal of the American Society of Nephrology,* 1993; 4:1028–1034.
11. Friend R, Singletary Y, Mendell NR, et al. Group participation and survival among patients with end-stage renal disease. *American Journal of Public Health,* 1986; 76:670–672.
12. Spiegel D, Bloom J, Yalom ID. Group support for patients with metastatic breast cancer. *Archives of General Psychiatry,* 1981; 38:527–533.
13. Yalom ID. *The Theory and Practice of Group Psychotherapy,* 3rd ed. New York: Basic Books, 1985.
14. Marmar CR. Brief dynamic psychotherapy of post-traumatic stress disorder. *Psychiat Ann,* 1991; 21:405–414.
15. Kiecolt-Glaser JK, Greenberg B. Social support as a moderator of the after-effects of stress in female psychiatric inpatients. *Journal of Abnormal Psychology,* 1984; 93:192–199.
16. Strang P. Emotional and social aspects of cancer pain. *Acta Oncologica,* 1992; 31:323–326.
17. Lewis FM, Hammond MA. Psychosocial adjustment of the family to breast cancer: a longitudinal analysis. *Journal of the American Medical Women's Association,* 1992; 47:194–200.
18. Pistrang N, Barker C. The partner relationship in psychological response to breast cancer. *Social Science and Medicine,* 1995; 40:789–797.
19. Ward S, Leventhal H, Easterling D, et al. Social support, self-esteem, and communication in patients receiving chemotherapy. *Journal of Psychosocial Oncology,* 1992; 9:95–116.
20. Mulder CL, van der Pompe G, Spiegel D, et al. Do psychosocial factors influence the course of breast cancer? A review of recent literature, methodological problems and future directions. *Psycho-oncology,* 1992; 1:155–167.
21. Spiegel D. Psychosocial intervention in cancer. *Journal of the National Cancer Institute,* 1993; 85:1198–1205.
22. Fawzy FI, Cousins N, Fawzy NW, et al. A structured psychiatric innovation for cancer patients: I. Changes over time and methods of coping in af-

fect of disturbance. *Archives of General Psychiatry*, 1990a; 47:720–725.

23. Fawzy F, Cousins N, Fawzy N, et al. A structured psychiatric intervention for cancer patients: II. Changes over time in immunological measures. *Archives of General Psychiatry*, 1990b; 47:729–735.

24. Spiegel D, Bloom J, Kraemer HC, et al. The beneficial effect of psychosocial treatment on survival of metastatic breast cancer patients: a randomized prospective outcome study. *Lancet*, 1989; 14:888–891.

25. Chochinov HM, Wilson KG, Enns M, Mowchun N, Lander S, Levitt M, Clinch JJ. Desire for death in the terminally ill. *American Journal of Psychiatry*, 1995; 152:1185–1192.

26. Taylor S. Adjustment to threatening events. *American Psychologist*, 1983; 38:1161–1178.

27. Derogatis LR, Morrow GR, Fetting J, Penman D, et al. The prevalence of psychiatric disorders among cancer patients. JAMA 1983; 249:751–757.

28. Greer S, Morris T, Pettingale TW. Psychological response to breast cancer: effect of outcome. *Lancet*, 1979; 2:785–787.

29. Greer S. Psychological response to cancer and survival. *Psychological Medicine*, 1991; 21:43–49.

30. Pettingale KW. Coping and cancer prognosis. *Journal of Psychosomatic Research*, 1984; 28:363–364.

31. Temoshok L, Heller BW, Sagebiel RW, et al. The relationship of psychosocial factors to prognostic indicators in cutaneous malignant melanoma. *Journal of Psychosomatic Medicine*, 1985; 29:139–154.

32. Pennebaker JW, Kiecolt-Glaser JK, Glaser R. Disclosure of traumas and immune function: health implications for psychotherapy. *Journal of Consulting and Clinical Psychology*, 1988; 56:239–245.

33. Neuhaus W, Zok C, Gohring UJ, Scharl A. A prospective study concerning psychological characteristics of patients with breast cancer. *Archives of Gynecology and Obstetrics*, 1994; 255:201–209.

34. Cooper CL, Faragher EB. Psychosocial stress and breast cancer: the inter-relationship between stress events, coping strategies and personality. *Psychological Medicine*, 1993; 23:653–662.

35. Vachon ML, Kristjanson L, Higginson I. Psychosocial issues in palliative care: the patient, the family and the process and outcome of care. *Journal of Pain and Symptom Management*, 1995; 10:142–150.

36. Cunningham AJ, Edmonds CV, Jenkins G, et al. A randomised comparison of two forms of a brief, group, psychoeducational program for cancer patients: weekly sessions versus a "weekend inten-

sive." *International Journal of Psychiatric Medicine*, 1995; 25:173–189.

37. Jarrett SR, Ramirez AJ, Richards MA, et al. Measuring Coping In Breast Cancer. *Journal of Psychosomatic Research*, 1992; 36:593–602.

38. Spiegel D. Facilitating emotional coping during treatment. *Cancer*, 1990; 66:1422–1426.

39. Holahan CJ, Moos RH. Personal and contextual determinants of coping strategies. *Journal of Personality and Social Psychology*, 1987; 52:946–955.

40. Spiegel D, Bloom JR, Gottheil E. Family environment of patients with metastatic carcinoma. *J Psychosoc Oncol*, 1983; 1:33–44.

41. Hilgard ER, Hilgard JR. *Hypnosis in the Relief of Pain*. Los Altos, CA: William Kauffman, 1975.

42. Zeltzer L, LeBaron S. Hypnosis and nonhypnotic techniques for reduction of pain and anxiety during painful procedures in children and adolescents with cancer. *Journal of Pediatrics*, 1982; 101:1032–1035.

43. Morrow GR, Morrell C. Behavioral treatment for the anticipatory nausea and vomiting induced by cancer chemotherapy. *New England Journal of Medicine*, 1982; 307:1476–1480.

44. Burish TG, Lyles JN. Effectiveness of relaxation training in reducing adverse reactions to cancer chemotherapy. *Journal of Behavioral Medicine*, 1981; 4:65–78.

45. Baider L, Uziely B, De-Nour AK. Progressive muscle relaxation and guided imagery in cancer patients. *General Hospital Journal of the American Medical Association*, 1994; 16:340–347.

46. Syrjala KL, Donaldson GW, Davis MW, et al. Relaxation and imagery and cognitive–behavioral training reduce pain during cancer treatment: a controlled clinical trial. *Pain*, 1995; 63:189–198.

47. Ferlic M, Goldman A, Kennedy BJ. Group counseling in adult patients with advanced cancer. *Cancer*, 1979; 43:760–766.

48. Gustafon J, Whitman H. Towards a balanced social environment on the oncology service. *Social Psychiatry and Psychiatric Epidemiology*, 1978; 13:147–152.

49. Wood PE, Milligan I, Christ D, et al. Group counseling for cancer patients in a community hospital. *Psychosomatics*, 1978; 19:555–561.

50. Turns DM. Psychosocial factors. In: Donegan WL, Spratt JS, eds, *Cancer of the Breast*, 3rd ed, Philadelphia: WB Saunders, 1988:728–738.

51. Forester B, Kornfeld DS, Fleiss JL. Psychotherapy during radiotherapy: effects on emotional and physical distress. *American Journal of Psychiatry*, 1985; 142:22–27.

52. Cain EN, Kohorn EI, Quinlan DM, et al. Psy-

chosocial benefits of a cancer support group. *Cancer*, 1986; 57:183–189.

53. Richardson JL, Marks G, Levine A. The influence of symptoms of disease and side effects of treatment on compliance with cancer therapy. *Journal of Clinical Oncology*, 1988; 6:1746–1752.

54. Richardson J, Shelton D, Krailo M, et al. The effect of compliance with treatment on survival among patients with hematologic malignancies. *Journal of Clinical Oncology*, 1990; 8:356–364.

55. Fawzy FI, Fawzy NW, Hyun CS, et al. Malignant melanoma: effects of an early structured psychiatric intervention, coping, and affective state on recurrence and survival six years later. *Archives of General Psychiatry*, 1993; 50:681–689.

56. Linn MW, Linn BS, Harris R. Effects of counseling for late stage cancer patients. *Cancer*, 1982; 49:1048–1055.

57. Gellert GA, Maxwell RM, Siegel BS. Survival of breast cancer patients receiving adjunctive psychosocial support therapy: A 10-year follow-up study. *Journal of Clinical Oncology*, 1993; 11:66–69.

58. Ilnyckyj A, Farber J, Cheang MC, et al. A randomized controlled trial of psychotherapeutic intervention in cancer patients. *Annals of the Royal College and Physicians and Surgeons of Canada*, 1994; 27:93–96.

59. Siegel B. *Love, Medicine and Miracles*. New York: Harper and Row, 1986:108.

60. Classen C, Koopman C, Angell K, Spiegel D. Coping styles associated with psychological adjustment to advanced breast cancer. *Health Psychology*, 1996; 15:434–437.

61. Goodwin PJ, Leszcz M, Koopmans J, et al. Randomized trial of group psychosocial support in metastatic breast cancer: the BEST (Breast-Expressive Supportive Therapy) Study. *Cancer Treatment Review*, 1996; 22:91–96.

62. Spiegel D. Mind matters: effects of group support on cancer patients. *Journal of the National Institutes of Health Research*, 1991; 3:61–63.

63. Rose RM. Overview of endocrinology of stress. In: Brown GM, ed, *Neuroendocrinology and Psychiatric Disorders*. New York: Raven Press, 1984:XXX–XXX.

64. Levine S, Coe C, Wiener SG. Psychoneuroendocrinology of stress: a psychobiological perspective. In: Brush FR, Levine S, eds, *Psychoendocrinology*. New York: Academic Press, 1989:341–377.

65. Kennedy S, Kiecolt-Glaser J, Glaser R. Immunological consequences of acute and chronic stressors: mediating role of interpersonal relationships. *British Journal of Medical Psychology*, 1988; 61:77–85.

66. Irwin M: Stress-induced immune suppression: role of the autonomic nervous system. *Annals of the New York Academy of Sciences*, 1993; 697:203–218.

67. Ader R, Felten D, Cohen N. Interactions between the brain the immune system. *Annual Review of Pharmacology and Toxicology*, 1990; 30:561–602.

68. Stones MJ, Dornan B, Kozma A. The prediction of mortality in elderly institution residents. *Journal of Gerontology*, 1989; 44:72–79.

69. Nemoroff CB, Wilderlov E, Bissette G, et al. Elevated concentrations of CSF corticotropin-releasing-factor-like immunoreactivity in depressed patients. *Science*, 1984; 226:1342–1344.

70. Levy S, Lippman M, d'Angelo T. Correlation of stress factors with sustained compression of natural killer cell activity and predictive prognosis in patients with breast cancer. *Journal of Clinical Oncology*, 1987; 5:348–353.

71. Kiecolt-Glaser JK, Fisher L, Ogrock P, et al. Marital quality, marital disruption, and immune function. *Psychosomatic Medicine*, 1987; 49:13–34.

72. Kiecolt-Glaser JK, Glaser R, Dyer C, et al. Chronic stress and immunity in family caregivers of Alzheimer's disease victims. *Psychosomatic Medicine*, 1987; 49:523–535.

73. Thomas PD, Goodwin JM, Goodwin JS. Effect of social support on stress-related changes in cholesterol level, uric acid level, and immune function in an elderly sample. *American Journal of Psychiatry*, 1985; 142:735–737.

74. Jensen AB. Psychological factors in breast cancer and their possible impact upon prognosis. *Cancer Treatment Reviews*, 1991; 18:191–210.

75. Ell K, Nishimoto R, Mediansky L, et al. Social relations, social support and survival among patients with cancer. *Journal of Psychosomatic Research*, 1992; 36:531–541.

76. Levy SM, Haynes LT, Herberman RB, et al. Mastectomy versus breast conservation surgery: mental health effects at long-term follow-up. *Health Psychology*, 1992; 11:349–354.

77. Waxler-Morrison N, Hislop TG, Mear B, et al. Effects of social relationships on survival for women with breast cancer: a prospective study. *Social Science and Medicine*, 1992; 33:177–183.

78. McNair PM, Lorr M, Drappelman L. *Profile of Mood States (POMS) Manual*. San Diego, CA: Educational and Industrial Testing Services, 1971.

79. Kelly JA, Murphy DA, Bahr GR, et al. Outcome of cognitive-behavioral and support group brief therapies for depressed, HIV-infected persons. *American Journal of Psychiatry*, 1993; 150:1679–1686.

80. Spiegel D, Yalom ID. A support group for dying patients. *International Journal of Group Psychotherapy*, 1978; 28:233–245.

81. Massie MJ, Holland JC. Depression and the cancer patient. *Journal of Clinical Psychiatry*, 1990; 51:12–17.

82. Bugenthal J. *The Search for Authenticity*. New York: Holt, Rinehart & Winston, 1965.

83. Fallowfield LJ, Hall A, Maguire GP, et al. Psychological outcomes of different treatment policies in women with early breast cancer outside a clinical trial. *British Medical Journal*, 1990; 301:575–580.

84. Spiegel D, Glafkides MC. Effects of group confrontation with death and dying. *International Journal of Group Psychotherapy*, 1983; 4:433–447.

85. De Stoutz ND, Glaus A. Supportive and palliative care of cancer patients at the Kantonsspital, St. Gallen, Switzerland. *Supportive Care in Cancer*, 1995; 3:221–226.

86. Breitbart W, Bruera E, Chochinov H, Lynch M. Neuropsychiatric syndromes and psychological symptoms in patients with advanced cancer. *Journal of Pain and Symptom Management*, 1995; 10:131–141.

87. Bonica JJ. Evolution and current status of pain programs. *Journal of Pain and Symptom Management*, 1990; 5:368–374.

88. Spiegel D, Bloom JR. Group therapy and hypnosis reduce metastatic breast carcinoma pain. *Psychosomatic Medicine*, 1983a; 45:333–339.

89. Brose WG, Spiegel D. Neuropsychiatric aspects of pain management. In: Yudofsky SC, Hales RE, eds, *American Psychiatric Press Textbook of Neuropsychiatry*. 2nd ed. Washington, DC: American Psychiatric Press, 1992:245–275.

90. Spiegel D. Cancer and depression. *British Journal of Psychiatry*, 1996; 168:109–116.

91. Speigel D, Bloom JR. Pain in metastatic breast cancer. *Cancer*, 1983b; 52:341–345.

92. Beecher HK. Relationship of significance of wound to pain experienced. *Journal of the American Medical Association*, 1956; 161:1609–1616.

93. Spiegel D. The use of hypnosis in controlling cancer pain. *Ca-A Cancer Journal for Clinicians*, 1985; 35:221–231. Reprinted in *Australian Journal of Clinical Hypnotherapy and Hypnosis*, 1986; 7:82–99.

94. Spiegel D. Hypnosis. In: Hales RE, Yudofsy SC, Talbott JA, eds, *American Psychiatric Press Textbook of Psychiatry*. Washington, DC: American Psychiatric Press, 1988:XXX–XXX.

95. Watson M, Greer S, Pruyn J, et al. Locus of control and adjustment to cancer. *Psychological Reports*, 1990; 66:39–48.

96. Daniolos PT. House calls: a support group for individuals with AIDS in a community residential setting. *International Journal of Group Psychotherapy*, 1994; 44:133–152.

PART IV
Pediatric Palliative Care

17

Psychiatric Care of the Terminally Ill Child

Margaret L. Stuber, M.D.
Brenda Bursch, Ph.D.

The dying child evokes powerful emotional responses from many caregivers. Some may feel a sense of injustice about a life so prematurely ended. Others may withdraw from the reminder of the vulnerability of their own children. Even experienced hospice workers who move from the care of adults to children may find the transition emotionally trying.

In addition to the emotional issues, however, there are a number of practical issues that differentiate the needs of a terminally ill child from those of adults. Age and developmental stage are significant variables for children, who change dramatically, physiologically and cognitively, as they mature. These variables have implications for their ability to understand what is happening, as well as for their response to medications and other interventions. Developmental concerns also change as a child grows from someone dependent on family to an adolescent who is preparing for independence. Thus, although many of the same issues arise in palliative care of children and of adults, one must always consider the age and developmental stage of the child in planning appropriate interventions.

The authors acknowledge the assistance of Edward Chen.

An additional issues to be considered is the role of the family. Although good palliative care of adults also requires consideration of the family's experience and wishes, work with the family is both essential and unavoidable when caring for children. Parents are usually functioning as the primary decision makers for young children and often are very involved in the day-to-day care. Although adolescents have more of a say in the decisions made about their care, the parents remain the legal decision makers while the adolescent is a minor. Siblings who live in the home also require consideration in many of the choices made about palliative care. Interactions with the families of terminally ill children often constitute a large part of the work of the palliative-care provider.

These basic issues of development, family concerns, and emotional impact on caregivers are major considerations in the psychiatric care of terminally ill children. In this chapter we discuss a number of practical issues raised by the developmental level of the terminally ill child or adolescent and the interaction of these issues with parental and sibling concerns. We then examine specific diagnostic and treatment approaches appropriate for palliative care of children and adolescents.

THE CHILD'S UNDERSTANDING AND CONCERNS

As Kastenbaum and Costa[1] note, until relatively recently it was believed that children did not comprehend death and that, even if they could understand, it would be harmful to them to attempt to discuss it with them. These beliefs formed the rationale for the general practice of hiding poor prognostic information from children.[2] Eventually, clinicians and researchers began investigating these beliefs and found that children appeared to sense the concern and anxiety of their doctors and parents, despite the adults' attempts to be cheerful.[3] It appeared to be the parental discomfort rather than a failure to understand that prevented seriously ill children from discussing death.[4] Spinetta[5] found that even children as young as 6 years understood the meaning and possible outcome of their leukemia.

Also contrary to the initial assumptions, open communication about death appears to be beneficial to children. Many concerns can be voiced, eliciting support, reassurance about unwarranted worries, and practical assistance with the immediate issues.[6] Such communication appears to help prevent depression[7] and reduce isolation.[3] Most clinicians now recommend open communication with children about their condition. While taking care not to force the children to deal with more than they are ready to handle, parents and caregivers are encouraged to bring up the topic rather than wait for the child to initiate questions, as was previously recommended.[8,9] Making it clear that these topics are open to discussion allows children to express their fears and to talk openly with their loved ones about their thoughts and feelings, without the constraints imposed by the supposedly protective silence. (For specifics on how to talk with children about death, see Spinetta[8] and Koocher.[9])

However, it is true that the ability to discuss death in the way that adults understand it may be limited in very young children. A child's understanding of the meaning of death normally varies significantly with the age of the child. Koocher[10,11] found that the Piagetian framework of cognitive development provides a reasonable explanation of the progression of the way a child thinks about death. Preschool-age children, in the preoperational or prelogical phase of thinking, are unlikely to see death as permanent and have a magical sense of things coming back to life. As children progress to the concrete operational thinking in their first years in school, they are more able to understand the permanence of death and begin to understand that death can be a consequence of serious injury or illness. Only in adolescence, when abstract thinking is obtained, is death understood in the ways that adults comprehend it.

The meaning of death and the child's concerns also vary significantly with age. Younger children focus on separation from parents and physical discomfort. School-age children are aware of being different from other classmates and unable to participate in the usual activities. As children reach junior-high or middle-school age, Piaget's stage of formal operational thinking, they may raise religious and philosophical concerns, which can sometimes be quite distressing or baffling to the parents and caregivers.

The loss of control is especially difficult for adolescents, who are trying to differentiate from their parents and establish an independent identity. The dependence inherent in palliative care is often extremely trying for these adolescents and difficult for their families. Allowing adolescents to make as many of their own decisions as possible (and as is appropriate to their medical status and their own wishes) while getting their input on other decisions helps them to feel more independent and less depressed.[12]

Assessment should thus include conversations with both child and parents, to ascertain both the level of understanding of the child and the types of communication that are going on between child and parent. Some education of the parent can be done at this point if parents are being unrealistically secretive or overwhelming the child with information. Such assistance generally is a relief to all parties and simplifies the task of the caregiver, as well as improving the quality of life for the child and family. Similarly, the amount of involvement of the child in decision making should be assessed and modified if it is inappropriate to the developmental level and medical status of the child.

In certain cases there may be significant disagreements as to the amount of medical intervention that is desired by the parents and by their child. With younger children, it is generally clear that, although the child has input, the decision is the parents'. However, as they approach the age of majority, the wishes of adolescent patients are typically given more weight, even when they involve choices about possibly life-sustaining treatment.[13] Palliative caregivers may wish to have psychiatric or even legal assistance under such circumstances, if the disagreements are serious.

FAMILY NEEDS IN
PALLIATIVE-CARE SITUATIONS

The response of the family to a child's terminal illness depends on a number of factors.[14] One is the meaning the illness has for the family. If the family feels guilty about the illness, this greatly complicates their responses to the terminal phase. Guilt can be the result of a realistic (or unrealistic) appraisal that earlier intervention would have resulted in less suffering or even an increased chance of survival for the child. Often the guilt stems from a belief that justice demands that such an unthinkable event happens for a reason and that the parents must have done something deserving of punishment. This interpretation is more likely if the family comes from a culture or religious background that encourages this way of understanding life events.

Prior experiences with death also influence the family's response to palliative care. Parents may be terrified that their child will suffer, as they may have seen others do in the terminal stages of illness. It is useful to inquire about other experiences early on so that misunderstandings or unwarranted assumptions can be addressed before they lead to conflict between parents and caregivers.

Secondary adversities, additional problems that complicate the situation, are common. These include the financial strain of the medical expenses and lost income if one parent must reduce hours worked or leave a paid position. Loss of enjoyed activities or even of the family home may result. There also may be significant struggles with insurance or with employers over the needs of the child, causing anxiety and stress for the parents. At times, practical assistance with these issues, such as recommending legal consultation with a parent advocate, may be indicated.

Balancing parental needs and the care of the child may at times be complicated. For example, the parents may be emotionally distraught if they are unable to interact with their child, but good pain management may cause the child to sleep for extended periods during the day. Palliative care often requires caregivers to balance sedation and pain control, but parents add an additional factor to consider in this titration.

The decision as to whether the child's final days will be spent in the home or hospital can arouse potentially conflicting needs. The child may prefer to remain in the comfortable and familiar surroundings of home, while the family may be apprehensive about managing the care themselves.[15] Some parents wish to protect their other children from the death, while others are frightened by the responsibility. Very few inpatient child hospice programs are available, and it is sometimes difficult to provide truly palliative care in a hospital setting. A good hospice home program can often allow family members to deal with their fears, while providing some time at home for the child.[16]

It is also difficult to balance the need for closeness and the need for protective withdrawal during the terminal period. Both parents and children will at times crave intimacy as they anticipate the upcoming separation, while at other times they will feel overwhelmed and need some time alone. Synchronizing these wishes is sometimes difficult and can create conflict within the family. This is also true for parents who find that their coping styles are not in synch, with one parent wishing to talk about the situation while the other prefers to concentration on the day-to-day tasks. Normalizing this type of conflict is often useful, helping parents understand that their marriage is not bad or unusual.[14] It is also useful to provide someone with whom parents may talk if they wish, such as the hospice social worker.

It has recently been recognized that learning of the life-threatening illness of yourself or your child is a traumatic event, capable of inspiring a posttraumatic stress response.[17] Symptoms typical of posttraumatic stress have been reported by survivors of life-threatening illnesses and their parents.[18,19] Parents as well as children may find that they are haunted by memories or reminded of the imminence of death by seemingly innocent objects or events, causing them distress. Others may feel numbed or blunted in response to the stress. Such responses are very normal but can lead to significant misunderstandings and conflict within the family. Facilitating communication about the types of things that stimulate anxious or painful memories can greatly aid the ability of family members to help each other during this stressful time.

Siblings often feel neglected in the midst of all the care that must be given to the sick child. Parents may expect the other children to take on responsibilities for which they are not yet ready or underestimate what the siblings are capable of comprehending. Either situation can cause difficulties and resentment. Siblings may rebel, leading to frustration from their already overburdened parents. Alternatively, siblings may attempt to accommodate, losing out on normal developmental processes, such as adolescent individuation. Palliative caregivers can assist parents to see that the siblings are usually not purposefully adding to their burden but are most often responding in developmentally normal ways to a highly stressful and demanding situation.

Preexisting family or marital conflict complicates all of these normal balancing problems.[20] Parental character pathology is especially challenging, as parents struggle with the narcissistic injuries of the loss of control or the symbolic meaning of the child, as well as the usual grief and mourning. Parents who devote their lives entirely to the dying child may lose not only the child but the rest of their family if they are emotionally unavailable for an extended time. Psychiatric intervention is usually warranted in such cases.

SPECIFIC DIAGNOSTIC AND TREATMENT APPROACHES

Although the basic psychiatric problems of terminally children and adolescents are similar to those of adults, the developmental and family considerations we have discussed result in the need for some modification of diagnostic criteria and treatment approaches. These are detailed in this section.

Anorexia

Common causes of anorexia include altered taste, pain, oral candidiasis, difficulty swallowing, chronic constipation, uninteresting food, meals not offered when the patient is hungry, unpleasant odors in the environment, nausea and vom-

iting, excessive medication, depression, metabolic problems, feelings of being full, and radiation therapy.[21,22] If eating is a topic of significant disagreement between the child and family, the anorexia may be an expression of independence or aggression by the child.

Assessment of the underlying cause of the anorexia requires inquiry into the various possible causes. General approaches to treatment include treating physical and emotional symptoms, providing a variety of the child's favorite foods as requested by the child, having small amounts of food available at all times, making meal time fun and free of tension, eliminating offensive odors, and offering foods that are an acceptable temperature. As patients approach death, they often enjoy foods that are cold, such as ice chips and ice cream,[22] and the types of food they want may change dramatically. It is sometimes necessary to coach parents regarding appropriate expectations for their child's food intake and/or ways to help their child express anger or independence in other ways. Such coaching can help reduce parents' disappointment, embarrassment, and feelings of guilt when their child does not eat. Finally, steroids may be used to stimulate the child's appetite if deemed worthwhile and when other methods have failed. If oral intake becomes too difficult, adequate hydration and nutrition may be maintained via nasogastric or intravenous methods.

Anxiety

Symptoms of anxiety among terminally ill children are not uncommon. Anxiety disorders requiring pharmacological intervention are less frequent. Many factors contribute to symptoms of anxiety in a dying child, including alarming physical symptoms, hospital environment, separation from parents, emotional response of parents, fear of death, dyspnea, and/or lack of accurate, age-appropriate, and consistent information. Extreme restlessness during the final 12 to 24 hours of life can result from unrelieved physical symptoms such as pain or hypoxia, with agitation being the only available means to communicate.[23]

Typically, the most effective treatment for symptoms of anxiety is intervention aimed at the cause of the anxiety. Such intervention can include explanation and treatment of physical symptoms, introduction of activities and personal belongings that make the environment more familiar, scheduling of predictable time to be spent with parents, ensuring continuity of medical care providers, offering support and education to the parents to aid in their coping, and providing consistent communication geared to the needs and abilities of the child. If it appears that these interventions are not sufficient or if the anxiety is acute, anxiolytics with the shortest half-lives should be prescribed. If pain is a central feature, effective pain management can also provide significant relief of anxiety if the pain medication is chosen with this dual goal in mind. For example, morphine can act as an analgesic, euphoriant, and anxiolytic.[22]

Delirium

Confusional states may be triggered by many physiological causes, including infectious processes, drug withdrawal, acute metabolic disturbances, trauma, increased intracranial pressure, CNS pathology, hypoxia, vitamin deficiencies, endocrinopathies, acute vascular incidents, toxins, medications, and heavy metals.[23,24] Additionally, children who have preexisting brain damage, who are drug addicted, who have been sleep deprived, or who have experienced sensory overload are at higher risk for a delirium. Mild delirium may be mistaken for regressive behavior in children and tends to be underrecognized.

Treatment of delirium depends on the cause of the syndrome. If a suspected etiology exists, assessment and intervention may be specifically targeted.[23] In general, the presence of familiar and soothing people who can reassure and orient the child can be very helpful. Family education regarding delirium may reduce family distress and support the family's efforts to provide the child with a soothing environment. Pharmacological intervention may be indicated, especially if the child is distressed by the delirium. Haloperidol and droperidol have been used successfully for delirium.[24] Both of these agents have negligible anticholinergic and hypotensive properties compared to the low-potency neuroleptics. When given intravenously, they also have minimal extrapyramidal side effects but must be carefully titrated. Steroids can be useful for delirium caused by increased intracranial pressure.[23] Benzodiazepines, while frequently used to manage the agitation of delirium, are contraindicated, as they

can exacerbate the confusional state by sedating or disinhibiting the child.

Depression/Suicidality

While terminally ill children may become depressed, few suffer from a major depressive disorder or require antidepressant medication. Depressive symptoms are appropriate and expected responses to progressive disease and impending death[23] and may most accurately be viewed as grieving. Considering the enormous number of losses faced by a dying child and his/her family, one would expect a significant grief response that includes periods of depression and even thoughts of suicide.

The diagnostic criteria for a depressive disorder are the same for a terminally ill child and for a healthy child. Generally, the child must present with a depressed or irritable mood or with diminished interest or pleasure in almost all activities for at least a 2-week period. Additionally, the child must have four of the following symptoms during the same time period: significant weight loss or change in appetite; insomnia or hypersomnia; psychomotor agitation or retardation; fatigue or loss of energy; feelings of worthlessness or inappropriate guilt; diminished ability to think or concentrate; or thoughts of suicide.[17] The most difficult diagnostic criterion to evaluate is that the requirement that the symptoms not be due to a general medical condition. Some argue that this criterion should be disregarded in order to avoid undertreating depressive disorders in physically ill children. Others suggest using the nonsomatic criteria to evaluate depression in the physically ill.

As with other children, assessment of suicidality includes inquiry into suicidal fantasies or actions, concepts of what the child thinks would happen if suicide were attempted/achieved, previous experiences with suicidal behaviors, circumstances at the time of the suicidal behavior, motivations for suicide, concepts and experiences of death, depression and other affect, family situations, and environmental situations.[25] Other risk factors include the child's being an adolescent, suicidal intent and plan, family history of suicide, the presence of a comorbid psychiatric disorder, intractable pain, persistent insomnia, lack of social support, inadequate coping skills, a recent improvement in depressive symptoms, and/or impulsivity. A recent study of suicide in childhood cancer patients failed to find any evidence that children are likely to commit "rational suicide," or suicide as a means to control the dying process.[26]

Treatment approaches should include opportunity and support for the patient and family to process their grief about the many losses imposed on them by the child's terminal condition.[23] Some children welcome the opportunity to discuss their thoughts and feelings about dying, death, and suicide. This is often true if the child's family is uncomfortable discussing these topics with the child. For some, the idea of suicide is an important source of control in the face of an unknown and uncontrollable illness course. Supporting the use of this coping device, while also abiding by legal and ethical mandates to protect the child, requires direct communication regarding one's obligation to protect and ongoing discussion and evaluation of suicidal ideation and plans. Social support systems should be activated as deemed helpful by the patient and family.

If a major depressive disorder appears to be present, pharmacological intervention should be considered. Current medications should be reviewed to ascertain whether pain management is optimal and whether any of the child's medications could be causing or exacerbating the depressive symptoms. Antidepressive medications have not proven to be very effective with young and latency-age children.[27,28] Special attention should be paid to the potential side effects of specific medications given the existing physical symptoms and vulnerabilities of the child. Tricyclic antidepressants can have significant cardiovascular side effects, as well as uncomfortable effects such as dry mouth or difficulties with urination. Monoamine oxidase inhibitors should generally be avoided because of their many potentially dangerous adverse interactions with foods and medications.[23] The specific serotonin reuptake inhibitors (SSRIs) appear to be the safest choices, although the data are primarily from experience with adults and may not be generalizable to children.

Fatigue

Fatigue can be a disturbing symptom as it is often the first visible sign of physical deterioration to patients and families.[23] Causes of fatigue include advanced disease, inactivity, poor nutrition, dehydration, anemia, pain, depression, insomnia, medication side effects, and radiation side effects.

Fatigue can be minimized early in the terminal phase by ensuring that the child is as active as possible and desired, nutrition and hydration are maintained, physical and emotional symptoms are well controlled, side effects are minimized, and insomnia is reduced. Physical therapy can help maintain functioning by increasing activity and reducing muscular atrophy. The use of steroids is sometimes useful to elevate mood and stimulate appetite.[23] As functioning decreases due to fatigue associated with advanced illness, assistance should be given to the patient, with attention given to maximizing the child's appropriate level of independence and control in other domains. Naps and the use of a stroller, walker, or wheelchair can help the child conserve energy for important activities.[29] Blood transfusions can be useful to temporarily increase energy level for a special event.[23] As the child approaches death, he or she may have a sudden burst of energy that can last for hours for an entire day.[29] Predicting this for the parents can be both reassuring and prevent unrealistic hope for a miracle.

Insomnia

Difficulty sleeping can be the source of much distress to both the patient and the patient's family. There are many potential causes of insomnia, including physical symptoms (particularly pain), anxiety (often subclinical), depression, reversal of the sleep pattern, bladder or bowel distention, frequent urination, night sweats, or withdrawal from barbiturates or benzodiazepines.[22,23] Environmental factors such as the position of the bed, noise, lighting, and room temperature should also be considered.

Because it is often difficult to identify the cause of insomnia, each of the possible factors requires investigation and attention. Treatment approaches include treating physical and emotional symptoms and altering potential environmental contributors to the insomnia. Subclinical anxiety may be treated simply by allowing the child to discuss his or her fears or nightmares, leaving a light on or a door open at night, or instituting another measure that was helpful to the child at a younger age. An intercom is sometimes helpful to reassure the child that the parent is within verbal contact.[29] Medication withdrawal symptoms may be addressed by resuming use of the agent, if not contraindicated. Interference with a reversal of sleep pattern (with daytime sleeping and nighttime wakefulness), is not always indicated, particularly if the patient and family can be reassured. If medication is prescribed to assist the patient with sleeping, long-acting benzodiazepines should be avoided. Some advocate the use of low doses of tricyclic antidepressants for children suffering from insomnia due to pain.[30]

Other Behavior Changes

Other common behavioral changes that may occur with terminally ill children include uncharacteristically negative, oppositional, aggressive, energetic, or emotional acting out and/or apathy and withdrawal from family and friends. As they approach death, they may talk more about death, carry on conversations with someone who has died or with God, or start picking at their bed or clothes.[29] Most of the time, these behaviors may be interpreted as the child's attempts to process what is occurring to them. Some children become very industrious, perhaps in an attempt to make the most out of their remaining time. Others withdraw from friends and family, perhaps to make the final good-byes easier. Negative, oppositional, and aggressive behavior can easily be viewed as the child's processing of anger. However, some behavior changes may be the direct result of physiologic changes in the child's body, particularly neurological changes.

Treatment of behavior changes is naturally dependent on the etiology of those changes. Physical contributions to undesirable behavior changes may be treated palliatively. Psychosocial approaches focus on helping the child emotionally process what is happening to him or her. They include providing opportunities to express feelings and fears through play, drawing, or other activity and allowing the child to talk about fears, concerns, losses, death, and beliefs. Some children benefit from completing unfinished business, such as saying goodbye, making amends, being absolved of perceived transgressions, writing letters, planning their memorial service, or deciding who gets particular belongings.[29]

Pain

Pain can be illness related, treatment/procedure related, or incidental to the illness. A thorough pain evaluation involves assessment of etiology, location, intensity, duration, and prior treatment of pain. The assessment of pain in children may be more complicated than in adults.[31] It is important to remember that children may not behave in the ways that we interpret as "pain behavior" in adults. Children are particularly good at distracting themselves with play or withdrawing into sleep when in pain. Children who lack verbal skills may be unable to express that they are in pain. Adolescents may not complain of pain because they assume their pain is being managed as well as possible, do not want to admit they have pain, and/or do not have the skills of assertion in the presence of adult strangers. Finally, children's exposure to antidrug campaigns can result in their reluctance to admit they are in pain for fear that they will become addicted to pain medication.

There are many psychosocial approaches to pain management. In general, those techniques that have been found to be soothing to the child in the past are helpful for pain reduction. This is true, in part, because of the relationship between anxiety and pain, with anxiety exacerbating perceptions of pain. Examples of techniques that are soothing to some children include increasing the child's sense of control/mastery over the experience, holding the child, encouraging the child to use distraction techniques (play, story telling, socializing), providing the child with activities and personal belongings that make the environment more familiar, arranging for predictable time to be spent with parents, providing consistent communication geared to the needs and abilities of the child, or engaging the child in physical activity. Procedural pain may be reduced by the cognitive-behavioral techniques of modeling, performing breathing or imagery/distraction exercises, and offering positive incentive and behavioral rehearsal.[32] Offering the child his or her choice of injection locations and the use of ice or another skin coolant is helpful for needle sticks.

The use of analgesics is determined by a number of factors associated with the patient's condition. In general, medication therapy should be provided along with introduction of physical and psychosocial approaches to pain reduction. Analgesic therapy should reflect the severity of the pain, with acetaminophen being used for mild pain, codeine or a nonsteroidal anti-inflammatory agent being added for moderate pain (minor surgery or trauma), and pure opioid agonists being added for acute pain. For cancer pain, postoperative pain, posttraumatic pain, and other acute pain, a stepwise approach called an analgesic ladder is recommended. This approach represents the standard of care followed by most pain teams. It is preferable to use the oral route of administration whenever possible. This may not be possible if the patient cannot take medication orally or at the dose and frequency required for pain control. Oral medication can be made to taste better if mixed with something sweet, such as honey, or when preceded by something cold, such as ice.[29] Medication for ongoing or chronic pain should be titrated for an effective dose schedule and then provided around the clock, at regular intervals, rather than on an "as needed" or PRN basis. Long-acting medications require less frequent dosing and result in better patient compliance.[30] Acute or procedural pain may require additional medication, which can be given PRN.

Preexisting Psychopathology

Typically, parents of children with preexisting psychopathology are aware of the psychopathology and effective modes of treatment. The primary things to remember for the family of a terminally ill child with preexisting psychopathology are that their emotional reserves may already be quite depleted, that the child's emotional or personality problems may become more pronounced, and that the parents may have a more difficult time with feelings of guilt about the condition of their child. Adding to the complexity is the higher likelihood that at least one parent also has preexisting psychopathology. Of course, some parents who have already had a difficult course with their child have acquired excellent coping skills, resulting in a more hardy and flexible ability to parent a terminally ill child.

Previously effective methods of the treating preexisting psychopathology should be used unless contraindicated. Previously undiagnosed psychopathology should be assessed and treated, if possible. The potential added impact of a comorbid psychiatric diagnosis on the child's illness course should be considered when responding to problems and making plans for the child and family. For example, a family with such a child may require more frequent respite, the child may require a more structured environment, or the medical team may need to alter its manner of communicating to better meet the needs of the child or family.

CAREGIVER ISSUES IN PEDIATRIC PALLIATIVE CARE

Even for the most experienced caregivers, caring for a terminally ill child can be very stressful and emotionally challenging. Although dying children have the potential to evoke the greatest anguish in their caregivers, relatively little literature and few social structures are focused on the care of the terminally ill child.[32,33] Perhaps two of the most difficult caregiver issues are how to make the transition from curative to palliative care of the child and how to deal with the occurrence of a terminal or life-threatening iatrogenic illness after another life-threatening medical condition has seemingly been treated successfully.

Making the Transition to Palliative Care

Anselm Strauss[34] describes seven critical junctures in the dying trajectory. These junctures are the patient is defined as dying, staff and family make preparations for the death, there seems to be nothing more to do to prevent death, the final descent, the last hours, the death watch, and death. Often, one of the most difficult junctures occurs when there seems to be nothing more to do to prevent death. There are several reasons why this juncture is particularly difficult. First, there is often much disagreement about whether or not the child is at this juncture. In general, the more caregivers the child has, the less agreement there is about this juncture. Second, even if there is agreement that there is nothing more to do to prevent death, it is extraordinarily difficult to do nothing, especially if the patient is a child. Strauss[34] suggests that when critical junctures occur unexpectedly, staff and family members are unprepared. Clearly, the realization that a *child* will die and that there is nothing more to be done about it is not the typical dying trajectory in developed countries. Added to the difficulty posed by this unexpected trajectory is the philosophy of traditional medicine, which is very action oriented, with the primary goal to save lives.

As the hospice movement has demonstrated, there is actually much to be done to optimize one's quality of life during the terminal phase of life. If staff and family can successfully focus on quality rather than length of life, feelings of helplessness can be somewhat attenuated. In fact, for some families, this period may be perceived as a relief because they and their child can stop "fighting" the dying process and focus on life. It is important, however, that the family's perception of which juncture their child is at be taken seriously by treating staff who may have differing opinions on the matter. For example, even if the staff believes nothing more can be done, family members will be unable to shift to palliative care and quality-of-life interventions if they do not share the staff's view. Some families need to "go down fighting" in order to feel that they have been good parents. Although it is important for families to be given accurate information about their child's condition and support as they cope with the information, active attempts to move families away from their desire for curative treatment can result in significantly strained provider-family relations and is not recommended.

Facing Life-threatening Iatrogenic Illness

Not often discussed, but becoming more of a salient issue, is the occurrence of a terminal or life-threatening iatrogenic illness following treatment of another life-threatening medical condition. It is devastating for parents to learn that their child has a life-threatening illness. Abstractly, however, most parents are aware that such illnesses occur and that there is a remote possibility that it could happen to their child. It is not usually seriously considered, or even known by most parents, that a second life-threatening illness may occur as a result of treatment. Nevertheless, the increasingly intensive treatments that have proven so successful in prolonging life for many pediatric illnesses can have serious long-term toxicity, much to the distress of both staff and families. Examples include secondary malignancies after intensive treatment for pediatric cancer and lymphomas that occur in response to the chronic immunosuppression needed by organ transplant recipients.

As questions are being raised regarding quality of life for children who go through life-saving or life-prolonging treatment protocols, the impact of life-threatening iatrogenic illness on the child and family must be examined. Both family and staff are likely to question prior decisions to treat the child and experience significant grief responses. It is also likely that these families and staff will be more vulnerable to effects of stress, given the number of losses, prolonged course, and unexpected nature of the child's trajectory.

References

1. Kastenbaum R, Costa PT. Psychological perspectives on death. *Annual Review of Psychology,* 1977; 28:225.
2. Evans AE. If a child must die. *New England Journal of Medicine,* 1968; 278:138.
3. Vernick J, Karon M. Who's afraid of death on a leukemia ward? *American Diseases of Children,* 1965; 109:393.
4. Kubler-Ross E. *On Death and Dying.* New York: Macmillan Publishing Co., Inc., 1969.
5. Spinetta JJ. Anxiety in the dying child. *Pediatrics,* 1973; 52:841.
6. Share L. Family communication in the crisis of a child's fatal illness: a literature review and analysis. *Omega,* 1972; 3:187.
7. Kellerman J, Rigler D, Siegal SE. Psychological effects of isolation in protected environments. *American Journal of Psychiatry,* 1977; 134:563.
8. Spinetta JJ. Disease-related communication: how to tell. In: Kellerman J, ed, *Psychological Aspects of Childhood Cancer.* Springfield, Ill: Charles C Thomas, 1980:190–224.
9. Koocher GP. Talking with children about death. *American Journal of Orthopsychiatry,* 1974; 44:404.
10. Koocher GP. Childhood, death, and cognitive development. *Developmental Psychology,* 1973; 9:369.
11. Koocher, GP, O'Malley JE. *The Damocles Syndrome: Psychosocial Consequences of Surviving Childhood Cancer.* New York: McGraw-Hill, 1981.
12. King NM, Cross AW. Children as decision makers: guidelines for pediatricians. *Journal of Pediatrics,* 1989; 115(1):10–16.
13. Leikin S. A proposal concerning decisions to forgo life-sustaining treatment for young people. *Journal of Pediatrics,* 1989; 115(1):17–22.
14. Koocher GP, MacDonald BL. Preventive intervention and family coping with a child's life-threatening or terminal illness. In: Akamatsu TJ, Parris Stephens MA, Hobfoll SE, Crowther JH,

eds, *Family Health Psychology. Series in Applied Psychology: Social Issues and Questions*. Washington, DC: Hemisphere Publishing Corp., 1992:67–86.

15. Brown P, Davies B, Martens N. Families in supportive care: II. Palliative care at home: a viable care setting. *Journal of Palliative Care*, 1990; 6(2): 8–16.

16. Armstrong-Dailey A, Goltzer SZ. *Hospice Care for Children*. New York: Oxford University Press, 1993.

17. American Psychiatric Association. *Diagnostic and Statistical Manual of Mental Disorders*. 4th ed. Washington, DC: American Psychiatric Association, 1994.

18. Stuber ML, Christakis D, Houskamp BM, Kazak AE. Post trauma symptoms in childhood leukemia survivors and their parents. *Psychosomatics*, 1996; 37:254–261.

19. Kazak AE, Barakat LP, Meeske K, Christakis D, Meadows AT, Casey R, Penati B, Stuber ML. Post traumatic stress symptoms, family functioning, and social support in survivors of childhood leukemia and their mothers and fathers. *Journal of Consulting and Clinical Psychology*, 1997; 65(1):120–129.

20. Davies B, Reimer JC, Martens N. Family functioning and its implications for palliative care. *Journal of Palliative Care*, 1994; 10(1):29–36.

21. DeWys W. Management of cancer cachexia. *Seminars in Oncology*, 1985;12(4):452–460.

22. Doyle D. Palliative symptom control. In: Doyle D, ed, *Palliative Care: The Management of Far-Advanced Illness*. Philadelphia: The Charles Press, 1984:95–116.

23. Levy MH, Catalano RB. Control of common physical symptoms other than pain in patients with terminal disease. *Seminars in Oncology*, 1985;12(4): 411–430.

24. Driscoll CE. Symptom control in terminal illness. *Primary Care*, 1987; 14(2):353–363.

25. Pfeffer CR. *The Suicidal Child*. New York: Guilford Press, 1986.

26. Kunin HM, Patenaude AF, Grier HE. Suicide risk in pediatric cancer patients: an exploratory study. *Psycho-oncology*, 1995; 4:149–155.

27. Kaplan CA, Hussain S. Use of drugs in child and adolescent psychiatry. *British Journal of Psychiatry*, 1995; 166(3):291–298.

28. Ryan ND. Pharmacological treatment of child and adolescent depression. *Encephale*, 1993; 19(2):67–70.

29. Gyulay J. Home care for the dying child. *Issues in Comprehensive Pediatric Nursing*, 1989; 12:33–69.

30. Shannon M, Berde CB. Pharmacologic management of pain in children and adolescents. *Pediatric Clinics of North America*, 1989; 36(4):855–871.

31. Amenta MO, Sumner L. Terminally ill children in hospice care. *Home Healthcare Nurse*, 1994; 12(4):66–67.

32. Jay SM, Elliot CH, Katz E, Siegal SE. Cognitive–behavioral and pharmacologic interventions for children's distress during painful medical procedures. *Journal of Consulting and Clinical Psychology*, 1987; 55(6):860–865.

33. Davies B, Eng B. Factors influencing nursing care of children who are terminally ill: a selective review. *Pediatric Nursing*, 1993; 19(1):9–14.

34. Strauss A. Dying trajectories, the organization of work and expectations of dying. In: Dickenson D, Johnson M, eds, *Death, Dying and Bereavement*. Newbury Park, Calif: Sage Publications, 1993: 122–145.

18

Psychotherapy with the Dying Child

Barbara M. Sourkes, Ph.D.

I was brought up to believe that life is a gift. God gives life as a gift with no strings attached. It should be a given, just to live. Then if you want to work to be different things, you work for that. But you shouldn't have to struggle just to live.

—adolescent

THERAPIST: Are you in any pain? Does anything hurt?

CHILD: My heart.

THERAPIST: Your heart?

CHILD: My heart is broken. . . . I miss everybody.

—Sourkes[1(p153)]

The distillation of anticipatory grief to its essence marks the imminence of death. At times imperceptibly, at other times dramatically, the child who has been living with a life-threatening illness is transformed into a dying child. He or she faces the ultimate leavetaking, the departure from all that is familiar and loved. A child or adolescent who is dying throws an assumed sequence out of order. In the normal course of events, there is the expectation of a period of role reversal when children will care for their dying parents. When parents instead find themselves watching their child face death, an overwhelming sense of tragedy prevails. Not only is time shortened, but its order is shattered. The dying child represents a premature separation to the family. Even before the child has become a differentiated individual through a natural developmental sequence, that child is wrenched away. There is little preparation for separation by death when a psychological separation has not yet been effected. The adolescent, who is just beginning to negotiate an independent existence, is often the hardest to face when that "moving forward" is disrupted and then halted. A child has not even had the chance to form life goals.[2(p27)]

Throughout the terminal phase, the child is often aware of the diminishing, or nonexistent, options that he or she faces. A 6-year-old child provided the following explanation for the death of another patient: "The doctors ran out of medicine, and when they ran out of medicine, they lost control of his disease." Although this child may have understood the loss of options in a concrete way (as if there were no bottles of medicine left

Much of this chapter is adapted from Armfuls of Time: The Psychological Experience of the Child with a Life-threatening Illness, by Barbara M. Sourkes, © 1995, by permission of the University of Pittsburgh Press.

on the shelf), he nonetheless captures a nightmarish experience. It is at this time that the child may ask anxiously: "What if this medicine doesn't work? What will you give me next?" The child experiences a profound sense of loss of control.

> An 11-year-old boy explained to the therapist: "One side of my head says: 'Think optimistic.' The other side says: 'What if this treatment doesn't work?' "

Decisions during the terminal phase are difficult, since there can no longer be any promise of prolonged time. The parents do not want their child to suffer more, yet they often cannot tolerate the thought of ending treatment, of "leaving any stone unturned." The physician's and the team's roles shift from leadership in recommending a treatment plan, to the clarification of remaining options and consequences. The choice between experimental treatment and cessation of treatment usually revolves around the child's quality of life and the family's comfort with the idea of terminating treatment. In most instances, the parents make the decision; however, to varying degrees, the child may be involved in such discussions.

> An 11-year-old girl was offered the option of radiation therapy for pain control. She confided to the therapist: "I'm scared because I'm not so good at making decisions. My parents want me to have radiation, but a little voice in me tells me not to. . . . My mother always said that if I die, she wants me to die happy and at home. If I had radiation, I'd have to come into the hospital every day. And I don't know if radiation will really help, or if I would die anyway."

A 7-year-old girl told her parents that she was too tired to fight anymore and that she wanted to give up. She added: "If I have to continue suffering, I would rather be in heaven." She repeated her words calmly in a session with a therapist. These statements were major determinants in the parents' choosing a palliative-care plan without any further treatment for her.

A 17-year-old boy cried: "Why don't you just tell me I'm dying—or tell me I'm living. . . . I have to have more treatment, or I'll die for sure, and I want to go to medical school."

The parents need information about how the child is likely to die and, in some instances, support in coming to a decision about a home or hospital death. Effective symptom control is a critical concern. The parents may be frightened at the prospect of the child dying at home and choose the security of the hospital, or, with sufficient preparation, they may want to keep him or her at home. The child may also express a preference in general terms about where he or she feels safe or likes to be, even if not referring explicitly to death. All these factors must be taken into consideration. Whatever the setting, the parents' presence and contribution to the child's care and comfort are crucial.

REVIEW OF THE LITERATURE

Discussion of psychotherapy with the dying child is still somewhat uncharted territory in the literature. There is a body of literature that identifies the clinical issues faced by the child with cancer and the family, providing a foundation for understanding the universalities of the entire illness experience. Coping strategies for particular milestones and stressors are delineated. However, in general, psychotherapy is not considered as a context for the child's adaptation.[3–11] Other authors focus more on psychological/psychiatric issues in the child with implications for psychotherapeutic or consultative intervention. To varying degrees, the vicissitudes of the therapeutic process with this population are addressed.[12–19] A few authors focus specifically on the psychotherapy of the child facing death.[20–22]

PSYCHOTHERAPY—A CONCEPTUAL FRAMEWORK

THERAPIST: Do you remember what we talked about last time?

CHILD: (without hesitation) About dying. . . . (A few minutes later) If I don't feel like talking about dying today, there will be other days.

Psychotherapy for the child or adolescent who is dying can provide the opportunity for the expression of profound grief and for the integration of all that he or she has lived, albeit in an abbreviated lifespan. Furthermore, even for a young child, considerations about remaining quality of life may be discussed. In working with a child facing death, the therapist must be able to enter the threat with the child, accompanying him or her down the road toward ultimate separation. The shared "knowledge" of the fine line that separates living from dying, whether implicit or explicit, becomes the containment of the psychotherapy.[23] The child can derive profound comfort from the safety and "ongoingness" afforded within the framework of the therapy. (For a detailed discussion of the psychotherapeutic framework and techniques, see Sourkes[1,2]).

> The therapist had seen a hospitalized 15-year-old girl for a session just prior to her receiving heavy sedation. When the therapist returned the next day, the girl said: "I've been asleep for a full day. I feel as if you were just here a few minutes ago, although I know it was really yesterday. It's as if you never left!"

A comment by Lindemann (in Coles[24(p101)]) referring to the polio epidemic of the 1950s, attests to the role of the therapist for the child facing death:

> These are young people who suddenly have become quite a bit older; they are facing possible death, or serious limitation of their lives; and they will naturally stop and think about life, rather than just live it from day to day. A lot of what they say will be reflective—and you might respond in kind. It would be a mistake, I think, to emphasize unduly a psychiatric point of view. If there is serious psychopathology, you will respond to it, of course; but if those children want to cry with you, and be disappointed with you, and wonder with you where their God is, then you can be there for them . . .

Lindemann thus reminds the therapist to "bear witness" to the child's extraordinary situation and to respond within the context of that reality.

With a psychodynamic conceptualization as the overarching framework, the concept of psychic trauma lends itself to understanding the experience of life-threatening illness in childhood. Terr[25] offers the following definition: " 'Psychic trauma' occurs when a sudden, unexpected, overwhelmingly intense emotional blow or a series of blows assaults the person from outside. Traumatic events are external, but they quickly become incorporated into the mind. A person probably will not become fully traumatized unless he or she feels utterly helpless during the event or events (p. 8)." This description certainly relates to the indelible imprint of the sustained assault on the body and psyche, and the overwhelming loss of control that the dying child has experienced throughout the course of the illness.

Winnicott (in Davis and Woodbridge)[26(p44)] defined trauma as "an impingement from the environment and from the individual's reaction to the environment that occurs prior to the individual's development of mechanisms that make the unpredictable predictable." While life-threatening illness does not literally originate in the environment, its devastating impact on the child more than qualifies it as trauma. In fact, the illness goes beyond what Winnicott referred to as "unthinkable anxieties" in its *actual* threat of death.[26(p44)] Winnicott further stressed the importance for the young child of the "presentation of the world in small doses . . . the preservation of a certain amount of illusion—an avoidance of too sudden insistence on the reality principle."[26(p108)] Certainly the experience of the dying child defies this recommendation: He or she stands unshielded from the terror of the ultimate reality principle—the recognition that life must end.

In child psychotherapy, play is the crucial vehicle of communication. Winnicott[27(p47)] differentiated between "to *play* at (thus coping with) rather than to *be in* the frightening fantasy." While the dying child is confronting reality rather than fantasy (or, reality in addition to fantasy), Winnicott's distinction highlights a definitive function of play. He further stressed that enjoyment of the play is an a priori condition of entering into the depth of the psychotherapeutic process. For the child whose very existence is suffused with gravity, such pleasure is intrinsically valuable.

The overwhelming nature of the illness cannot be approached by reality alone. Paradoxically, the illusion afforded by play is what allows reality to be integrated. Through play, the child can advance and retreat, draw near and pull away from the intense core. These tentative forays allow the child to contain and master the experience. Illusion is not to be construed as avoidance; on the contrary, play is the essence of a child's expression. Furthermore, illusion is translucent, if not transparent, and thus reality shines through for both the child and the therapist even when not addressed directly by either.

Inextricably linked with play is the child's use of symbolic language and images. The words themselves (not simply the thematic content) often reveal images that are idiosyncratic to a particular child, and consistent over time. They provide windows into his or her experience.

> During the previous night, a 6-year-old boy's temperature and blood pressure had dropped precipitously. Although he was revived quickly, he had been blue, hard to rouse, and very cold. In a session the next day, the child reported that: "Poly Polar Bear [his "therapeutic stuffed animal"[1]] is very sad now because he didn't swim. The water was ice." Through this image, the child reiterated his own traumatic experience of being "cold." From then on, he always associated images of cold with death. For example, in a story about an alligator, he recounted: "The alligator died. The ice came. The ice ages came."

AWARENESS OF IMPENDING DEATH

During the terminal phase, the child's awareness of dying becomes more focused. No longer an abstract threat in the distance, death takes on an identity of its own. Rather than being a possible outcome, death is *the* outcome, its time of occurrence the only unknown. References to its proximity can be quite direct and explicit. If an open climate has been established from the beginning of the illness, it will be reflected in how the child talks about death.

> An 11-year-old girl commented matter-of-factly: "Some of my friends have died. I wish I could talk to those kids' parents to see what their symptoms were, so that I would know what is happening to me."

The awareness may also be expressed symbolically, although no less powerfully, through words, play, and art (examples of children's drawings may be found in Sourkes[1]).

> A 13-year-old girl with widespread disease recounted to the therapist: "I know how to read palms, and I read my own. I'll be famous. I'll be married once. I see a break in my life when I'm about 17. I wonder what that is. . . . "

> A 3-year-old boy played the same game with a stuffed duck and a toy ambulance each time he was hospitalized. The duck would be sick and need to go to the hospital by ambulance. The boy would move the ambulance, making siren noises.

> THERAPIST: How is the duck?
>
> CHILD: Sick.
>
> THERAPIST: Where is he going?
>
> CHILD: To the hospital.
>
> THERAPIST: What are they going to do?
>
> CHILD: Make him better.
>
> THERAPIST: Is he going to get better?
>
> CHILD: Yes, better.

> During what turned out to be the boy's terminal admission, he played the same game with the duck. However, the ritual changed dramatically in its outcome:

> THERAPIST: How is the duck?
>
> CHILD: Sick.
>
> THERAPIST: Is he going to get better?
>
> CHILD: (shook head slowly) Ducky not get better. Ducky die.

Catastrophic images often emerge in the child's language and stories during the terminal phase. Fear, desperation, and the sense of disaster are all evident, even if in derivative form.

> A 6-year-old boy recounted the following story to the therapist in the months before his death: "The TV fell off the wall and the IV pole crashed on the dinosaur and then the lights turned out and then the bed turned back to the wall. The door slammed, the walls fell, and the hospital broke down on the dinosaur."

ANTICIPATORY GRIEF

Loss of relationships, expressed through fears of separation, absence, and death, is paramount in anticipatory grief: "grief expressed in advanced when the loss is perceived as inevitable."[28] Anticipatory grief may show itself as the child's increased sensitivity to separation, without any specific reference to death; comments or questions related to death that may be seen as a type of preparation or rehearsal; and the undiluted and unmistakble grief of the terminal phase of the illness.

> THERAPIST: What does it mean to be alive?
>
> CHILD: That your family doesn't miss you. They miss you if you die. When you're alive, you don't miss people because they are right here.

I don't want to be out of the picture.

—adolescent

Themes of presence and absence, disappearance and return, may be evident in the child's play, mirroring the concerns of "not being here," the crux of anticipatory grief. The child is also testing whether his or her absence will be noticed and whether he or she will be missed.

A 6-year-old boy proposed a game to the therapist: "When I snap my fingers, I'll disappear." He would hide somewhere in the office with several small toy animals. While the child was "invisible" to the therapist, she would do a monologue wondering where he could be, progressing from innocuous to more threatening possibilities: "I wonder whether he is in school and that's why I can't find him. . . . Maybe he went down to the cafeteria. . . . Maybe he's not feeling well. . . . I wonder whether something happened to him. . . . I would be sad if something happened to him. . . . Everyone would miss him. . . . " The child would listen intently to her words, without answering. At a certain point he would throw a small animal out of his hiding place for the therapist to question about his whereabouts. Eventually, one of the animals, through the therapist's voice, would "tell" where the child was hiding. He would reappear with a bound, and the therapist would greet him with enthusiasm and relief. The child played this ritual over many sessions.

In another manifestation of anticipatory grief, the child projects concern about him or herself onto a significant adult, usually a parent or the therapist. On one level, the child recognizes his or her extreme dependence on the adult and panics at the thought of something happening to that person. This reaction may be particularly pronounced in the child of a single parent. On another level, the child is expressing fear about his or her own situation through this mirror image. At least initially, the projection is best left untouched, as the child is clearly communicating extreme vulnerability.

After a discussion about his bad dreams, the therapist asked a 6-year-old child what else he felt scared about.

CHILD: I am scared of what if my mother dies. Then there will be no one to take care of me.

THERAPIST: I know that your mother takes good care of herself and is healthy so that she can take good care of you.

CHILD: Yes. She is trying very hard to stay alive. She eats all the time and she kisses me a lot.

THERAPIST: What else are you scared about?

CHILD: I am scared that when I come back to the hospital, you will not be here.

The child's grief related to the possibility of his or her own dying may be cloaked in symbolic terms or in questions about others. As in all other communications, the therapist must stay close to the immediate concern, leaving the child in control of how far to pursue the topic. Often he or she will make an isolated statement or pose one question and then, without further comment, turn to other subjects. The most powerful disclosures are those in which the child makes reference to the possibility of his or her own dying. Whether through the weight of the sadness or through the actual words or images, the dying child's anticipatory grief is palpable, as he or she lives the intensity of separation in its ultimate form.

A 5-year-old child animatedly told the therapist: "Wally Skubeedoo Walrus's [one of his stuffed animals] birthday is November 14." The therapist asked the child the date of *his* birthday. He answered: "November 14. All my animals' birthdays are on November 14. Too bad you're not also." The therapist then asked him how old he would be on November 14. The child's affect changed markedly, and he responded very quietly: "Six. . . . " His excited anticipation collapsed into sadness when the birthday was personalized to his own growing up into the future.

An 18-year-old boy was dying in the hospital. His parents had a long history of marital problems. Normally quite taciturn, he responded explosively to the therapist's question about how he felt about his parents' conflict: "That's what's killing me—not the disease. I don't want to live if they aren't together. Some nights I cry all night."

—Sourkes[23]

The fear of being replaced looms for the child and may find expression either directly or through play. To replace makes explicit the fact that something has been lost or has ceased to exist. Thus, for the child, replacement carries with it the recognition of his or her own mortality. The fear is often manifested through an upsurge in resentment toward a younger sibling perceived as being in line to take his or her place.

Some parents, recognizing the hopelessness of their own child's situation, demonstrate an intensified interest in another patient, particularly one who is "doing well." This is a manifestation of anticipatory grief gone awry and causes inordinate suffering. In the eyes of the child, being replaced by another patient is the ultimate betrayal. Furthermore, the child feels that in "failing" the treatment, he or she has failed the parents, and thus the replacement is perceived as punishment.

As the child confronts impending death, he or she may show signs of preparation. The child's actions or words are often quite matter of fact; their significance is not necessarily elaborated.

> A 7-year-old girl had a recurrent dream: "In the dream, I want to be with my mother, and I can never quite get to her." The girl recounted the dream in a joint therapy session with her mother. Whereas the mother found the dream "excruciating," her daughter stipulated that "even though the dream is very sad, it's not a nightmare." The dream eventually provided the focal image for mother and child to work through the anticipatory grief process.

The endpoint of the terminal phase is often marked by a turning inward on the part of the child, a decathecting from the external world. Cognitive and emotional horizons narrow, as all energy is needed simply for physical survival. A generalized irritability is not uncommon. The child may talk very little and may even retreat from physical contact. Although such withdrawal is not universal, a certain degree of quietness is almost always evident. The child is pulling into him or herself, not away from others. If the parents understand this behavior as a normal and expectable precursor to death, they do not interpret it as rejection. In certain instances, the therapist can play a crucial role in turning around the child's withdrawal and thus "returning" him or her to the parents.

> A 6-year-old boy had been exceedingly withdrawn over several days. He hardly talked, except to say, "I am in such discomfort," and lay with his back to everyone. The parents and therapist talked in his room about this dramatic change from his usual outgoing behavior. The child yelled: "Get out if you are going to talk." The therapist told him that it was important that he hear the discussion, even if he didn't feel like joining in. The therapist then began a monologue: "I wonder if you are just fed up

with all this hospital stuff and treatments and that you still don't feel well. . . . I wonder if you feel kind of angry that nothing seems to be really helping you to feel much better. . . . " After making several more statements about how he might possibly feel, and how children in general feel, the therapist asked casually: "Do you think you feel a little like that?" The child said: "I guess so." The parents were startled and immediately pleased by his verbal acknowledgment. The therapist continued: "Kids sometimes feel mad . . . mad at doctors, nurses, even their psychologist, and *even* their mother and father. . . . I wonder if you feel a little like that. . . ." The child said clearly: "Yes." The therapist was then called out of the room for a few minutes. On her return, his mother reported that he had reached over and hugged her for the first time in days.

Withdrawal from the therapeutic relationship is also common. The child may not want to see the therapist or may be content simply for the therapist to stay with him or her, without much interaction. Frequently, at this point, the therapist sees the child only in the presence of the parents. Therapeutic intervention can be critical at this ultimate point. The therapist may invite the child to say or ask anything that has remained unspoken. An adolescent's statement to her parents illustrates the power of this simple and unobtrusive intervention:

> I don't want to leave you. I'm not supposed to have cancer at my age. You both took such good care of me at home. You came faster than the nurses when I called. Everyone is crying—why is everyone crying here? Something very tragic must be happening.

While such a dramatic epilogue is rarely forthcoming, the opportunity for disclosure should be made available if the child is alert. However, under no circumstances may the therapist ever attempt to force the expression of "final words".

WORK WITH PARENTS

> My parents and I are in this together.
>
> —adolescent

With the intrusion of the illness, from the moment of diagnosis, the relationship between the child and parents organizes around the pivot of potential loss. Thus, it is critical that the therapist not intercede as a divisive wedge between them. From the outset, an ongoing alliance between the child's therapist and the parents diminishes this threat and optimizes the outcome of the work. The nature of the alliance will of course differ depending upon the age of the child. Terr[25(p30)] in her work with traumatized children, comes to similar conclusions: "It is almost impossible for a . . . [therapist] to treat a child without providing some access to parents . . . who participate in the child's life." Without the respect of an established alliance, the therapeutic work with the child will be compromised and, during the terminal phase, probably rendered impossible.

During the terminal phase of the illness, the therapist must be vigilant about the danger of overinvolvement with the child. In such circumstances, the parents can begin to feel estranged and supplanted just at the time when they are desperately trying to "keep" their child. Parents' pervasive guilt about their dying child (whether conscious or unconscious) will only be exacerbated if they feel that the therapist is "better" than they are at achieving closeness with the child or at eliciting secrets that cannot be shared.

The child may become frightened by an inordinate amount of closeness to the therapist, while simultaneously needing the relationship. During this critical time, a sense of threat arises from the child's guilt at being close to an adult other than the parents. He or she may feel trapped: "having to choose" between parents and therapist, with the simultaneous fear of alienating either. However, if the child senses a strong alliance between the therapist and parents, he or she can feel secure in the therapeutic relationship.

Throughout the illness, the range and depth of work with parents can vary greatly, from a concentrated focus on child-management issues to more traditional psychotherapy of the individual or the couple. Whatever the framework, the parents' reactions to the child's illness and the impact on their marriage and family are the organizing themes. A focus on the well siblings must be an aspect of the work, including, at times, meetings between the therapist and these children. Too often, the siblings stand outside the spotlight of attention, even though they have lived through the illness experience with the same intensity as the patient and parents.[29,30] Although these parameters do not change once the child is dying, they do intensify and come into even sharper focus. The therapist can also enhance the parents' understanding of and competence with their child so that they can become associates in the therapeutic process. Any means of intervention that the therapist can provide for the parents to use with the child is an antidote for their helplessness.

The therapist can facilitate and empower the parents' interaction with medical professionals. In addition, and with the parents' consent, the therapist may share selective aspects of the therapeutic material that bear directly on the care of the child. In promoting the parents' interactions with the medical team, and through these direct communications, the therapist plays a pivotal role in the integration of the child's total care.

References

1. Sourkes B. *Armfuls of Time: The Child's Psychological Experience of Life-Threatening Illness*. Pittsburgh: University of Pittsburgh Press, 1995.
2. Sourkes B. *The Deepening Shade: Psychological Aspects of Life-Threatening Illness*. Pittsburgh: University of Pittsburgh Press, 1982.
3. Adams D, Deveau E. *Coping with Childhood Cancer*. Hamilton, Ontario, Canada: Kinbridge Publications, 1988.
4. Chesler M, Barbarin O. *Childhood Cancer and the Family*. New York: Brunner/Mazel, 1987.
5. Ettinger R, Heiney S. Cancer in adolescents and young adults. *Cancer Supplement*, 1993; 71:3276–3280.
6. Gibbons M. Psychosocial aspects of serious illness in childhood and adolescence. In: Armstrong-Dailey A, Goltzer S, eds, *Hospice Care for Children*. New York: Oxford University Press, 1993:60–74.
7. Katz E, Dolgin M, Varni J. Cancer in children and adolescents. In: Gross A, Drabman R, eds, *Handbook of Clinical Behavioral Pediatrics*. New York and London: Plenum Press, 1990:129–146.
8. Kellerman J. *Psychological Aspects of Childhood Cancer*. Springfield, Ill: Charles C. Thomas, 1980.
9. Rowland J. Developmental stage and adaptation: child and adolescent model. In: Holland J, Rowland J, eds, *Handbook of Psychooncology*. New York: Oxford University Press, 1989:519–543.
10. Spinetta J, Deasy-Spinetta P. *Living with Childhood Cancer*. St. Louis: C.V. Mosby, 1981.
11. Van Dongen-Melman J, Sanders-Woudstra J. Psychosocial aspects of childhood cancer: a review of the literature. *Journal of Child Psychology and Psychiatry*, 1986; 27:145–180.
12. Adams-Greenly M. Psychosocial interventions in childhood cancer. In: Holland J, Rowland J, eds,

Handbook of Psychooncology. New York: Oxford University Press, 1989:562–572.

13. Emanuel R, Colloms A, Mendelsohn A, Muller H, Testa R. Psychotherapy with hospitalized children with leukaemia: is it possible? *Journal of Child Psychotherapy*, 1990; 16:21–37.

14. Glazer J. Psychiatric aspects of cancer in childhood and adolescence. In: Lewis M, ed, *Child and Adolescent Psychiatry: A Comprehensive Textbook*. Baltimore: Wilkins and Wilkins, 1991:964–977.

15. Koocher G, Gudas L. Grief and loss in childhood. In: Walker C, Roberts M, eds, *Handbook of Clinical Child Psychology*. New York: John Wiley, 1992:1025–1034.

16. Lansky S, List M, Ritter-Sterr C, Hart M. Psychiatric and psychological support of the child and adolescent with cancer. In: Rizzo P, Poplack D, eds, *Principles and Practice of Pediatric Oncology* 2nd ed. Philadelphia: JB Lippincott, 1993:1127–1139.

17. Pfefferbaum B. Common psychiatric disorders in childhood cancer and their management. In: Holland J, Rowland J, eds, *Handbook of Psychooncology*. New York: Oxford University Press, 1989: 544–561.

18. Stuber M. Psychotherapy issues in Pediatric HIV and AIDS. In: Stuber M, eds, *Children and AIDS*. Washington, DC: American Psychiatric Association Press, 1992:213–223.

19. Wiener L, Fair C, Pizzo P. Care for the child with HIV infection and AIDS. In: Armstrong-Dailey A, Goltzer S, eds, *Hospice Care for Children*. New York: Oxford University Press, 1993:85–104.

20. Bertoia J. *Drawings from a Dying Child: Insights into Death from a Jungian Perspective*. London and New York: Routledge, 1993.

21. Kubler-Ross E. *On Children and Death*. New York: Macmillan, 1983.

22. Lewis M. Dying and death in childhood and adolescence. In: Lewis M, ed, *Child and Adolescent Psychiatry: A Comprehensive Textbook*. Baltimore: Wilkins and Wilkins, 1991:1051–1059.

23. Sourkes B. The child with a life-threatening illness. In: Brandell J, ed, *Countertransference in Psychotherapy with Children and Adolescents*. Northvale: Jason Aronson, 1992:267–284.

24. Lindemann E. Quoted in: R. Coles, *The Spiritual Life of Children*. Boston: Houghton-Mifflin, 1990.

25. Terr L. *Too Scared to Cry*. New York: Basic Books, 1990.

26. Davis M, Wallbridge D. *Boundary and Space: An Introduction to the Work of DW Winnicott*. New York: Brunner/Mazel, 1981.

27. Winnicott DW. *The Piggle: An Account of the Psychoanalytic Treatment of a Little Girl*. New York: International Universities Press, 1977.

28. Aldrich CK. Some dynamics of anticipatory grief. In: Schoenberg B, Carr A, Kutscher A, Peretz D, Goldberg I, eds. *Anticipatory Grief*. New York and London: Columbia University Press, 1974:3–9.

29. Sourkes B. Siblings of the pediatric cancer patient. In: Kellerman J, ed, *Psychological Aspects of Childhood Cancer*. Springfield: Charles C Thomas, 1980:47–69.

30. Sourkes B. Siblings of the child with a life-threatening illness. *Journal of Children in Contemporary Society*, 1987; 19:159–184.

PART V
Family and Staff Issues

19

Family Issues and Palliative Care

David K. Wellisch, Ph.D.

Patients with terminal cancer are profoundly influenced by their family relationships and interactions; conversely, patients are major sources of influence on the lives and interactions of their family members, especially as they become more gravely ill. This chapter is an attempt to look at some of the issues, themes, mutual influences, and potential interventions in relation to the family of the end-stage cancer patient.

This chapter focuses on one family with a member who had metastatic breast cancer and presents it as a model for many of the themes, issues, and interventions that may be relevant for families dealing with terminal cancer. Of particular importance for this chapter and for work with all such families is the consideration of the "family" as a series of subunits and not simply as a unitary entity. In practical terms, this may mean assessing the interactions, functioning, and conflicts of the marital unit, the parent-child unit(s), the sibling subsystem, the grandparent-grandchild unit, and the complex system formed by the health-care-provider team and the family. In the family to be discussed in this chapter, every one of these parts had a distinct life of its own that required understanding, consideration, time, and separate as well as overlapping interventions. To have evaluated them as a whole entity or to have intervened with them only as a whole group would have essentially missed or circumvented the emotional life of this family.

THE PATIENT

The patient in the family, Mrs. S, was 65 years old by the time she died. She had metastatic breast cancer. She died in October 1994. She had been diagnosed in 1986 with infiltrating lobular carcinoma, with 17 of 22 lymph nodes positive for tumor involvement at diagnosis. She underwent a complete mastectomy and subsequently was treated with adjuvant chemotherapy. She had a course of radiation therapy and was also placed on Tamoxifen for period of 24 months. The patient was referred to me for treatment of depression late in 1989. By that time she had bony metastases and was undergoing periodic "spot" radiation courses. Pain ranged from mild to profound, depending on the progression of her disease. Early in 1991 she was admitted to UCLA for intractable pain, as well as for severe nausea and vomiting possibly related to narcotics. She was treated with intravenous Dilaudid and with intravenous Compazine, with satisfactory results. She was soon readmitted with fevers and chills secondary to external jugular thrombophlebitis. In that hospitalization, MRI studies showed multiple skull metastases but no brain metastases. In the summer of 1991 she was then readmitted with dyspnea and found to have bronchitis. She was treated systematically during that period with a variety of agents, including 5-FU, Leucovorin, Megace, and Tamoxifen. None of these stemmed the slow progression of her disease. She was not readmitted to the hospital until early in 1993. At that time she had chronic obstructive pulmonary disease, as well as further progression of her metastatic disease. Her next hospitalization, in fall 1993, was for lethargy, fatigue, and agitation. No brain metastases were found, nor did a lumbar puncture show malignant cells. Her last hospitalization occurred late in 1993 for severe bony pain. CT scan of the pelvis at that time revealed a healed right pubic fracture and a more recent extra-articular right iliac pathologic fracture. A diffuse series of osteolytic metastases were also seen in the pelvis and proximal femurs. She was placed in a brace and once again given a course of radiation therapy. She was never readmitted to the hospital after that admission and was maintained at home for the next 11 months by licensed vocational nurses and, later (from May to October 1994), a home hospice agency. For purposes of this chapter, the period of time from the last hospital stay until her death (November 1993 to October 1994) will be the main focus. It should be understood that the preceding medical report is a summary and focuses mainly upon her hospitalizations. The main issue is that she was ill and under continuous treatment with a large variety of interventions from the time of her diagnosis until home care began. The types of interventions changed in the final 11 months, but the expense, intensity, and stress related to the interventions did not change for her or for the family. Thus, by the time palliative care formally began, Mrs. S had been treated continuously for almost 7 years. Additionally, by the time of her death, her psychotherapy with me had continued at least weekly for almost 5 years. Treatment for depression and associated stresses, including chronic anxiety, occasional panic attacks, and sleep disorder, involved extensive psychopharmacological interventions plus psychotherapy. The psychotherapy included elements of support, relaxation training, cognitive-behavioral interventions, and ultimately family therapy. The family therapy largely occurred in the last 11 months of her illness, in the homebound palliative phase.

The psychopharmacological interventions were coordinated by a psychiatric colleague who made a series of home visits to reassess Mrs. S over the last 11 months of her life at home.

THE FAMILY

The extended family unit consisted of a total of 13 people in three generations (Figure 19.1). In the process of family therapy interventions, I came to know and interact with virtually everyone in this family system except one person. These interventions/interactions were more frequent with some members and subunits than with others.

In the patient's generation were three members, plus the patient herself. One sister (sister #1), age 75, who lived in an eastern city, visited at least four times per year, was an extremely successful businessperson, and clearly was in a matriarchal/maternal role for the entire family. She inspired a mixture of respect, fear, and anxiety in the family system. A second sister (sister #2), age 70, who also lived in an eastern city, visited at least four times per year, was primarily a homemaker, and had a "softer," more relaxed presence than sister #1. Mr. S, the husband of the patient, had been married to her for 40 years. He was a highly successful sales representative who was affable but was anxious and compulsive about many aspects of his life, including work, alcohol use, and smoking. He lived a high-pressure existence and continually complained about being harassed and bedeviled by work pressures and paperwork requirements. The patient was the youngest child of the three sisters. She had been a successful businesswoman in her own right for several years. Her parents were both dead, with her mother also having died from breast cancer.

In the children's generation, there were four members. Daughter #1 had been married for about 20 years to a man who had had a steady series of business failures. During the patient's illness, Daughter #1 decided to separate and divorce her husband. As I closely evaluated her circumstances, it became clear that she had lived in gross denial and that her family's finances were a shambles. In the midst of her mother's dying process, she and her three children were forced to turn to Mr. and Mrs. S for economic survival. This necessity was understood and embraced by Mr. and

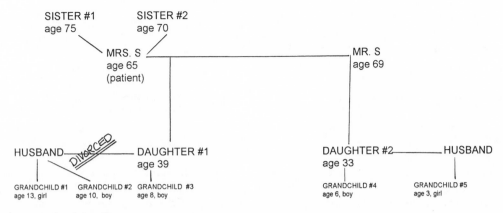

Figure 19.1 The S Family

Mrs. S, but added considerably to family stress. Daughter #1 had always had the role of "overcompetent" child, which shifted substantially during this period to "harassed" child. During this period she returned to work and vigorously pursued a sales business. The husband of Daughter #1 was the only family member that this writer never met. He was a peripheral figure during this time but one who nevertheless commanded substantial family attention and affect, mainly of a hostile, negative nature because of his inadequate and manipulative behaviors. Daughter #2 had been married about 8 years to a professional man who worked enormously hard, only to achieve modest success. It was a work pattern strikingly similar to that of Mr. S, but with less material success. Daughter #2 had a life history of separation anxiety with regard to her mother and had a role in the family as "anxious, undercompetent child." This role shifted dramatically during her mother's dying process, where this daughter's coping was far steadier and more competent than she or the family ever expected. Much to her surprise, she essentially changed roles with her sister during this period. She was not elated by this, however, as it left her without the big sister to lean on as a future maternal substitute. The husband of Daughter #2 had a warm, quiet, steady presence and was close to Mrs. S in the same reassuring fashion he was close to his wife.

There were five members in the grandchildren's generation. Daughter #1's children were faced during this period with parental separation and changes in their living environment, as well as in the dying process of their beloved grandmother. They were also faced with their mother's

being split among earning a living, parenting, trying to have a social life, and spending time with her mother. Clearly, these conflicting demands imposed almost overwhelming stress on this family unit. Grandchild #1, a teenage girl, took over many maternal functions and partially parented her brothers. Grandchild #3 had a severe reading disability, which became a major concern for the patient, Mrs. S, and for the whole family during this period.

Daughter #2's children had a steadier family course and a more stable family unit during this period. Grandchild #4, a boy, was the most sensitive, articulate, and reactive of the grandchildren. Although all were close to the patient, he was perhaps the closest. Grandchild #5 was the youngest, named after her grandmother. Conceived and born during her grandmother's illness, she was less articulate than her brother (mainly due to her age/developmental level) but highly reactive to the situation, especially to separations from her mother and her mother's attention to and preoccupation with Mrs. S.

FUNDAMENTAL FAMILY ISSUES

Three key family system interactional concepts have been presented as fundamental in the assessment of the family with a terminally ill cancer patient. These include homeostasis, bonding, and basic type of family system.[4,5]

Homeostasis reflects the relative constancy of the family internal emotional environment and the ability of the family to maintain that constancy when presented with severe and destabilizing stresses, such as the terminal illness of a member. I tend to rate families grossly as "good," "fair," or "poor" in this area. The S family was fair. It had enjoyed good family stability in the past, but by the time Mrs. S. was in her palliative phase, two factors threatened the family's usual stability besides her illness. One was Daughter #1's marital crisis, which competed for resources, time, and support with the cancer. A second was Mr. S's fatigue, burnout, and depression in relation to his job performance, which he brought into this phase. His insecurity about his earning capacity also competed for family resources, time, and support. Family homeostasis in the S. family was bolstered, however, by the strong attempts to maintain continuity and homeostatic interactional balance in continuing family situations such as Friday night dinners, socialization with friends at members' homes, and family planning and participation in important events such as Grandchild #1's Bas Mitzvah. These things were important counterbalances in this process. The maintenance of family rituals and usual interactions such as these can be very important interventions to restore family emotional/interactional homeostasis.

Bonding reflects family maintenance of its territory within the larger community space by regulation of incoming/outgoing people, objects, and ideas.[5] Here again, I rate family capacities grossly as "good," "fair," or "poor." The S family was good in this respect. For example, members quickly integrated the licensed visiting nurse (LVN) into their home and interactions. They also integrated equipment such as Mrs. S's hospital bed, her morphine pump, and her oxygen tank. They accepted, worked with, and benefited from the concept of the hospice team model. Some families feel "invaded" by such professionals and equipment and are continuously stressed by the inability to feel like a family when surrounded by such people or things. The S family was the opposite and optimized such resources.

The concept of *family system* is closely related to the concept of bonding. Kantor and Lehr have identified three styles of basic family system, labeled "opened," "closed," and "random."[5] The closed family is characterized by a strong need for fixed space, regular time, and steady interactions. The open family has relatively stable structure, yet has the flexibility of moveable space, variable time, and flexible energy. The random family has dispersed space, irregular time, and fluctuating energy as an interactional style. These are characteristic styles of functioning, and no one style is better or worse in an absolute sense than the others. The S family was a blend of open and random. It was able to move schedules, structure, and space and even to cope with variable spaces and times for interaction. For example, Mr. S was able to continue necessary business trips during Mrs. S's palliative period, with her sisters entering and leaving their home to replace his functions without conflict or crisis. The family often included members of the home-care team at the dinner table if they were present, seeing them as an enhancement rather than as an intrusion or invasion. Mr. S was able to cycle between his own and another bedroom to sleep when he was awakened by Mrs. S too many nights in a row. In this writer's experience, some families are not nearly as able to accept these modifications in their structure and routines. With less flexible families, a type of cognitive-behavioral family intervention has seemed helpful in which the family may be helped to evaluate whether a certain change is as frightening or disastrous as it seems. For example, a well spouse commonly must sleep in a separate room for respite when a partner is terminally ill. This can be perceived as "the end" of the relational intimacy, or it can be used as a stimulus to increase quality time and emotional intimacy at other times. Mr. and Mrs. S faced this fear and did learn to have structured quality time together during the evening.

I would add two other concepts to the three already mentioned for basic assessment purposes. They are mutuality and joint problem solving.

Mutuality has been defined as the flexible, adaptive pattern of relational continuity that incorporates change.[6] This involves the ability to communicate and the ability to cope with distancing, disengagement, and reengagement in a constructive fashion. Mrs. and Mrs. S were seasoned veterans at this process, having moved several times to different cities and reestablished themselves. They also had tolerated Mr. S's countless lengthy business trips, after which they constructively reengaged. This writer has seen several couples, by contrast, who lacked the communicational skills or the ability to come back from periods of distancing or disengagement. Cancer for these couples leaves them isolated and increasingly insecure with each other. A basic and important intervention for such couples is facilitation of basic communication about shared aspects of cancer so that reengagement is possible after an episode of hospitalization or after the crisis is over.

Joint problem solving involves shared engagement in tasks that create the potential for relational growth.[7] Cancer usually presents a series of couple and family problems to solve, both in technical areas (i.e., pain management) and in situational areas (i.e., redistributing family tasks such as bill paying or other chores). A basic intervention can have the family participate in such technical and/or situational areas and feel a sense of joint participation and mastery. The benefits of this participation are enhancement of feelings of relatedness and reduction of family-based anxieties over the experience of helplessness. The S family ceded areas such as pain management to the home-care staff but persisted up to the end of Mrs. S's life in working on other problems, such as Grandchild #3's reading disability. This grandchild, two weeks before Mrs. S's death, came to her home and read to her at her bedside.

In assessing a family with an end-stage cancer patient for interventional possibilities, a few basic questions are relevant.[1] These might include:

1. Who is in the family, and who constitutes the family unit? In the S family, the 13 people in Figure 19.1 constituted the unit. However, several friends were significant participants and supporters in the unit; they helped as much or more than Mrs. S's sisters. Thus, the unit was actually larger than the 13 people in Figure 19.1.

2. What is the ethnic, cultural, and religious background of the family? Cultural beliefs may characterize and influence patterns of grief and mourning as well as styles of expressing other affects. The S family was Jewish, with strong links to the network of their temple. The temple family network was highly important in providing social and emotional support during the long period of this patient's illness. I have seen other families and couples who had no such network and who consequently were significantly more isolated, stressed, and depressed. The presence of social support in dealing with cancer has been shown to be a buffer to stress; lack of social support reduces support coping[8].

3. Where is the family in the developmental life cycle? The problems of a young adult couple in which one partner has cancer are potentially very

different from those of an elderly couple where one partner has cancer. It has been shown, for example, that the younger couple is more likely to experience relationship stresses stemming from the psychodynamic shifts in dependence/independence imposed by cancer. By contrast, older couples experience stresses from situational factors such as exhaustion, fatigue, and guilt (e.g., the patient's feelings of being a burden).[9] The S family was complicated in this regard. Although there were two adult children, at a deeper level both children still had financial and emotional dependencies on the parents that presented important issues to consider and understand. These were some of the key stresses within the family system besides the cancer itself.

4. How does the family communicate? Communication patterns affect family members' ability to discuss the diagnosis, make decisions jointly, and ultimately support one another. Assessment can involve probing the following questions: Who talks to whom? Is communication direct or indirect? Is communication partially or heavily nonverbal? Is one member a "go-between" or "gatekeeper" in the family in regard to communication?[10]. When there is a "go-between," communication moves from a health-care team member through one member of the family to the rest of the family. This, to a degree, was the process in the S family, where communication went through Mrs. S to the children and the grandchildren, with Mr. S being more peripheral. As Mrs. S became more ill, Mr. S learned gradually to step in and communicate directly with his family. This was an important and adaptive shift in this family, one that became a focus of family therapy interventional efforts during this period. Closely tied to communication is the family's ability to make decisions as a unit, rather than have one person make decisions. This is linked to the concept of joint problem solving, If families are communicating and making joint decisions, they are then likely to cope more effectively. An obviously high-risk family situation is one in which the sole decision maker, on whom the rest of the family has always depended to make decisions, now has terminal cancer. Such a family may rise to the occasion and begin to take on the decision-making responsibilities, or it may not, thereby requiring very intensive professional intervention and resources.

5. What was the role of the ill member, and what is it now? All family members have various in-

dividual roles and tasks. Some families are more rigid and inflexible about these roles and tasks; others are more flexible and adaptable. It has been shown that families with mid-range (rather than high or low) adaptability experience less global distress in coping when a member develops cancer.[11] Families that are too low on this variable are likely to be rigid, and those that are too high are likely to be chaotic in their attempts to adapt. An analysis of the ill member's activities of daily living and his or her emotional tasks and meaning in the family will reveal how much distress and anxiety the illness is likely to bring to the family. In the S family, Mrs. S was the "pivot" or emotional hub of the family. While she was not the chief wage earner, her illness had a significant effect on the capacities of the family to organize, plan, problem solve, and interact.

THE MARITAL RELATIONSHIP

The functioning of the spouse of an end-stage cancer patient is related to many variables, some current and some historical in the marriage. Generally, the majority of spouses, possibly as many as 80%, are able to be supportive and persist in this supportive role throughout the patient's illness.[12] Differences have been found in what affects husbands and wives when their partners are ill with cancer. When the wife is the ill partner, the husband's distress is almost completely related to her condition; his individual characteristics (e.g., socioeconomic status, and own health) do not contribute or explain his distress. When the husband's the ill partner, the wife's distress is affected by and moderated by his condition as well as by individual factors such as her own health (if it is poor, she will feel more distress) and level of outside social support (less support leads to more distress). However, the more distress she feels, the more likely the wife is to seek support outside the family.[13] Studies of the relationship between stage of disease and spousal emotional distress have consistently shown that an advanced or metastatic stage of disease has been associated with greater mood disturbance, depression, and feelings of being overwhelmed than localized disease. [14-17] It is cautioned, however, that stage and prognosis alone may not totally predict spousal distress or even match spousal perceptions. Variables such as patient restrictions in role performance, increased patient demands related to the illness, and severity of symptoms (especially pain) may better predict spousal distress than objective medical data alone.[17] Several studies have shown that spousal emotional distress, especially for spouses or breast cancer pateints, is correlated with the patient's level of emotional distress.[18,19] The overall conclusion is that spouses of patients with compromised psychological functioning appear to be at higher risk of poor adjustment. This may actually be an old pattern of the relationship that is now being played out in the cancer arena. Nevertheless, research suggests that affective states, especially depression, may be "contagious" and that depressed patients will generate depressed spouses, who then have less to give, further deepening the depression and guilt of the patient. This argues heavily for joint treatment, or at least serious consideration of the spouses' coping status and symptomatology.

Turning to Mr. and Mrs. S, it was evident that Mr. S was represented in the 80% of spouses who manage to be supportive. This is not to say, however, that his ability to cope was robust. In fact, it grew quite strained at times. As the literature suggests, he was very responsive to his wife's medical and psychological condition. For example, ongoing difficulties with her pain management were clearly distressing to him, so much so that he asked various members of the team, "When will this be over—can't it be sooner rather than later?" Difficulties in managing Mrs. S's depression also appeared to depress him. He felt, at times, that no amount of giving on his part was enough to bring her "out of the dumps." One of his characteristic modes of self-regulation was to use alcohol. He periodically drank more as her illness wore on, particularly in the final 11 months. As he drank more, his functioning declined, and his irritability and sleep problems predictably worsened. The dam burst when he became enraged at one of his grandchildren one evening over a relatively minor provocation. The entire family then insisted that he accept antidepressant medication and urged that he undergo formal alcohol treatment. Mr. S was willing to accept the medication immediately but felt he needed to defer the alcohol treatment. He did recognize and acknowledge the reality of his problems with alcohol but felt overwhelmed by his wife's illness and argued that he could not take on a major treatment involvement in the midst of her terminal illness period. He did have consultation for psychopharmacologic treatment by a specialist, who prescribed the selective serotonin reuptake inhibitor (SSRI) Zoloft. Several things changed when he started taking Zoloft. He was less irritable; had a reduced feeling of being in chaos; was more able to work, organize, and get paperwork done; and felt a modest elevation in his mood state. He promised to and did limit his alcohol consumption for the remainder of his wife's illness. Of note, he did enter an outpatient alcohol treatment program after his wife's death. In the program he stopped his use of alcohol and tobacco. He has continued to abstain from smoking and now drinks in moderation.

Mr. S changed his familial role dramatically during the period of Mrs. S's terminal illness. He became a central rather than a peripheral member of the family. Behaviorally, he coordinated the LVNs, did cooking (especially in the evenings), and was directly involved with and responsive to his daughters' emotional concerns. All of this had previously been the domain of Mrs. S. More important, he changed in his emotional reactivity to the situation. Whereas previously he had used hyperactivity as a coping mechanism and defense against his feelings, at this point he could not and would not do this. Rather, he began to openly grieve his wife's illness and imminent death through bouts of crying. This was totally uncharacteristic of his previous mode of functioning. On several occasions when I was at the family home in the evenings, he went into the backyard, either alone or with a daughter, and wept openly. In a sense, the disequilibrium of the relationship homeostasis allowed him to change to other modes of functioning. Mrs. S did not ever really withdraw from the family interaction, but she became increasingly less central and pivotal. This allowed Mr. S to shift to a more central role and to increase his competence in the family arena. It seemed as if family members had previously cooperated to make Mrs. S overcompetent in the family arena and less so in the work arena; Mr. S's role had been the opposite. Now this situation was reversed, and Mr. S became much more competent in the family arena and actually lost one of his major sales lines during this period. In our work, he was facilitated in reassessing whether this loss was truly catastrophic. He decided that he would regroup after Mrs. S's

death, without being absolutely sure he wanted to remain in his field of sales. Thus, the sense of catastrophic change was reconceptualized as a period of semiretirement, necessary to apply his attention to the family, and as a time to reconsider the future. After Mrs. S's death, he entered alcohol treatment, recommitted to his sales area, entered a new relationship (within 6 or 8 months), and again became semiperipheral to his daughters and grandchildren. When he met for a follow-up with this writer, 6 months after Mrs. S's death, he looked 10 to 15 years younger than he had previously.

Several key decisions must be made when a therapist is beginning family intervention with the spouse of a terminally ill cancer patient. The clinician must answer these questions:

1. Would it be preferable to see the spouse together with the dying partner or separately, or would some combination be best? In the case of Mr. and Mrs. S, doing both seemed reasonable. Some joint counseling around communication and stress reduction needed to be facilitated. This was especially true when Mr. S needed to sleep separately, inducing separation anxiety in Mrs. S. However, Mr. S was more likely to vent his feelings, pressures, and fears in individual counseling sessions. This required a shift for Mrs. S and this writer, as I had been her therapist alone for several years. She was able to handle this and give Mr. S the time with me, recognizing that she would get back what she was giving as Mr. S settled down.

2. Is the spouse as depressed or perhaps more depressed than the ill partner and therefore in need of antidepressant medication to "go the distance"? In a study that systematically evaluated emotional symptoms of couples who had been together before, during, and since the male partner's cancer, depression was found to be the *only* symptom that in which there was a significant correlation between the spouses. In addition, partners experienced a level of depression 64% higher than the patients two years after the patients' initial diagnoses.[20]

3. Is the level of communication and support adequate for the patient's need? If it is not, joint intervention is necessary. However, the clinician must carefully determine whether this couple was able to communicate and be mutually supportive in the past. If the answer is no, then expectations for couples therapy need to be drastically reduced. Some relationships can grow in the face of such a stimulus; others cannot.

4. What are the well spouse's obligations and commitments? A detailed inventory, including economic, parental, business, and social responsibilities, should be compiled and, if necessary, revised and negotiated. The well spouse can rarely keep all his or her external responsibilities while the ill spouse is dying, but some retention of external ties and obligations is anchoring for the well spouse. These indicate a continuity, a future, and a capacity to avoid being totally immersed in the partner's illness. For elderly spouses, this may be difficult as most or all external ties may have already been relinquished. Reestablishing a few of these may be vital for the elderly well spouse.

5. Is the well partner able to tolerate the emotional and sexual deprivation that comes with having a dying partner, or has the spouse looked elsewhere to have these needs met? If the well spouse has gone outside the marriage before the ill spouse's death, he or she may feel intense shame, guilt, and even self-loathing but need to do it nevertheless. The therapist's maintenance of a nonjudgmental stance is crucial in such situations. For the spouse to admit this kind of activity to the therapist indicates a high degree of pain and potentially a high degree of trust in the therapist. This writer explores at least three questions when this arises, which include:

- Does this behavior seem to be part of an historical pattern in the relationship for one or both spouses, or was it generated by the illness?
- Does the well spouse feel that the behavior impacts on his or her ability to give to and support the ill spouse?
- Does the well spouse feel that the behavior may impact his or her own self-appraisal in the bereavement period or beyond? The spouse needs to be reminded that he or she will have to continue to live with this self-appraisal and that there will be no opportunity to "edit" or "redo" interactions with the spouse. (This is the central theme of a recent stage play, titled *Skylight*, by David Hare, in which the male protagonist is tormented by his dying spouse's discovery of his affair during her terminal phase.) If the well spouse is conflicted about such an affair, it is likely that the conflict will prolong and complicate the bereavement process, with attendant problems of depression, guilt, and inability to enter into a relationship with a new partner after the spouse's death. Thus, such a revelation by a well spouse can be understood, but it is a complicated matter to discuss in the therapeutic relationship.

PAIN AND THE FAMILY OF THE DYING CANCER PATIENT

The family relationship to pain management is complex and intense and has an effect on both the patient and the family. Professional, family, and even patient ignorance about pain management and fear of addiction can present a significant barrier to good pain management.[21–22] Closely tied to this is the issue of patient pain ratings by caregivers. It has been found that concordance of ratings between caregivers and patients is good at low and moderate levels of pain but this agreement breaks down at high levels (above 7 on a visual analog scale of 0 to 10).[23] Thus, the possibility of undermedication for pain, especially when it is most needed, arises. Even experienced professionals have a hard time perceiving accurately the need for medications; family members may find it close to impossible. It may therefore be unwise for family members to have sole responsibility for pain management, especially if the patient is dying at home.

Associated with this function is the often complex interplay of denial by both the well spouse and the ill spouse. I once saw a couple where the wife was very ill and was obviously in pain. The husband had assumed the role of dispensing her pain medication, including determining when and how much medication she should get. He was terrified that her illness would progress, she would die, and he would be left alone. She recognized this and tried to soothe him by cooperating with his need to deny. He reasoned that if her disease was not progressing, she could cope without an increase in the pain medications. She tried to cooperate with this contorted reasoning by not asking for medications and living (however uncomfortably) in chronic pain. This interaction, based on the husband's need to deny reality, required urgent couple-based interventions. He required more help and support with his fears; she had to learn to be appropriately assertive; and the treating physician was required to step in and take more control of the pain management function.

Associated with these issues are family (and sometimes professional) fears about hastening death by increasing patient narcotic levels. These matters are worth exploring with the family. The family may be in denial about where the patient is physically and psychologically. In addition, family members may feel they are not being adequately supported by the physicians and nurses in terms of education and direction about pain management. All too frequently, when the patient is dying at home, the physician becomes a distant, isolated, seemingly inaccessible person who communicates only through the home-care nurses, leaving the family feeling adrift and abandoned. Reconnecting the family directly to the physician can reverse this feeling for the family. A third issue is the question of whether the concerns about killing the patient are a defense against underlying wishes that the patient hurry up and die. Such underlying wishes are usually unacceptable to the family and are therefore unable to be tolerated or discussed. The normalization of such feelings and thoughts can sometimes help normalize the pain management situation for the family and the health-care deliverers.

The S family was happy to turn the pain management function over to the hospice nurse agency. They did not express conflicts about escalating Mrs. S's narcotics level. In fact, Mr. S, when his depression level was high and his coping ability was low, expressed a wish to hasten the process of her dying. This request ceased when he became restabilized himself. Mrs. S was placed on a morphine pump a few months prior to her death. It always worked well, with one noteworthy exception. One Saturday the pump repeatedly malfunctioned despite numerous attempts to fix it and numerous hospice nursing visits. Needless to say, Mrs. S was in acute distress during this day. I received multiple phone calls that day from the family, starting at 9:00 A.M. and continuing until 11:30 P.M.. Visiting the family home the next day, I found family members exceedingly exhausted and the children regressed in alarming ways. There was no question that lack of pain management in the patient dramatically affected the family system in direct, observable ways. In all three generations of the family, coping was not possible until pain management was restored. The problem with the pump was a pin-hole-size leak in the tubing leading into the pump itself. That pin-hole-size leak put a massive hole in the family structure around coping with anxiety. Thus, for the family as well as for the patient, pain management is a first-order priority to support coping and to reduce psychological symptomatology. One study showed that a patient in significant pain was twice as likely to have a psychiatric diagnosis as a patient without significant pain.[21] This finding probably extends to family members as well, to extrapolate from previously cited data.[20]

CHILDREN IN THE FAMILY OF THE DYING CANCER PATIENT

The category "children" includes both adult children and dependent children, a category that itself encompasses a wide range of developmental levels. For example, in the S family, there were two adult children and five grandchildren, ranging from a toddler to an early adolescent. This section focuses on the impact of a dying cancer patient on both adult and dependent children.

For adult children, at least four issues are preeminent, while many others remain in the background. First is the issue of *role fragmentation*. Adult children are pulled simultaneously in many directions, a result of their multiple roles as spouses, parents, friends, and wage-earners. In this writer's experience, the role of caretaker/organizer for the ill parent usually (not always) falls on the female adult children. This caretaker role becomes a priority, thus capturing the very essence of "role stress."

A second issue is that of *role reversal*. Adult children are likely to reverse roles with the sick parent, and possibly with the well parent as well. For some adult children this may hardly be a novel experience, while for others it may be the first time such a reversal has occurred. The key issue is that it is occurring just exactly when the adult child is also probably most frightened and in need of some bolstering and parenting. This is especially true during the acute dying process, when the ill parent becomes totally dependent on the significant and professional others. Some parent-child relationships have the flexibility to incorporate role reversals, while others cannot. Role reversal can precipitate role tensions and struggles with the well parent.

A third issue is that of *sibling rivalry*, growing out of a "sealed-over" conflict that may or may not have reached true resolution in earlier years. The imminent death of a parent may powerfully reactivate these conflicts. One stimulus, as noted, may be a role reversal, which can raise the question of which adult child has more power and authority and receives the most respect. Another stimulus can be a frantic attempt to grab the last fragments of parental attention, approval, and affection as the ill parent is dying. Such a parent may have little energy to give, setting off an acute struggle for some precious last moments. Mixed up in this rivalry may be old or renewed conflicts about equal sharing of responsibilities; less competent adult children can feel pushed aside or denigrated by siblings for failing to "do the right thing," while more competent children can feel overburdened and unappreciated by their siblings. If these tensions erupt at the dying parent's bedside, they are likely to make the parent feel desperate; the parent may feel like a failure and be anxious about dying before these issues are unresolved.

A fourth issue is that of *burn out*. The role stresses when a parent is dying are so intense that they pose the threat of overload, burnout, and psychological withdrawal. This can come in the form of detachment, doing things in a robotic fashion without genuine emotional involvement.[25] To avoid burnout, siblings must interact functionally enough to have a schedule, coordinate responsibilities, and share the burden. When there is only one adult child, the likelihood that burnout will occur reaches nearly 100%, in this writer's experience.

For adult-daughters of the S family, all four of these issues were in evidence, some more than others. The daughters were severely fragmented, with one setting up a new business to support herself and her children and the other having two children under 6 years of age. I was present one evening when the younger daughter had to choose whether to go home with her children or to stay with her mother (who was less than 2 weeks away from dying). She chose to stay with her mother, and we witnessed her children literally screaming for her as they were taken to the car by their father. We reasoned together she would have a lot more time with her kids but little left with her mother. She, however, looked literally stricken by the pull between these two immutable forces. Facilitating some balance and resolution between these forces can be a vital function of a mental health professional at such times.

Both daughters did well and were graceful in the role-reversal process. I sat with the daughters at Mrs. S's bedside in her final days, balancing support and resolution of "unfinished business." A great deal got accomplished in the context of

Mrs. S's severely limited energy and emerging delirium. Mr. S, without feeling threatened, gave his daughters space to become their "mother's mother" during this time.

Sibling rivalry between the sisters was actually minimal at this point. The younger sister faced the reality that her older sister would not become a maternal substitute, and the older sister appeared to respect the competence of her sister to perform all the functions with their mother that she consistently did perform. This allowed the older sister to see to the development of her business, which was so essential to her survival. The sisters were able to seal over their several unresolved conflicts during this period. Each also seemed gratified by what she got from her mother during this time.

Both daughters struggled with burnout and were successfully able to coordinate their schedules together and with the heath-care staff. Each struggled with multiple role demands; on follow-up, this writer found that the struggle remained a major factor in both sisters' lives.

Dependent children face a variety of issues when a parent or a grandparent is dying of cancer. Some of the issues reflect the child's age and developmental level. A key variable in achieving a healthy adaptation to parental loss in dependent children is familial relationships characterized by sharing of information.[26] This includes allowing open expressions of guilt, anger, and sadness,[27] as well as preparing the child for the death and providing the opportunity for the child to ask questions.[28] In some families, communication about death is avoided, unrealistic, or inadequate. This pattern has been shown to produce children who have unresolved and pathological mourning or acting-out behaviors, which lead to emotional complications later in adult life.[29–31] It has also been suggested that children take their cues about talking about difficult issues from parental behaviors and that some families may avoid talking about them so as to avoid questions that will force them to deal with them before they themselves are ready.[32,33] In a recent study of 91 families, with 136 children, in which one parent was terminally ill, several conclusions were reached:

1. In the vast majority of families (95%), discussion regarding the parental illness did occur.
2. The length of time between parental diagnosis and the first discussion varied, with two peaks,

at 2 months or less (34%) and more than 1 year (44%).

3. Disclosure about the possibility of parental death was split (44% no, 56% yes), with the well parent being the most likely discloser of this information (43%) and the length of time from first discussion of probable death to actual death being relatively short (67% within 2 months or less of the death).

4. The age of the child was related to the probability of discussing possible death, 50% of children ages 7–11 were told; 61% ages 12–18 were told.[34]

I have noted certain implications of parental death for children at different developmental ages. Role reversals, the end of childhood, and increased child care/homemaker responsibilities are more likely for adolescents, especially for adolescent girls. Teenagers are sometimes treated as (young) adults who no longer have childhood needs. Latency-age children may not be attended to unless they begin a pattern of acting out.[35] Prelatency-age children are faced with separation-anxiety problems of a fundamental nature, which can induce alarming levels of regression (this is also true for older children, but usually with less profound levels of regression). Separation anxiety is a ubiquitous issue, but is especially prominent in dependent children.

In the S family, many of these issues were present for the children. For the adolescent granddaughter, her mother's role fragmentations left her frequently in charge of her two latency-age brothers. One of her brothers had a long-term reading disability. This drew and held family attention, especially from Mrs. S, even during her terminal period. When he sat at her bedside and read to her shortly before her death, it seemed to visibly release her from a chronic worry and help reduce her death anxieties. Perhaps the most expressive grandchild of all (Grandchild #4, Figure 19.1) was Daughter #2's 6-year-old son. The day after Mrs. S's morphine pump malfunctioned, I visited with the family and found this boy in a frankly regressed, clingy state with his parents. He was uncharacteristically uncommunicative and was asked to draw a picture of anything to begin the process of communicating. He drew a picture (see Figure 19.2), which he described as "a thin woman with a fat dress and huge feet getting ready to go on a very long trip." When asked to say who the woman was or to tell more about the picture, he had no idea. This took place as we sat in his grandparents' living room with one wall separating us from Mrs. S's sick room. I interpreted to him that the woman might be his grandmother and that he had felt helpless to help her yesterday and that she was much sicker and pos-

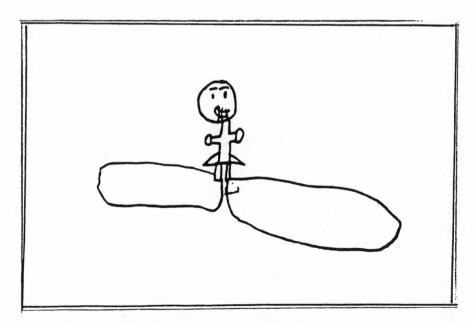

Figure 19.2 6-Year-Old Grandson's Drawing

sibly would die and therefore take "a long trip." This appeared to decrease his agitation, and he was able to open up a bit and talk about yesterday's disturbing events. What came through as especially troubling was seeing his own parents in a helpless state. For me, the bottom line in this interaction was that all family members, including very young children, need to feel some sense of control and some sense of empowerment. This child's solution was to equip his emaciated grandmother with huge shoes to help her on her big trip from life to death.

Two years after Ms. S's death, this child wrote his grandmother a note, which his mother shared with me. In the letter, at age 8, he wrote:

Dear Grandma,

I want to know if you can see me right now because I would like to know if you are looking at me. I youused to tell you this after you died and slowly stopped. . . . I would also like to say that I wish I would go to your funirle because I wasn't there for you when you died and Mommy was. I wasn't there for your funurle either, but I know I was younger but I still think it is unfair. But right know I am taking trumet [trumpet], piano and tennis lessons. In the future I hope to be a chemist, a cemedian, and the president of the USA. I think the part of me that makes me redd [haired and complexioned] comes from you. . . . We miss you, send you love. Did you meet god yet?

This letter highlights several important aspects of childhood grief resolution, including these:

1. Because of the presence of necessary and powerful repressive and suppressive defense mechanisms, grief resolution in children proceeds slowly and takes years to process.
2. Children can maintain strong bonds and identifications ("that the part of me that makes me redd") with the dead relative, even while making slow progress in separating ("I youused to tell you this after you died and slowly stopped").
3. Adult wishes to protect the child may create barriers to working through childhood grief ("I was younger [at the time of your death] but I still think it is unfair" [that I wasn't allowed to attend your funeral]).
4. Children may exhibit a continuing need to please the lost figure possibly out of unresolved guilt over perceived unmet expectations, especially around the time of death ("I wasn't there") ("I hope to be . . . president of the USA").

5. Children continue to feel an ongoing attachment to the perceived power of the lost figure; for example, Mrs. S was actually powerful and central to the family and is still obviously powerful in her grandson's emotions ("Have you met God yet?").

THERAPIST COUNTERTRANSFERENCE ISSUES WITH TERMINAL PATIENTS AND FAMILIES

A classic definition of countertransference is: "Countertransference reactions arise in the therapist as a result of the patient's influence on the therapist's unconscious feelings and have their origin in the therapist's identification and projections."[36] Shneidman, in bringing this into the psycho-oncology context, comments:

There is a well-known caveat: Where there is transference there will[37] be countertransference—the flow of feeling from the therapist to the patient. The therapist invests himself in the patient's welfare and is thereby made vulnerable. When the patient dies, the therapist is bereaved. And during the dying process the therapist is anguished by the prospect of loss and sense of impotence. . . . The therapist would be well advised to have good support systems in his or her own work life—loved ones, dear friends, a congenial work situation, and peer consultants."[37]

The mental health professional, in working with the patient, family, and health delivery team, can be expected to be barraged with emotions, transference reactions, and demands from any or all of these people. The therapist, in turn, may respond in ways that range from the reasonable to the irrational, depending, at least partially, on the effect of countertransference issues. Holland suggests several aspects of the work life of the psycho-oncologist that must be examined, including:

1. Isolation from colleague peers, the very thing that Shneidman[34] offers as a primary necessity in this area of work
2. Role ambiguity
3. Absence of a primary "tool" other than psychological support
4. The wish to solve what are sometimes unsolvable problems
5. Maintenance of functional distance

6. Personal loss history reactivated by the present situation.[38]

I view all six of Holland's concerns as important in work with families of dying cancer patients but would particularly emphasize role ambiguity, maintenance of functional distance, and personal loss history in the context of the S family. Role ambiguity played an unexpected and dramatic presentation during work with the S family after the introduction of the home-care hospice team, particularly the hospice RNs. When they came into the S family home, they defined their role as including mental health care, in fact *all* mental health care. They then proceeded to create a boundary between Mrs. S and me, essentially ignoring the fact that we already had a 5-year therapeutic relationship. The conflict came to a head when one RN saw herself as needing permission to discuss "confidential" information about Mrs. S with me. Although I wished to work as a team with the hospice nurses, seeing them as cotherapists, clearly they did not reciprocate. The nurse related that she could share such "confidential " information only with the approval of the patient's medical oncologist. I felt quite irritated by this behavior. I saw it as a systems problem created by a blurring of role functions and workgroup boundaries. A significant concern for me was that this problem not become a problem for the S family, so I immediately discussed the situation with Mrs. S's oncologist (to whom I had initially referred Mrs. S). He immediately clarified the situation for the home-care hospice agency. The net result was a level of coexistence between me and the RN team, which did accept my suggestions but certainly did not engage in a collegial or cotherapy relationship. I was told that the agency staff had never previously had an on-site mental health professional engaged in therapeutic work with a dying patient and family. Thus, the potential role ambiguity suggested by Holland became inevitable.[35] In retrospect, it appears that these team conflicts did not become a problem for the family. Rather, the professionals agreed to provide two avenues of psychological support to the patient and family.

I view the maintenance of functional distance, Holland's fifth concern, as a fundamental problem, heavily complicated and reinforced when the therapist is working in the family home directly with all of the family members. I dined with the family at least twice during the end-stage period of Mrs. S's illness. Such a wide departure from usual therapeutic activities requires careful thought and self-scrutiny to determine whether one has become more like a family member than a therapist. I was not asked by the family about personal reactions or feelings about Mrs. S's approaching death, nor did I discuss them. I thus avoided looking to the family for support. I am in fundamental agreement with Shneidman that spousal *and* (not *or*) peer support are essential for the therapist in such stressful and potentially confusing circumstances. However, in this case, my working in the family home was necessary to the family and the patient during the phase of end-stage care.

Issues surrounding the reactivatin of the therapist's personal loss history by the present situation seem to emerge directly from the need to maintain functional distance. Working with the entire family, in the home setting, makes family reactions and interactions far more intense than they would be in an office or even an inpatient hospital setting. This increases the likelihood that unresolved therapist losses and unresolved mourning will be reactivated. The therapist may need to "make things right," as may well have been impossible in the therapist's own family, and the therapist may push family members too hard out of his or her own unresolved countertransferential feelings. In another powerful potential therapist countertransference issue, the therapist may compete with the spouse and/or the adult children to be the most supportive, best spouse, or best child.

Holland presents isolation from peers as a major issue. This too is magnified in a home-care setting where the psycho-oncologist is ostensibly physically removed from his or her peers. Group case discussion and/or peer individual supervision are essential components of work done in such a context. Additionally, therapists who are considering working in such a setting should give strong consideration to personal therapy to work through their own losses.

Finally, the wish to solve what are unsolvable problems must be carefully considered in such work. Coming into a family milieu at a time of terminal illness creates a strong impetus and a sense of urgency to finish up all "unfinished business" in the family. Some unfinished business is unfinished precisely because it is unfinishable.

Supervision may help the therapist stay targeted on reasonable primary goals and objectives, and to avoid trying to manage his or her sense of impotence or desperation about the dying process by attempting to solve age-old family problems. This allows maximum energy to remain with the key issue—that of increased family and patient comfort with the immediate problem of the dying process. This remains the bottom-line mandate with family interventions with dying cancer patients.

References

1. Kristjanson LJ. Validity and reliability testing of the FAMCARE scale: measuring family satisfaction with advanced cancer care. *Social Science and Medicine*, 1993; 36:693–701.

2. Kristjanson LJ, Leis A, Koop PM, Carriere KC, Mueller B. Family members' care expectations, care perceptions, and satisfaction with advanced cancer care: results of a multi-site pilot study. *Journal of Palliative Care*, 1997; 13:5–13.

3. Kristjanson LJ, Nikoletti S, Poruck D, Smith M, Lobchuk M, Pedler P. Congruence between patients and family caregivers' perceptions of symptom distress in patients with terminal cancer. *Journal of Palliative Care*, 1998; 14:24–32.

4. Gordon A, Rooney A. Hospice and the family: a systems approach to assessment. *American Journal of Hospice Care*, 1984; Winter:31–33.

5. Kanter D, Lehr W. *Inside the Family: Toward a Theory of Family Process.* New York: Harper Calophon Books, 1974.

6. Wynne LC, Wynne AR. The quest for intimacy. *Journal of Marital and Family Therapy*, 1986; 12: 383–394.

7. Wynne LC. Communication disorders and the quest for relatedness in families of schizophrenics. *American Journal of Psychoanalysis*, 1970; 30:100–114.

8. Bloom JR, Kang SH, Romano P. Cancer and stress: the effects of social support on a resource. In: Cooper C, Watson M, eds, *Cancer and Stress: Psychological, Biological, and Coping Studies.* New York: John Wiley, 1991:95–124.

9. Wellisch DK, Wolcott DL, Pasnau RO, et al. Evaluation of psychosocial problems of the homebound cancer patient. III. Family problems as a variable in patient adjustment. *Journal of Psychosocial Oncology*, 1989; 7(1/2):55–76.

10. Zuk G. The go-between process in family therapy. *Family Process*, 1965; 5:162–178.

11. Heinz-Schultz K, Schultz H, Schultz O, Von Kerekjarto M. Family structure and psychosocial stress in families of cancer patients. In: Baider L, Cooper CL, Kaplan-De-Nour A, eds, *Cancer and the Family.* New York: John Wiley, 1996:225–256.

12. Wellisch DK, Jamison KR, Pasnau RO. Psychosocial aspects of mastectomy. II: The man's perspective. *American Journal of Psychiatry*, 1978; 135: 543–546.

13. Keller M, Heinrich G, Sellschopp A, Beutel M. Between distress and support: Spouses of cancer patients. In: Baider L, Cooper C, Kaplan-DeNour A, eds, *Cancer and the Family.* New York: John Wiley, 1996.

14. Gotay C. The experience of cancer during early and advanced stages: The views of patients and their mates. *Social Science and Medicine*, 1984; 18(7):605–613.

15. Ell KO, Nishimoto RH, Mantell JE, et al. Psychological adaptation to cancer: A comparison among patients, spouses, and non-spouses. *Family Systems Medicine*, 1988; 6(3):335–348.

16. Cassileth BR, Lusk EJ, Strouse TB, et al. A psychological analysis of cancer patients and their next-of-kin. *Cancer*, 1985; 55:72–76.

17. Friedman LC, Baer PE, Nelson DV, et al. Women with breast cancer: perception of family functioning and adjustment to illness. *Psychosomatic Medicine*, 1988; 50:529–540.

18. Lewis FM. The impact of cancer on the family: A critical analysis of the research literature. *Patient Education and Counseling*, 1986; 8:269–289.

19. Northouse LL. Social support in patients' and husbands' adjustment to breast cancer. *Nursing Research*, 1988; 37(2):91–95.

20. Gritz ER, Wellisch DK, Siau J, et al. Long term effects of testicular cancer on marital relationships. *Psychosomatics*, 1990; 31(3)301–312.

21. Macaluso C, Weinberg D, Foley KM. Opiod abuse and misuse in a cancer pain population. *Journal of Pain and Symptom Management*, 1988; 3:54 (abstract).

22. Charap AD. The knowledge, attitudes, and experience of medical personnel treating pain in the terminally ill. *Mount Sinai Journal of Medicine*, 1978; 45:561–580.

23. Grossman SA, Sheidler VR, Swedon K, et al. Correlations of patient and caregiver ratings of cancer pain. *Journal of Pain and Symptom Management*, 1991; 6:53–57.

24. Derogotis LM, Morrow GR, Fetting J, et al. The prevalence of psychiatric disorders among cancer patients. *Journal of the American Medical Association*, 1993; 249:751–757.

25. Maslach C. The burnout syndrome and patient care. In: Garfield CA, ed, *Stress and Survival: The Emotional Realities of Life-Threatening Illnesses*. St. Louis Missouri: Mosby, 1979:111–120.

26. Cohen P, Dizenhuz IM, Wingit C. Family adaptation to terminal illness and death. *Social Casework*, 1977; 58:223–228.

27. Vollman RR, Ganzert A, Picher L, et al. The reactions of family systems to sudden and unexpected death. *Omega*, 1971; 2:101–106.

28. Bowlby J. *Loss*. New York: Basic Books, 1980.

29. Rosenthal PA. Short-term family therapy and pathological grief resolution with children and adolescents. *Family Process*, 1980; 19:151–159.

30. Becher D, Margolin F. How surviving parents handled their young childrens' adaptation to the crisis of loss. *American Journal of Orthopsychiatry*, 1969; 37:753–757.

31. Soler L, Skolnick N. Childhood parental death and depression in adulthood: Roles of surviving parent and family environment. *American Journal of Orthopsychiatry*, 1992; 62:504–516.

32. Knight-Birnbaum N. Therapeutic work with bereaved parents. In: Altschul A, Pollock GH, eds, *Childhood Bereavement and Its Aftermath*. Madison, CT: International Universities Press, 1988:107–144.

33. Silverman SM, Silverman PR. Parent-child communication in widowed families. *American Journal of Psychotherapy*, 1979; 33:428–441.

34. Siegel K, Raveis VH, Karus D. Pattern of communication with children when a parent has cancer. In: Baider L, Cooper CL, Kaplan-De-Nour A, eds, *Cancer and the Family*. New York: John Wiley, 1996:109–128.

35. Wellisch DK. Adolescent acting-out when a parent has cancer. *International Journal of Family Therapy*, 1979; 1:230–241.

36. Noyes AP, Kolb LC. *Modern Clinical Psychiatry*. Philadelphia: W.B. Saunders Co., 1963.

37. Shneidman ES. Some aspects of psychotherapy with dying patients. In: Garfield C, ed, *Psychosocial Care of the Dying Patient*. New York: McGraw Hill Co., 1978.

38. Holland J. Stresses on mental health professionals. In: Holland JC, Rowland JH, eds, *Handbook of Psycho-oncology*. New York: Oxford Press, 1989.

20

Communication with Terminally Ill Patients and Their Relatives

Peter Maguire, M.D.

Recent research has emphasized the importance of effective communication in ensuring the adequate care of cancer patients, including those with terminal illness, and their relatives. However, it has also found that serious deficiencies in communication occur in practice. The nature of these deficiencies and the reasons for them are described in this chapter, along with possible solutions.

COMMUNICATION AND PSYCHOLOGICAL ADAPTATION

Longitudinal studies of the psychological reactions of patients with cancer have found that two aspects of communication best predict later psychological adjustment. Patients who perceive that they are given too little or too much information about their diagnosis and treatment are more likely to develop a major depressive illness, generalized anxiety disorder, or adjustment disorder than are patients who feel that their information needs are met appropriately.[1] Similarly, patients who experience a recurrence of their cancer and feel that the information offered is confusing or inadequate are also at risk of developing these affective disorders (Fallowfield, Hall, Maguire, and Baum, personal communication).

A recent 2-year follow-up study of more than 600 patients with newly diagnosed cancers found a strong relationship between the number and severity of patients' concerns about their predicament and the later development of an affective disorder. Patients who had more unresolved concerns, both moderately severe and severe, were much more likely to become clinically anxious or depressed.[2] Patients most at risk were also more likely to perceive that there was nothing they could do to resolve their concerns.

A major question, then, is how successful health professionals are in identifying and responding appropriately to cancer patients' needs for information at key phases in their illness and how well they elicit their patients' concerns, whether physical, social, psychological, or spiritual in nature.

Problems with Giving Information

Objective study of consultations between doctors and patients when the doctor had to impart bad news found that, regardless of disease status, doctors made little attempt to tailor information to patients' needs. Instead, doctors tended to assume that they knew what patients wished to know about their disease and possible treatments and responded accordingly.[3] This often conflicted with patients' needs for information. Moreover, doctors tended to assume that they knew what the patients' resultant concerns would be. Immediately after breaking the bad news, they gave advice or information about diagnosis and treatment in a bid to reassure their patients that something could be done. When faced with patients with terminal illness, they assumed that patients were preoccupied with fears of suffering, especially pain. They tried to reassure them that the doctors should be able to alleviate the pain.

Patients given bad news usually have some idea of the nature of their predicament and are appropriately concerned. The giving of bad news often provokes additional concerns. Instead of identifying these concerns and giving patients the chance to talk about them, most doctors move into advice and information giving immediately. Consequently, as doctors are giving information about what might be done to treat or palliate the disease, patients remain preoccupied with their preexisting and new concerns. They register little of the newly offered information and attend selectively to negative aspects of the communication. Thus, a patient who was informed that her cancer had recurred and was metastatic but that it could be controlled for some time remembered only the word "metastatic." She continued to be plagued with thoughts that she was dying.

Seale studied relatives of adults dying in England in 1987 to determine their perceptions of what cancer patients knew about their diagnosis and prognosis. In a fifth of cases[4] relatives were confident that patients did not know they were terminally ill at the time of death. Some 12% of doctors admitted they avoided discussing the prognosis with patients; instead, they put the burden on the relatives. Overall, health-care professionals thought that only half of the patients realized their true diagnosis and prognosis. Yet, in the west it is estimated that 80% or more of patients who are dying are aware of their predicament and would welcome information about what is happening, along with the opportunity to disclose and discuss their concerns.

Problems in Identifying Patient Concerns

Wilkinson[5] tape-recorded assessment interviews between 57 cancer nurses and three types of newly admitted patients: those with newly diagnosed cancer, those with recurrent disease, and those with terminal illness. Coverage by the nurses of psychological or social concerns was judged to be very poor or absent. Even assessment of important physical problems like pain was often poor. The nature, severity, and duration of any pain often remained vague. The nurses were least confident in talking to patients with recurrent disease.

Higginson, Wade, and McCarthy[6] asked support teams looking after terminally ill patients in the community to complete an assessment schedule to determine patients' needs. In the last assessment before death, 50% of patients reported uncontrolled pain and 70% of patients had problems with anxiety. Anxiety in family members was also considered to be a major problem. Yet, these concerns were not known beforehand to the support team.

Hockley et al.[7] examined the care given to 26 patients dying in a hospital without a palliative-care team. They used a 16-item checklist to determine patients' current needs. Patients reported needs in many physical areas, including anorexia and pain. Nineteen of the 26 had depression but had not disclosed this. Bergen[8] evaluated the care given by 18 district nurses to nine terminally ill patients. All the nurses identified pain as being a problem, but patients' concerns about mobility, tiredness, swelling, and constipation were underreported by the district nurses. There was also serious underreporting of mood disturbance.

Heaven and Maguire[9] assessed the ability of hospice nurses to elicit the concerns of newly admitted terminally ill patients. They recorded each of the nurses' interviews to permit later rating of the concerns elicited from the patients. An independent research nurse then used a checklist to elicit patients' concerns. Only two in every five of patients' main concerns (a sum of those elicited by the nurse and the research nurse) were elicited, although most of the patients had only a few weeks to live. Patients who were clinically anxious and depressed as judged by their scores on the Hospital Anxiety and Depression Scale were least likely to disclose their concerns to the nurses.

Current evidence suggests, therefore, that doctors and nurses involved in caring for the terminally ill have difficulty determining the information needs of patients, eliciting their concerns, and responding to them appropriately. Recent work also indicates that relatives' concerns often go undisclosed.[10] The reasons for these deficiencies need to be considered.

REASONS FOR DEFICIENCIES IN DOCTOR-PATIENT COMMUNICATIONS

Patient-Led Reasons

Patients do not disclose their concerns because they believe that any problems that develop are an inevitable consequence of their disease and treatment[3] and that nothing can be done to remedy them. Hence, there is no point in mentioning them to a doctor or nurse.

Paradoxically, the more patients grow to like and respect the health-care professionals looking after them, the more they are concerned about burdening them and upsetting them unnecessarily. So, they actively avoid disclosing problems. They fear that they will be judged inadequate if they admit that are struggling to cope with their predicament. They claim that they would have disclosed their problems if the health professional had talked to them in a way that indicated it was legitimate to disclose their concerns. They reported that questions about how they were feeling and reacting to their predicament were asked only rarely. When faced with this lack of appropriate questioning, some patients tried to give verbal and nonverbal cues about their concerns. They said that their cues were met by responses that made them feel that health professionals were not interested in pursuing these concerns any further (i.e., by distancing strategies).

Relatives give similar reasons for nondisclosure. They also feel that their concerns have less priority than those of the patients and that they have no right to bother anyone with their concerns.[10]

Health Professionals—Led Problems

Doctors and nurses admit readily that they are reluctant to ask cancer patients questions that would encourage patients and relatives to disclose their concerns.[3] In a longitudinal study of 186 mastectomy patients, no doctors or nurses asked any woman how she had felt about losing a breast. Faced with this lack of inquiry, the women believed, albeit wrongly, that doctors and nurses were not interested in their reactions to surgery. This reluctance to ask appropriate questions has also been found in terminal care.[9] Nurses working in two hospices were loathe to ask the kinds of questions that would educate patients that it was legitimate to mention concerns about psychological or social issues. Patients were reluctant to disclose problems that they believed lay outside the areas the nurses were interested in. Patients believed that the nurses were primarily interested in hearing about physical symptoms like pain and bowel function. They actively withheld giving information about problems like anxiety and depression and concerns about the future, how they might die, becoming a burden to the family, loss of role, and changes in body image. They explained that they wished they could have discussed their concerns and the associated feelings, even when they realized that their concerns, like the fear of dying, were not resolvable.

Wilkinson[5] examined the ability of cancer nurses to determine patients' concerns. She found that more than half of the nurses' utterances had the function of blocking patient disclosure and avoiding getting into patients' feelings. These findings applied as much to patients who were terminally ill as to patients with good prognoses.

To determine how well they could elicit patients' problems,[11] 206 doctors and nurses attending workshops in communication and counseling skills were asked to interview patients.[12] Their interviews were tape-recorded to permit rating of their interviewing behaviors. They used a high proportion of blocking strategies and asked few of the kinds of questions that encourage patients to disclose their concerns. The use of blocking strategies and other inhibitory behaviors bore no relationship to the health professionals' age, experience, or prior training unless that training had addressed specific communication skills directly. Doctors and nurses working in palliative and hospice care exhibited the same profile of interviewing behaviors as doctors and nurses involved in general cancer care. They used interviewing behaviors that inhibited patient disclosure as much or more often than behaviors that promoted it. There are a number of such inhibitory behaviors that discourage patient communication, including normalization, premature reassurance, switching the topic, selective attention, and avoidance.

Inhibitory Behaviors

Normalization. In normalization, the health professional may note correctly that a patient is distressed but, instead of acknowledging the distress and exploring the reasons, dismiss it as understandable and claim it will lessen over time. For example, a 32-year-old mother of two children who was dying of breast cancer was admitted to a hospice for respite care. While the nurse was taking her history, the patient became very distressed and started crying. The nurse responded by saying "You are bound to be distressed. Most people are when they come here at first. I'm sure you'll settle in over the next few days." Her response prevented the patient from disclosing her terrors of how she might die and concerns that her children and husband would be unable to cope without her. This intensified her emotional distress and interfered with pain control.

Premature reassurance. Most doctors and nurses enter their profession because they wish to reduce patients' suffering. They like to "fix" any problem they elicit by offering advice and information immediately. However, if they offer advice and information before they have identified the nature and extent of their patients' current concerns, this will be inappropriate and unhelpful. For example, a woman with terminal cancer explained that she was very worried that her cancer had recurred so soon and spread. She realized that it meant she was dying. She was frightened she might not be able to cope. She was told by a doctor in a hospice, "There is every chance we can keep your disease at bay for some years." The doctor said this because he wished to help the patient feel better in what he perceived to be a terrible predicament. His reassurance was premature and ineffective because he did not first find out what she was worried about. She remained very frightened.

Switching the topic. Objective scrutiny of consultations has shown that health professionals sometimes switch the topic when a patient asks an important but potentially distressing question. Sometimes, this switching is automatic. The health professional is unaware that the topic has been switched. More commonly, health professionals are aware that they changed the subject deliberately. In this example, a social worker met a patient some weeks after she had undergone a mastectomy. When she asked the patient how she was feeling, she said she

"felt terrible." The social worker clarified what she meant by "terrible." The woman said that she could not tolerate the loss of a breast. It had made her feel "ugly and repulsive." It had caused serious problems in her relationship with her husband. Instead of exploring these issues further, the social worker asked the patient, "Have you told your children about your mastectomy?" Although the consultation continued for another 15 to 20 minutes, the social worker did not return to the subject of the patient's body image problems. Consequently, when her disease recurred and became progressive, her body image problems remained.

Selective attention. When patients are asked how they are coping with their predicament, they give verbal and nonverbal cues about any current problems. Health professionals tend to selectively hear and register cues related to physical symptoms that they feel confident they can deal with. When patients also disclose important information about social, psychological, or spiritual problems, these are not heard and recorded.[12]

Avoidance. Health professionals may worry so much about the problems they may encounter if they communicate effectively with dying patients or their relatives and about the distress frank talk might cause that they put off seeing them for as long as possible.

If communication between health professionals and terminally ill patients and their relatives is to be improved, we need to understand why professionals use these distancing strategies so frequently and find other approaches.

REASONS FOR DISTANCING STRATEGIES

Health professionals involved in cancer care have been interviewed to establish why they avoid asking questions that would elicit patients' concerns and information about the impact of the disease and treatment on patients' daily lives, relationships, and mood.[13,14] Three main factors were identified: fear of harming patients psychologically, inadequate training in how to assess patients' concerns and feelings, and lack of available practical and emotional supports.

Fear of harming a patient. Health professionals worry that if they ask questions about how patients feel about their diagnosis and treatment, how the illness is affecting them, and how they see things working out, it will cause psychological harm from which patients will not recover. They fear that patients will become so distressed that the professionals will not be able to help the patients "put the lid back on." They also fear that it will take up too much time and interfere with the smooth running of clinics and wards. Establishing an effective dialogue with patients could lead patients to trust professionals with difficult questions like "Am I dying?," "Will I suffer too much pain?," or "Why was my cancer not diagnosed sooner?" Professionals are also concerned that if they elicit information on the impact of the diagnosis, treatment, and prognosis on patients, this will reveal how much the patients are suffering in their daily lives. This could impair their ability to make crucial decisions about treatment and survive emotionally.

Lack of training. Health professionals involved in palliative and terminal care often acknowledge that they have had little training, if any, in how to assess patients' concerns, perceptions, and reactions. They also feel ill equipped to deal with common but difficult communication tasks like breaking the news that the cancer is incurable, dealing with denial, handling angry patients or relatives, communicating with withdrawn patients, and trying to break collusion when a relative has insisted that the patient should not be told the truth.[15] Few medical schools include formal training in these interviewing skills and communication tasks at either the undergraduate or the postgraduate level. Consequently, health professionals have relied on role models who had no formal training in communication skills.

Lack of practical and emotional support. Wilkinson[5] sought to determine what factors determine whether or not cancer nurses use blocking strategies. Blocking was used significantly less when nurses felt they were being given practical and emotional support by their supervisors. Nurses needed to feel cared for as persons before they were willing to fully assess their patients' problems and associated feelings.

Booth and Maguire,[14] in their study of how well hospice nurses assessed patients, also confirmed that nurses' perception of the support they were receiving was paramount. Unless nurses felt valued as persons by those supervising them, they avoided communicating effectively with patients, even if they had the relevant interviewing skills.

Thus, it can be concluded that if health professionals involved in terminal care are to be effective in identifying patients' and relatives information needs, eliciting their concerns and feelings, and dealing with the difficult situations they encounter, they need help to reduce their fears, relinquish their distancing strategies, acquire the relevant interviewing skills and communication strategies, and know that they will be supported in their endeavors.

IMPROVING PROFESSIONALS' COMMUNICATION SKILLS

Workshops were established to help doctors and nurses involved in cancer, palliative, and hospice care acquire the relevant communication skills and relinquish distancing behaviors.[15] These were limited to 16 to 20 participants and were multidisciplinary in nature. It was hypothesized that helping different health professionals train together would allow barriers resulting from poor communication between members of different disciplines to be discussed and resolved. The workshops were of 3 or 5 days' duration and were residential so that health professionals could devote all their attention to communication.

After the inception of these workshops, participants questioned whether specific communication skills were as important as a nonspecific caring attitude. A study was, therefore, conducted to test hypotheses about which specific skills promoted patient disclosure and which behaviors inhibited it.[11] Those doctors and nurses who were best able to promote patient disclosure could be distinguished from those who obtained the least disclosure on the basis of the number of open directive questions they asked ("How have you been feeling since you have been in the hospital?"); their use of questions with a psychological focus ("How do you see things working out from here?," "How do you feel about being in the hospice?," "How has all this been affecting you in yourself?"); their efforts to clarify cues given by the patient ("You say you are devastated that no more active treatment is available; could you tell me exactly what you mean?"); their expressions of empathy ("No wonder you are so frightened."); and their use of educated guesses ("As we are talking I get the feeling you are much more distressed about knowing your disease is back than you are willing to admit; could I be right?"). In response to such educated guesses the patient can confirm ("Yes, you are right."), refute ("No, that is not right."), or correct ("It is not so much distress as anger. I blame the doctors for not diagnosing it sooner."). Behaviors like offering advice and reassurance before all problems had been elicited and understood were confirmed as inhibiting patient disclosure of key concerns.[11]

While these workshops helped health professionals acquire positive skills and relinquish inhibitory behaviors, they did not eradicate blocking behaviors. While participants obtained much more significant information about patients' problems and feelings, they responded to patients' greater disclosure of concerns and associated feelings by using blocking strategies.[16]

When the reasons for this further blocking were explored in interviews, participants suggested that insufficient attention had been paid to their fears and attitudes about exploring patients' concerns. They remained unconvinced that active inquiry about patients' perceptions and reactions would enhance patients' psychological adjustment. They still worried that it would take up too much time and prevent them giving effective care.[13]

The workshops were modified, therefore, to allow participants more opportunity to practice their skills by reducing the group size to four or five participants plus a trained facilitator. They focused on their feelings and attitudes when blocking and on how to integrate questions about physical and psychological aspects. It has been found that the longer a doctor or nurse spends asking questions about the physical aspects of illness (for example, pain) before asking a question focused on the psychological aspects, the more patients assume that the doctor or nurse is not interested in hearing about psychological, social, or spiritual aspects.

This new style of workshop proved more capable of changing skill levels, attitudes, and feelings in the desired direction than the original format. Feedback from participants at 6-month follow-up confirmed that the strategies being taught worked in daily practice. However, their feedback also highlighted the importance of practitioners' receiving personal and practical support in their work setting if they were to apply their newly acquired skills with patients and relatives.

Razavi and colleagues have also developed communication skills workshops. They restricted members to one discipline (cancer nurses) and paid particular attention to participants' attitudes and feelings about dying. They were able to improve the attitudes of those with negative ideas about dying patients but had little impact on their communication skills.[17] The key question, therefore, is what should be the optimal balance between the attention paid to skills and the attention paid to participants' fears and feelings in communication skills training.

Bandura's theories about changing behavior have suggested that two specific variables merit attention.[13] "Self-efficacy" refers to health professionals' belief that they have the skills to deal with the task. "Outcome expectancy" refers to the belief that using the skill will have a helpful or harmful outcome. Training should, therefore, seek to increase both self-efficacy and outcome expectancy. It should do so by helping health professionals learn strategies that will enable them to deal effectively with the main communication tasks that arise within palliative care.

Key Strategies for Effective Communication

Checking patients' awareness. Most patients with advanced and terminal disease realize the seriousness of their predicament. But it is important, while taking a history of their presenting problems, to check what they perceive to be going on. Thus, you might ask the patient, "Have you any thoughts about what might be the cause of your symptoms?" It is useful to doublecheck by asking "Are there any other reasons why you should think that?" This allows patients who find it too painful to admit that they are aware of their predicament to move back into denial. Most will signal that there are other good reasons why they believe they have a terminal illness. Your task is then to confirm that the patients' perceptions are correct.

From 10% to 20% of patients with a recurrence of cancer or terminal disease are unaware of the gravity of their situation. They may have been misled deliberately about the prognosis by family or professional careers, or they may be in denial. The key task is to decide whether a patient is willing to face the truth without pushing him or her into denial or overwhelming distress. You should proceed, therefore, with the truth-telling process as far as patients indicate they can tolerate it.

Using a hierarchy of euphemisms. First, you can fire a warning shot ("I am afraid that it looks as though things are not so straightforward any more.") The patient can indicate that he does *not* want more information by saying, "I don't want the details. Just tell me if you can do anything for me." Most patients respond by asking, "In what way do you mean not straightforward?" You can reply by saying, "Your tumor is no longer responding to treatment." Your patient may indicate that he or she is not interested in further details but wishes to know whether anything can be done. Most will ask, "What does that mean?" This signals that they are willing to hear that treatment will now be palliative, rather than curative.

In considering how to tailor information to what a patient is ready to know, it is important to avoid being misled by information given in referral letters from other health professionals or by relatives about what they believe the patient has been told or knows. Patients' knowledge of their predicament is dynamic and can change from day to day. It is their perceptions that are all-important and that govern their behavior. So, it is important to check out with patients what their perceptions are rather than ask, "Why did the doctor tell you was going on?"

Pausing after bad news is confirmed or broken. After giving bad news or confirming that the patients' awareness is correct, it is crucial to pause. This allows patients time to assimilate the news and become distressed. You should acknowledge this by saying, "I can see that what I have told you has made you very distressed." This explicit acknowledgment may seem banal and unhelpful. However, it indicates to the patients that it is legitimate for them to talk about their reactions. You should then negotiate with patients whether they are prepared to disclose why they are distressed ("Can you bear to tell me exactly what is making you distressed?"). This invitation educates patients that it is legitimate to disclose any concerns that are contributing to their distress but that they also have permission not to talk about their feelings.

Eliciting patients' concerns and feelings. You should then summarize any concerns that are disclosed and determine their true nature and extent before checking whether there are any other concerns. When patients are able to share their concerns and associated feelings, they feel less distressed. Once all the patients' concerns have been elicited, you should summarize them and negotiate the order in which these concerns should be dealt with.

Focusing on the patient's agenda rather than on the doctor's or nurse's agenda has been found to be more productive in terms of promoting disclosure. Henbest and Stewart[18] found that "patient centeredness" was associated with greater disclosure and resolution of patients' concerns. In practice, patients' concerns usually match those that the doctor would have wished to identify and help with.

Acknowledging patients' distress and eliciting the concerns that are causing it before discussing what can be done to help patients with their problems transforms what might have been be overwhelming distress to distress of tolerable levels. Most patients understand that their disease cannot be cured. It helps to acknowledge this by saying, "In discussing your concerns, I have to acknowledge that the one thing I am unable to do is to eradicate your disease. You may, therefore, feel that dealing with your other concerns is a waste of time. However, I suggest we look at each of your concerns to determine how we might deal with them."

However well patients' information needs are established and responded to and their resulting concerns and associated feelings elicited and resolved, the health professional will still encounter communication tasks that are difficult to deal with.[19] These include the following:

Difficult Communication Tasks

Handling Difficult Questions

Doctors and nurses who work with patients with advanced and terminal cancer often worry that they will be asked difficult questions, for example, "Am I dying?" Does the patient want reassurance that death is not imminent (because he wants to deny the reality of the illness) or the truth? Only the patient can indicate the direction he or she wishes to follow. You can check this by asking, "I will answer your question, but would you first mind telling me why you are asking me that question?" It should then become clear whether the patient is asking the question because he or she has guessed what is going on and wants confirmation of it or wishes to remain in denial.

When patients realize that they have a poor prognosis, they are likely to be concerned about the uncertainty of their predicament. The problem is how to help them cope with this without becoming demoralized.

Handling Uncertainty

When asked "How long have I got,?" it is tempting to give a finite answer ("Oh, 3 months.") or a range ("Anything from 1 month to 6 months."). These predictions are inaccurate, usually err on the optimistic side, and can cause serious problems. Patient pace themselves according to the time they believe is left. If they deteriorate earlier than expected and are prevented from dealing with unfinished business, they may feel cheated. Relatives can find an unexpectedly prolonged survival (borrowed time) hard to cope with because they have used up all their physical and emotional resources. So, it is best to acknowledge the uncertainty.

DOCTOR: You asked me how long he has. The trouble is I just don't know. This uncertainty must be awful for you.

MRS. W: It is. It is terrible knowing that he is going to die but not knowing when. Could it be before Christmas?

DOCTOR: That's the trouble. I don't know how long it will be. I wish I could tell you.

Then check whether the relative or patient wishes to know more about the signs and symptoms that might herald further deterioration.

DOCTOR: What I could do, but only if you agree, is tell you what changes could suggest he is beginning to deteriorate further and approaching death.

MRS. W: I think that would help me.

DOCTOR: He will probably complain of feeling more breathless and weak, go off his food, and lose weight.

You can then encourage the relative to put the time before these markers emerge to good use.

DOCTOR: As long as there are no signs like that, I think you can take it his illness is static. So, try to make the most of this time if you can. Is there anything in particular you would like to do with the time?

You should also provide a lifeline by adding that you are prepared to check the patient regularly and negotiate the frequency of checkups.

You can then explain that if any of these potential markers occur, you can be contacted immediately. This gives patients and relatives confidence that they have rapid access to expert help. Few patients or relatives will abuse this offer. Some patients and relatives who face this uncertainty indicate that they do not want any markers. They are able to put their concerns to the back of their minds until events occur that trigger further worry.

Breaking Collusion

It is claimed that relatives withhold the truth from patients because they cannot face the pain of what is happening and wish to deny it. More commonly, it is an act of love. Relatives cannot bear to cause anguish to their loved ones. Approaching collusion from this perspective makes it possible to respect relatives' reasons and work positively with them. The first step is to acknowledge the collusion, then explore and validate the reasons for it.

DOCTOR: You have told me that you don't feel Richard ought to know that he is dying. Why do you feel that?

MRS. P: I am terrified he will fall apart and give up. I couldn't bear that.

DOCTOR: You know him best, and you could be right. Are there any other reasons why you feel he shouldn't be told?

MRS. P: No, I don't think so.

DOCTOR: So, you have good reasons for keeping the truth from him?

MRS. P: Yes.

You should next check out if there are any emotional costs being incurred because of the collusion.

DOCTOR: Can I ask what effect this has been having on you personally?

MRS. P: It has been a terrible strain. I am feeling extremely tense and getting a lot of nightmares.

DOCTOR: Would you like to tell me about your nightmares?

MRS. P: He seems to be wasting away.

DOCTOR: That is what could happen, isn't it, given that he is dying?

MRS. P: (In tears) Yes, it is. I am very worried about it.

DOCTOR: It sounds like you are finding it a great strain.

MRS. P: Yes, it is. It is a big strain. I worry he's going to guess. He has already commented that I seem quieter than usual.

DOCTOR: Just how tense have you been?

MRS. P: At times I feel I am at screaming point. I am taking it out on the children. I'm so irritable.

DOCTOR: Are you experiencing any other problems because of not telling him?

MRS. P: Yes. We're not talking together like we used to. I would like to be extra-loving to him, but if I am, he will guess. He says I am backing off. It is horrible. Just when I want to be close to him, a great barrier is growing between us.

DOCTOR: So, there are two good reasons for us trying to consider together if there is some other way of dealing with this—first, the emotional strain on you, and, second, its effect on your relationship with your husband.

MRS. P: Yes.

DOCTOR: So, would you like me to suggest how we might be able to do something about it?

MRS. P: But you are not going to tell him, are you?

DOCTOR: No. What I am going to discuss does not involve telling him. Would you like to go into it with me?

MRS. P: Yes, I would.

You should now indicate you would like to chat with her partner to check whether he has any idea of what is happening to him. You should emphasize that you have no intention of telling him and enter a contract to this effect.

DOCTOR: Let me emphasize that I have no intention of telling him. I would simply like to check how he sees his situation. This may reveal that he knows that his cancer is untreatable. If that is the case, there is no reason to maintain the pretense.

MRS. P: But you're not going to tell him, are you?

DOCTOR: No, I am not. I will simply check whether he knows.

Your next task is to establish her partner's level of awareness. You should ask an appropriate directive question that elicits his view of what is happening and then explore the cues he gives.

DOCTOR: I wanted to have a chat with you to see how you feel things are going.

MR. P: Not very well.

DOCTOR: Not very well?

MR. P: Isn't it obvious! They are not giving me any treatment. I have less and less energy. I'm losing weight and am even more breathless.

DOCTOR: What are you making of this?

MR. P: It's the end, isn't it?

DOCTOR: Are there any other reasons why you think it is the end?

MR. P: I have always known I had cancer, even though they didn't tell me. Now I am beginning to think I haven't long to live.

DOCTOR: It sounds as though you have known for some time what is happening?

MR. P: Yes, but I didn't want to upset my wife by talking about it. She has enough on her plate with me being ill and the children to cope with.

You should confirm that the patient is right in his perception ("I am afraid you are right") and seek permission to convey this awareness to his wife. You can then negotiate with the couple to see if they wish to talk with you to share their current concerns or wish to be left alone.

Breaking collusion is painful because you witness the love between a couple and the emotional impact of the threatened loss. It is important to break collusion as soon as it becomes a problem. Otherwise, important unfinished business will be left unresolved, and patients are likely to become morbidly anxious and depressed. This mental suffering lowers the threshold at which patients experience physical symptoms like pain and sickness and can hinder symptom relief. Being left with important practical and emotional unfinished business makes it more difficult for relatives to resolve their grief. They may then develop major psychiatric morbidity.

Challenging Denial

Patients use denial as a defense when the truth is too painful to bear. So, it should not be challenged unless it has created serious problems for the patient or relative. In challenging denial, it is important to be gentle so that fragile defenses are not disrupted but to be firm enough that any awareness can be explored and developed. Begin by asking patients to give an account of what has happened since their illness was first discovered, and explore how they felt at each key point, for example, when they first developed symptoms, saw a specialist, were tested, and were informed about the results. You should also explore their perceptions about what is wrong. This may provide glimpses of doubt: "I was certain it was just an ulcer; at least I am pretty sure it is." By repeating "pretty sure?" you may prompt the patient to say, "Well, I suppose there could be some doubt. It may mean my cancer is back." Sometimes patients are ambivalent about whether they want to face reality. It is useful to confront this by saying, "It looks as though part of you prefers to believe that it is not serious, but another part of you is willing to consider your cancer is back and not responding to treatment. Which part of you should I relate to?"

If this strategy fails, it is important to challenge any incongruence between the patient's experiences and perceptions.

> DOCTOR: You say you are far bigger in this pregnancy than your two previous ones. Have you considered why this might be?
>
> MRS. J: I thought it was one of those things. I didn't think any more about it.
>
> DOCTOR: Are you sure?
>
> MRS. J: Yes, I am sure it is a normal pregnancy.

This patient had advanced ovarian cancer, and no active treatment could be offered. She was in denial and insisted that the symptoms were normal sequelae of pregnancy.

If challenging inconsistencies fails to dent denial, check whether there is a "window" on it. "I can understand that you think it is an infection. Is there any time, even a moment, when you consider it may not be so simple?" If the patient says no, you should accept that the patient finds it too painful to accept what is happening. Alternatively, the patient may admit, "Yes, there is. Sometimes I feel it could be something sinister." Exploring what the patient means by "sinister" may help him or her acknowledge that something more serious than an ulcer is present. This will help the patient shift from denial into relative or full awareness of the illness or prognosis. Any concerns can then be elicited.

CONCLUSION

If health professionals who work with the terminally ill wish to validate or improve their communication skills, they need opportunities to assess how well they elicit patients' concerns and deal with difficult communication tasks. This can be done by asking them to practice these tasks in role play or by having them interview simulated or real patients and relatives and recording these interviews on audiotape or videotape and offering constructive feedback about their performance.[16] As discussed earlier, training also needs to focus on any blocking behaviors, the attitudes and feelings that underlie these, and the health professionals' perceptions of their "self-efficacy" and outcome expectancy.[13] Such training may also reduce the risk of burnout (high emotional exhaustion, low personal accomplishment, and high depersonalization), which has been linked to health professionals' feeling their lack of key communication skills.[19]

References

1. Fallowfield LJ, Hall A, Maguire GP, Baum M. Psychological outcomes of different treatment policies in women with early breast cancer outside a clinical trial. *BMH*, 1990; 301:575–580.
2. Parle M, Jones B, Maguire P. Maladaptive coping and affective disorders in cancer patients. *Psychological Medicine*, 1996; 26:735–744.
3. Maguire P. Barriers to psychological care of the dying. *British Medical Journal*, 1985; 291:1711–1713.
4. Seale C. A comparison of hospice and conventional care. *Social Sciences and Medicine*, 1991; 32(2);147–152.
5. Wilkinson S. Factors which influence how nurses communicate with cancer patients. *Journal of Advanced Nursing*, 1991; 16:677–688.
6. Higginson I, Wade A, McCarthy M. Palliative care: views of patients and their families. *British Medical Journal*, 1990; 301:277–281.
7. Hockley J, Dunlop R, Davis R. Survey of distressing symptoms in dying patients and their families. *British Medical Journal*, 1988; 296:1715–1717.
8. Bergen A. Evaluating nursing care of the terminally ill in the community: a case study approach. *International Journal of Nursing Studies*, 1992; 29(1):81–94.
9. Heaven CM, Maguire P. Training hospice nurses to elicit patients' concerns. *Journal of Advanced Nursing Studies*, 1996; 23:280–286.
10. Harrison J, Haddad P, Maguire P. The impact of cancer on key relatives: a comparison of relative and patient concerns. *European Journal of Cancer*, 1995; 31A:1736–1740.

11. Maguire P, Booth K, Elliott C, Hillier V. Helping cancer patients disclose their concerns. *European Journal of Cancer*, 1996; 32A:78–81.

12. Heaven C, Maguire P. Disclosure and identification of concerns by hospice patients and their identification by nurses. *Palliative Medicine*, 1997; 11:283–290.

13. Parle M, Maguire P, Heaven C. The development of a training model to improve health professionals skills, self-efficacy and outcome expectancies when communicating with cancer patients. *Social Science and Medicine*, 1997; 44:231–240.

14. Booth K, Maguire P, Butterworth A, Hillier V. Perceived professional support and the use of blocking behaviours by hospice nurses and professional support. *Journal of Advanced Nursing*, 1996; 24:522–527.

15. Maguire P, Faulkner A. How to improve the counselling skills of doctors and nurses involved in cancer care. *British Medical Journal*, 1988; 297:847–849.

16. Maguire P, Booth K, Elliott C, Jones B. Helping health professionals involved in cancer care acquire key interviewing skills: The impact of workshops. *European Journal of Cancer*, 1996; 32:1486–1489.

17. Razavi D, Delvaux N, Farvacques C, Robaye E. Immediate effectiveness of brief psychological training for health professionals dealing with terminally ill cancer patients: a controlled study. *Social Science and Medicine*, 1988; 27:386–375.

18. Henbest RJ, Stewart M. Patient centeredness in the consultation. 2: Does it really make a difference? *Family Practice*, 1990; 7:28–33.

19. Ramirez AJ, Graham J, Richards MA, Cull A, Gregory WM. Mental health of hospital consultants. *Lancet* 1996; 347:724–728.

21

Burnout and Symptoms of Stress in Staff Working in Palliative Care

Mary L. S. Vachon, R.N., Ph.D.

From the early days of the hospice/palliative-care movement, stress in staff members was identified as a potential problem,[1,2] and mechanisms, particularly staff support,[3] were put into place in order to decrease staff stress. A recent review of the literature[4] has shown that, in part as a result of organizational policies and support mechanisms, levels of stress and burnout among workers in palliative care probably lower than those experienced by caregivers in other specialty areas, but that is not to say that stress and burnout are not issues that merit attention in order to manage stress in the future. Studies have shown that approximately one-quarter of palliative-care staff report symptoms that indicate psychiatric morbidity and burnout.[5–7] Although the levels of stress may be lower than those of caregivers in oncology and other medical specialties,[5,8,9] nevertheless the sources of stress must be addressed in order to maintain palliative-care staff functioning at the highest possible level.

OVERVIEW

Caregiver stress can derive from many sources but can be seen to be the result of the interaction between the person and the environment.[10] The underlying principle of this model is that adap-

tation is a function of the "goodness of fit" between the characteristics of the person and those of the work environment. "Fit" is the mesh between the needs of the individual and the supplies or resources available within the environment and/or the abilities of the individual and the demands made by the work environment. In part, fit is determined by the extent to which environmental supplies are available to meet individual needs and values; it is also determined by the ability of the person to manage the environment.[11]

PERSONAL VARIABLES

Demographic Variables

Younger caregivers have been found to perceive more stress,[12] to report more stressors, to exhibit more manifestations of stress and fewer coping strategies,[13] and to be more prone to burnout.[14,15] In a study, done in the United Kingdom, that compared clinical oncologists (formerly known as radiotherapists), medical oncologists, and palliative care specialists, burnout was associated with being under age 55.[5] When this study was expanded to include other hospital consultants (gastroenterologists, surgeons, radiologists, and oncologists), being age 55 or younger was identified as an independent risk factor for burnout.[16] Increased job satisfaction was found to be associated with older age,[17] although older staff members may be more sensitive to a gap between their real and their ideal work situation, and, if such a gap occurs, older caregivers might be more vulnerable to stress reactions.[9]

Being married and having more children was associated with better job satisfaction in a Swedish Study,[17] although those with more responsibility for dependents, either children or elderly parents, reported more stress in an American study.[12] Being single was an independent risk factor for burnout in the study of consultants in the United Kingdom.[16]

There is some evidence that female physicians may be more at risk of mental health problems,[18] although male, but not female, oncologists were at more risk of burnout in a Finnish study of physicians from many specialties.[19]

Personality Variables

Hospice workers have been found to be more deeply religious than other caregivers[20] and to ground their work in self-awareness and a clear personal philosophy.[21] Working with dying patients has been found to shape one's attitude toward death and dying.[22] Those who coped adequately with death were found to have a tendency to live in the present, rather than the past or future. They scored higher on inner-directedness, self-actualizing value, existentiality, spontaneity, self-regard, self-acceptance of aggression, and capacity for intimate contact.[23]

The death anxiety of hospice workers was found to be within the norm for the general population, and those who exhibited a "higher sense of purpose in life" tended to score lower on death anxiety.[24] Death anxiety was found to correlate significantly with the severity of job stress for medical-surgical but not for hospice nurses[25] and was negatively correlated with time competence, inner-directedness, self-regard, and self acceptance.[23]

Psychological characteristics such as self-esteem and a sense of mastery have been shown to be effective in sustaining staff against the emotional distress associated with palliative work.[26,27] The personality characteristic of hardiness[28,29] does not appear to have been studied in hospice work, but

has been found to be associated with decreased rates of burnout in oncology nurses[30] and was associated with improved coping in house officers at Memorial Sloan-Kettering Cancer Center.[31] Hardiness is said to lead to perception, interpretation, and successful handling of stressful events which prevent excessive activation of arousal and therefore result in fewer symptoms of stress.[32] Nurses who experienced higher degrees of burnout reported a lack of a sense of control over external events.[30]

Social Support

Social support was identified early as crucial to survival in palliative-care work, and the existence of a good support system was seen as one of the qualities of the ideal palliative-care nurse.[33] Hospice nurses have been found not to differ significantly in social support from critical-care nurses.[8] High levels of mental ill health in hospice nurses were, however, found to be predicted by a lack of social support.[34] A reciprocal relationship between hospice nurses and patients has been found to be crucial to the development of an empathic relationship.[35] Such reciprocal relationships could place staff at an increased risk of difficult grief reactions.

Stressful Life Events

Stressful life events may serve as a source of strength as well as act as stressors. Caregivers have been found to have higher than average levels of deprivation in their childhood.[36] Successful resolution of previous stressful life events can give one strength to bring to the workplace. However, unresolved previous stressful life events, such as the death of a parent, a history of sexual abuse, or family alcoholism, can leave the caregiver vulnerable to stress reactions in his or her professional practice.[37]

Recent personal bereavement and unresolved grief from deaths that occurred prior to the worker's coming into a children's hospice were associated with high stress on the General Health Questionnaire,[7] and a study of palliative-care nurses and administrators found a significant correlation between job satisfaction and absence of loss in the preceding year.[12] Concurrent stressors of caregivers[13] included illness or bereavement in the caregiver's personal support system, problems within marriage or other relationships, and personal concerns such as divorce, health problems, and family problems. Caregivers reported that sometimes these personal stressors interfered with their ability to perform their work, while at other times they felt that the work situation allowed them to avoid thinking about their personal problems.

ORGANIZATIONAL VARIABLES

Constant exposure to death and loss may leave caregivers with grief overload and considerable distress. Caregivers may be more vulnerable to feelings of loss, grief, and distress because they identify with particular patients or families, because they are experiencing concurrent stressors or previous unresolved losses in their own life, because they invest too much in the work situation or because they experience problems within the work environment resulting from work overload, team conflict, administrative problems, or role conflict. Yet, problems related to patient/family interaction are generally not the major problem of those working in palliative care.

Work Environment

A recent review of the literature on worker stress in palliative care found that environmental stressors are generally more common than stressors related to caring for dying persons and their families.[4] Team communication problems were identified early in the field and continue to be an ongoing problem. The problems included a lack of support from colleagues,[26,27] which has been implicated in high levels of depression.[34] Colleagues have been found to be a major source of stress as well as a major stress reducer.[12–14,26,27,34]

Communication problems with others in the health-care system, including workers in other departments, general practitioners, and staff at other hospices, have been a recognized problem and may become worse with the current economic climate.[37] Internationally, caregivers report problems in trying to position their hospice/palliative-care programs within the changing health-care environment. Rivalries are encountered as programs try to determine with which agencies, if any, they will have preferred partner arrangements. The aggressive marketing techniques of

some hospice programs have resulted in conflicts among the programs existing in and/or developing within some communities. This problem is undoubtedly more pronounced in the United States, given the current climate of rapid changes in health care imposed by managed care and other economic forces.[37]

Hospital-based palliative-care physicians reported more stress and less satisfaction from their management than did their colleagues working in hospices.[18] Other environmental stressors included communication problems with administration, the nature of the system, with its constant exposure to dying patients, and inadequate resources. Communication problems with administration involved conflicts between nursing staff and administration reported by hospice matrons;[38] problems dealing with bureaucracy;[12] a lack of management support;[38] and participation on management committees and administrative duties (reported by hospice matrons and medical directors).[39]

The struggle around decision making in the British context is reflected in the fact that hospice medical directors rated their relationships with the matron as being most problematic.[39] "Encountering difficulties in relationships with nurses" was the only aspect of work in which palliative-care physicians reported more stress than their colleagues in other specialties. This was hypothesized to derive in part from the lack of role clarity in the roles of consultants and senior nurses in palliative care, since historically some charity-funded hospices were run by matrons.[18] Hospice matrons report a lack of participation in decision making and planning,[38] and a lack of decision-making authority was implicated in high levels of depression among British hospice nurses.[34]

On a more positive note, no organizational factors tested were related to burnout in a large American study,[14] and both hospice and hospital nurses reported *less* stress than nurse managers on two workload measures.[34]

Role Stressors

The role of the hospice nurse has been described as consisting of primary and secondary work effort.[40] Primary work effort consists of providing supportive care to patients and families and facilitating the work of other professionals. The impediments to preserving one's own integrity in the primary work effort of the palliative-care support team nurse are seen as being the limitations of the system, intrapersonal conflict, interpersonal conflict, and the characteristics of palliative care. The secondary work effort of palliative-care nurses involves attempting to overcome the impediments to preserving one's own integrity through role adaptation, intrapersonal conflict management, and interpersonal conflict management.

Role strain, or difficulty in performing various aspects of one's professional role, for the most part, involved difficulty dealing with the constant effort to cope with the needs of dying persons and their families.[13] Staff reported difficulty in fulfilling their own performance expectations and felt pressured into a continuous commitment of time and energy to care for the dying because of the belief that the time to care is brief and the process happening at the moment is the only meaningful measure of having cared well for this patient.[40] They reported struggling to narrow the gap between "real" and "ideal" as well as straddling the caring-versus-curing dilemma, the stress flowing from the diffuse demands of home care, and the challenge of being both a professional and a friend.[41]

Role strain was experienced by palliative-care physicians, 35% of whom felt insufficiently trained in communication skills and 81% of whom felt insufficiently trained in management skills. Burnout was more prevalent among consultants who felt insufficiently trained in communication and management skills.[18]

Role strain also involved feelings of isolation reported by matrons;[38] the burden of working with volunteers, who were seen as extra people;[23] the sense of status ambiguity experienced by volunteers;[42] and feelings of being inadequately prepared for one's role.[22,42] Feeling inadequately prepared to deal with the emotional needs of patients and families and feeling that the nursing care offered was purposeless was associated with high stress scores.[43] Burnout in medical specialists, including palliative-care physicians, was associated with feeling insufficiently trained in communication and management skills.[16]

Role overload and its effect on home life made the greatest contribution to the job stress of palliative-care physicians. However, palliative-care physicians reported less stress from overload then did other specialists.[18]

Role ambiguity exists when there is a lack of clear, consistent information about what is expected of a person in a role or when an individual does not understand what others expect of someone in that role.[13,44] Role ambiguity can result when professional roles and responsibilities are not defined clearly enough or when the boundaries between the role of professional and that of friend in relationships with palliative-care patients and families are not clearly understood. In general, the more ambiguity one experiences in one's role, the more one is subject to tension and anxiety. Furthermore, most people want less role ambiguity than they have.[13,45]

Role conflict can result when a person holds two or more roles and the demands of one role conflict with the demands of the other. Such conflict was found between hospice work and family obligations in several studies.[12,13,22,34] Feeling overloaded and the effect of such feelings on the physician's home life has recently been found to have the greatest impact on the work stress of palliative-care physicians.[18]

Patient/Family Stressors

Not unexpectedly, stress can be associated with caring for dying patients,[1,2,13,33,41] although stress may now be somewhat reduced composed to levels in the early days of the palliative-care movement. Palliative-care physicians report less stress than other consultants from aspects of work involving communicating with patients and relatives in difficult situations, and having good relationships with patients, relatives, and staff was regarded as their greatest source of job satisfaction.[18]

The need to deal with death and dying and inadequate preparation to deal with the emotional needs of patients and families was associated with higher stress scores in nurses,[43] while for palliative-care physicians and oncologists, increased risk of burnout was associated with feelings of being inadequately trained in communication skills.[5] The final relationship and death trajectory were related to higher depression scores in nurses.[34] In a study comparing ICU, hospice, and medical-surgical nurses, hospice and ICU nurses perceived significantly more stress related to death and dying.[46] When hospice nurses were compared with medical-surgical nurses, hospice nurses were significantly higher on the death and dying dimension of the Nursing Stress Scale. For medical-surgical but not for hospice nurses, death

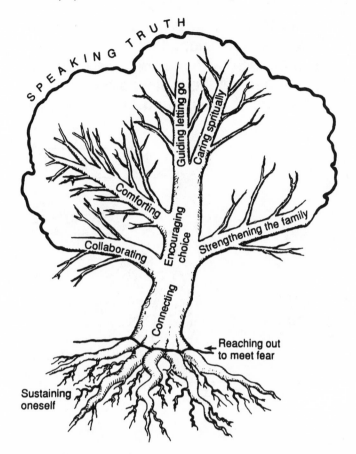

Figure 21.1 A Visual Model of Hospice Nursing

anxiety was significantly correlated with death and dying as a source of stress.[25]

Zerwekh has recently identified nursing practice competencies of hospice nurses and developed a visual model that uses a tree with roots to represent the practice of hospice nursing (see Figures 21.1 and 21.2).[47] At the root of hospice care giving is Sustaining Oneself as a Nurse (Figure 21.1). Reaching Out to Meet Fear grows out of these roots into the crown of the tree where it emerges from the ground. Reaching Out to Meet Fear involves the process of showing courage in facing the turmoil and apprehension that so often accompany dying. "Connecting with patients and loved ones is visualized as the trunk extending upwards, Encouraging Choice extends out of the trunk, and all other competencies spring from this center. Speaking Truth determines all branches of competencies. Collaborating, Strengthening the Family, Comforting, Spiritual Caring,

and Guiding Letting Go are the major competencies that branch from Encouraging Choice."[47] Figure 21.2 illustrates sources and processes by which hospice nurses can sustain themselves and continue to be the root of hospice care. As hospice caregivers struggle to define what they are doing in the process of caring, knowledge is gained, understanding can be improved, and skills can be taught to enable caregivers to be involved without being destroyed by constant exposure to death and grief.

BURNOUT AND SYMPTOMS OF STRESS

Caring does have its costs. The constant exposure to death and to the grief of terminally ill persons and their families; the need for caregivers to care and to let go while experiencing their own

The root is below ground and holds the tree in position. It draws sustenance from the soil. The crown is the neck of the root where it emerges above ground.

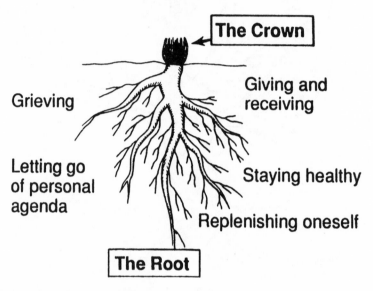

Grieving

Giving and receiving

Letting go of personal agenda

Staying healthy

Replenishing oneself

The Crown

The Root

Figure 21.2 The Root of Hospice Caregiving

grief and coping with the stressors of the work environment can lead to stress and burnout among palliative-care workers, particularly for vulnerable caregivers. It is important to recognize one's own vulnerability to burnout and to recognize the signs of stress if one hopes to avoid burning out.

Burnout

Burnout* is the most common outcome variable used to measure stress in palliative care.[48] Burnout has been characterized as "the progressive loss of idealism, energy, and purpose experienced by people in the helping professions as a result of the

---

*The section on burnout is adapted from MLS Vachon, Staff stress in hospice/palliative care: a review, *Palliative Medicine*, 1995; 9:91–122, and MLS Vachon, Stress and burnout in oncology, in A Berger, MH Levy, RK Portnoy, DF Weissman (Eds.), *Principles and Practices of Supportive Oncology*. Philadelphia: JB Lippincott Company, in press.

conditions of their work."[49(p14)] Burnout has also been described as a syndrome of responses involving increased feelings of emotional exhaustion, negative attitudes toward the recipients of one's service (depersonalization), a tendency to evaluate oneself negatively with regard to one's work, and a feeling of dissatisfaction with one's accomplishments on the job.[30,50]

Burnout is generally seen to result from the interaction between the needs of a person to sacrifice himself or herself for a job and a job situation that places inordinate demands on an individual (see Table 21.1). The person who is likely to develop burnout may well have unrealistically high personal expectations for satisfaction in a given area of life. The phenomenon can occur not only in an individual but also within a system.[49,51]

Pines[52] proposed a social-psychological model of burnout in which certain characteristics of the work environment are seen as contributing to burnout. According to her model, professionals with a high level of motivation can either achieve

Table 21.1   The Burnout Personality

Thrives on intensity
Sets self up to lurch from crisis to crisis
Functions best under pressure
   Crisis occurs
   Girds for action
   Adrenalin flows
   Senses come to life
   Feels alert, powerful, acutely tuned,
     unconquerable
   After triumph, feels deep melancholy

peak performance if working within a positive environment or develop burnout symptoms if the individual continues to confront a stressful, discouraging environment. Individual differences determine how soon an individual develops burnout and how extreme the experience may be.[53]

The most commonly used instrument to measure burnout is the Maslach Burnout Inventory [MBI],[54] which measures emotional exhaustion, depersonalization, and a lack of personal accomplishment on two dimensions, frequency (how often a feeling occurs) and intensity (the strength of that feeling). Using the MBI in the study of hospital consultants in the United Kingdom,[5,16,18] researchers found that the burnout rate was lower for palliative-care specialists than for other specialists. Radiologists reported the highest level of burnout in terms of personal accomplishment. Both burnout and psychiatric morbidity were found to be associated with feelings of being overloaded and the effect of this feeling on palliative-care providers' home lives, a sense of being poorly managed and resourced, and the need to deal with patients' suffering. Burnout was also associated with low levels of satisfaction derived from relationships with patients, relatives and staff; low levels of satisfaction derived from professional status/esteem; and low levels of satisfaction derives from intellectual stimulation.[16]

The largest study of burnout in hospice staff was conducted in the early days of the movement and involved 1281 hospice staff surveyed in the National Hospice study.[14,15] The burnout rate was low but was found to be higher in those under 40, those with higher levels of education, those with long tenure, and those who worked full-time. Demographic variables were found to account for nearly 15% of the variance in burnout scores, and occupational characteristics added only 6%.[14]

Turnipseed studied 65 registered nurses and licensed practical nurses working full-time and with patient care responsibilities in hospices in seven states and found they had a low burnout rate, both absolutely and compared to the Maslach Burnout Inventory normative means and standard deviations.[6] Turnipseed suggests and quotes from Pines and Aronson[55] that the reasons for low burnout rates in hospice may be that burnout is the result of "chronic stress of consistent or repeated emotional pressure associated with an intense involvement with people over long periods of time."[66(p112)] He hypothesizes that this may well not be the case for hospice nurses, who report organization or staff support stress more often than stress arising from patients and families.[6] Burnout has also been found to be "associated with work overload, role ambiguity, role conflict, time and staffing limitations, lack of advancement opportunities, poor working relationships, lack of chairperson and peer support, head nurse leadership style, increased demands by patients and families, and frequent exposure to death and dying."[30,p.188]

A comparison of hospice and oncology nurses by Bram and Katz showed that hospice nurses had significantly lower burnout scores than oncology nurses who cared for the terminally ill on hospital-based oncology units.[9] Hospice nurses perceived a greater opportunity to express work-related feelings and to discuss problems in the workplace. A positive relationship was noted between perceived social support at work and lower burnout scores. While hours of direct patient contact have been found to be associated with role overload and thus with burnout, in this study the opposite was found to be true; the fewer the hours of direct contact with patients, Bram and Katz reported, the higher the burnout scores for hospice nurses. The authors hypothesized that hospice nurses were less stressed when they had more time to spend with patients and families.

Other authors have found that, while the stressors involved in the care of the dying and bereaved are undeniable, the major stressors identified as leading to burnout involved relationships with other professionals.[56–59] Table 21.2 lists the signs and symptoms. Compared with critical-care nurses, hospice nurses were less likely to report burnout as reflected in lower levels of emotional exhaustion, less utilization of the technique of depersonalization, and a greater sense of personal

Table 21.2   Signs and Symptoms of Burnout

Fatigue
Physical and emotional exhaustion
Headaches
Gastrointestinal disturbances
Weight loss
Sleeplessness
Depression
Boredom
Frustration
Low morale
Job turnover
Impaired job performance (decreased empathy, increased
    absenteeism)

accomplishment; in addition, they reported less occupational stress and death anxiety.[8]

Distress

Distress* has been measured using the General Health Questionnaire (GHQ).[60] One of the earliest studies in the field found that 3 months after the Royal Victoria Hospital Palliative Care Unit opened, the nursing staff had GHQ scores that were twice as high as those of the nurses on two control units.[1] At 3 months, more than 50% of the Palliative Care Unit nurses reported scores of 10 or more on the 30-item GHQ, on which a score of 5 indicates "caseness." The staff stress declined over the next 10 months, in part because those with the highest GHQ scores tended to leave the unit. The scores of the nurses on the PCU were only slightly lower than those of new widows and were considerably higher than scores of women beginning radiation treatment for a new diagnosis of breast cancer.[2] The scores reported in the RVH study were among the highest reported in the literature and probably reflect the fact that the study was conducted in the early days of the movement and before issues of staff selection and vulnerability were clearly understood.

Using the 60-item GHQ, researchers found no differences between hospice and mental handicap nurses,[43] and three-quarters of the staff in a children's hospice were under little stress as measured by the 60-item GHQ, but a subgroup was under considerable distress, with anxiety, insom-

*The section on distress is adapted from MLS Vachon, Staff stress in hospice/palliative care: a review, *Palliative Medicine*, 1995; 9:91–122.

nia, somatic symptoms, and social dysfunction.[7] In a study of hospice nurses, a "caseness" rate of 10% was reported using the 28-item GHQ, and the length of time working in palliative care was found not to be related to the GHQ score.[22]

Most recently, Ramirez et al.[5,16,18] used the 12-item GHQ in their study of medical consultants. The estimated prevalence of psychiatric disorder from the GHQ was 27% and was not significantly different among the four specialist groups. As noted previously, three specific factors were related to both psychiatric disorder and burnout. These included feelings of being overloaded and the effects of this on home life, feelings of being poorly managed and resourced, and the need to deal with patients' suffering. Job satisfaction significantly protected the consultants' mental health against the adverse effects of job stress.[16]

Overview of Anxiety and Depression

Caregiver anxiety and depression have most often been measured using the Hospital Anxiety and Depression Scale (HAD).[61] Hospice matrons had scores similar to those of other nurse groups, and they were less anxious than policemen. They were slightly more depressed, however, than two other groups. Those with the highest Nursing Stress Scores were more likely to have higher HAD scores.[38] Using the Crown-Crisp Experiential Index,[62] Cooper and Mitchell found that high levels of mental ill health among hospice nurses were predicted by a lack of social support, deep involvement at work, and high workload.[34]

Anxiety has been measured in a number of studies. Researchers found that hospice nurses did not reveal levels of anxiety significantly different from those of mental handicap nurses.[43] Hospice nurses did, however, approach significance on somatic anxiety and were significantly higher than nurse managers on free-floating anxiety and somatic anxiety. Predictors of free-floating anxiety were staff support and involvement in decision making, the nature of the final relationship between the nurse and the dying patient, and employment as a lower-status nurse with fewer postbasic qualifications. Somatic anxiety was correlated with high workload, lack of staff support, and low involvement in decision making.[34]

One study found a tendency to self-medicate; 10% of hospice medical directors and matrons used psychotropic medications, 29% of medical directors and one matron used hypnotics, and one-third used alcohol to relieve stress.[39]

Depressive symptoms were found in many of the hospice medical directors and matrons studied by Finlay et al.[39] Of particular concern in that study was the fact that 16% of the physicians reported suicidal thoughts of more than 2 weeks' duration; 11% of the matrons and 8% of the physicians acknowledged suicidal thoughts of 2 weeks' duration or less.

Depression, Loss, and Grief

Self-reported feelings of depression, grief, and guilt were found to be closely intertwined[13] and were often experienced in response to a loss that involved bereavement. This loss could be the death of a patient but might also reflect a loss of self esteem or the loss of support from one's significant others. The individual meaning that is consciously or unconsciously ascribed to the particular loss determines whether an individual will experience grief.

Identifying strongly with the patient and/or family member can cause the caregiver to become wrapped up in the patient's illness and distress and to experience what Weisman calls "caregiver plight."[63] In this situation the caregiver is so overwhelmed by what is happening to the patient that he or she is no longer able to be objective. Caregivers often identify with patients who remind them of themselves or of people from their past or present life.

Larson has described a similar concept, the Helper's Pit,[64] in which the caregiver can imagine the person being helped as being in a pit with the caregiver on the edge of the pit. If the person on the edge of the pit identifies with the person in the pit, the caregiver can fall into the pit. "If you empathize, you feel *with* the person in the pit and get inside his or her experiential world. If you sympathize, you stand on the edge of the pit and are concerned and compassionate—sympathy is *feeling for* the person in distress" (p. 38).

The multiple losses in hospice are such that if one were to allow oneself to feel the pain of each grief, one would never get beyond acute grief. Data from the AIDS field suggests that the flooding of emotion involved in grief may lead to incapacitation, rather than healing. To defend against this flooding, some people become emotionally numb. Grothe and McKusick[65] suggest

that the alternatives to coping with massive loss may be similar to two phases common in post-traumatic stress syndrome, intrusive-repetitive and denial-numbing. Caregivers may find themselves experiencing feelings of failure if the patient did not receive inadequate pain control or did not have a "good time" before the end; they may become preoccupied with images of those who did not have a "good death," feel overwhelmed by highs and lows of emotion, feel burdened by a sense of responsibility for the quality of life of patients, feel drained of energy because of their desire to reach out to multiple needs, or feel saturated with grief and guilt.[41]

Depression and Burnout: Do They Differ?

Feelings of depression must be distinguished from burnout.* Maslach states that one phase of the burnout syndrome involves a sense of reduced accomplishment and a loss of self-esteem, which is a central characteristic of depression. The loss may be of original ideals or of "good people" to work with. A professional's sense of self-worth and self-esteem may be threatened by the inevitable outcome of patients' deaths and the physical, psychological, and social pain of terminal illness.[54] Caregivers may also feel they have failed at their work or have failed to live up to their original standards.[54] Burnout is generally regarded as being associated with overinvolvement in any one area of life to the exclusion of all others. Usually this is the occupational role.[51]

While the burned-out person may be depressed, the symptoms expressed are not primarily intrapsychic but are at least partially situationally induced. An appropriate evaluation of burnout requires that the possibility of a clinical depression be ruled out. A clinical depression might be suspected if the person has had a recent loss, has the vegetative symptoms of depression, has had a previous history of depression, or has a family history of depression.[66] If the symptoms are worse in the work situation, are associated with conflict or feelings of being misunderstood by colleagues, or are present in a person who tends to work long hours

---

*The section on depression and burnout is adapted from MLS Vachon, Stress and burnout in oncology, in A Berger, MH Levy, RK Portnoy, DE Weissman (Eds.), *Principles and Practices of Supportive Oncology*. Philadelphia: Lippincott, in press.

and/or always takes work home and has no time for outside interests or support from others, then the problem may well be burnout.

Ramirez et al.[5] attempted to distinguish between the phenomenon of burnout and psychiatric disturbance using the MBI and the 12-item GHQ. They found that clinical oncologists were significantly more likely to be identified as burned out than as depressed. The estimated prevalence of psychiatric disorder from the GHQ was 28% and was not significantly different among the three oncology specialty groups. These findings were in accordance with those from other studies.[5] The researchers concluded that, although clinical oncologists experience the greatest amount of work-related stress and had the least satisfaction from work-related sources, they are not at any greater risk of psychiatric disorder than their colleagues. No demographic or job characteristics predicted psychiatric disorder as measured by the GHQ. However, high GHQ scores indicative of psychiatric disorder were associated with high levels of stress from feeling overloaded, and from being involved with treatment toxicity and errors, and with low levels of satisfaction related to having professional status and esteem.[5]

Feelings of helplessness, uselessness, and insecurity may be a part of both burnout and depression but may also occur as temporary symptoms. These feelings often derived from caregivers' unrealistic expectations of themselves and their roles.[13] Those symptoms and situations that left nurses feeling helpless and useless were the most stressful.[22] Staff in a children's hospice experienced a sense of impotence when unable to relieve patients' perceived needs or distress.[7]

COPING

The research on coping with job stress is still limited.* There have been few long-term longitudinal studies of coping. Studies have found that in-

*The section on coping is derived from MLS Vachon, Staff stress in hospice/palliative care: a review, *Palliative Medicine*, 1995; 9:91–122, MLS Vachon, The stress of professional caregivers, in D Doyle, GW Hanks, and N McDonald (Eds.), *Oxford Textbook of Palliative Medicine*, 2nd ed. Oxford: Oxford University Press, in press; In: MLS Vachon, Stress and burnout in oncology, in A Berger, MH Levy, RK Portnoy, DE Weissman, *Principles and Practices of Supportive Oncology*. Philadelphia: Lippincott, in press.

dividual coping is repetitive for certain kinds of fixed stimuli but is flexible in the face of new challenges.[67] The effectiveness of strategies for handling stress and burnout have generally not been studied with reference to their impact on performance, productivity, or client outcome.[59] The work of Graham, Ramirez, et al. is, therefore, helpful in identifying burnout as more prevalent among consultants who feel insufficiently trained in communication and management skills;[18] These respondents reported deriving low satisfaction from relationships with patients, relatives, and staff, low satisfaction related to professional status or esteem, and low satisfaction from intellectual stimulation.

Dealing with job stress is not solely the responsibility of either the individual or the organization. Effective coping strategies require the use of both personal and environmental coping mechanisms. In a multidisciplinary, multispecialty study, caregivers were twice as likely to report that personal coping strategies rather than environmental strategies were helpful in dealing with and preventing occupational stress.[13]

A Sense of Competence, Control and Pleasure from One's Work

In a large international study of occupational stress in caregivers,[13] a sense of competence, control, and pleasure in one's work was the most common coping mechanism for physicians and the second most common for the group as a whole and for those working in palliative care. This sense of competence, control, and pleasure in one's work was often associated with belonging to a team "which knew what it was doing." Through team affiliation, one may derive an ongoing sense of personal worth that survives even if individual patients die.[13]

When asked what it was that motivated them to be able to continue in their stressful jobs, caregivers often said, "The bottom line is that I know what I am doing, and I am good at it." This sense of competence developed through a series of stages in which caregivers developed their professional skills, set goals for themselves, had frequent tests of their competence, proved their competence in many situations, learned that because they were secure in their own competence they could share their competence with others, and eventually were able to report being comfortable living with a sense that they were competent in their work situation.

Along with this sense of competence came the realization that one had a certain degree of control in one's work situation and that one could derive pleasure from work. The sense of competence and control is very similar to Kobasa's Hardy Personality,[28,29] which has been found to be associated with decreased rates of burnout in oncology nurses[30] and improved coping in oncology house officers,[31] as already noted.

The recent findings of Ramirez's group that job satisfaction significantly protected consultants' mental health against the adverse effects of job stress[16] and that palliative-care physicians reported that having good relationships with patients, relatives, and staff made the greatest contribution to their job satisfaction[18] are similar to the earlier findings. In addition, Papadatou et al.[30] have recently suggested that the challenge of working with cancer patients may serve as the reward that counterbalances the stressful aspects of practice in oncology.

In their study comparing oncologists with palliative-care specialists, Ramirez et al.[5] studies 20 sources-of-satisfaction items, which were aggregated into four factors. The satisfaction factor "dealing well with patients and relatives" contributed most to overall job satisfaction; it was followed by "having professional status and esteem," "deriving intellectual stimulation," and "having adequate resources." Overall, clinical oncologists reported the lowest levels of satisfaction for all the factors. Medical oncologists reported higher levels of satisfaction from "deriving intellectual stimulation" than either of the other two groups. Palliative-care specialists reported the highest levels of satisfaction from "dealing well with patients and relatives" and "having adequate resources."

Team Philosophy, Team Building, and Support

When palliative-care staff were compared with those in other specialties, it was found that team philosophy, team building, and team support were the primary coping mechanisms of palliative-care workers, and team conflict was less of a stressor for this group than it was for those in other specialties.[4,13] Research has suggested that there is a relationship between these two findings—that the work hospice caregivers had put into team

building since the inception of the specialty, might have been responsible for the fact that the hospice team buffered more effectively the other stressors caregivers confronted than was the case in other specialties.[68] Help and support from others on the team and a cooperative effort were found to contribute to role fulfillment.[26,27]

Effective teamwork involved belonging to a team that knew what it was doing (team philosophy), knew how to get team members to work toward defined professionals and personal goals (team building), and knew how to support team members through professional and personal stressors (team support).[13]

The environments in which teams work can produce uncertainty, anxiety, and frustration. The inability to manage these feelings can lead to a downward spiral with increasing anxiety and declining job performance. If team members can learn to communicate, support one another, and problem solve, the team will be self-renewing or autotherapeutic. If they fail to communicate and support one another, there will be more anxiety, which will drain team energy and spirit and lead to a downward spiral.[69]

Regular team meetings have been found to be important.[7,41] Such meetings served to set goals for the team, provided a time of evaluation and reflection on the work being accomplished, and allowed for shared decision making. As has already been noted, team dynamics are an ongoing problem. While good relationships with staff were a major source of job satisfaction to palliative-care physicians, difficulties in relationships with nurses was the only aspect of work in which palliative-care physicians had more difficulties than their colleagues in other specialties.[18] Involvement in decision making was of greater consequence to hospice nurses than to nurses in other specialties, possibly because they needed greater emotional support because of the nature of their work.[34] An alternative explanation is that hospice nurses have had a more independent role than those in hospital settings and may resist any action that seems to threaten this role.

The need to work through team dynamics and decision making is crucial, but the process is often not easy. A quote attributed to Dr. Cicely Saunders in the early days of the hospice movement still is true—"If you say you work in a hospice team, you have to be willing to show your battle scars."

Each setting must develop its own approach to dealing with team building and education. One such approach involves continuous education and an organization that stimulates the staff's own initiative but is also capable of support the staff when necessary.[17] Another setting uses the concept of initiating educational meetings whenever there is an issue that causes difficulty for staff. The session allows for an intellectual approach to dealing with the issue and often then leads to discussions of a more personal nature (E. Bruera, personal communication, 1994). Staff support groups have been suggested by many authors,[41,42,70] but for the most part their efficacy has not been evaluated. Other approaches to maintaining effective teams include ongoing monitoring of staff stress to assess the intensity of issues such as stress, satisfaction, and morale, and sharing of nonwork-related social activities as a team.[13,33]

Dealing with Loss and Grief

Both as individuals and as team members, caregivers must learn to deal with their grief. Memorial services and death rounds where caregivers can share what happened at the time of the death reflect on the car given, and lessons learned can be helpful. Memory books, grief and loss seminars and groups,[71] journaling, and participation in memorial projects such as the AIDS quilt can be helpful.

Other techniques that have been shown to be effective in helping staff to deal with multiple losses include:

- Witness the pain—tell the story and express the pain to allow catharsis and healing.
- Help the person to stay involved in something outside himself or herself.
- Assist in the creation of meaningful rituals.
- Provide structure and support when emotional flooding is overwhelming, and utilize action instead of retreating into immobility and fear.
- Refocus on the elevating emotions of joy and hope.[65]

Support from Colleagues

Support from colleagues is very important for hospice workers.[7,13,22,41] In the early days of the hospice movement, support from colleagues, family, and friends was considered to be important, but more recently support from colleagues has been found to be more effective in helping staff deal with work-related stress. Sixty-seven percent of palliative-care nurses used "talking things over with a colleague" as a coping mechanism, compared with 18% of palliative-care nurses who talked with people at home.[22] The overall mental health of hospice nurses was in part predicted by the level of staff support.[34] The association between support from colleagues and low burnout scores for hospice nurses shows the value of providing staff support within the work setting.[9]

Administrative Policies

Inadequate preparation for dealing with communication and management responsibility has been found to be associated with burnout in medical specialists, including those in palliative care and oncology.[5,16,18] Direct observation of doctors and nurses talking with real, simulated, or role-played patients suffering from terminal illness has shown that caregivers consistently use distancing tactics that prevent them from getting close to their patients' psychological suffering. Such techniques are used to ensure the caregiver's emotional survival but serve to discourage patients from disclosing their psychological concerns.[72] Organizations need to consider either providing education in dealing with these issues or making it possible for caregivers to pursue such educational opportunities by providing time off and/or tuition assistance for such programs. Specific attention may need to be directed to younger caregivers.[14,41] Recent publications give specific approaches for dealing with many of these issues,[73,74] as well as for teaching others.[75]

Attempts should be made to clarify the unrealistic expectations that staff members may have of themselves,[76] of hospice care, and of the organization. A need for clear and practical recruitment policies for both volunteers[42] and staff has also been identified.[12] For older hospice nurses, the importance of a congruence between professional ideals and the philosophy of the health care setting has been noted. This factor should be emphasized in the organization's hiring practices.[9]

Clearly defined job descriptions are needed for volunteers;[42] there should be reasonable workloads and on-calls, and overwork should be avoided.[7,12,34] Determining appropriate workloads is particularly important in the current climate of diminishing resources. There is already some evidence that the stressors on those in oncology are changing and that in the 1990s work overload, lack of resources, and staff shortages became the biggest stressors,[77] although caregivers in oncology had earlier been identified as the group most likely to report difficulty with role overload.[13]

As those in palliative care define their role as being involved at an earlier time in the illness trajectory and as they are called on to reduce the pressures on acute-care beds, the issue of work overload may become a bigger stressor and will need to be addressed. The fact that palliative-care physicians working in hospital settings report more stress and less satisfaction from their management and resources than their colleagues working in hospice settings[18] may reflect the economic pressures that currently confront acute-care institutions in many countries.

Administrative policies to address the issues of appropriate workloads will need to be addressed. This might be accomplished in part through a work environment designed to stimulate the staff's own initiative[17] and to allow for shared decisionmaking.[34] It is important that organizational structures, policies, and values at both the institutional and the unit levels support nursing practices that facilitate nurses' engaging in empathic relationships.[35]

There is some evidence that effective administrative policies have been developed in hospice; hospice nurses report significantly higher satisfaction with supervision, coworkers; and pay, although they have significantly lower satisfaction with opportunities for promotion than do mental handicap nurses.[43]

Sustaining Oneself

In order to be able to develop effective relationships with clients without becoming engulfed in their difficulties, it is important for caregivers to have insight into their own personal dynamics and potential areas of difficulty. Personal knowledge can nurture one's empathic capacity.[35] However, caregivers need to learn to avoid excessive involvement with particular clients, which can preclude objective counseling, advice giving, and medical care.

Davies and Oberle speak of the importance of helping hospice nurses to preserve their own integrity. They define this as the ability to maintain feelings of self-worth and self-esteem and to maintain energy levels. Nurses maintain self-esteem by looking inward, by valuing personal worth, and by acknowledging and questioning personal behaviors, reactions, and needs. They maintain energy levels by using particular strategies of distancing to regain self-control, using humor, protecting the self by hiding personal feelings, learning from mistakes, and sharing frustrations.[78] Maintaining a positive attitude in the face of random suffering promotes coping by increasing self-esteem and maintaining a sense of power.[65]

Caregivers needed to recognize that it takes a "total person" to respond day after day to the "total needs" of other people. They need to recognize that they must assume responsibility for meeting their own holistic needs and for recognizing their increased need for nurturing relationships and diversified interests.[41] The recognition of one's own needs requires acknowledging the responsibility to avoid having one's occupational role dominate one's life. Caregivers must be aware of personal needs for overwork and overinvolvement that might lead to emotional exhaustion and burnout.

A personal philosophy regarding illness, death, and one's role in caring for dying persons and their families is essential for the mature caregiver in this field. This philosophy may or may not be related to one's religious and/or spiritual beliefs.[13,21] A factor related to burnout for older, married, more experienced, and more academically educated hospice nurse was the congruence between their professional ideals and the goals, philosophy, and environment of hospice.

Lifestyle Management

Lifestyle management includes having outside activities;[13] engaging in physical activities and diversions;[41,13] organizing nonjob-related social interaction;[33] taking time off; attending to one's needs for nutrition and adequate sleep;[12] and utilizing meditation and relaxation techniques.[13] There is some evidence from AIDS caregivers that "escapist" leisure engagements—those that involve high levels of distraction and allow little capacity for reflection—appear to be ineffective solutions for preventing burnout, particularly the aspect of attentional fatigue that is associated with continued, focused caring. Such escapist leisure activities actually appear to incur negative psychological effects. In contrast, restorative activities—those that engage attention but still provide room for reflection (e.g., walking, gardening)—influence functioning in a positive way and provide for restoration and renewal.[79]

DISCUSSION AND IMPLICATIONS OF FINDINGS

Stress was identified as a problem early in the hospice movement.* Caregivers were found to have GHQ scores that were only slightly lower than those of newly widowed women and higher than those of women with a new diagnosis of breast cancer.[2] The first study to assess burnout found that it was lower than anticipated and suggested, even at that time, that supports, such as team meetings, that had been put into place might have served to decrease the staff stress.[14]

This overview has shown that staff in palliative-care settings have less burnout than do professionals in mental health,[14] oncologists,[5] other medical specialists,[18] oncology nurses,[9] and critical-care nurses.[8] Several studies have used the GHQ to measure distress. While more than 50% of hospice nurses initially reported high GHQ scores,[1] later studies have found from 11%[22] to about one-quarter of hospice nurses[7] experienced high levels of distress. Twenty-seven percent of medical specialists, including palliative-care physicians, had high levels of distress, and there were no significant differences across medical specialties.[16] Nurses in hospice were found to experience less job stress than CCU, ICU, and oncology nurses and had less difficulty dealing with issues of death and dying than did their colleagues in the hospital.[34] Palliative-care physicians had less job stress than did physicians in oncology[5] and other medical specialties,[18] and they were found to have greater job satisfaction.[18] Job satisfaction was found to protect consultants' mental health against the adverse effects of job-related stress.[16] However, consultants who felt insufficiently trained in communication and management skills were at higher risk of burnout.[16]

*The section on discussion and implication of findings is adapted from MLS Vachon, Staff stress in hospice/palliative care: a review, *Palliative Medicine*, 1995; 9:91–122.

Hospice staff were generally found not to be significantly different from other populations with regard to symptoms of anxiety and depression; however those with the highest Nursing Stress Scores were also found to have higher HAD scores.[38] High levels of mental ill health were predicted by a lack of social support, high level of involvement at work, and high workload.[34]

Some areas of concern were the use of drugs and alcohol by and the presence of suicidal ideation in hospice medical directors and matrons.[39] Free-floating anxiety in hospice nurses was found to be associated with job-related issues involving staff support, involvement in decision making, the nature of the relationship between the nurse and the dying patient, and workload.[34] When compared with other medical/surgical nurses, hospice and ICU nurses perceived significantly more stress related to death and dying,[46] and they were higher on the death and dying dimension of the Nursing Stress Scale.[25] Caregivers in hospice may be at higher risk for the experience of loss and grief. Suggestions for dealing with multiple losses were given.

While stress exists in hospice/palliative care, it is by no means a universal phenomenon. That this is the case may in large measure result from the fact that, from the earliest days of the hospice movement, staff support programs and team development were seen as integral to effective palliative care. It was hypothesized even in the early research that these buffers might serve to mitigate the stress that would otherwise be more evident.[13,14,68] The fact that the levels of stress and burnout recorded are not particularly high compared with those of normative groups does not mean that team development, education, and team support mechanisms should be dropped but rather that they should continue and be seen as important buffering mechanisms. In addition, individual caregivers have long realized that they have a responsibility to care for themselves physically, emotionally, and spiritually and to monitor their own reactions to palliative care in order to continue to be able to practice in the field and even to grow and thrive. This realization has probably led many caregivers to do palliative care for a limited period of time or on a part-time basis in order to ensure that they are able to maintain their own mental health. This trend may shift as palliative care becomes a specialty.

The stress that exists currently in palliative care results in large measure from organizational issues, but there is still some difficulty in dealing with issues of death and dying. The phenomenon of burnout in palliative care generally seems not to be a big problem at this point, but some staff members do have problems with anxiety and depression, some of which are probably work related and some of which may reflect personal issues such as problems with low self-esteem, a tendency to become overly involved and to make one's work life the center of one's existence, death anxiety, unresolved previous or concurrent stressors, and difficulty managing loss.

There are probably some caregivers who are at higher risk for having difficulty with stress and burnout in the area of palliative care. These may be those who are younger, have unresolved personal losses, or have low self-esteem and a tendency to derive their identity from their job or career. Those who have more education may be at higher risk,[12,14] but so too may be older staff members who are in settings that are not congruent with their value systems.[9]

The stress of dealing with dying people and their family members is a part of palliative care, and some staff may need additional assistance to deal with the issue. It is important to ensure that caregivers are well educated in communication as well as in management skills.[5,16,18] In service education, the opportunity to have good supervision in early intense relationships with dying patients and their family members, attendance at conferences, and the opportunity to grieve appropriately and to mourn multiple losses are helpful in dealing with issues related to death and loss.

The major problems in palliative care today are probably more related to issues of reimbursement, social problems and economic pressure, government and insurance intervention into the provision of palliative care and the development of services and expectations, conflict and rivalry with other specialties, referral practices, how "active" palliative care should be, team conflict, and the role of hospice in the current health-care environment. While these issues are not totally new to the field, they are assuming increasing importance as we enter the twenty-first century.

Good team communication, team building, and team support remain essential to underpin the work that needs to be done in palliative care. Support from colleagues will be essential as caregivers experience the changes in hospice imposed by increasing fiscal constraints. The time to build bridges to other disciplines and specialties and to work collaboratively is now.

Future research in the area of stress in palliative care might concentrate on the following issues:

- Which types of programs are most effective in buffering stress for which individuals or which types of hospice organizations?
- What is the impact of the changing hospice environment on the experience of staff stress?
- How can "appropriate" workloads be determined in today's health-care environment?
- Given the sensitivity of hospice caregivers to work overload, how can caregivers effectively cope with the changing hospice environment?
- Does extra support for those new to palliative care influence their ability to practice effectively and for longer periods of time?

References

1. Lyall WAL, Rogers J, Vachon MLS. Report to Palliative Care Unit of Royal Victoria Hospital regarding professional stress in the care of the dying. In: *Palliative Care Service Report*. Montreal: Royal Victoria Hospital, 1976:457–468.
2. Vachon MLS, Lyall WAL, Freeman SJJ. Measurement and management of stress in health professionals working with advanced cancer patients. *Death Education*, 1978; 1:365–375.
3. Beszterczey A. Staff stress on a newly developed palliative care service: the psychiatrist's role. *Canadian Psychiatric Association Journal*, 1977; 22: 347–353.
4. Vachon MLS. Staff stress in hospice/palliative care: a review. *Palliative Medicine*, 1995; 9:91–122.
5. Ramirez AJ, Graham J, Richards MA, Cull A, Gregory WM, Learning MS, Snashall DC, Timothy AR. Burnout and psychiatric disorder among cancer clinicians. *British Journal of Cancer*, 1995; 71:1263–1269.
6. Turnipseed DL. Burnout among hospice nurses: an empirical assessment. *Hospice Journal*, 1987; 3: 105–119.
7. Woolley AH, Stein A, Forrest GC, Baum JD. Staff stress and job satisfaction at a children's hospice. *Archives of Disease in Childhood*, 1989; 64:114–118.
8. Mallett K, Price JH, Jurs SG, Slenker S. Relationships among burnout, death anxiety, and social support in hospice and critical care nursing. *Psychological Reports*, 1991; 68:1347–1359.

9. Bram PJ, Katz LF. Study of burnout in nurses working in hospice and hospital oncology settings. *Oncology Nursing Forum*, 1989; 16:555–560.

10. French JRP, Rodgers W, Cobb S. Adjustment as person-environment fit. In: Coelho GV, Hamburg DA, Adams E, eds, *Coping and Adaptation*. New York: Basic Books, 1974:316–333.

11. Harrison RV. Person-environment fit and job stress. In: Cooper CL, Payne R, eds. *Stress at Work*. Chichester: John Wiley, 1979:175–205.

12. Krikorian DA, Moser DH. Satisfactions and stresses experienced by professional nurses in hospice programs. *American Journal of Hospice Care*, 1985; 2(1):25–33.

13. Vachon MLS. *Occupational Stress in the Care of the Critically Ill, the Dying and the Bereaved*. New York: Hemisphere, 1987.

14. Masterson-Allen S, Mor V, Laliberte L, Monteiro L. Staff burnout in a hospice setting. *Hospice Journal*, 1985; 1:1–15.

15. Mor V, Laliberte L. Burnout among hospice staff. *Health and Social Work*, 1984; 9:274–283.

16. Ramirez AJ, Graham J, Richards MA, Cull A, Gregory WM. Mental health of hospital consultants: the effect of stress and satisfaction at work. *Lancet*, 1996; 16:724–728.

17. Beck-Friis B, Strang P, Sjoden P-O. Caring for severely ill cancer patients: a comparison of working conditions in hospital-based home care and in hospital. *Supportive Care in Cancer*, 1993; 1:145–151.

18. Graham J, Ramirez AJ, Cull A, Gregory WM, Finlay I, Hoy A, Richards MA. Job stress and satisfaction among palliative physicians. *Palliative Medicine*, 1996; 10:185–194.

19. Olkinuora M, Asp S, Juntunen J, Kauttu K, Strid L, Aarimaa M. Stress symptoms, burnout and suicidal thoughts in Finnish physicians. *Social Psychiatry and Psychiatric Epidemiology*, 1990; 25:81–86.

20. Amenta MM. Traits of hospice nurses compared with those who work in traditional settings. *Journal of Clinical Psychology*, 1984; 40:414–419.

21. Zerwekh J. Transcending life: the practice wisdom of nursing hospice experts. *American Journal of Hospice and Palliative Care*, 1993; 5:26–31.

22. Alexander DA, Ritchie E. "Stressors" and difficulties in dealing with the terminal patient. *Journal of Palliative Care*, 1990; 6(3):28–33.

23. Robbins RA. Death anxiety, death competency and self-actualization in hospice volunteers. *Hospice Journal*, 1991; 7(4):29–35.

24. Amenta MM, Weiner AW. Death anxiety and purpose in life and duration of service in hospice workers. *Psychological Reports*, 1981; 54:979–984.

25. Bene B, Foxall MJ. Death anxiety and job stress in hospice and medical-surgical nurses. *Hospice Journal*, 1991; 7(3):25–41.

26. Yancik R. Sources of work stress for hospice staff. *Journal of Psychosocial Oncology*, 1984; 2(1):21–31.

27. Yancik R. Coping with hospice work stress. *Journal of Psychosocial Oncology*, 1984; 2(2):19–35.

28. Kobasa SC. Stressful life events, personality and health: an inquiry into hardiness. *Journal of Personality and Social Psychology*, 1979; 37:1–11.

29. Kobasa SC, Maddi SR, Kahn S. Hardiness and health: a prospective inquiry. *Journal of Personality and Social Psychology*, 1982; 42:168–177.

30. Papadatou D, Anagnostopoulos F, Monos D. Factors contributing to the development of burnout in oncology nursing. *British Journal of Medical Psychology* 1994; 67:187–199.

31. Hansell PS. Stress on nurses in oncology. In: Holland JC and Rowland JH, eds, *Handbook of Psychooncology*. New York: Oxford University Press, 1989:658–663.

32. Kash KM, Holland JC. Special problems of physicians and house staff in oncology. In: Holland JC & Rowland JH, eds, *Handbook of Psychooncology*. New York: Oxford University Press, 1989:647–657.

33. Gotay CC, Crockett S, West C. Palliative home care nursing: nurses' perceptions of roles and stress. *Canadian Mental Health*, 1985; 33:6–9.

34. Cooper CL, Mitchell S. Nursing the critically ill and dying. *Human Relations*, 1990; 43:297–311.

35. Raudonis B. The meaning and impact of empathic relationships in hospice nursing. *Cancer Nursing*, 1993; 16:304–309.

36. Raphael B. *The Anatomy of Bereavement*. New York: Basic Books, 1983.

37. Vachon MLS. The stress of professional caregivers. In: Doyle D, Hanks GW, and MacDonald N, eds, *Oxford Textbook of Palliative Medicine*, 2nd ed. Oxford: Oxford University Press, 1998:919–932.

38. Alexander DA, MacLeod M. Stress among palliative care matrons: a major problem for a minority group. *Palliative Medicine*, 1992; 6:111–124.

39. Finlay IG. Sources of stress in hospice medical directors and matrons. *Palliative Medicine*, 1990;4:5–9.

40. McWilliam CL, Burdock J, Warmsley J. The challenging experience of palliative care support-team nursing. *Oncology Nursing Forum* 1993; 20:770–785.

41. Munley A. Sources of hospice staff stress and how to cope with it. *Nursing Clinics of North America*, 1985; 20:343–355.

42. Paradis LF, Usui WM. Hospice staff and volunteers: issues for management. *Journal of Psychosocial Oncology*, 1989; 7:121–139.

43. Power KG, Sharp GR. A comparison of sources of

nursing stress and job satisfaction among mental handicap and hospice nursing staff. *Journal of Advanced Nursing*, 1988; 13:726–732.

44. Kahn RL, Wolfe DM, Quinn RP, Snoek JD. *Organizational Stress: Studies in Role Conflict and Ambiguity*. New York: Wiley, 1981 (reprint). Malabar, FL: Krieger, 1964.

45. French JRP. Person role fit. *Occupational Mental Health* 1973; 3:15–20.

46. Foxall MJ, Zimmerman L, Standley R, Bene' B. A comparison of frequency and sources of nursing job stress perceived by intensive care, hospice and medical-surgical nurses. *Journal of Advanced Nursing*, 1990; 15:577–584.

47. Zerwekh JV. A family caregiving model for hospice nursing. *Hospice Journal*, 1995; 10:27–44.

48. Vachon MLS. Stress and burnout in oncology. In: Berger A, Levy MH, Portnoy RK, Weissman DE, eds, *Principles and Practices of Supportive Oncology*. Philadelphia: Lippincott, in press.

49. Edelwich J, Brodsky A. *Burn-out: Stages of Disillusionment in the Helping Professions*. New York: Springer, 1980.

50. Maslach M. *Burnout—The Cost of Caring*. New York: Prentice Hall, 1982.

51. Vachon MLS. Battle fatigue in hospice/palliative care. In: Gilmore A, Gillmore S, eds, *A Safer Death*. New York: Plenum, 1988:149–160.

52. Pines AM. Who is to blame for helper's burnout? Environmental impact. In: Scott CD, Hawk J, eds, *Heal Thyself: The Health of Health Care Professionals*. New York: Brunner/Mazel, 1986.

53. Freudenberger HJ, Richelson G. *Burnout: the High Cost of High Achievement*. New York: Anchor Press, 1980.

54. Maslach M. *Burnout—The Cost of Caring*. New York: Prentice Hall, 1982.

55. Pines AM, Aronson E. *Career Burnout: Causes and Cures*. New York: Free Press, 1988.

56. Nash A. A terminal case? burnout in palliative care. *Professional Nurse*, 1989; 4:443–444.

57. Ward AWM. *Home Care Services for the Terminally Ill: A Report for the Nuffield Foundation*. Sheffield: University of Sheffield Medical School, 1985.

58. Lunt B, Yardley J. *A Survey of Home Care Teams and Hospital Support Teams for the Terminally Ill*. Southampton: Cancer Care Research Unit, 1986.

59. Cohen MZ, Haberman MR, Steeves R, Deatrick JA. Rewards and difficulties of oncology nursing. *Oncology Nursing Forum*, 1994; 21(8):9–17.

60. Goldberg D, Williams P. *A Users Guide to the General Health Questionnaire*. Windsor, Berkshire: NFER-Nelson Publishing, 1988.

61. Zigmond AS, Snaith RP. The hospital anxiety and depression Scale. *Acta Psychiatrica Scandinavica*; 1983; 67:361–370.

62. Crown S, Crisp AH. *Manual of the Crown-Crisp Experiential Index*. London: Hodder and Stoughton, 1979.

63. Weisman AD. Understanding the cancer patient: the syndrome of caregiver plight. *Psychiatry*, 1981; 44:161–168.

64. Larson DG. *The Helper's Journey*. Champaign, IL: Research Press, 1993.

65. Grothe T, McKusick L. Coping with multiple loss. *Focus* 1992; 7(7):5–6.

66. Vachon MLS. Are your patients burning out? *Canadian Family Physician*, 1982; 28:1570–1574.

67. Heim E. Job stressors and coping in health professions. *Psychotherapy and Psychosomatics*, 1991; 55:90–99.

68. Vachon MLS. Myths and realities in palliative/ hospice care. *Hospice Journal*, 1986; 2(1):63–79.

69. Wise H, Beckhard R, Rubin I, Kyte G, eds. *Making Health Care Teams Work*. Cambridge, MA: Ballinger, 1974.

70. Hunsberger P. Creation and evolution of the hospice staff support group: lessons from four long-term groups. *American Journal of Hospice Care*, 1989; May/June:37–41.

71. Hinds PS, Puckett P, Donohue M, Milligan M, Payne K, Phipps S, Davis SEF, Martin GA. The impact of a grief workshop for pediatric oncology nurses on their grief and perceived stress. *Journal of Pediatric Nursing*, 1994; 9:388–397.

72. Maguire P. Barriers to psychological care of the dying. *British Medical Journal*, 1985; 291:1711–1713.

73. Faulkner A, Maguire P. *Talking to Cancer Patients and Their Relatives*. Oxford: Oxford University Press, 1994.

74. Faulkner A. *Effective Interaction with Patients*. Edinburgh: Churchill Livingstone, 1992.

75. Faulkner A. *Teaching Interactive Skills in Health Care*. London: Chapman and Hall, 1993.

76. Killeen ME. Getting through our grief: for caregivers of persons with AIDS. *American Journal of Hospice and Palliative Care*, 1993; 10(5):18–24.

77. Wilkinson SM. The changing pressures for oncology nurses 1986–93. *European Journal of Cancer Care*, 1995; 4(2):69–74.

78. Davies B, Oberle K. Dimensions of the supportive role of the nurse in palliative care. *Oncology Nursing Forum* 1990; 17:87–94.

79. Canin LH. *Psychological Restoration among AIDS Caregivers: Maintaining Self-care*. Ph.D. dissertation, University of Michigan, 1991.

22

Understanding and Managing Bereavement in Palliative Care

Sidney Zisook, M.D.

It has been estimated that for every person who dies, at least five close friends, relatives, and loved ones are left behind.[1] Thus, anyone involved in palliative care will encounter considerably more grief reactions than dying patients. Most often, these grief reactions, although gut wrenching, acutely painful, and disruptive to the lives of the bereaved, lessen in intensity over time and do not require professional attention. At times, however, grief can become unrelenting and chronic and may set the stage for the onset, exacerbation, or persistence of a number of medical or psychiatric complications in vulnerable individuals. Thus, it is important for palliative-care providers to learn the boundaries and dimensions of "normal" grief, to be familiar with risk factors for complicated grief, and to be able to intervene promptly and appropriately when indicated.

with a known etiology and relatively predictable symptoms and course that causes distress and dysfunction and may be associated with several potentially severe complications.

Whether considered a normal reaction to loss or a disease state, grief has manifestations that vary from person to person and from moment to moment and that involve all aspects of the bereaved's being. Defined as the emotional, behavioral, social, and functional responses to loss, grief is not specific for loss via death. Individuals faced with any real or threatened loss can be expected to grieve. In palliative care, clinicians deal with multiple grief reactions: grief over loss of health, function, mobility, potential. When the loss is the result of the death of a loved one, the term "bereavement" is used. Thus, a bereavement reaction is grief following loss through death.[3]

NORMAL GRIEF

Is the very concept of "normal" grief an oxymoron? In his classic and provocative paper aptly titled "Is Grief a Disease?," Engel[2] argues that grief shares many pathognomonic features of other diseases: Grief is a well-defined syndrome

STAGES OF GRIEF

Several investigators have proposed "stages" of grief or bereavement.[4-7] Such a staging of grief is not meant to be taken too literally; grief is not a linear process with concrete boundaries but rather a composite of overlapping, fluid phases that vary from person to person and ebb and flow over time. Thus, the "stages" are meant to be general guidelines that are not intended to prescribe where a bereaved individual "ought" to be at any period of time during grief.

Most stagings of grief include an initial period of *shock* or *numbness* lasting moments to hours to weeks and characterized by varying degrees of disbelief and denial. Statements such as "it can't be" or "I don't believe it" are ubiquitous, and the accompanying feeling of numbness pervades much of the initial period. Mourning rites and the gathering of family and friends often help facilitate passage through this stage, but, in certain circumstances, such as when the deceased's body is missing or unrecognizable, uncertainty may be prolonged. In palliative care, when dying generally is recognized long before death occurs, some of the shock may occur when the diagnosis and prognosis are given and is therefore attenuated by the time of the actual death.

As the death is acknowledged both cognitively and emotionally, the grief slips into the next phase, *acute mourning*. This period, measured in weeks to months, generally includes intense feeling states occurring in periodic waves of emotional and somatic discomfort. This distress often is accompanied by social withdrawal, a preoccupation with thoughts of the deceased, and, not infrequently, identification with the deceased.[8]

In the *restitution* phase, bereaved individuals know that they have grieved and now can begin to shift attention to the world around them. Memories are, and loneliness may be, part of that world, but the deceased, with their ills and problems, are not. The hallmark of this phase is the ability of the bereaved to recognize that they have grieved and now can resume old roles and acquire new ones as necessary, reexperience pleasure without guilt, and seek the companionship and love of others.[5]

DURATION OF GRIEF

It is probably a mistake to put an arbitrary limit on the duration of grief. Early investigators measured grief in terms of weeks to months.[2,8] However, most contemporary investigators have emphasized the chronicity of grief. Parkes,[9] for example, reported that after 13 months of bereavement, only a minority of widows could look at the past with pleasure or to the future with optimism; most widows described themselves as sad, poorly adjusted, depressed, often thinking of their husband, having clear visual images of them, and still grieving much of the time. Thus, Parkes concluded that the question of how long grief lasts is still unanswered. Similarly, Bornstein et al.[10] found that a significant minority of widows and widowers meet criteria for major depression 13 months after their spouses' death and that symptoms of crying spells, weight loss, and insomnia are particularly frequent. Others have extended the period of distress to 2 years[11,12] or beyond.[13] Moreover, an interminable duration of grief is not necessarily pathological, prompting Goin et al.[14] to state, "You don't get over it, you get used to it." Many individuals maintain a "timeless" emotional involvement with the deceased, and the attachment often represents a healthy adaptation to the loss.[14,15]

MULTIDIMENSIONAL APPROACH TO BEREAVEMENT

Considered to be among the most disruptive of all events of ordinary life,[16] bereavement has the capacity to perturb all aspects of the bereaved's life. Yet, when conceptualizing grief, many clinicians focus only on the intense and painful feeling states that pervade the early weeks to months of the bereavement period and perhaps on the bereaved's efforts to cope with or minimize the pain. But grief's impact extends far beyond affective turmoil and coping strategies. For one thing, grief work demands a reconfiguration of one's relationships to the deceased.[17] Grief also affects interpersonal relationships—those within the individual's prebereavement circle of friends, family, and acquaintances, as well as the development of new relationships over time. In addition, grief often affects one's ability to function medically, psychologically, socially, and occupationally. Finally, grief forces bereaved individuals to reassess their view of themselves, the work around them, and their futures. Thus, Shuchter and colleagues[15,17] have proposed a multidimensional approach to bereavement that comprehensively provides assessment,[18] outlines prevention,[19] and guides treatment[20] of clinical problems that might arise.

Mental and Emotional Disruptions

As shock, denial, and detachment dissipate, a sense of loss accompanied by yearning, pining, and searching behavior ensues.[21] The loss extends beyond the deceased person to a loss of intimacy, companionship, security, lifestyle, roles, and meaning of future visions. Loneliness, often increasing in severity over time, may be felt even when the bereaved person is not alone.[22] Along with the disruption of attachment bonds, intense forms of insecurity, fear, and anxiety may emerge. Vivid and intrusive images of the deceased often arise, particularly at times when the individual's mind is not actively engaged, such as when the person is home alone or is in bed but not yet asleep. These intrusive images may be especially pronounced when the death is sudden and unexpected.[23–25]

Pangs of intense psychological and somatic anguish are common.[8] These are described as painful eruptions of autonomic explosions: a wrenching of gut, shortness of breath, chest pain, lightheadedness, weakness, rapid welling up of tears, and uncontrollable crying. During the early days and weeks, these responses tend to erupt often, suddenly, and unexpectedly. Over time, they become more often associated with reminders of the deceased. While the intensity and frequency of these pangs of grief generally subside as time passes, they may reemerge in response to reminders of the loss, such as anniversaries, birthdays, or other special occasions.

Myriad other feelings and thoughts also are common. Anger may be experienced as irritability, hatred, resentment, envy, a sense of unfairness, or not at all. It may be directed at the deceased, the bereaved person, the deceased's physician, the hospital, God, or the world in general. Especially if the deceased endured prolonged illness with much suffering, relief may be felt. However, the cost of such relief, even when genuinely felt, may be feelings of guilt for being relieved. When guilt is experienced, it often is associated with perceptions that the bereaved person may have contributed to the death or suffering of the deceased by improper feeding, inadequate support, failing to prevent unhealthy behavior or lifestyle, or not pushing the physician hard enough to detect or treat the disorder. Survival guilt is particularly tenacious when the bereaved person has concrete reasons to feel responsible for the loss, for example, if he or she was the driver in a fatal vehicle accident.

Especially within the early weeks after bereavement, mental disorganization, manifested by poor concentration, confusion, forgetfulness, and a lack of clarity, is common. The cumulative effect of the number of upheavals in the mental, emotional, and cognitive lives of the bereaved persons often leads to a sense of being overwhelmed, out of control, helpless, and powerless. These regressive pulls result in what Horowitz et al.[26] have termed "negative latent self-images."

As the pain and disorganization subside and individuals begin to function again, they often are surprised at how well they do. Adapting to the loss may demand mastery of new tasks; a bereaved husband may now need to learn, for the first time, to bottle-feed a child or iron clothes, or a wife may be faced with the need to handle the finances and maintain the automobile. Mastery of such tasks can bring pride, independence, or wisdom.[7] Bereaved persons often are surprised at their capacity to feel pleasure or to grow.

Coping

The thrust toward homeostasis places the bereaved in an enormous conflict between powerful and opposing forces. On the one hand, there is the reality of the loss and the associated pain and anguish; on the other hand, there is the equally compelling psychological reality of the need to shut off such pain. Facing the reality of the loss initiates pain, which, in turn, sets off a variety of mechanisms to mitigate against it. Throughout the grieving process, adaptation operates in highly idiosyncratic ways to allow survivors to face reality while simultaneously protecting against too great an onslaught of affect at any one time. Most bereaved individuals find a way to regulate, or "dose," the amount of pain they can bear and divert the rest, using defensive operations of the most mature as well as the most regressive nature.

One of the most pervasive coping measures is the numbness and disbelief described earlier. Protecting individuals from the immediate impact of the loss, disbelief becomes a significant force within their protective operations. Individuals may choose to suppress or defer their grief to moments of greater convenience, support, or privacy. While "being strong" often is necessary when important decisions must be made or tasks must be completed, such overcontrol can also interfere with individuals' need to feel their grief. Intellectualization and rationalization may allow survivors to transform an awful truth into a better or more acceptable one, dampening the pain of the former. Humor is another adaptive means of achieving distance from the pain of a loss while not necessarily removing the bereaved from the reality they face. One of the most frequently used and effective means of coping with death, faith facilitates the acceptance of death as part of a plan. Religious beliefs and rituals can provide survivors with the sense that there is someone to help them cope with the suffering as well as to support them in facing the difficult tasks ahead. There may be reassurance that the deceased will be provided for in the hereafter and that the deceased and the bereaved may be reunited in heaven.

Avoidance behavior may help the bereaved stay away from "triggers" that set off pangs of anguish, but it may also limit the bereaved's contact with otherwise supportive people or gratifying experiences. Exposure to reminders may facilitate grief and a sense of loyalty or attachment but may also place the bereaved in situations where they are constantly bombarded by painful reminders. As a rule, people who have usually faced other stresses in their lives with avoidance behaviors will do so when bereaved, while more active problem solvers may be more likely to use exposure as a focus of adaptation to their loss. If a particular coping strategy has served someone well in the past, it likely will also serve that person well in times of bereavement.

Another effective and adaptive coping mechanism is keeping busy, particularly involvement in useful activity. Such efforts provide a respite from suffering, and are sanctioned by their usefulness. Similarly, involvement with others may help focus survivors on things other than their pain while simultaneously providing a means for them to obtain support from others. More passive forms of distraction, such as watching television or listening to music, also can take one's mind off the pain and may even provide human faces and voices, helping the bereaved stave off a sense of isolation and loneliness. Certainly, direct verbal and emotional expressions of inner experiences can be a highly adaptive means of coping with the painful aspects of grief. Most survivors experience some sense of relief through direct catharsis.

One of the least adaptive coping strategies is indulgence in food and alcohol or other unhealthy activities. Bereavement is a time when powerful, deeply felt cravings for nurturance and security can be transformed into needs for food, alcohol, tobacco, or sex. Sanctions against such cravings may be overridden by a strong sense of entitlement relating to the loss or by fatalistic or apathetic responses. Unfortunately, when these cravings are indulged to excess, they have the potential to compound the challenges of bereavement. Especially in vulnerable persons with preexisting problems in these areas, prompt treatment intervention should be considered.

The Continuing Relationship with the Deceased

Perhaps the most powerful means of mitigating the anguish of losing a loved one is to maintain a continuing relationship with the deceased person. Although this at first may seem contradictory, all students of human nature recognize that relationships can be as powerful in their nonmaterial forms—dissociated with time, place, and even person—as they are in their material forms. While the bereaved have lost their loved ones in a real and substantial fashion, they have formed attachment bonds to the deceased at emotional levels so deep that they persist beyond the person's physical death.[21,27]

Bereaved individuals face a dilemma. On the one hand, there is the demand of reality to accept the loss; on the other hand, there is an equally strong demand to maintain the lost relationship, which, although now technically illusory, is nevertheless emotionally quite real and thus requires working through for the survivor to approach emotional homeostasis.[17] The psychological purpose of the latter demand and its effects are likely to be comforting. The usual course of bereavement includes some fluctuations between each of these states, mediated by the survivor's shifting needs and capacities.

These continuing relationships exist in many forms, including location, continuing contact, symbolic representations, living legacies, rituals, memories, and dreams. Most survivors experience their deceased loved ones as having an existence either in a spiritual form, often locating them in heaven, or with some material elements located at the site of their burial if in a cemetery or where ashes have been scattered. Continuing contact with the deceased is maintained in several ways. During the early weeks and months, survivors often anticipate the abrupt return of the deceased; they may search in crowds or hear the voice of the deceased in otherwise nondescript sounds. Even frank hallucinatory experiences are common, most often in the form of sensing the presence of the deceased person. The bereaved may feel their departed loved ones hovering, watching out for and protecting them. There is frequent communication with the deceased; survivors may discuss or recount the events of the day, ask for advice, or reprimand the deceased for their betrayal and abandonment.

Symbolic representations of the deceased often are experienced in a highly ambivalent manner, as painful reminders of the deceased and simultaneously as valued sources of continued contact. Symbolic items may include the person's favorite possessions, pictures, writing, toys, rings, hobbies, and the like. Living legacies are less symbols than living "extensions" of the personality, ideas, appearance, or other features of the deceased that are borrowed and incorporated into the life of the survivor. Thus, identification with the deceased through ideas, traits, and mannerisms or even symptoms creates continuity. Efforts to "carry on" the works or traditions of the deceased through individual activities, naming others after the deceased, or memorial donations may play a role in perpetuating the relationship.

Every culture's unique beliefs, customs, behaviors, and other mourning rituals that attend to the deceased also contribute to the continuing relationship. In prevailing North American culture, for example, the funeral is an important public acknowledgment and display. The funeral presents reality and finality, countering the effects of denial; it garners support for the survivors; it pays tribute and initiates memorialization. Other ceremonies are initiated through visitations with their continued show of support; confrontations with reality, and stimulation of memories. The funeral and memorial service as well as subsequent holidays, birthdays, and anniversaries become intensified foci for the relationship, at times exacerbating powerful affective states that may seem as fresh as the original experience. Over time, these reminders may become attenuated, but they are generally present in some form and to some degree.

Dreams of the deceased are quite common. The dreamer may often be disturbed when, upon waking, he or she must face the reality of the loss. As time passes, memories become the most powerful means of continuing the relationship. As with all the connecting links, they are bittersweet: They provide comfort in bringing the deceased back to life and stimulate pain as a reminder of what is lost. Memories are often selective, tending to idealize the deceased, especially in the early months after the death. In palliative care, distortions of memory can be enhanced by prolonged illness or deterioration where the "shadow" of illness may block certain memories of better times together. It may be useful to help such individuals free themselves from these distorted images by encouraging their discussions of times before the person became ill.

Changes in Function

The impact of bereavement on health is well documented. Bereaved individuals are at risk not only for mental illness[11] but also for medical morbidity,[3,28,29] increased mortality rates,[30] and other health-damaging activities such as alcohol and substance use.[31] Both accident and suicide rates are elevated among the bereaved,[32] and general well-being often is compromised.[33] Similarly, both social and work functioning may be impaired for protracted periods. As the supportive social interactions resulting from visitations and other mourning rituals wear off, individuals often find themselves experiencing varying degrees of social inhibition, withdrawal, and isolation; loneliness, even when the person is not alone, becomes one of the most dysphoric and unrelenting phenomena many bereaved individuals will face. In addition, numerous changes in role functioning may be precipitated by the death of a loved one. For example, a widower may have to learn for the first time to cook his own meals, iron shirts, or care for the emotional needs of young children; a widow may need to find employment outside the home, care for the car, or balance the budget for the first time ever. The challenge of filing insurance claims or obtaining social security benefits may appear overwhelming to a grieving person who has never before carried out such tasks. In palliative care, some of these new roles may be anticipated and their mastery facilitated by appropriate social service referrals before the death.

Changes in Relationships

The death of a loved one alters the dynamics of many relationships.[34] Complex changes occur within the family and close friendships. If the survivor is to blame for the fatal illness or terminal event (e.g., if he or she was the driver in a fatal automobile accident), guilt feelings and anger may distance these relationships that now more than ever need to be experienced as close and supportive. Survivors may have to contend with grief of surviving parents, children, in-laws, friends, and siblings as well as with efforts to enlist support for themselves. While there is an opportunity to achieve greater intimacy and repair old wounds, there also is the converse potential to exacerbate conflict and disruption. For widows and widowers, the additional challenge of dealing with the interactions of single life may be difficult. This task may be complicated by continued devotion to the deceased spouse, societal and familial reactions, imputations of disloyalty from the children, and fears of recurring loss.[34,35]

Identity

It should not be surprising that people living through what is likely to be the most profoundly disruptive experience of their lives are subject to dramatic changes in the ways they perceive themselves and the world around them.[16] During the earlier phases of grief, there may be intense regression as survivors feel on the verge of being overwhelmed by the constant bombardment of anguish, images, confusion, and disorientation. Self-perceptions emerge of hopelessness, inadequacy, and incapacity—childlike regressive states that are experienced as all enveloping and internal.[23] The perspective of family, friends, and counseling that these states are transient and that bereaved people will emerge from them can help the bereaved endure even the most difficult periods. As time goes on and survivors "survive"—

that is, learn of their capacity to tolerate grief, carry on tasks, and discover new ways of dealing with the world—new feelings and self-images may emerge. Often, these are in the direction of an evolving sense of strength, autonomy, assertiveness, and maturity.[7] Frequently, the bereaved become more appreciative of daily living and perhaps even more patient, accepting, and giving. They may start careers or change old ones, enjoy themselves with more gusto, or find new outlets for their creativity.

In a parallel way, they may shift from viewing their world as rational, just, or safe. Personal views of control and invincibility may evolve toward greater flexibility and vulnerability. While many bereaved individuals credit their faith in God with getting them through the difficult period, others may lose faith or remain bitter. Since the death of a loved one evokes such powerful and fundamentally existential issues, religious counseling often is appreciated.

ANTICIPATORY GRIEF

The concept of "anticipatory grief" is used to describe the separation anxiety experienced by patients' families and friends as they witness the patients' terminal illnesses and slow deaths.[36] While it is painful to watch someone die, individuals can become part of the comfort-giving team, complete unfinished business, say good-bye, clarify misunderstandings, and anticipate and prepare for social adjustments to come. Thus, they may be more ready for bereavement when it occurs. Some investigators have found that emotional preparation may ease the intensity of grief after death and diminish the risk of serious medical, psychological, and social reactions,[22,29,36–38] but the findings are not totally consistent in this regard.[39]

Other investigators have challenged the very notion of anticipatory grief if the relative stays actively involved with the patient throughout the illness.[40,41] Parkes differentiates the reactions of friends and relatives who spend time with a person who is dying from those that emerge after the death. First, he suggests that the emotional reaction to discovering the prognosis is not grief, with its attendant sense of loss and utter desolation, but rather a feeling of intense separation anxiety or fear. Unlike the separation anxiety seen in grief, however, the characteristic despair and "giving up" do not occur. In contrast, the anticipation of loss intensifies attachment. Thus, anticipated loss has emotional implications different from those of bereavement.[41]

The resurgence of attachment behavior that commonly follows the discovery that a loved one is nearing the end of life may have immediate value for the relationship and later value for the survivor. For example, relationships often get closer and more honest. Even though awareness of impending loss makes for great pain, the concluding period of closeness often is treasured afterward. In addition, forewarning permits certain kinds of anticipatory preparation. There is learning to live with the prospect of loss, so when the loss in fact occurs, it is at least not unexpected.[41] There is the opportunity to make plans for the future, to the extent that such plans are not seen as a betrayal of a dying person. But it is only after the actual loss that grief occurs.

One of the risks of forewarning is "premature" grief. In this scenario, the physician, friends, or family begin acting as if the person has died before the actual event, and withdrawal rather than attachment occurs. This does no good either for the dying person or for the eventual survivors. It deprives individuals of the opportunity to provide support to their dying loved ones and to prepare emotionally for the loss. To accept the death while the person still lives is to become vulnerable to later self-accusations of having abandoned the person before death has occurred. Preventing premature grief is one of the difficult tasks of terminal care. It can best be accomplished by giving open and honest information about diagnosis and prognosis, confirming that the information has been understood, and ensuring that family members get every opportunity to come to terms themselves with the impending death. Thus, honest and effective communication is the antidote for premature grief.

COMPLICATIONS OF GRIEF

Zisook et al.[42] has postulated separate categories of grief complications: those that arise directly from the process of grief itself (too little, too much, too long) and those general medical or psychiatric conditions whose onset, exacerbation, or persistence are affected by bereavement.

Complications in the Process of Grief

Grief can occur later than expected (absent, delayed, or inhibited grief),[43] be more severe than considered healthy (hypertrophied grief), or last too long (chronic grief). Of these, only chronic grief has any experimental validation or is generally agreed on as a "real entity."[44] It is defined as a protracted preoccupation and idealization of the deceased person along with protracted intense dysphoria and pining.[41,44,45] Although there is no consensus regarding how long grief should last before it can be called chronic, it is more than unmodulated, intense preoccupation with the deceased and its interference with other relationships or functioning that define its essence. Risk factors for chronic grief are loss of a child,[46] a dependent or clinging relationship with the deceased,[41] or an unnatural death.[24,47–49] We have rarely seen chronic grief except after sudden and traumatic losses, lending some experimental validation to Prigerson et al.'s postulate that complicated grief may be a variant of posttraumatic stress.[50] Treatment often is protracted and difficult, possibly reflecting the close association of chronic grief with both major depression and posttraumatic stress.

High-Risk Medical and Psychiatric Complications

Although there still is controversy over the nature and extent of morbidity associated with bereavement, several studies suggest that at least some bereaved individuals are vulnerable to a decline in general medical health[3,28,51] and possibly to certain cancers,[52,53] cardiovascular disease,[2,54–56] and poor self-care.[57] In addition, as reviewed by Stroebe and Stroebe,[58] bereaved individuals are at risk for dying; the highest risk is in weeks to months following the loss; men are relatively more vulnerable than women; younger bereaved adults (especially men) are at particular risk, as may be the socially isolated; and the best-established excesses are for heart diseases, suicides, accidents, and liver cirrhosis. By far the greatest risk factor for morbidity and mortality after bereavement is preexisting poor general medical and psychiatric health.

Psychiatric complications are even better documented than are general medical problems. The best-studied and most frequently cited complication of bereavement is depression. Depressive symptoms,[12,46,59–64] subsyndromal syndromes,[65,66] minor depression,[67] and major depression[11,63] all have been reported to be highly prevalent and relatively persistent after bereavement. Major depressive syndromes are present in about 50% of all widows and widowers at 1 month after their spouse's death,[63] 25% at 2 months after the death, 16% at 1 year,[63] and 14–16% at 2 years.[11,12] Similar rates have been found in children[68] and in the elderly.[66] According to the DSM-IV, if a full major depressive syndrome has its onset within the first 2 months of bereavement and does not last beyond the second month, and if the depression is not too severe (i.e., no melancholia or psychotic features, no suicidal ideation, and mild impairment), the diagnosis should be Bereavement rather than Major Depressive Episode. However, Zisook and Schuchter[11] have found that by the second month, bereavement-related depressions tend to be chronic, lead to protracted biopsychosocial dysfunction, and are associated with impaired immunological function. Thus, all severe major depressive syndromes, at any time, and all full major depressive syndromes beyond the second month of bereavement should be taken seriously, considered legitimate medical concerns, and treated as aggressively as other nonbereavement-related depressions. Major risk factors for depression 1 year after the death include having a major depressive syndrome at 2 months, having had intense depressive symptoms earlier in life, personal and family history of depression, youth, and poor general medical health.[11]

Anxiety symptoms also are prevalent and long lasting after bereavement.[39,69] While most longitudinal studies on bereavement emphasize symptoms rather than syndromes of anxiety, Jacobs et al.[70] found higher than expected rates of both panic and generalized anxiety disorder throughout the first year of spousal bereavement, agoraphobia in the first 6 months, and social phobia in the second 6 months. Risk factors for anxiety symptom intensity at 7 months include intense depression and anxiety at 2 months, nonresolution of grief, lower income, younger age, being female, and less environmental/social support.[57] Although not as relevant in palliative care, posttraumatic-like states also have been found during bereavement, particularly when the death is "traumatic"[71] or occurs after a disaster;[49,72] when the cause of death is suicide, homicide, or other unnatural cause;[47,73] when the death is unex-

pected;[74] or when the cause of death is AIDS.[75] Prigerson et al.[50] has suggested that much of what we call complicated grief may be a variant of posttraumatic stress. When posttraumatic stress disorder and bereavement coexist, the treatment of the trauma must take precedence.[49]

TREATMENT

General Principles

Palliative care allows ample opportunity for clinicians to help families and loved ones deal with impending death as adaptively as possible. It is important that the physician convey the seriousness of the illness to patients as well as to their families. Because bad news often is met with denial and numbness, it is important to have follow-up discussions, anticipate and encourage questions, and answer all queries honestly. Such information must be given in a way that is heard but that does not constitute an overwhelmingly traumatic confrontation with the impending loss.[41]

Although there is no general consensus about the concept of "anticipatory grief," there is some support for the value of counseling families and loved ones before the death of a terminally ill family member.[76] It is important that this counseling not encourage a sense of helplessness or premature withdrawal. Honest and open communication builds trust and allows the family to address unresolved conflict, repair miscommunication, and begin to prepare for inevitable changes. It may be important to ensure that family members caring for a dying person do not neglect their own needs. Such neglect could add to the already heightened risks of medical and psychiatric complications after the death of a loved one. For example, it is known that bereaved individuals are at risk for premature death from cardiovascular disease or cirrhosis.[30,32] Family members should be encouraged to maintain healthful behavior themselves, eat and sleep well, take their medicines, and visit physicians for routine medical care. Similarly, the risk for protracted and disabling depressive and anxiety disorders are greatest for individuals with preexisting problems in these areas. Individuals on maintenance medication or in psychotherapy should continue; individuals who have had two or more past major depressive episodes who are not on medication may want to consider prophylactic treatment to prevent the onset of a new episode or the worsening of an ongoing one.

In most cases, grief does not require professional intervention. Although painful and distressing, it is a normal reaction to loss, and most men and women reveal remarkable adaptive capacities. However, nowhere is the adage "a sorrow shared is a sorrow halved" more true than in bereavement. Thus, it almost always helps for individuals to use their customary social support—friends, family, clergy, and physician—for a friendly ear or shoulder while the healing process unfolds. Support groups, especially when other social supports are not readily available, after a particularly traumatic death (e.g., from Sudden Infant Death Syndrome), or in high-risk groups, may facilitate healing.[77–80] In general, professional intervention should be reserved for individuals with chronic grief or who have experienced grief-related psychiatric disorders.

We do not recommend treatment for absent or delayed grief. Suppression and denial are not illnesses or in themselves pathological; they may be quite adaptive for individuals dealing with life adversity. Clinicians used to think that it was unhealthy to suppress grief,[43] but several studies of normal bereavement have found that those who were most disturbed earlier in the bereavement remained most disturbed later and that absent or attenuated grief did not lead to later problems.[4,11,27,39,81] Thus, minimal expressions of affect should not be regarded as pathologic, and it is not necessarily beneficial to talk about feelings and emotions that follow the death of a close person.[39] On the other hand, prolonged grief that interferes with functioning and does not allow for the painful preoccupation with the deceased to abate is never healthy. When it occurs, it often is a complication or unrecognized major depression and will be ameliorated as the depression lifts, although, on occasion, additional grief-specific psychotherapy is necessary.[82]

When psychiatric disturbances—depressive disorder, anxiety disorder, substance abuse and dependence—occur, they should be treated as aggressively as they would be in any other circumstance. When such disorders occur after the loss of a loved one, they are no less virulent and destructive than when they occur after other stressors, such as divorce, financial ruin, or a diagnosis of cancer, or when they occur spontaneously.

The real questions when deciding when and how to treat are not whether or when someone died but, rather, past history, severity and persistence of symptoms, and degree of impairment. Historically, physicians have been reluctant to treat depression or anxiety in the context of bereavement, feeling that such treatment interferes with grief and with nature's restorative properties. But the reverse is true; depression and anxiety interfere with grief. If anything, treatment of these pathologic conditions helps facilitate grieving.[61,83] Thus, we advocate active treatment of major depression and anxiety disorders that occur in the context of bereavement.

Hospice Care

One of the unique characteristics of hospice care is a commitment to the comprehensive care of dying patients and their families during the terminal stage of illness and continuous bereavement care for the survivors after the death.[84] At St. Christopher's Hospice in Britain, trained volunteers visit all "high-risk" widows and widowers in their homes 10 to 14 days after their spouse's deaths and then provide whatever counseling and support seems needed. In a small study to evaluate this service, individuals who received the intervention had better health scores and lower use of drugs, alcohol and tobacco at follow-up than the "high-risk" group that did not receive the intervention.[85] On the other hand, results of the National Hospice Study on caregivers' postbereavement status are equivocal.[86] Before and after bereavement, caregivers from hospital-based hospices were less distressed emotionally, felt less burdened by patient care, and reported greater satisfaction with patient care than survivors managed in home-care hospices. Following the deaths, however, home-care family members, although more disturbed, scored significantly better on a scale of social reengagement than did hospital-based caregivers.

Despite the relative lack of well-designed outcome studies on hospice-care bereavement services, many of the principles of hospice care are rightfully being integrated into general hospital and palliative-care practices. Thus, the use of multidisciplinary teams, ongoing to support for families before and after the patient's death, provision of educational and community resource material, explanation of all procedures and findings, and family conferences on request should aid bereaved individuals cope with their loss.[87]

Group Psychotherapy

Short-term, interactive group treatment may help promote grief work and potentially attenuate its complications. Reporting on 8-week bereavement groups whose members comprised individuals who had lost a spouse to cancer and were undergoing "normal" grief, Yalom and Vinogradov[88] observed several important themes: the transition from "we" to "I," loneliness and aloneness, freedom and growth, personal change necessitated by new responsibilities and roles, questions about the proper length of time to grieve, formation of new relationships, and existential themes such as lack of justice in nature and the dissolution of a belief in personal omnipotence and immortality. Although formal outcome data were not gathered, at 1-year follow-up 34 of 36 subjects gave high testimonials to the group. Similarly, Summers et al.[89] reported lower levels of anxiety and depression at 6-month follow-up in "high-risk" men who had received 12 weeks of group therapy for AIDS-related losses when compared to bereaved counterparts who had not received therapy. However, Leiberman and Yalom[90] did not find marked differences between experimental and control groups of bereaved spouses after 1-year follow-up. Clearly, more study needs to be done on this potentially efficient preventive intervention.

Individual Psychotherapy

In his classic study on bereavement following the Coconut Grove fire in Boston, Lindemann[8] stated that brief psychological management aimed at facilitating the bereaved's "grief work" could prevent prolonged and serious psychosocial and medical disturbances. According to Lindemann, clinicians must help the bereaved accept the pain of bereavement, review the relationship with the deceased, and find new patterns of rewarding interactions. Lindemann felt this could be done in 1 to 10 interviews.

Two controlled studies were unable to provide strong support for the efficacy of brief therapy to prevent long-term complications.[91,92] However, Raphael[93] found significant benefits for widows given 6 to 8 sessions of individual psychotherapy 3 to 12 weeks after their husbands' deaths. Treatment was geared to providing support for grieving processes, including encouragement of expression of various grief affects, reviewing the positive and negative aspects of the lost relationship, providing supportive interaction with the widow's social network, and working through old unresolved losses that interfered with the pres-ent grief. Follow-up assessment at 13 months showed significant benefits for the interactive group in terms of decreased risk for general medical and psychological complications. In particular, widows whose risk had been defined by the perceived nonsupportiveness of their social networks benefited in terms of reduced health-care utilization, while widows at risk because of ambivalent relationships with their husbands experienced a significant decrease in the severity of depressive symptoms.

Other investigators have reported the usefulness of a variety of individual therapeutic approaches to bereaved individuals with "complicated" grief [94–98] or with grief-related adjustment disorders[99] or depression.[82] Worden[100] and Shuchter and Zisook[17,101] advocate an individualized, task-specific form of treatment that may involve multiple modalities of care. Shuchter and Zisook[101] emphasize an approach that follows directly from the multidimensional model of bereavement that was described earlier. In this approach, the therapist has several therapeutic tasks, including helping the patient to develop the capacity to experience, express, and integrate painful affects; use of the most adaptive means possible of modulating painful affects; integrate a meaningful and acceptable continuing relationship with the deceased spouse; maintain health and continued functioning; achieve a successful reconfiguration of altered relationships and the capacity to develop new ones; and achieve an integrated, healthy self-concept and a stable world view. Shuchter and Zisook also emphasize the chronicity of grief—just as the dead do not reawaken, grief never fully ends—and the need for the therapist to remain available, often in the background, as old conflicts reemerge or new issues arise.

Medications

Grief per se should not be medicated. Even though bereaved individuals often feel overwhelmed by their anguish, despair, sadness, loneliness, sense of loss, and other emotional pains, most do not require, or desire, medication. However, there are circumstances when medication should be considered.

For individuals who develop a substantial sleep disorder, short-term intervention with hypnotic agents may be both helpful and humane. A persistent and continuous sleep disruption with features of early, middle, or both types of insomnia may herald the onset of a major depression.[102]

When grief-related anxiety disorders become a source of ongoing distress or interfere with functioning, pharmacologic treatment should be considered. Unfortunately, there are not yet any studies on the benefits or risks of pharmacologic treatment of any of the anxiety disorders—generalized anxiety, phobias, panic, or posttraumatic stress disorder—that have been associated with bereavement.

Depression is the best documented complication of bereavement. Although always a serious problem, major depression is woefully underdiagnosed and rarely treated when it occurs in the context of bereavement.[103] There are no controlled studies of pharmacologic treatment of bereavement-related major depression. However, two open studies support their safety and efficacy.[61,83] In each of these studies, tricyclic antidepressants ameliorated symptoms of depression in widows and widowers with major depressive episodes; such treatment did not interfere with grief. Zisook et al. reported preliminary results that suggested bereaved HIV-seropositive men with major depression responded better to treatment than nonbereaved men and that active medication (fluoxetine) appeared more affective than placebo in these individuals. Reynolds[104] is currently conducting a study to compare interpersonal therapy, antidepressant medications, and no treatment for bereaved individuals with major and minor depression and has reported preliminary findings that suggest psychotherapy may be more helpful for separation distress, while medication may be of greater benefit for treating the depression. It will be important to follow these ongoing studies as they are completed.

SUMMARY

Bereavement is an important component of palliative care. While some individuals begin to deal with separation issues prior to death, grief and bereavement begin when a loved one actually dies. A multidimensional process, bereavement not only creates emotional pain and turmoil but also elicits attempts to modify the pain, requires a reconfiguration of the relationship to the person who has died, affects medical as well as psychological and social functioning, perturbs ongoing interpersonal relationships, and challenges the bereaved to integrate their sense of self and the world around them with the loss of their beloved. Grief doesn't go away but remains a part of one's life for as long as one lives. Despite the pain and disruption caused by the death of a loved one, most bereaved individuals ultimately do well, learn to live with their loss, may grow from the experience, and never require professional intervention. However, a certain percentage of individuals may need help with their grief or with psychiatric complications for which the bereaved are at risk. A variety of self-help, group and individual psychotherapy, and pharmacologic interventions are available.

References

1. Cleiren MPHD. *Adaptation after Bereavement.* Leiden: Leiden University, DSWO Press, 1991.
2. Engel GL. Is grief a disease? *Psychosomatic Medicine,* 1961; 23:18–22.
3. Osterweis M, Solomon F, Green M, eds. *Bereavement: Reactions, Consequences, and Care.* Washington, DC: National Academy Press, 1984.
4. Glick IO, Weiss RS, Parkes CM. *The First Year of Bereavement.* New York: John Wiley, 1974.
5. DeVaul RA, Zisook S, Faschingbauer TR. Clinical aspects of grief and bereavement. *Primary Care,* 1979; 6:391–402.
6. Bowlby J. *Attachment and Loss.* Vol 3. *Loss: Sadness and Depression* New York: Basic Books, 1980/1981.
7. Pollock GH. The mourning-liberation process in health and disease. *Psychiatry Clin North America,* 1987; 10:345–354.
8. Lindemann E. Symptomatology and management of acute grief. *American Journal of Psychiatry,* 1944; 101:141–148.
9. Parkes CM. Psychosocial transitions: a field study. *Soc Sci Med,* 1971; 5:101–115.
10. Bornstein PE, Clayton PJ, Halikas JA, et al. The depression of widowhood after thirteen months. *British Journal of Psychiatry,* 1973; 122:561–566.
11. Zisook S, Shuchter SR. Uncomplicated bereave-

ment. *Journal of Clinical Psychiatry*, 1993; 54:365–372.

12. Harlow SD, Goldberg EL, Comstock GW. A longitudinal study of the prevalence of depressive symptomatology in elderly widowed and married women. *Archives of General Psychiatry*, 1991; 48:1065–1068.

13. Zisook S. Unresolved grief. In: Zisook S, ed, *Biopsychosocial Aspects of Bereavement*. Washington, DC: American Psychiatric Association, 1987:23–34.

14. Goin MK, Burgoyne RW, Goin JM. Timeless attachment to a dead relative. *American Journal of Psychiatry*, 1979; 136:988–989.

15. Shuchter SR, Zisook S. Multidimensional approach to widowhood. *Psychiatric Annals*, 1986; 16:295–308.

16. Holmes T, Rahe R. The social readjustment rating scale. *Journal of Psychosomatic Research*, 1967; 11:213–218.

17. Shuchter SR, Zisook S. Widowhood: the continuing relationship with the dead spouse. *Bulletin of the Menninger Clinic*, 1988; 52(3):269–279.

18. Shuchter SR, Zisook S. The course of normal grief. In: Stroebe MS, Stroebe W, Hansson RO eds, *Handbook of Bereavement: Theory, Research and Intervention*. Cambridge: Cambridge University Press, 1993:23–43.

19. Zisook S, Shuchter SR, Summers J. Bereavement risk and preventive intervention. In: Raphael B, Burrows GD, eds, *The Handbook of Studies on Preventive Psychiatry*, 1995:203–223.

20. Zisook S, Shuchter SR. Bereavement. In: Dunner DL, ed, *Current Psychiatric Therapy II*, 1996: 248–252.

21. Bowlby J. Attachment and loss. In: *Separation: Anxiety and Anger* (Vol 21). New York: Basic Books, 1973.

22. Lund DA, Caserta MS, Dimond MF, et al. Impact of bereavement on self-conceptions of older surviving spouses. *Symbolic Interaction*, 1986; 9: 235–244.

23. Horowitz MJ. *Stress Response Syndromes*. Northvale, NJ: Aronson, 1986.

24. Rynearson EK. Pathologic grief: the queen's croquet ground. *Psychiatric Annals*, 1990; 20:295–303.

25. Jacobs S. *Pathologic Grief*. Washington, DC: American Psychiatric Association, 1993.

26. Horowitz MJ, Wilner N, Marmar C, Krupnick J. Pathological grief and the activation of latent self images. *American Journal of Psychiatry*, 1980; 137: 1157.

27. Parkes CM. *Bereavement: studies of grief in adult life*. 2nd ed. New York: International Universities Press, 1972.

28. Klerman GL, Izen J. The effects of bereavement and grief on physical health and general well being. *Advances in Psychosomatic Medicine*, 1977; 8:63–104.

29. Sanders CM. Risk factors in bereavement outcome. In: Stroebe MS, Stroebe W, Hansson RO, eds, *Handbook of Bereavement: Theory, Research and Intervention*. Cambridge: Cambridge University Press, 1993:255–267.

30. Kaprio J, Koskenvuo M, Rita H. Mortality after bereavement: a prospective study of 95,647 widowed persons. *American Journal of Public Health*, 1987; 77:283–287.

31. Zisook S, Shuchter SR, Mulvihill M. Alcohol, cigarette and medication use during the first year of widowhood. *Psychiatric Annals*, 1990; 20:318–326.

32. Helsing KJ, Comstock G, Szklo M. Causes of death in a widowed population. *American Journal of Epidemiology*, 1982; 116:524–532.

33. Clayton PJ. The sequelae and nonsequelae of conjugal bereavement. *American Journal of Psychiatry*, 1979; 136:1530–1534.

34. Lund DA, Caserta MS, Dimond MF. The course of spousal bereavement in later life. In: Stroebe MS, Stroebe W, Hansson R, eds, *Handbook of Bereavement: Theory, Research and Intervention*. Cambridge University Press: Cambridge, 1993:240–254.

35. Schneider DS, Sledge PA, Shuchter SR, Zisook S. Dating and remarriage over the first two years of widowhood. *Annals of Clinical Psychiatry*, 1996; 8:51–57.

36. Sanders CM. Risk factors in bereavement outcome. *Journal of Social Issues*, 1988; 44:97–112.

37. Parkes CM. Determinants of outcome following bereavement. *Omega*, 1975; 6:303–323.

38. Vachon MLS. Predictors and correlates of adaptation in conjugal bereavement. *American Journal of Psychiatry*, 1982; 139:998–1002.

39. Clayton PJ. Bereavement. In: Paykel ES, ed, *Handbook of Affective Disorder*. London: Churchill Livingston, 1982.

40. Silverman PR. Widowhood and prevention intervention. *Family Coordinator*, 1972; 21:95–102.

41. Parkes CM, Weiss RS. *Recovery from Bereavement*. New York: Basic Books, 1983.

42. Zisook S, Shuchter SR, Summers J, Grant I, Hutchin S, Burns K. *Adult Bereavement and Depression*. Presented at the 1995 Annual Meeting of the American Psychiatric Association, Miami, Florida, May 20–25, 1995.

43. Deutsch H. Absence of grief. *Psychoanalytic Quarterly*, 1937; 6:12–22.

44. Raphael B, Middleton W. What is pathologic grief? *Psychiatric Annals*, 1990; 20:304–307.

45. Raphael B, Middleton W, Martinek N, et al. Counseling and therapy of the bereaved. In: Stroebe MS, Stroebe W, Hansson RO, eds, *Handbook of Bereavement: Theory, Research and Intervention*. Cambridge, England: Cambridge University Press, 1993:427–453.

46. Raphael B. *The Anatomy of Bereavement*. New York: Basic Books, 1983.

47. Rynearson EK. Psychotherapy of pathologic grief: revisions and limitations. *Psychiatric Clinics of North America*, 1987; 10:487–500.

48. Rynearson EK, McCreery JM. Bereavement after homicide: a synergism of trauma and loss. *American Journal of Psychiatry*, 1993; 150:250–261.

49. Pynoos RS, Nader K. Children's exposure to violence and traumatic death. *Psychiatric Annals*, 1990;20:334–344.

50. Prigerson HG, Frank E, Kasl SV, Reynolds CF, Anderson B, Zubenko GS, Houck PR, George CJ, Kupfer DJ. Complicated grief and bereavement-related depression as distinct disorders: preliminary empirical validation in elderly bereaved spouses. *American Journal of Psychiatry*, 1995;152(1):22–30.

51. Stroebe W, Stroebe MS. *Bereavement and Health*. New York: Cambridge University Press, 1987.

52. Schmale A, Iker H. Hopelessness as a prediction of cervical cancer. *Social Science and Medicine* 1971; 5:95–100.

53. Schmale A, Iker H. The psychological setting of uterine cervical cancer. *Annals of the New York Academy of Sciences*, 1965; 125:794–801.

54. Chambers WN, Reiser MF. Emotional stress in the precipitation of congestive heart failure. *Psychosomatic Medicine*, 1953; 15:38–60.

55. Weiner A, Gerber IE, Battin D, et al. The process and phenomenology of bereavement. In: Schoenberg B, Berger I, Weiner A, et al, eds., *Bereavement: Its Psychosocial Aspects*. New York: Columbia University Press, 1975.

56. Parkes CM, Benjamin B, Fitzgerald RG. Broken heart: a statistical study of increased mortality among widowers. *British Medical Journal*, 1969; 1:740–743.

57. Zisook S, Mulvihill M, Shuchter SR. Widowhood and anxiety, *Psychiatric Medicine*, 1990a; 8:99–116.

58. Stroebe MS, Stroebe W. The mortality of bereavement: a review. In: Stroebe MS, Stroebe W, Hansson RO, eds, *Handbook of Bereavement: Theory, Research and Intervention*. Cambridge: Cambridge University Press, 1993:175–195.

59. Parkes CM. Bereavement and mental illness. *British Journal of Psychology*, 1965; 38:388–397.

60. Gallagher-Thompson DE, Breckenridge J, Thompson LW, et al. Effects of bereavement on indicators of mental health in elderly widows and widowers. *Journal of Gerontology*, 1983; 38:565–571.

61. Jacobs SC, Nelson JC, Zisook S. Treating depression of bereavement with antidepressants: a pilot study. *Psychiatric Clinics of North America*, 1987; 10:501–510.

62. Bruce M, Kim K, Leaf P, et al. Depressive episodes and dysphoria resulting from conjugal bereavement in a prospective community sample. *American Journal of Psychiatry*, 1990; 147:608–611.

63. Clayton PJ. Bereavement and depression. *Journal of Clinical Psychiatry*, 1990; 51:34–40.

64. Zisook S, Shuchter SR. Depression through the first year after the death of a spouse. *American Journal of Psychiatry*, 1991; 148:1346–1352.

65. Pasternak RE, Reynolds CF, Miller MD, et al. The symptom profile and two-year course of subsyndromal depression in spousally bereaved elders. *American Journal of Geriatric Psychiatry*, 1994; 2:210–219.

66. Zisook S, Shuchter SR, Sledge P, Paulus M, Judd LL. The spectrum of depressive phenomena after spousal bereavement. *American Journal of Psychiatry*, 1994b; 55(4):29–36.

67. Zisook S. Death, dying and bereavement. In: Kaplan HI, Sadock BJ, eds, *Comprehensive Textbook of Psychiatry*. 6th ed. Baltimore: Williams & Wilkins, 1995a.

68. Weller RA, Weller EB, Fristad MA, Bowes JM. Depression in recently bereaved children. *American Journal of Psychiatry*, 1991; 148(11):1536–1540.

69. Zisook S, Schneider D, Shuchter SR. Anxiety and bereavement. *Psychiatric Medicine*, 1990b; 8(2):83–95.

70. Jacobs SC, Hansen F, Kasl S, et al. Anxiety disorders in acute bereavement: risk and risk factors. *Journal of Clinical Psychiatry*, 1990; 51:267–274.

71. Raphael B, Maddison D. The care of bereaved adults. In: Hill OW, ed, *Modern Trends in Psychosomatic Medicine*. London: Butterworth, 1976.

72. Lindy JD, Green BL, Grace M, Titchener J. Psychotherapy with survivors of the Beverly Hills Supper Club Fire. *American Journal of Psychotherapy*, 1983; 37:593–610.

73. Parkes CM. Psychiatric problems following bereavement by murder or manslaughter. *British Journal of Psychiatry*, 1993; 162:49–54.

74. Ludin T. Morbidity following sudden and unexpected bereavement. *British Journal of Psychiatry*, 1984; 144:84–88.

75. Martin JL, Dean L. Bereavement following death from AIDS: unique problems, reactions and special needs. In: Stroebe MS, Stroebe W, Hansson RO, eds, *Handbook of Bereavement: Theory, Research and Intervention*. Cambridge: Cambridge University Press, 1993:317–330.

76. Cameron PM, Leszcz M, Bebchuck W, Swinson RP, Antony MM, Azim HF, Doidge N, Korenblum MS, Nigam T, Perry JC, Seeman MV. The practice and roles of the psychotherapies: a discussion paper. Working group of the Canadian Psychiatric Association Steering Committee. *Canadian Journal of Psychiatry*, 1999; 44:185–315.

77. Vachon MLS, Sheldon AR, Lance WJ, et al. A controlled study of self-help intervention for widows. *American Journal of Psychiatry*, 1980; 137:1380–1384.

78. Constantino RE. Comparison of two group interventions for the bereaved. *Image*, 1988;20:83–87.

79. Lieberman MA, Videka-Sherman L. The impact of self-help groups on the mental health of widows and widowers. *American Journal of Orthopsychiatry*, 1986; 56:435–449.

80. Marmar CR, Horowitz MJ, Weiss DS, et al. A controlled trial of brief psychotherapy and mutual-help group treatment of conjugal bereavement. *American Journal of Psychiatry*, 1988; 145:203–212.

81. Wortman CB, Silver RC. The myths of coping with loss. *Journal of Consulting and Clinical Psychology*, 1989; 57:349–357.

82. Miller MD, Frank E, Cornes C, et al. Applying interpersonal psychotherapy to bereavement-related depression following loss of a spouse in late life. *Journal of Psychotherapy Practice and Research*, 1994; 3:149–162.

83. Pasternak RE, Reynolds CF, Schlernitzauer M, et al. Acute open-trial nortriptyline therapy of bereavement-related depression in late life. *Journal of Clinical Psychiatry*, 1991; 52:307–310.

84. Mor V. *Hospice Care Systems*. New York: Springer Press, 1987.

85. Parkes CM. Evaluation of a bereavement service. *Journal of Preventive Psychiatry*, 1981; 1:179–188.

86. Greer DS, Mor V. An overview of national hospice study findings. *Journal of Chronic Diseases*, 1986; 39:5–7.

87. Moseley JR, Logan SJ, Tolle SW, Bentley JH. Developing a bereavement program in a university hospital setting. *Oncology Nursing Forum*, 1988; 15:151–155.

88. Yalom ID, Vinogradov S. Bereavement groups: techniques and themes. *International Journal of Group Psychotherapy*, 1988; 38:419–446.

89. Summers J, Zisook S, Atkinson JH, Patterson T,

Chandler J, Malone J. *Bereavement and Unresolved Grief in Seropositive Men and Men at High Risk for HIV*. New Research Program and Abstracts of the One Hundred Forty-Five Annual Meeting of the American Psychiatric Association, New Orleans, Louisiana, May 11–16, 1991.

90. Lieberman MA, Yalom I. Brief group psychotherapy for the spousally bereaved: a controlled study. *International Journal of Group Psychotherapy*, 1992; 42:117–132.

91. Gerber I, Weiner A, Battin D, et al. Brief therapy to the aged bereaved. In: Schoenberg B, Gerber I, eds, *Bereavement: Its Psychosocial Aspects*. New York: Columbia University Press, 1975:310–313.

92. Polak PR, Egan D, Vandenburgh R, et al. Prevention in mental health: a controlled study. *American Journal of Psychiatry*, 1975; 132:146–149.

93. Raphael B. Preventive intervention with the recently bereaved. *Archives of General Psychiatry*, 1977; 34:1450–1454.

94. Volkan VD. "Regrief" therapy. In: Schoenberg G, Gerber IE, eds, *Bereavement: Its Psychosocial Aspects*. New York: Columbia University Press, 1971:334–350.

95. Lazare A. Unresolved grief. In: Lazare A, ed, *Outpatient Psychiatry*. Baltimore, MD: Williams & Wilkins, 1979:498–512.

96. Paul N, Grosser G. Operational mourning and its role in conjoint family therapy. *Community Mental Health Journal*, 1965; 1:339–345.

97. Melges FT, DeMaso DR. Grief resolution therapy: reliving, revising and revisiting. *American Journal of Psychotherapy*, 1980; 34:51–61.

98. Mawson D, Markes IM, Ramm L, et al. Guided mourning for morbid grief: a controlled study. *British Journal of Psychiatry*, 1981; 138:185–193.

99. Horowitz MJ, Marmar C, Weiss DS, et al. Brief psychotherapy of bereavement reactions. *Archives of General Psychiatry*, 1984; 41:438–448.

100. Worden JW. *Grief Counseling and Grief Therapy: A Handbook for the Mental Health Practitioner*. New York: Springer, 1991.

101. Shuchter SR, Zisook S. Hovering over the bereaved. *Psychiatric Annals*, 1990;20:327–333.

102. Reynolds C, Hoch CC, Buysse DJ, et al. Electroencephalographic sleep in spousal bereavement and bereavement-related depression of late life. *Biological Psychiatry*, 1992; 31:69–82.

103. Zisook S. Bereavement, depression and immune function. *Psychiatry Research*, 1994a; 52:1–10.

104. Reynolds C. *The Post-treatment Course of Depression in Bereaved Elders*. Presented at the 2nd International Conference on New Directions in Affective Disorders, Jerusalem, Israel, September 7, 1995.

PART VI
Ethical and Spiritual Issues

23

Ethical Issues in Palliative Care

Edmund D. Pellegrino, M.D.

It is as much the business of the physician to alleviate pain and
smooth the avenues of death, when inevitable, as it is to cure
disease.
> —John Gregory (1725–1773), *On the Duties and Qualifications
> of Physicians*

The care of incurably ill persons has always presented moral challenges to those who attend them. For families, friends, and society, those challenges reside in the burdens of ministering to the decline of a fellow human being. To the physician, the challenges lie in the impotence of the medical art to forestall death and in turning the focus of that art from seeking cure to providing care and comfort and to smoothing the "avenues of death," as John Gregory so pithily put it. Today, these ethical challenges often devolve on the collective responsibilities of a team of specialists engaged in the practice of intensive comprehensive palliative care (ICPC).[1]

Generically, the ethical issues surrounding the care of patients who need palliation in dying are no different from those encountered in the care of any sick person. What is different is the existential predicament of the incurably ill. Their existence as sick persons is markedly altered when the possibility of cure has been supplanted by the realization of the reality of their impending confrontation with finitude. Then, if the good of the patient is to be served, technical proficiency must yield to compassion, comfort, and consolation.

Accordingly, this discussion of the ethical issues in palliative care proceeds as follows: It begins with a phenomenological description of the existential state of the terminally ill patient; it moves from this to the special needs of such patients, the ethical issues encountered by those who care for them, and the resolution of ethical conflicts that emerge from their special needs.

HISTORICAL PROLOGUE

It is difficult to discern historically when the moral obligation to care became as important as the obligation to cure. The evidence from the Hippocratic era is somewhat equivocal. The primacy of beneficence in the Oath,[2] the exhortation to "do away with sufferings of the sick"[3] and to avoid "doing harm by useless efforts[4,5] seem to require the care of incurable cases. Yet, elsewhere, there is the suggestion that a physician ought to refuse to treat hopeless cases lest they reflect negatively on his reputation. Edelstein thinks this latter opinion was not the dominant one.[6]

However, when the nobler moral precepts of the Hippocratic ethic were adopted and given spiritual sanction by the teachings of the three great monotheistic religions, care for the suffering and the dying became both a moral and a religious obligation. This synthesis is epitomized in the parable of the Good Samaritan and actualized in succeeding centuries in the traditional commitment of Christian religious orders and foundations to the care of the sick, the poor, and the dying.[7,8] Hospitals were founded at a time when their major function could only have been care of the dying, since physicians then offered little in the way of truly effective therapeutics. They provided the only refuge for those who had no other place in which to suffer or to die.

John Gregory's view reflects this fusion of the Christian tradition of solicitude for the sick and the Hippocratic ethics. It is a combination that dominated eighteenth-century medical ethics in England and subsequently shaped the ethical code of the American Medical Association.[9] This integration of care and cure is also now the prevalent note in nonreligious, humanistic, holistic theories of therapeutics for both dying and nondying patients.

SOME DEFINITIONS

At the outset, it is essential to define the way I shall use the term *intensive comprehensive palliative care* (ICPC).

Palliative implies the fact that cure—that is, return of the patient to a former or a better state of health—is not possible and that the patient is fatally ill and death foreseeable as a result of the presenting disease. The patient need not be terminal; death may not be foreseeable in the immediate future, but it is firmly established that whatever disease the patient suffers from is an ultimately fatal disease that will cause death unless some other cause intervenes.

To *palliate* in these circumstances means to ease or lessen the violence of a disease while not yet curing it. It means to recognize the physician's or other caregiver's inability to change the natural course of events. To palliate is to follow the Hippocratic injunction to "lessen the violence" of disease and to "do away with suffering."[3] This requires much more than relief of pain, though this is the first step in palliation.

Providing comfort must be *comprehensive*. It must take into account the highly individualized, personal, and unique response of *this* patient to the predicament of *this* sickness—a predicament never the same for any two persons. It must be comprehensive in that it encompasses physical but also psychosocial comfort. Nursing care, attention to spiritual and emotional needs, and elaboration of a suitable support structure all must

be included and integrated if comprehensiveness is to be a reality.

In a sense, CPC is *healing even while the patient is dying*. This may seem at first a contradiction, since healing means "to make whole to restore."[10] Manifestly this is not possible in any ordinary sense, since by definition a terminal or fatal illness is one in which a dying patient has progressed beyond the point of no return. But, if we regard healing in a broader sense of establishing a new balance, a new accommodation between the progress of the disease and the patient's adaptation to the course of that disease, then healing may occur even when the patient is dying. Healing here means to recompose the person as person within the confines imposed by the knowledge, inevitability, and actuality of dying.

Comprehensive palliative care is also *intensive care*—that is, it brings all the capacities of medicine and medical care to focus on the end of palliation. Palliative care must be pursued just as energetically, purposefully, and forcefully as care in the intensive-care unit. The difference is that the end of cure is replaced by the end of comfort, of easing and preparing for death. In the palliative hierarchy of patient good, the medical good takes a lesser place, while primacy is given to other dimensions of patient good—his own assessment of the good, his notion of quality of life, his good generically as a human being, and his spiritual good.[11]

This definition of CPC specifies the end or *telos of medicine* as it applies to the care of the dying patient. This telos is what determines what actions and treatments are to be taken, as well as the duties incumbent on the physician, nurse, and other health professionals. It unites them as a team, determines how conflicts among them are to be resolved, and defines the virtues each must exhibit. Conscious commitment to this telos constitutes the act of profession, the promise implicit in it, and the covenant that binds the health professional when he voluntarily offers or agrees to care for a dying patient.

Hospice programs are the place in which comprehensive palliative care is usually practiced in its most intensive form. They may be free standing, hospital based, hospital affiliated, or community based. It is a mistake, however, to confine palliative care to these settings and thereby to relieve others of this responsibility. Any patient with a fatal illness, whether or not in a terminal state, is entitled to the kind and range of ministration included under CPC. Indeed, CPC is, in essence, holistic medicine. It is holistic care of the patient as a human person in whom disease and illness are complex, multifaceted phenomena that generate a wide spectrum of needs. If these needs are unmet, true healing cannot occur. To be sure, CPC, like holistic medicine in general, is an ambitious and even in some ways a presumptuous ideal. But it is an ideal that should guide the caregiver—a standard to work toward even if it is not totally achievable. Palliative care, in fact, in its elements, is the kind of care owed to every patient regardless of whether he or she is in a terminal state or in a hospice. It is simply optimum care fitted to the special requirements of individual incurably ill patients.[12]

THE EXISTENTIAL STATE OF INCURABILITY

The Changing Societal Context

The ethical issues in palliative care occur within the societal and personal contexts of death as it is perceived in modern society. In recent years, much attention has been given by sociologists and historians to our changed attitudes toward death. We have moved in Western civilization from death as an inevitable, public, social event in which all play a central role one day to death as a technological failure in the march of modern medicine toward immortality. As Aries and others have so well documented, we no longer practice the *artes moriendi*, the arts of dying, which, from the late Middle Ages until the twentieth century portrayed death as the drama that prepares a person and her soul for communion with God.[13,14] The dying person then played the leading role, summoning all to the bedside, issuing dying statements, giving orders to his family or forgiveness to his foes. Friend, priest, doctor, family each had a prescribed but secondary role among the dramatis personae of dying.

Modern society has "deprived man of his death."[15] The patient still plays a role, of course. But now the dying person is an autonomous agent who decides when treatment should be stopped and ordains how she should be treated when she loses the capacity to make decisions. She may insist on treatment even when it is opposed by the physician. The patient remains central in one sense, but in a very different way from previously. He or she no longer accepts death as inevitable, since modern medicine holds promise for defeating so many serious diseases. While surrounded by an ever-expanding health-care team, the patient may well fear more than anything else the prospect of dying alone, isolated by her autonomy. She must make her own decisions, whereas previously those decisions were made in conformity with a supporting societal matrix of custom, ritual, and belief.

Today's patient dies, too, in a social milieu in which being ill is a defeat, an automatic ejection from the cult of youth and health. The dying person intrudes on everyone else's pursuit of business or pleasure. In the modern world, dying is an obscenity, an experience to be avoided at all costs, (whether via pharmacology or euthanasia).

Within this milieu of isolation, alienation, devaluation, and rejection, the dying person must confront his own mortality. Modern societal attitudes toward dying materially add to and accentuate the experiential modalities of being ill, being a patient, and being on the way to personal extinction.

Becoming a Patient

An ill person becomes a patient when she decides that whatever symptoms or signs she has experienced have reached a state that requires that she seek help from a health professional. Being a patient signals one's entrance into a new form of existence, one that forces a special kind of relationship with another human being. Being a patient is being in a special state of vulnerability. This vulnerability results from several things, as follows.

The patient is in an unequal relationship with the caregiver: She is dependent on the caregiver's knowledge, skill, and character. The patient has little choice but to enter this relationship if she wishes to be healed. She must trust that what is recommended and what is done are in her best interests and that she is not being exploited to the doctor's advantage. The doctor, for his part, in offering or agreeing to help makes a promise that the good of the patient, in all its dimensions, will be his primary concern—that is, that the medical good, the good as perceived by the patient, and the good of the patient as a human being and spiritual good will all be served.

In his healing, the doctor is obliged to respect the patient's dignity as a human being capable of reasoned choice according to her own values and beliefs. Not to do so is to violate the humanity of the sick person, an act per se maleficent. That is why respect for autonomy is consistent with, and not antagonistic to, beneficence. Strong paternalism violates autonomy, but it violates beneficence, as well.

When, in addition to becoming a patient, a person is confronted with a diagnosis and a prognosis of fatality, a new order of magnitude is added to her vulnerability.[16,17] The usual phenomena of vulnerability that accompany any illness are exaggerated. This, in turn, accentuates the obligations of the physician to mitigate the impact of that vulnerability. As a result, the usual ethical duties and obligations of the healing relationship are rendered much more urgent and complex. The already existing inequality of power is tipped far in the direction of the doctor, but so, too, is the weight of obligations to protect the patient's vulnerability.

Dying patients must confront their own finitude, not simply as a future, remote possibility but as an actual, foreseeable, and immediately palpable reality. For most humans, this is the greatest anxiety they will ever confront. They often fear the process of dying, perhaps more than death itself. The fatally ill person faces the anticipation of pain, the loss of her value in the sight of others, and a sense of guilt for being a burden to others. She suffers an assault on her self-image and alienation from her own body, which is now seen as a mortal enemy. Every progress or regress of symptoms is a portent of the rate at which death is advancing.

Whether or not one has been a believer, there is a spiritual challenge in dying. The dying patient must come to some terms with the inevitability of her finitude. She can no longer ignore the challenge to accept or reject the question of God's existence and of life after death. Every ill person, and, most acutely, every fatally ill person, asks Job's questions: Why? Why me? Why now? Some will deny, others will affirm, a religious belief. Some will seek atonement; some, reconciliation. None will be indifferent.

Hope, on which so much of the human capacity to face the future depends, is concomitantly compromised. By definition, there is no chance for cure. Hope must be redirected to living the last days as well as possible, to spiritual and moral growth, and to entering new and enriched relationships with friends, families, and foes.[18] Hope is transformed or extirpated, depending on how the emotional and spiritual crisis is addressed. To go from being a patient, even one with a serious illness to being a patient whose disease has been pronounced as incurable to being a patient who has been told that her death is imminent is to go through progressive stages of existential change. These substantially alter the degree if not the kind of obligations owed to that person by caregivers, whether doctor, nurse, social worker, family member, friend, or minister.

CONCRETE ETHICAL ISSUES IN INTENSIVE COMPREHENSIVE PALLIATIVE CARE

It is against this social and personal existential and experiential backdrop that the specific, practical, concrete, everyday ethical issues of CPC must be examined.

Pain Relief

The first moral obligation of any palliative-care program is to be competent in the optimal relief of pain.[19] This is so obvious as hardly to need mention were it not for the fact that many physicians still do not treat pain properly. Measures for pain relief are available today such that no patient need die in pain.[20,21] Not to use pain medication well is a moral failure that is inexcusable and tantamount to legal malpractice, as well.

Pain medications should be used in doses sufficient to control pain. They should not be withheld or used sparingly for fear of making the patient an addict. This is surely not a problem of consequence in patients whose death is imminent. Nor is the danger of suppressing respiration as a side effect. So long as the intention is not to cause death but to relieve pain, if no other measure is available to relieve pain, if the patient's relief of pain is not dependent on the death of the patient and there is a proportionate reason for running the risk, then high doses of narcotics can be used.[22] The moral principle of double effect would be operative under these conditions.[23] We knowingly run risks of serious side effects with any potent medication. Moreover, the fact of the matter is that patients given increasing doses of narcotics develop considerable tolerance to their respiration-depressing effects.

Pain relief alone is not sufficient. There is a concomitant moral obligation to relieve suffering, a much more complex phenomenon whose elements have already been outlined. Optimal relief of pain and suffering are the first two morally mandatory obligations of any physician who cares for the incurably ill.

These obligations must be more judiciously approached with patients who have a fatal or incurable disease but whose death is not imminent. Such patients may suffer from chronic pain. They surely deserve optimal treatment. But if there are many years yet to be lived in the natural history of the disease, fear of addiction is a justifiable reason for caution in the administration of addictive drugs. Chronic pain is a subject of its own, a nexus of psychosocial and physiological interacting factors that requires the most careful evaluation and treatment. In these patients, the dangers of addiction cannot lightly be dismissed. The physician's moral obligation is to refer such patients to experts in pain management and not to fall into the trap of escalating doses of opiates.

Freedom to Choose, Refuse, and Request

A major ethical issue is the capacity of fatally ill patients to make choices and to give ethically valid consent. An ethically valid consent must meet several criteria: (1) It must be informed, (2) it must be free of coercion, and (3) it must be made by a mentally competent person. This is not the place to review the requirements for an ethically valid informed consent.[24] Rather I wish to underscore the ethical issues in informed consent peculiar to the existential state of being fatally ill. In this state, for example, patients are exceedingly vulnerable to the suggestions of those around them. The family and the doctor assume central roles of power, which they must exercise with careful regard for patients' personal wishes and values.

The assumption is too easily made by the comprehensive palliative-care team that the patient implicitly understands or accepts the full program of care offered in a comprehensive-care setting or a hospice program. This may not be the case at all. As with other treatment, consent must be explicit before the patient enters the program. Special attention is necessary to such things as the degree of sedation a patient may wish in the relief of his pain or suffering. Some patients accept and want any degree of sedation required to attain relative comfort. Others want to preserve a certain degree of consciousness and are willing to trade off some pain to remain in conscious contact with family and friends or to preserve decision-making ability.

Another example is the depth, if any, to which patients may want their psychological, personal, or sexual lives probed by a team intent on ferreting out the causes of a patient's suffering. This is a particularly sensitive problem in the realm of spiritual conflicts and values. Any fatal illness entails grappling with spiritual issues. Fear of eternal punishment, confrontation with the question of God's existence, and desire for reconciliation or atonement may play a role in the patient's fear of dying. For many if not most patients the religious as well as the psychological aspects of dying are important to recognize. But others reject and resent probing into their spiritual lives as unwarranted intrusions. It is a mistake to assume that entry into a hospital program implies acceptance of every facet of that program for the duration of the illness.

These are some of the personal matters examination of which the palliative-care teams must not assume will be welcomed by every patient. Respect for patient autonomy requires the patient's suitably informed consent, particularly before the team begins an examination of psychosocial or religious causes of suffering. For some patients, the religious dimension may be the most important way to find meaning in suffering.[25] Regardless of the caregiver's own views on religion, there is an obligation, therefore, to offer the patient the opportunity of receiving help in confronting these issues or rejecting them as she sees fit. There is an equal obligation not to use the patient's vulnerability as an opportunity to convert him or her to the caregiver's belief system. One may offer such help, but only if the patient wishes it and requests it.

In an era in which there is a tendency to psychologize all of life from birth to death, the same respectful attention is necessary in probing the inner psychic life of the dying patient with the patient or with family members. The dividing line between the licit exploration of the psychological aspects of suffering and the illicit imposition of such probing is especially difficult to locate. There is no clear, bright line that divides unwelcome and offensive psychological paternalism from beneficent identification of a treatable or ameliorable cause of depression.

Similarly difficult is the question of what treatments to offer to the dying patient. On a strong view of autonomy, all treatments, including those that are of the most marginal benefit, or that are futile, should be offered. This is the consumer view of the autonomy of the patient. On a more moderate view of autonomy, futile treatments, those that are ineffective in altering the natural progress of the disease or are excessively burdensome, ought not to be offered. Presumably, a patient who has entered a hospice program understands that its purpose is to ease the process of suffering and dying, not to effect a miraculous cure.

Cardiopulmonary resuscitation, under ordinary circumstances, frustrates this acceptance of the inevitability of death. Yet, there are patients who may see personal benefit in living a few days or a week longer, for example, to see a relative, a baby born, a child graduate. Under such circumstances, patients must be warned of the dangers of cardiopulmonary resuscitation, such as the vegetative state, rib fractures, spleen rupture, and other conditions that may result. Except in unusual circumstances, cardiopulmonary resuscitation should not be offered.

Telling the Truth

Truth telling poses a problem in the patient's last days, when consciousness and cognitive capacity may wax and wane or be lost entirely. Presumably, the patient who enters a hospice program knows he has a fatal and terminal illness. Clearly, he knows his diagnosis and his likely prognosis. This should be the case with dying patients in similar circumstances outside the hospice program. There is no way patients can participate authentically in their own dying without knowing the truth. With some exceptions, to be mentioned later, truth telling is a requisite for comprehensive palliative care in any setting.

The major problems with truth telling arise from two sources: how the truth is communicated and cultural differences that affect the care of dying patients.[26]

As far as the method of truth telling goes, no formula can be prescribed. Communication is a highly personal interaction in which the value and the psychological convictions of doctor and patient meet and interact. Each meeting is a unique event. The language and level of detail used in telling the truth should be fitted to the patient's culture, educational background, and age. In general, it is wise to allow patients to direct the rate and depth of information by their questions. Patients should be given room enough to navigate their way through the details in their own way. Poor timing, abruptness, impatience, failure to listen, and insensitivity to the gravity and impact of the truth, are lapses of the ethical obligation of truth telling.

In some cultures, it is customary not to give a patient bad news or the full truth on the ground that this destroys hope and only makes the patient more miserable.[27] Some physicians, particularly older ones, stubbornly hold to this view for all patients. Cultural differences should be respected when it is clear that the patient has not requested information, is not desirous of violating his cultural mores, and is not harmed by dying within the formulae prescribed by his own culture. Patients need not die the Anglo-American way, which places much more emphasis on personal autonomy than do other cultures.[28]

Sometimes a patient requests in advance that the truth, or at least all its details, be not revealed. Provided such a choice is genuine and that it is made by a fully competent patient, it ought to be respected so long as it does not so impair the process of care in a way that causes identifiable harm to the patient. Physicians who cannot, in good conscience, take patient autonomy this far should so inform the patient. They should decline to enter the therapeutic relationship or withdraw respectfully. To insist on telling the whole truth over a patient's objections seems a contradictory violation of autonomy to preserve autonomy.

Similarly, however good the doctor's intent may be, it is a breach of trust to shape a vulnerable patient's decision by withholding essential facts, selecting or shaping them to achieve what the doctor thinks best. The vulnerability of the patient and the inequality in knowledge, physical stamina, and power between patient and physician must always be a moral brake on doing harm so that good may come of it.

In any case, most experienced clinicians agree that there are very few instances in which patients are genuinely harmed by knowing the truth. Rather, it is the way truth is communicated and the attitudes the doctor exhibits in telling the truth that cause problems. With respect to truth telling and respect for autonomy, the key ideal is to make decisions *with* and *for* the patient. To this end, clinical decisions, especially in the case of fatally ill patients, are best when they arise somewhere between doctor and patient. If decisions veer too strongly to the side of the doctor's estimate of what is "good" for the patient, those decisions can be harmful to the patient; if they are too far from the physician's estimate, they may pose moral conflicts for the physician. In their zeal to do good, or in their enjoyment of the satisfaction of doing so, physicians may unconsciously be tempted to intimidate the patient or to "take over" in the name of relieving the patient of the anguish of decision making.

Surrogate Decision Making

When patients lose the capacity for self-governance, their moral right to make decisions is transferred to surrogates. This surrogate may be designated by the patient before he loses his capacity to decide. Surrogates can be designated by word of mouth, by execution of a durable power of attorney for health, by legal definition in some states of the United States, or de facto by virtue of being the available next of kin.

However designated, the surrogate is vested with the moral authority to make decisions in the place of the patient. This authority is not absolute.[27] For one thing, the physician remains morally bound to protect the welfare of the patient. Physicians cannot abrogate this fiduciary responsibility. The physician must write the order that affects the patient and thus cannot escape moral complicity. As a result, the physician has an obligation, within reasonable limits, to ascertain the moral validity of a surrogate, regardless of the way that surrogate is designated. The physician must assess whether the surrogate actually knows the patient's wishes or values, has a financial or emotional conflict of interest in the decision, or is making the decision as if she were the patient and not as the patient himself would have made it.

Conflicts may occur between surrogates and physician or between both and an advance directive, such as a living will. Few people (in-cluding physicians) can so accurately predict the clinical circumstances of their final days that they are able while still competent to write precise orders to for others to carry out when the time arrives. Doctor, patient, surrogate, and advance directive may in the actual moment of decision making conflict with one another. If this occurs, the determining factor should be the best interests of the patient, determined among and between those who have a fiduciary obligation to protect the patient's interest, including doctors, nurses, chaplains, family, friends, and surrogates. If discussion and dialogue fail to resolve disagreements, an ethics committee often can be useful. Its purpose is not to substitute for the valid decision makers but to assist them to resolve differences. The use and abuse of ethics committees are separate topics too large to be examined in this chapter.

Physician and Surrogate Autonomy

Like the autonomy of the patient, the autonomy of surrogates is not absolute. Autonomy is limited when it is patently not in the interest of an incompetent patient, when it results in injury to third parties, when it violates the physician's moral integrity or her perception of what is scientifically valid medicine, or when the criteria for a decision are themselves not morally defensible, for example, when quality-of-life or economic criteria are used to decide the fate of a patient in a permanent vegetative state who has not previously expressed preferences on these matters.

Economic and quality-of-life criteria are valid if employed by the patient in her living will or transmitted to a morally valid surrogate. They are not valid if used as reason to withhold a palliative treatment that would be of benefit to the patient. In our era of concern for rising health expenditures and the dominant cult of youth and health, there is great danger of devaluing the lives of whole segments of society (the elderly, the handicapped, or the terminally ill) because of a "poor" quality of life. If assisted suicide and euthanasia are legalized or socially tolerated, as in the Netherlands, the danger is accentuated, and involuntary and nonvoluntary euthanasia became realities.[28,29]

Intensive comprehensive palliative care is the rational alternative to euthanasia and assisted suicide. It is an inescapable moral obligation for anyone who oppose assisted suicide and euthanasia as immoral to provide such care. Hospices in particular must be exceedingly careful not to permit any kind of assisted suicide or euthanasia within their programs. They can too easily become society's designated agents of death, not its haven for fully human, sympathetic, truly compassionate care and dying.

This does not in any way imply that ICPC is inconsistent with the cessation of care that is futile—that is, ineffective, nonbeneficial, and/or excessively burdensome. Nor does it imply that pain relief and comfort are in any way to be compromised, even if the use of narcotics or sedatives intended to relieve pain and suffering results in unintended death. Intentional hastening of death and withdrawal of noneffective life-sustaining care must be distinguished carefully.[30] Preserving the distinction is particularly important when dealing with the vulnerability of patients with fatal and terminal illnesses. The moral philosophy of intention is a neglected subject in ethics, where utilitarianism is the dominant theory, yet intention is an essential element in evaluating the moral status of any human act.[31]

Alternative and Experimental Treatment

Patients in whom the diagnosis of a fatal or terminal illness has been made are understandably desperate for some alternative to standard or scientific medicine. Families and friends in an effort to be helpful may urge nonstandard therapies on patients. These may range from relatively innocuous high-dosage multivitamin, herbal, dietary, or behavioral therapies to toxic, highly expensive, or burdensome treatments.

The ethical obligation of the physician, mindful of the desperation of family, friends, and patient, is always to present the scientific viewpoint, nonjudgmentally and respectfully. In general, alternate therapies that are not positively harmful can be tolerated. But, alternative therapies that are harmful or interfere with proven beneficial therapy should always be refused. Physicians will vary in where they draw the line. Neither absolute capitulation to patient requests nor absolute rejection seems justifiable in light of the aims of comprehensive palliative care.

Similarly, patients in a clinical state that requires palliative care are often eager to be experimental subjects in hopes that an untried treatment might alter the fatal thrust of their illness. Fully competent patients can legitimately participate as experimental subjects if they give informed consent, if the procedure is relatively safe, and if it is potentially of value for the patient or for others similarly afflicted. For reasons already outlined, the complexities of informal consent for experimental care in patients receiving palliative care require particular attention.

With patients who cannot give consent, research is admissible only in the most narrowly defined conditions—if danger and discomfort are nonexistent and the benefits to others significant. For such subjects, consent must be given by morally valid surrogates, as well as by an institutional review board. Anticipatory declarations made by patients while competent that give unspecified permission for research are too easily susceptible to abuse to be morally admissible.

Conflicts between the physician's role as care provider and his role as clinical scientist are complicated with any kind of human subject research.[32] These conflicts are yet to be resolved in any definitive way. With terminally ill patients and patients in vegetative states, they are magnified. The caregiver physician's role is primarily to serve as guardian of the patient, given the enormous possibility for abuse in research with terminally ill patients. If any such research is undertaken under rigorous control, the investigator must not be the caregiver physician.

Heroic treatments are sought by some patients and physicians who hope with one throw of the dice to reverse the expected course of the disease. This is a scenario more imagined than actualized. Under rigorously controlled conditions, where preliminary results are promising, where death is inevitable, where the patient is fully competent, and where conflicts of interest on the part of the investigator are minimal, such research may be allowable. On the whole, the danger of turning a fatally ill human being into a test object is sufficient great to make heroic treatments allowable only if ever under the rarest of circumstances.

Ethics of the Palliative-Care Team

Intensive palliative care of necessity requires a team of caregivers, and this introduces the special ethical issues that arise in collective activity.[33] No one physician or nurse can possibly meet the requirement to be "comprehensive" in the sense the term is used—that is, to designate care aimed at meeting the combined physical, psychosocial, spiritual, and personal needs of the dying person. The advantages of cooperative team care bring with them a variety of ethical issues, some general to team care and some specific to the care of incurably ill persons.[34–36]

To begin with, there is the question of how accountability is to be divided. Three possibilities exist: Responsibility may reside in one team member; responsibility may be assigned to each member relative to his or her function in the team; and there may be true collective responsibility in which each team member shares responsibility for the whole team's actions. There seems no clear way to disentangle them entirely.

The physician writes the orders and is ultimately responsible for the patient's care, since those orders affect the welfare of the patient even if they are recommended and agreed to by other members of the team. On the other hand, nurses, chaplains, social workers, and psychiatrists are professionals in their own right; all have a code of ethics that makes them responsible for that part of care they provide. They cannot be asked to violate their professional ethics by any other member, even the doctor. Any member who cooperates in, or fails to object to, any harmful act is a moral accomplice. Every team member in that sense shares in the collective responsibility of the whole team for the care provided.

Another complicating factor is the considerable overlap of roles and responsibilities in palliative care. To be sure, each member has special expertise that defines his profession, and each is responsible for applying that expertise to achieving the ends of palliative care. But it would be artificial to confine the physician to the realm of technical expert and to assign the work of caring and advocacy to the nurse, the psychosocial aspect to the social worker and the psychiatrist, or the spiritual aspect solely to the chaplain. Each team member has a responsibility for palliative care, which, unlike medical or other technical procedures, can never be discontinued or abandoned or neglected by any team member. All team members must apply their expertise humanely, sensitively, and compassionately.

An additional issue in team ethics is when to "blow the whistle"—to object if harm is being done or incompetence is observed. Everyone is obliged to be on the patient's "side"—to be an advocate. Team members must beware of seeing themselves as the only ones who understand the patient's plight and needs. Each must also feel responsible for the total team effort and refuse to let territorial prerogatives interfere with a patient's access to necessary care no matter who makes it available. Each must remember that intrateam conflict has moral implications because it affects the care the patient receives.

Another set of issues revolves around team dynamics. In the interest of team harmony, members can become too compliant. Members can be enveloped in the satisfaction of their own personal needs, in doing "good." Others may complain of the "anguish of the caregiver" manifested in themselves and their colleagues.[37] Self-pity and self-righteousness are subtle tendencies in those who attend dying and suffering patients. Some may be so infatuated with the superiority of group wisdom that the patient's wisdom about his own body and psyche are ignored.

Finally, there is the proper exercise of the role of team leader. This is becoming less the role of a "captain" or leader and more that of facilitator or convener. Patient and family members have roles to play as members of the palliative-care team. As always, the ethical imperative must be the impact of any decision on the comprehensive care of the patient, keeping the goal of palliation always in view.

Too often the palliative-care team develops such a conviction that it is "doing good" that it becomes self-justifying, in a way invading the privacy as well as the autonomy of the patient. Dying patients fear dying alone. They also fear "do-gooders" who appropriate patients' misfortunes to serve their own psychological needs. This is a distorted notion of beneficence that reduces patient to projects of others' need for expressing their own altruism. The result is infantalized patients who are smothered by a "system" that can all too easily become standardized in just the situation where individualized, personalized, and differentiated care is most urgently needed.

Comprehensive Palliative Care Ideologized

As a concept and as a moral obligation, ICPC is an admirable and necessary method for the care of the terminally and incurably ill patient. Its ethical status is firmly grounded in the existential and experiential predicament of patients who are directly confronting their finitude. Yet, as with any powerful concept, ICPC can become an ideology, a self-justifying way to deal with a ubiquitous human problem. This "ideologization" is manifest in several ways.

First of all is the medicalization of care for the dying, which is both a unique and a universal human experience. For centuries caring for the moribund was the responsibility of families, friends, and family doctors and nurses. Now it has become a professional specialty. There are obvious advantages to such a transformation but also some dangers. Where there are specialists, we tend to turn the task over to them and relieve ourselves of responsibility. This is unfortunate and may not at all serve the needs of the sick.

All the needs encompassed by comprehensive palliative care cannot be met, since the number of specialists is limited. But even if they were available, the crucial aspects of palliative care rely on humane, compassionate, and sensitive responses to the predicament of suffering. These are not necessarily technical skills. They depend on qualities of personal commitment that belong to those who have a genuine, friendly interest in the patient. A professional relationship cannot substitute for nor even approximate this kind of commitment. While family and friends are usually incorporated into a ICPC program, they are necessarily under control of the team. This may result in a tendency to manipulate patients, family, and friends so that they conform to a formularized way of dying. When ICPC is ideologized, it can tyrannize and psychologize every aspect of dying, not always beneficently, it then discourages and displaces those other nonprofessionals to whom the patient has turned in other life crises.

A certain amount of denial, depression, and alienation accompanies the knowledge one is dying. Some of this is quite normal. Many patients can deal with this knowledge informally, allowing a certain amount of denial or a certain degree of wanting to "hang on" rather than give in. Some patients want to protect their privacy against invasion and probing by zealous professionals determined to do "their thing," to make the patient die according to formula. Some patients want to die 'facing the wall' and not the team. This was once "normal" and may still be for some patients.

None of this is to contravene the enormous value of ICPC. It points, rather, to the frustration of the ends and purposes of palliative care if it is applied mindlessly or more for the satisfactions of those who have made it their specialty than for those whom it is meant to serve. Like every other powerful therapeutic tool, ICPC used within ethical constraints is a great help to the dying person. Used inappropriately, it becomes a travesty, a distortion of the compassion and comfort it so proudly promises and the patient so desperately needs.

Food and Hydration

Withholding or withdrawing food and fluid from dying patients is a much-debated ethical dilemma.[38] That debate can be touched on only sketchily here. Some of the disputed issues are these: Are food and fluids similar in all respects to medical treatments and therefore to be withdrawn under the same conditions as respirators? Are they symbolically and actually such ordinary measures and signs of care as rarely to be discontinued? These questions may be answered differently when the patient is fully competent, when he is in a permanent vegetative state, when he is in a state of waxing and waning consciousness.

These questions also occur, of course, outside the perimeters of palliative care, although, as with the other ethical issues we have been discussing, they take on special urgency when death is imminent and unavoidable. For the purposes of this chapter, can only summarize the ethical issues that I have discussed in more detail elsewhere.[39]

Anorexic patients who refuse food by mouth or take it in small and insufficient quantities should not be forced to eat more; nor should they be fed artificially against their wills. On the other hand, a lax and negligent attitude that makes no reasonable effort to help the patient take in food and fluids is not defensible, particularly if there is an intention of hastening death.

With patients who are in a permanent vegetative state, food and hydration should be maintained unless the process becomes overly burdensome—for example, if aspiration pneumonia, esophageal or nasal ulcerations, or pulmonary edema occur. These may distort the balance between putative harm and benefit to such an extent that the normal presumption in favor of sustaining nutrition and hydration becomes injurious.

CONCLUSION

Intensive comprehensive palliative care is, in essence, the extension of the comprehensive and holistic care all patients are entitled to. It is revised to meet the special needs of the incurably ill. In meeting those needs, palliative care presents ethical issues similar to those encountered in the care of any seriously ill patient. But these ethical issues taken on special dimensions and emphases because of the existential realities of modern-day societal attitudes toward dying and the predicament of the dying patient within that social context.

References

1. Canadian Palliative Care Association. *Palliative Care: Toward a Consensus on Standardized Principles of Practice.* (Ottowa: Canadian Palliative Care Association, 1995.

2. Hippocrates. *The Oath.* English translation by W. H. S. Jones. Loeb Classical Library, vol. 1, Cambridge: Harvard University Press, 1972:299.

3. Hippocrates. *The Art.* English translation by W. H. S. Jones. Loeb Classical Library, Vol. 2. Cambridge: Harvard University Press, 1981:193.

4. Hippocrates. *On Joints LVIII.* English translation by W. H. S. Jones. Loeb Classical Library, vol. 3. Cambridge: Harvard University Press, 1968:339.

5. Hippocrates. *On Diseases I–IV.* English translation by W. H. S. Jones. Loeb Classical Library, Vol. 5. Cambridge: Harvard University Press, 1988:113.

6. Edelstein L. *Ancient Medicine: Selected Papers of Ludwig Edelstein,* Temkin O, Temkin CL, eds, Temkin CL, trans. Baltimore: Johns Hopkins University Press, 1967:97–98.

7. Amundsen DW. *Medicine, Society, and Faith in the Ancient and Medieval Worlds.* Baltimore: Johns Hopkins University Press, 1996.

8. Temkin O. *Hippocrates in a World of Pagans and Christians.* Baltimore: Johns Hopkins University Press, 1991.

9. Pellegrino ED. Percival's medical ethics: the moral philosophy of an 18th-century English gentleman. *Archives of Internal Medicine* 1986; 146:2265–2269. Also reprinted in Barondess JA, Roland CG, eds, *The Persisting Osler II: Selected Transactions of the American Osler Society 1981–1990* Malabar, FL: Krieger Publishing Company, 1994:9–21.

10. Healing. In *The Oxford English Dictionary.* Vol 5. (Oxford: Clarendon Press, 1961, p.153.

11. Pellegrino ED, Thomasma DC. *For the Patient's Good: The Restoration of Beneficence in Health Care.* New York: Oxford University Press, 1987.

12. Woodruff R. *Palliative Medicine: Symptomatic and Supportive Care for Patients with Advanced Cancer.* Melbourne, Australia: Asperula, 1993.

13. Aries P. The reversal of death: changes in attitudes toward death in western societies. In: Stannard DE, ed, *Death in America.* Philadelphia: University of Pennsylvania Press, 1974:137–138.

14. Aries P. *The Hour of Our Death.* New York: Alfred A. Knopf, 1981.

15. Aries P. The reversal of death: changes in attitudes toward death in western societies. In: Stannard DE, ed, *Death in America.* Philadelphia: University of Pennsylvania Press, 1974:143.

16. Cacanan M, Kelly P. *Final Gifts.* New York: Bantam Books, 1993.

17. Strauss AL, Glaser BG. *Anguish: A Case History of a Dying Trajectory.* Mill Valley, California: The Sociology Press, 1970.

18. Kraus K. *Hoping in the Healing Process: An Integral Condition in the Ethics of Care.* Ph.D. Dissertation, Georgetown University, 1993.

19. Randall F, Downie RS. *Palliative Care Ethics: A Good Companion.* New York: Oxford University Press, 1996.

20. Agency for Health Care Policy and Research, Public Health Service, Department of Health and Human Services. Acute pain management: operative or medical procedures and trauma. In: *Clinical Practical Guidelines.* Washington, DC: U.S. Government Printing Office, 1992.

21. McGuveny WT, Crooks GM. The care of patients with severe chronic pain in terminal illness. *Journal of the American Medical Association,* 1984; 251: 1182–1188.

22. Pius XII. Allocutio. *Acta Apostolicae Sedis,* 1957; 49:129–147.

23. Griese ON. *Catholic Identity in Health Care.* Braintree, Mass: Pope John XXIII Center, 1987:246–299.

24. Faden RR, Beauchamp TL. *A History and Theory of Informed Consent.* New York: Oxford University Press, 1986.

25. Kreeft P. *Making Sense Out of Suffering.* Ann Arbor, MI: Servant Books, 1986.

26. Pellegrino ED. Is truth-telling a cultural artifact. *Journal of the American Medical Association,* 1992; 268(13):1734–1735.

27. Surbone A. Information, truth, and communication: for an interpretation of truth-telling practices around the world. In: Surbone A, Zwitter M, eds, *Communication and the Cancer Patient: Information and Truth*. New York: New York Academy of Sciences, 1997.

28. Royal Dutch Medical Society. *Euthanasia in the Netherlands*. 4th ed. Utrecht: Royal Dutch Medical Society, 1995.

29. Van der Maas PJ, et al. Euthanasia and other medical decisions concerning the end of life, an investigation performed upon request of the commission of inquiry into the medical practice concerning euthanasia [Special issue]. *Health Policy*, 1992; 22.

30. Sulmasy DP. *Killing and letting die*. Unpublished doctoral dissertation, Georgetown University, Washington DC, 1995.

31. Donagan A. *Choice: The Essential Element in Human Action*. London and New York: Routledge and Kegan Paul, 1987.

32. Guttentag O. The physician's point of view. *Science*, 1953; 117:207–208.

33. Pellegrino ED. The ethics of collective judgments in medicine and health care. *Journal of Medicine and Philosophy*, 1982; 7(1):3–10.

34. Clark D, ed. *The Future of Palliative Care: Issues in Policy and Practice*. Philadelphia: Open University Press, 1993.

35. Higby DJ, ed. *Issues in Supportive Care of Cancer Patients*. Boston: Martinus Nijhoff, 1986.

36. Jeffrey D. There Is Nothing More I Can Do. In *Introduction to the Ethics of Palliative Care*. Cornwall: Petten Press, 1993.

37. Nash A. A terminal case? Burnout in palliative care. *Professional Nurse*, 1989; June:443–444.

38. Tuohey JF. *Caring for Patients with AIDS and Cancer*. St. Louis, Missouri: Catholic Health Association of America, 1988:157–169.

39. Pellegrino ED. Withholding and withdrawing treatments: ethics at the bedside. *Journal of Clinical Neurosurgery*, 1989; 35:164–184.

24

Addressing the Needs of the Patient Who Requests Physician-Assisted Suicide or Euthanasia

Margaret V. McDonald, M.S.W.
Steven D. Passik, Ph.D.
Nessa Coyle, R.N., M.S., FAAN

The ethical and legal debate over physician-assisted suicide and euthanasia has gone on and will likely continue for quite some time. Serious consideration is being given to legalizing these practices, as can be seen in a growing number of legal decisions and state referenda.[1-3] Some of the central issues discussed are whether euthanasia and physician-assisted suicide are morally acceptable practices, whether legalization of these practices would produce a "slippery slope" effect, causing wrongful deaths, and whether individuals have the right to control the timing and manner of their deaths. Issues of patient autonomy and the "right to die" are at the cornerstone of the public debate for the proponents of euthanasia and assisted suicide. Opponents to legalization argue that our current health-care system is not providing adequate palliative care, thorough psychiatric evaluations, or appropriate interventions to many dying patients. These opponents believe that, until these causes of concern are addressed, any discussion of legalizing euthanasia or assisted suicide is premature.

As the debate goes on, clinicians continue to be left to face the practical concerns and problems of managing the care of dying patients. Advocates for the "right to die" base their views on the assumption that a request to hasten death in a terminally ill patient represents a "rational act" that in not all instances has been influenced by distressing physical symptoms or comorbid psychiatric conditions. While this may be true in a small minority of situations, the majority of patients who request hastened death are facing untreated psychiatric conditions and poorly controlled physical symptoms.[4] Advocates for the "right to die" usually highlight the shortcomings in the care of terminally ill and chronically ill patients, leaving already vulnerable dying patients more frightened. Recognition and management of the influence of public opinion and media coverage of this issue on dying patients is just one of many challenges health-care professionals must deal with in working with terminally ill patients who request euthanasia or physician-assisted suicide.

Several researchers have attempted to study attitudes toward euthanasia and physician-assisted suicide among the lay public, medical professionals, and terminally ill patients. Among the general public, more than 60% favor the legalization of voluntary euthanasia for patients with terminal illness.[5,6] In recent surveys of physicians, 28–40% of those responding reported that in some circumstances they would perform euthanasia if it were legal.[7-10] Patient attitudes have also been reported. Owens et al.[11] surveyed cancer patients and found that a third of the patient sample indicated that suicide and/or euthanasia would play some role in their future. Pain was the most common reason reported for considering suicide. In a 1988 survey, 57% of California physicians responding reported that they had been asked by terminally ill patients to hasten death. The primary reasons for such requests for physician-assisted suicide were persistent pain and terminal illness.[12] Chochinov et al.[13] found that pain, low levels of family support, and depression were correlated with a pervasive desire to die in terminally ill inpatients.

Similarly, in a study of ambulatory AIDS patients,[14] depression and psychological distress were significant correlates to favorable attitudes toward physician-assisted suicide. Tindall et al.[15] found in a study of persons with severe HIV disease that approximately 90% of the sample would personally like to have the option of euthanasia available if they were given a life-threatening diagnosis. In this same group, 86% stated that they were afraid of physical suffering, but only 19% stated that they were afraid of death. Pain and physical suffering seem to be paramount factors leading to favorable attitudes to euthanasia and physician-assisted suicide, but other important variables mentioned in these reports are fear of dependency, of other distressing symptoms, of loss of dignity, and of loss of ability to lead a purposeful life (see Table 24.1).

As the public attitude toward euthanasia and physician-assisted suicide grows more favorable, clinicians involved in the primary or palliative care of patients with cancer, AIDS, and other chronic illnesses will be confronted with requests from patients and their significant others for assistance in hastening death. In such situations, the ethical and legal debates are transformed into

existential and clinical challenges. Clinicians need to have sufficient knowledge and understanding of end-of-life issues to ensure that the debate over patients' right to die does not obscure patients' right to quality palliative care. Physicians and other health-care providers also need to be aware of the intense emotional connection that they can develop with patients, especially if the relationship is long and their identification with the patient is strong.[4] Sharing the responsibilities of care for the terminally ill patient with a multidisciplinary team allows for the best care of the patient.

UNDERSTANDING AND ADDRESSING THE NEEDS OF PATIENTS WHO REQUEST EUTHANASIA OR PHYSICIAN-ASSISTED SUICIDE

Thoughts of death and dying, along with fleeting thoughts of hastening death, are common among terminally ill patients. But it should not be assumed that thoughts of ending one's life or requests to hasten death are part of the ordinary experience of these patients or that these requests are rational expressions of patient autonomy. The complex nature of such requests and the multiple factors that go into them can never be captured in one-dimensional surveys; rather, these requests need to be explored and understood in the context of the individual patient experience. How symptoms and suffering have been addressed in the past has set up the patient's expectations and concerns about the future. Requests for euthanasia or physician-assisted suicide should be viewed as a call for help; they are an indication that something is not going right, that the patient's pain, suffering, and/or fears are not being adequately treated or have not been resolved.

Throughout this chapter, statements of terminally ill patients about their personal experiences and emotions are presented. These statements were recorded verbatim by one of the authors (NC) working in the Supportive Care Program of the Pain Service at Memorial Sloan-Kettering Cancer Center.[16] They do not express the speakers' feelings about euthanasia or physician-assisted suicide but rather contain expressions of the suffering that patients go through in our society, suffering that often goes unrecognized or untreated because the resources and the com-

Table 24.1   Desire-to-die Vulnerability Factors

Advanced illness, poor prognosis
Uncontrolled pain
Depression, hopelessness
Delirium, disinhibition
Loss of control, helplessness
Preexisting psychopathology
Exhaustion, fatigue
Lack of social support
Perceived loss of dignity
Loss of purpose and meaning of life

Adapted and modified from Breitbart, 1990

mitment necessary for the care of the terminally ill are not adequate in our current health-care system. The act of listening to these personal narratives helps ameliorate suffering. When not attended to, this suffering can influence patient requests for euthanasia and assisted suicide.

Pain and Symptom Management

The pain was so bad yesterday, if I had had a gun I would have shot myself. It's better now.

Acute, overwhelming pain can cause desperation in patients and push them to desire death. Adequate pain management must address the actual physical pain, as well as the fear of having intractable pain. People learn to trust that pain will be relieved by their experience of pain relief. Dying patients, along with the general public, are exposed to newspapers, television programs, and perhaps, experiences with other family members or friends that can give them a preconceived notion of how their illnesses may progress. One of the most popular television dramas of the 1990s, ER, in one episode depicted a dying cancer patient who lived her final few days with severe, unrelenting pain. This portrayal is very one sided, but it reached a large audience and undoubtedly left a long-lasting impression. Unfortunately, many of patients' concerns (especially cancer and AIDS patients) about pain and its undertreatment are legitimate.

Prevalence studies report that one-third of cancer patients in active therapy and two-thirds of cancer patients with far-advanced disease have significant pain.[17,18] Pain in AIDS is also often severe and highly prevalent, affecting 40% to 60% of patients.[19-21] The World Health Organization Cancer and Palliative Care Unit has reported that 4.5 million patients from developing and developed countries die each year with uncontrolled pain.[22] Pain in AIDS is also dramatically undertreated; a recent study indicated that 49% of AIDS patients in the sample who were experiencing moderate to severe pain were not receiving any analgesic therapy.[23] Uncontrolled pain is repeatedly cited as an important contributing factor among patients who have suicidal ideation[11,24] and is the primary reason cancer patients request physician-assisted suicide or euthanasia.[12,25]

There have been great advances in the management of pain in the past decade. New method-

ologies for diagnosing and assessing pain, the identification of various pain syndromes, and the development of guidelines for a therapeutic approach to the management of pain have all contributed to a comprehensive body of knowledge. It has been demonstrated that more than 90% of cancer pain can be managed with uncomplicated drug therapies.[26] Yet, there still remains an unacceptable level of undertreatment. Barriers to effective pain management include a lack of knowledge and training among health-care professionals in the use of pharmacological approaches to cancer pain management; fears of addiction by physician and patients; and current restrictions in the health-care system that interfere with the delivery of effective pain management.[27]

Although there is a growing number of hospice programs, dying patients are cared for in large part by primary-care physicians and nurses, most of whom have had no formal educational training in pain management or symptom control in terminally ill patients. There needs to be a greater commitment to educate and train the practitioners who work with these patients so that clinicians acquire knowledge of and training in all methods of pharmacological interventions. The use of opioids is the mainstay of therapy for cancer patients with pain, but fears of addiction have prevented patients from receiving adequate treatment. Patients need to be educated about the difference among physical dependence, tolerance, and psychological dependence or addiction. Clinicians who are familiar and comfortable with the use of opioids and adjuvant analgesics are able to convey to their patients an assurance that their pain and comfort needs will be met. Availability of palliative-care interventions should be explained. Often patients and families do not know the questions to ask, and it is helpful for clinicians to start the conversation. Clinician should take an active role early on in treatment to identify patients' concerns and to make a commitment to patients that their pain and other distressing symptoms will be aggressively treated. Patients will then feel more supported and gain more confidence in their treatment. Thoughts of suicide and requests for euthanasia may be diminished by greater attention to palliative care.

Physicians also need to be able to distinguish, for patients as well as for themselves, between pain control and euthanasia. The intent of pain control is to relieve pain and/or suffering. The administration of opioids, barbiturates, and other adjuvant medications may be necessary to provide comfort. Treatment of pain is never a form of euthanasia. Aggressive and appropriate treatment will be curtailed if physicians do not accept this differentiation. When issues of pain and symptom management are discussed, physicians should also explore patients' feelings about diminished alertness in the event that medications that induce drowsiness or sedation are required to relieve suffering. Any limitation in providing appropriate pain management interventions can leave patients susceptible to suffering and exacerbate thoughts of suicide and requests for euthanasia.

Depression and Other Psychological Symptoms

I've had a weekend of real fatigue and depression. It makes me feel very lonely, like there's no one who really understands what it's like, feeling that your options are running out. Cancer appearing all over the media, radio, TV, magazines, terminal cancer a major element, puts me into a gray, gray mood.

Depressed mood and sadness can be appropriate responses as patients with life-threatening illnesses face death. These emotions can be manifestations of anticipatory grief over the impending loss of one's life, health, connections to loved ones, and autonomy. At times, however, they signal the presence of a major depressive syndrome. As several studies have demonstrated, depression often influences a person's request to die.

In a recent study of 200 terminally ill inpatients, Chochinov et al.[13] found that occasional wishes that death would come soon were common (reported by 44.5% of the patients), with 8.5% of the patients acknowledging a serious, pervasive desire to die. Pain and low levels of family support were correlated with the desire for death in this population, but the most significant correlate with the desire for death was depression. Similarly, in a study of ambulatory AIDS patients[14] that examined predictors of favorable attitudes toward physician-assisted suicide, depression and psychological distress were the most statistically significant correlates. Given these

findings, the accurate identification of depression is crucial when working with terminally ill patients, yet the diagnosis of depression is often missed in the medical setting.[28,29]

It is a challenge for clinicians to recognize the symptoms of depression in patients with advanced disease. The presence of neurovegetative signs and symptoms of depression, such as fatigue, loss of energy, and other somatic symptoms, confounds a diagnosis of depression. The clinician needs to rely more on the psychological and cognitive symptoms of major depression, such as worthlessness, hopelessness, loss of social interest, and suicidal ideation. The issue is further complicated by the association between high rates of symptoms and depression[30] and the overlapping symptoms of normal sorrow and depression. How is the clinician to interpret feelings of hopelessness in the dying patient when there is no hope of recovery? While many patients never hope for a cure, they are able to maintain hope that pain can be controlled and quality of life can be maintained. Hopelessness that is pervasive and accompanied by a sense of despair or despondency is likely a symptom of a depressive disorder.

The patient with life-threatening illness presents with a complex mixture of physical and psychological symptoms, which makes the recognition of symptoms of anxiety that requires treatment challenging. Patients with anxiety complain of tension or restlessness, or they exhibit jitteriness, autonomic hyperactivity, vigilance, insomnia, distractibility, shortness of breath, numbness, apprehension, worry, or rumination. Often the physical or somatic manifestations of anxiety overshadow the psychological or cognitive ones and are the symptoms that the patient presents.[31] The clinician must use these symptoms as a cue to inquire about the patient's psychological state, which is commonly one of fear, worry, or apprehension. The assumption that a high level of anxiety is inevitably encountered during the advanced phases of illness is neither helpful nor accurate for diagnostic and treatment purposes. Intervention and initiation of treatment can curtail problematic patient behavior, such as noncompliance due to anxiety, and improve family and staff reactions to the patient.

Organic mental disorders are also common in patients with advanced disease. The presence of these syndromes in patients voicing requests for hastened death, assisted suicide, and euthanasia, perhaps more than any other psychiatric complication, tempers the rationality of such requests with these patients. While virtually all forms of organic mental syndromes can be present in patients with advanced disease, the most common include delirium, dementia, and organic mood and anxiety disorders. Yet, the diagnosis of organic mental syndrome is often overlooked. The earliest symptoms of dementia are often mistaken for functional psychiatric disturbance. Patients often react with disbelief, denial, numbness, irritability, feelings of hopelessness, and, occasionally, suicidal ideation. These symptoms are common in major depression, anxiety disorders, and adjustment disorders and are easily misconstrued as understandable reactions to the diagnosis of a life-threatening illness rather than as signs of early encephalopathy.[32] As dementia progresses, the organic nature of the psychiatric symptoms becomes more obvious. Formal neuropsychological testing can be quite helpful in accurately documenting AIDS dementia complex and in distinguishing it from depression or an adjustment disorder.

The presence of an organic mental syndrome complicates the assessment of the desire to hasten death in patients with terminal illnesses. It can be difficult to determine whether the organic mental syndrome is transient or permanent, whether it affects the patient's competence, and whether the attitudes expressed by the patient are similar to those the patient held prior to the development of cognitive problems.

Dependency and Loss Issues

I've thought of suicide, and yet I love life. It's boring and a chore to be sick. I'm afraid of starving to death. I'm afraid of losing Lucy. I'm deeply in love with life and I'm deeply in love with my wife, and I want to retain that state of being. Lucy gave me hope. I'm afraid I won't like the food she makes and she will be disgusted. Life depends on eating. I'm afraid people are planning my death and not telling me about it. I'm scared shitless. I'm an anxious person. I've felt the void and emptiness of not existing.

The sense that they are a burden on family members can be very distressing to chronically and ter-

minally ill patients. Results of a survey published in 1994[25] found that for noncancer patients (i.e., patients with ischaemic heart disease, strokes, other circulatory respiratory diseases, and Alzheimer's), the feeling that an earlier death would have been better, as well as requests for euthanasia, was related predominantly to issues of dependency. The dying patient's relationships with family and significant others are frequently pushed to the limit. The family members are dealing with their own feelings of anger, confusion, anticipatory grief, and hopelessness while trying to meet the needs of the sick person. Relatives may find themselves overwhelmed. Patients can see this and become concerned for the family, which is in fact carrying an increased burden in our current health-care system. Patients also often take on the responsibility of not wanting to disappoint the health professionals involved in their treatment; as the illness progresses and there is less hope of a cure or prolongation of life, patients may feel guilty for failing to get better. Patients' requests for euthanasia or assisted suicide may be seen as an appropriate decision in the attempt to protect the family and clinicians against the despair, financial expense, and sacrifice involved with taking care of a terminally ill patient.

Options should be made available to patients and their families when there is concern about the burden of care. Additional resources, such as home health aides and visiting nurses, may be offered. Moving the patient from the home to the hospital or providing respite care are further possibilities. Reassurance given to family members and other caretakers that their stress and disappointment are natural reactions because they love and care for the patient can also alleviate some of the concern the patient may be feeling.

I have no control, my adulthood has been taken away from me, I'm told what to take and when, when I can and cannot go out, I make no decisions, no one knows how I feel. I want to learn what I can and cannot do through trying.

Loss of autonomy, which is often equated with loss of dignity, is commonly cited by advocates for euthanasia and assisted suicide as reason to favor these practices. There are numerous examples of how patients' individual needs and rights are subjugated by our health-care system. This description of a patient's experience demonstrates the way that patients are assigned the subordinate role while receiving medical care:

> In the Admitting Office to which he went with overwhelming fear, [the patient] signed innumerable forms, including permission for all kinds of possible surgery. He also indicated his next of kin and signed all his valuables and identification over to the hospital safe. He was given a wrist label which could not be removed easily.... The patient was given a gown which did not quite close in the back, making it embarrassing to leave his room.... In some cases, the patient is put to bed with the siderails up as an infant is kept in a crib for his own protection. Such patients must ask permission even to go to the bathroom.[33]

Patients are asked to make accommodations for the "practical" needs of the health-care system, such as having various people going in and out of their rooms at all hours without knocking, being examined in front of large groups of strangers during clinical rounds, eating meals at assigned times, and being routinely disturbed in the middle of the night for temperature and blood pressure checks. These are just a few examples of how people's lives are changed when they become patients. Patients' adjustment can be facilitated by the caregiver's acknowledgment that these changes can be difficult and by discussions about how to make the experience better.

Isolation and Abandonment

I wasn't invited anywhere for July 4th; I wouldn't have gone, but I would have liked to have been invited.

Thoughts of being left to face illness alone can be extraordinarily frightening to patients. Feelings of isolation and abandonment often lead to the development of hopelessness. In the general population, hopelessness is a key variable linking depression and suicide.[34] It can be taxing for family members and health-care providers to continue to earnestly offer support to the dying patient. The prolongation of life through modern technology often includes a number of hospitalizations, multiple procedures, and high expenses. Throughout treatment, there can be a number of advances and a number of setbacks. Both family members and health-care providers may suffer from feelings of anticipatory grief, apprehension,

and guilt brought on by a belief that the illness might have been prevented or at least made more comfortable.[35] Family members, friends, and care providers may start to withdraw from the patient in response to these feelings. This "emotional quarantine," as Weisman calls it, often causes the patient to experience additional suffering and despair. Clinicians need to continue to restore feelings of attachment to others. Strong support systems can provide patients some distraction from their illness at times, can allow patients to express their feelings and emotions, and can add meaning to their life.

Existential Suffering

I am not complete because my body does not function now. Before I was almost a normal person; everything functioned even though I had pain for many years. I'm so impotent now I can't do what I want to. Yesterday my grandchild fell on a broom. I felt so bad I couldn't run to save her. I feel so inadequate in this world.

Patients may feel that their lives are so changed that they have little meaning. When patients feel this way, requesting euthanasia or assisted suicide may be a way for them to ask for their caregiver's "opinions" about whether their lives continue to have value. If physicians, nurses, or others agree to provide euthanasia, this may validate patients' fears that their lives are meaningless. Patients may question whether continued treatment and the tasks of care are worthwhile. Existential care concentrates on reestablishing the meaning and sense of purpose of life, while cognitive therapies can help patients strengthen their coping abilities.[36] If patients view their situations as horrible tragedies and are deeply despairing, they need to be introduced to new strategies of adaptation. While acknowledging their despair, cognitive restructuring can help patients learn to approach potentially stressful events believing that they have the ability to successfully endure the situation. For example, patients who fear loss of control and dependency can learn to appreciate that by receiving help they are permitting others to express their love and feelings of loss.

Patients should be encouraged to identify achievable short-term objectives. Depending on patients' level of functioning and need, they might set goals of increasing their mobility or resuming responsibility over their personal care needs; they might wish to resolve family conflicts or aim help others through patient-to-patient counseling programs or other voluntary activities.

RESPONDING WHEN A PATIENT REQUESTS ASSISTED SUICIDE OR EUTHANASIA

Ideally, physicians and other caregivers should discuss end-of-life issues with their patients early in treatment. Requests for euthanasia and assisted suicide are best dealt with before the intensity of emotions and the severity of the illness become too overwhelming and stressful. Early discussions about how the disease progresses, what the patient should expect, and options for care and treatment can alleviate much of the anxiety and fear related to uncertainty of the future.

A good physician-patient relationship needs to be established if the patient is to openly express concerns and anxieties. Patients need to have confidence in their caregivers, and they need to feel that they will not be abandoned as their disease progresses.

If a patient does request euthanasia or assisted suicide, a comprehensive evaluation of vulnerability factors is appropriate (see Table 24.2). Con-

Table 24.2   Evaluation of the Patient Who Desires Death

Establish rapport with an empathic approach.
Obtain patient's understanding of illness and present symptoms.
Assess mental status.
Assess pain and symptom control.
Obtain history of prior emotional problems or psychotic disorders.
Obtain family history.
Assess family issues and burden of care.
Assess suffering component/quality-of-life issues for patient.
Assess suffering component/quality-of-life issues for family.
Assess suicidal thinking, intent, plans.
Ask the patient what can be done to help him or her the most.
Ask the patient what he or she fears the most.
Evaluate need for one-to-one nurse in hospital or companion at home.
Formulate treatment plan, immediate and long term.

Adapted and modified from Breitbart, 1990

sultations with experts in palliative care or psychiatric care is advisable. Clinicians need to commit themselves to their patients and to provide continuity of care, which gives patients some confidence that their needs will be acknowledged and treated.

SUMMARY

There is an increasing likelihood that legislative proposals to legalize euthanasia and assisted suicide as a means of ending suffering of patients with terminal illness will be accepted in some states. This chapter does not attempt to debate whether requests for assisted suicide is rational or ethical but rather emphasizes the importance of understanding the complexities involved in a request for hastened death. Understanding the desire to hasten death demands that clinicians improve their appreciation of a number of psychiatric, social, and medical factors. At present, these factors are poorly recognized and treated in the clinical situation, and they have not been well studied by researchers.

References

1. Altman LK. Jury declines to indict a doctor who said he aided in a suicide. *New York Times,* July 27, 1991:1,10.
2. Mathews J. Washington state confronts euthanasia. *The Washington Post,* February 6, 1991:A1,A7.
3. Annas GJ. Death by prescription: the Oregon initiative. *New England Journal of Medicine,* 331: 1240–1243.
4. Breitbart W (1993). Suicide risk and pain in cancer and AIDS patients. In: Chapman CR, Foley KM, eds, *Current and Emerging Issues in Cancer Pain: Research and Practice.* New York: Raven, 1993:49–65.
5. Blendon RJ, Szalay US, Knox RA. Should physicians aid their patients in dying? the public perspective. *Journal of the American Medical Association,* 1992; 267:2658–2662.
6. Genuis SJ, Genuis SK, Chang W. Public attitudes toward the right to die. *Canadian Medical Association Journal,* 1994; 150:701–708.
7. Kuhse H, Singer P. Doctors' practices and attitudes regarding voluntary euthanasia. *Medical Journal of Australia,* 1988; 148:623–627.
8. Kinsella TD, Verhoef MJ. Alberta euthanasia survey, I: physicians' opinions about the morality and

legalization of active euthanasia. *Canadian Medical Association Journal*, 1993; 148:1921–1926.

9. Fried TR, Stein MD, O'Sullivan PS, et al. Limits of patient autonomy: physician attitudes and practices regarding life-sustaining treatment and euthanasia. *Archives of Internal Medicine*, 1993; 153: 722–728.

10. Shapiro RS, Derse AR, Gottlieb M, et al. Willingness to perform euthanasia: a survey of physician attitudes. *Archives of Internal Medicine*, 1994; 154:575–584.

11. Owens C, Tennant C, Levi J, et al. Suicide and euthanasia: patient attitudes in the context of cancer. *Psycho-oncology*, 1992; 1:79–88.

12. Helig S. The San Francisco Medical Society euthanasia survey. Results and analysis. *San Francisco Medicine*, 1988; 61:24–34.

13. Chochinov HM, Wilson KG, Enns M, et al. Desire for death in the terminally ill. *American Journal of Psychiatry*, 1995; 152:1185–1191.

14. Breitbart W, Rosenfeld BD, Passik SD. Interest in physician-assisted suicide among ambulatory HIV infected patients. *American Journal of Psychiatry*, 1996; 153:238–242.

15. Tindall B, Forde S, Carr A, et al. Attitudes to euthanasia and assisted suicide in a group of homosexual men with advanced HIV disease (letter). *Journal of Acquired Immune Deficiency Syndromes*, 1993; 6:1069–1070.

16. Coyle N. Suffering in the first person. In: Ferrell, BR, ed, *Suffering*. Boston: Jones & Bartlett, 1996: 29–64.

17. Foley KM. The treatment of cancer pain. *New England Journal of Medicine*, 1985; 3:84–95.

18. Daut RL, Cleeland CS. The prevalence and severity of pain in cancer. *Cancer*, 1982; 50:1913.

19. Lebovits AK, Lefkowitz M, McCarthy D, et al. The prevalence and management of pain in patients with AIDS: A review of 134 cases. *Clinical Journal of Pain*, 1989; 5:245–248.

20. Singer EJ, Zorilla C, Fahy-Chandon B, et al. Painful symptoms reported for ambulatory HIV-infected men in a longitudinal study. *Pain*, 1993; 53: 15–19.

21. O'Neill WM, Sherrard JS. Pain in human immunodeficiency virus disease: a review. *Pain*, 1993; 54:3–14.

22. World Health Organization. *Cancer and Palliative Care*. Geneva: WHO, 1990.

23. Breitbart W, Rosenfeld B, Passik S, et al. The undertreatment of pain in ambulatory AIDS patients. *Pain*, 1996; 65:243–249.

24. Breitbart W. Cancer pain and suicide. In: Foley KM, Bonica JJ, Venatafridda V, eds, *Advances in Pain Research and Therapy*. Vol 16. New York: Raven, 1990:399–412.

25. Seale C, Addington-Hall J. Euthanasia: Why people want to die earlier. *Social Science and Medicine*, 1994; 39:647–654.

26. Ventafridda V, Tamburini M, Caraceni A, et al. Validation study of the WHO method for cancer pain relief. *Cancer*, 1987; 59:350–356.

27. Foley KM. The relationship of pain and symptom management to patient requests for physician-assisted suicide. *Journal of Pain and Symptom Management*, 1991; 6:289–297.

28. Knights EB, Folstein MF. Unsuspected emotional and cognitive disturbance in medical patients. *Annals of Internal Medicine*, 1977; 87:723–724.

29. Moffic HS, Paykel ES. Depression in medical in-patients. *British Journal of Psychiatry*, 1975; 126:346–353.

30. Hays RB, Turner H, Coates TJ. Social support, AIDS-related symptoms, and depression among gay men. *Journal of Consulting and Clinical Psychology*, 1992; 60:463–469.

31. Holland JC. Anxiety and cancer: the patient and family. *International Journal of Psychiatry in Medicine*, 1985–1986; 15:75–79.

32. Perry SW. Organic mental disorders caused by HIV: Update on early diagnosis and treatment. *American Journal of Psychiatry*, 1990; 147:696–712.

33. Fisher D. The hospitalized terminally ill patient: an ecological perspective. In Germain C, ed. *Social Work Practice: People and Environments*. New York: Columbia University Press, 1979; 25–44.

34. Kovacs M, Beck AT, Weissman A. Hopelessness: an indication of suicidal risk. *Suicide*, 1975; 42: 98–103.

35. Weisman AD. Misgivings and misconceptions in the psychiatric are of terminal patients. *Psychiatry*, 1970; 33:67–81.

36. Cherny NI, Coyle N, Foley KM. The treatment of suffering when patients request elective death. *Journal of Palliative Care*, 1994; 10:71–79.

25

Spiritual Care of the Dying Patient

Michael Kearney, M.D.
Balfour Mount, CM OQ M.D., FRCPC

Does a chapter on spiritual care belong in a textbook on psychiatry in palliative medicine? How do we understand the term "spiritual" in this secular age? The reader may well feel at one with our colleague who commented, "When you use terms like *spirit*, you lose me. I really just do not understand what we are talking about!" Alternatively, you may feel that the answers to these questions are self-evident, that all of life may be seen in spiritual terms, and you may respond with the observation of Irvin Yalom, professor of psychiatry at Stanford University, who has written, "There are ... domains where knowledge must remain intuitive. Certain truths of existence are so clear that logical argument or empirical research corroboration seems highly gratuitous. Karl Lashley, the neuropsychologist, is said to have once commented: 'If you teach an Airedale to play the violin, you don't need a string quartet to prove it.' "[1] Perhaps you would respond that the spiritual in life has to do not with knowledge but with experience.

Our goal is to discuss spiritual care in a manner that is relevant to those who hold each of these perspectives, since spiritual issues, as we

conceive them, have a relevance beyond personal world view, for they lie at the very center of the existential crisis that is terminal illness. When our approach to health care ignores the spiritual, we seriously limit our understanding of, and our response to, the patient's illness.

Case Examples

MHM, a youthful, dynamic octogenarian, leaned forward, her face betraying the well of tension and controlled urgency within. Her eyes filled with tears. "How do you prepare to die? How do you?" The perennial optimism that had colored her full, productive life had been eroded by the sequelae of her slowly advancing small bowel sarcoma. She quietly gave voice to her anguish, her most intimate fears. "I have more questions than answers. I thought I had a faith. Now I'm not so sure. . . . I worry about H [her husband] and about you all [her family]. How will you get along without me? . . . You know, I just can't imagine being dead."[2]

CD was 30 years old when he presented with a widely disseminated germinal testicular tumor. Radical surgery and chemotherapy resulted in the serum markers of disease reverting to normal and the hope of cure, but within months his cancer progressed, with ensuing extreme cachexia leading slowly to death over a 12-month period. CD had

The alphabetical listing of authors for this chapter reflects equality of input and gratitude of the collaborative process involved.

always stood out from his peers. He has always been a winner. Outgoing. Gracious. A world-class athlete, he was a member of the national ski team; he was successful in business and engaged to be married. Now dying! **CD, dying!** To his family, friends, and many admirers, it seemed unbelievable. Then, just days before he died, he married his fiancee and said goodbye to those he loved. To his physician he remarked, "This last year has been the best year of my life." That year? The best year? Of that life? CD confided that the source of this sense of quality time was a new awareness of the spiritual dimension of human existence. Physical agony had been transcended through a journey inward that came to be characterized by grace and a sense of growth he had not previously known.[3]

Mrs. C, a widow born in Eastern Europe and now in her seventies, was admitted to a palliative-care ward with uncontrolled bone pain associated with metastatic breast carcinoma. Assessment suggested that the pain should have been easy to control with routine measures, but all attempts failed. A daughter was her closest relative. Palpable tension hummed between them. A conversation with her doctor shed light on the texture of the mother's life. "When were you last well?" "Do you mean physically?" "No, I mean in yourself." "Doctor, I've never been well a day in my life." "Really! Well, if we are body, mind, and spirit, where do you think the problem has been?" "I've been sick in mind and spirit every day of my life." Her anguish persisted until death, a by-product, perhaps, of her well-established life script rather than the cancer that ended her suffering.[3]

Palliative care is said to attend to the needs of the whole person, including the physical, psychological, social, and spiritual aspects of suffering[4]—the needs of body, mind, and spirit. Yet, in this postreligious age, what does this statement mean? In discussing the *physical* needs of patients and the pathophysiology of their diseases, we have the advantage of a shared vocabulary. We agree on the meaning of concepts such as neuropathic pain and the cachexia-anorexia syndrome. Similarly, we discuss their *psychological* status with a common understanding of terms such as anxiety, depression, identification, and denial. But, concerns, considered by some to be issues of the *spirit*, are raised and language loses its precision, more often acting as an obstacle to communication than a vehicle for shared understanding. We stumble on barriers of semantics and concepts

erected by religious and cultural tradition. What exactly is "the spirit" if not simply a mythical construct born out of our search for meaning? What is meant by "soul"? What are the components of personhood implied by those speaking of the "spiritual domain"? What mechanisms are involved in healing this part of our being? Are there approaches to care that may foster such healing? Can these questions be discussed in terms that bridge the wide spectrum of beliefs held in our pluralistic society? In order to examine spiritual care of the dying patient, let us start by defining relevant terms.

BASIC CONCEPTS

Spiritual is defined as "of, or pertaining to, affecting or concerning the spirit or higher moral questions."[5] *Spirit*, from the latin *spiritus*, meaning breathing, breath, air, life, soul, pride, courage,[6] has been defined as "the animating or vital principle in persons; the soul of a person, as commended to God, or passing out of the body, in the moment of death."[5] It is widely understood to be the aspect of our reality that is independent of matter; unconfined by the constrictions of time and space. In the modern Western view, the body contains the spirit, while a more ancient wisdom conceives the spirit as being the highest evolution of consciousness and containing the body. Spirit is matter incandescent.[7] While some have drawn sharp distinctions between "spirit" and "soul,"[8] in this chapter we use the term *spirit* as inclusive of both terms.

While the existence of the spirit cannot be proven, it can be experienced. From earliest recorded time, persons have thought themselves to be something more than body and mind. That "something more" is spirit.[9] It is, in this conception, the essential self. Thus, spirituality refers to that which is deepest and most genuine in us, the ground of our being, and what we, and others,[10,11] refer to as spiritual pain is the experience of alienation from this depth. Spirit cannot be directly observed and tested, as can the mind and body, but provides evidence of its well-being indirectly through both.

Spirit may be conceived analogously as healthy, well-nourished, and mature or as neglected, stunted, compromised. Discussions with the third patient described earlier suggested that the latter might describe her plight. Like mind and body, the spirit may experience health or ill health. Being part of an indivisible whole, its state of well-being may be expected to impact on the well-being of the other components of personhood. As seen with CD, also described earlier, it may be the source of dynamic new life, even in the face of crippling physical decline.

Spirit is relational in its expression. That is, it is expressed in relationship, love, and community[12]—in dialogue, in communion with others, including God, the Other, however conceived. It is the agent involved in our most profoundly meaningful interactions, those deeply personal meetings in which contact is made at a "spirit" level, meetings described by the Viennese Jewish religious philosopher Martin Buber as I-thou relating.[13] Acceptance of the existence of the spiritual dimension thus commits us to a relational view of human existence and challenges the atomistic individualism, so common in our relating, that leads to seeing others as objects, separate from self, defined by labels that act as a numbing buffer against our experience of their transcendent self (Ormont LR, Ormont J, personal communication).

The nature and capacity of the spirit has been expressed in religious thought. In the Judeo-Christian tradition, Jesus, a Jew, observed that "the Kingdom of Heaven is within you."[14] The spirit is the *pneuma* of Christian writings.[15] The Hindu Upanishads speak of Atman, the Spirit of man, the Self in every one and in all.[16] In the Buddhist tradition, Nirvana, as experienced by Buddha, is the Nirvana described in the *Bhagavad Gita* as "the peace supreme that is in me."[17]

The Taoist philosopher Chuang-tzu advocates, "Don't listen with your ears, listen with your mind. No, don't listen with your mind, but listen with your spirit. Listening stops with the ears, the mind stops with recognition, but spirit is empty and waits on all things. The Way gathers in emptiness alone."[18]

Plato said, "If the head and body are to be well, you must begin by curing the soul."[19] Now, 2,400 years later, conditioned by Cartesian dualism and analytical science with its reductionist perspective, our perception of personhood and health has narrowed[20] so that "soul," in either the Platonic sense, as mind, or as "the spiritual part of man in contrast to the purely physical,"[5] is often neglected. We tend to focus on the bi-ology of disease rather than on the patient's experienced illness;[21] to interpret the rich, mysterious whole in terms of the more understandable specific.[22]

This limited perspective is now, however, being challenged by a call to whole-person care, a perspective that posits that "man, as man, supersedes the sum of his parts," that is, that man cannot be understood from a scientific study of part functions.[23] Physicians now recognize that pain must be understood as "total pain," in terms of aetiologic components beyond the noxious physical stimulus, including emotional, social, financial, and spiritual factors,[24] while suffering must be seen as potentially having its origins in any dimension of human experience.[25]

Similarly, some psychotherapists have come to recognize the need to consider issues beyond the confines of scientific behaviorism and Freudian psychoanalysis, a stance that embraces antideterminism, with an emphasis on freedom, choice, purpose, values, meaning, responsibility, and commitment to appreciating the unique experiential world of each individual.[26] Existential psychotherapy adopts these goals.[26] It addresses the inner conflict and anxiety born out of our awareness of the vulnerability we experience as a product of the existential "givens" that frame our lives. These givens, our ultimate concerns, include **death** (existential obliteration), **freedom** (the absence of external structure), **isolation** (the final unbridgeable gap separating self from all else), and **the question of meaning** (the dilemma of meaning-seeking creatures who recognize the possibility of a cosmos without meaning). The existential position challenges the Cartesian view of a world full of objects and of subjects who perceive those objects, seeing the person instead as a consciousness who participates in the construction of reality; who is at the same time the meaning giver and the known.[26]

Finally, what is the relationship between the spiritual and religion? The spirit is a dimension of personhood, as is the mind or pancreas, a part of our being. Religion, on the other hand, is a construct of human making that, for some, enables conceptualization and expression of spirituality. Religion is "a system of faith and worship, a recognition on the part of man of some higher unseen power as having control of his destiny and as being entitled to obedience, reverence and worship.[5]

THE EXPERIENCE OF THE SPIRIT

Aboriginal people see their world and the cosmos in spiritual terms. In responding to an 1852 offer from Washington to buy their land, the Indian chief Seattle of the Puget Sound tribe commented:

> Every part of this earth is sacred to my people. Every shining pine needle, every sandy shore, every mist in the dark woods, every meadow, every humming insect. All are holy in the memory and experience of my people. . . . If we sell you our land, you must remember that it is sacred. . . . One thing we know: our god is also your god. The earth is precious to him and to harm the earth is to heap contempt on its creator.[27]

For many today, however, the experience of the spiritual is a foreign concept, a quaint notion, a holdover from a superstitious age. The Pulitzer Prize–winning essayist Annie Dillard has described our situation with great clarity:

> God used to rage at the Israelites for frequenting sacred groves. I wish I could find one. Martin Buber says: "The crisis of all primitive mankind comes with the discovery of that which is fundamentally not-holy, the a-sacramental, . . . , a province which steadily enlarges itself." Now we are no longer primitive; now the whole world seems not-holy. We have drained the light from the boughs in the sacred grove and snuffed it in the high places and along the banks of sacred streams. We as a people have moved from pantheism to pan-atheism. Silence is not our heritage but our destiny; we live where we want to live.[28]

And yet Ghandi observed, "If we have listening ears God speaks to us in our own language, whatever the language be."[29] "If we have listening ears"? How do we *hear* the spirit domain? However understood, we have all had experiences of that dimension of our being, a sense of oneness, unity, or transcendence; a sense of profound awareness, connectedness, silence, and peace. Elijah sensed the spirit not in wind, earthquake, or fire but in a still small voice.[30] The Psalmist found the spirit everywhere and wrote, "Whither shall I go from thy Spirit? Or whither shall I flee from thy presence? If I ascend to heaven, thou art there! If I make my bed in Sheol, thou art there!"[31]

For some, the catalyst for an awareness of the spiritual may be the mystery and splendor of nature. Thomas Berry sees the universe, by definition, as a "single gorgeous celebratory event" and exclaims, "If we have a wonderful sense of the divine, it is because we live amid such awesome magnificence."[32] A theology of nature, suggested by such a stance, "does not solicit the help of science to provide a basis for or to confirm faith, but uses the contemporary picture of reality from the science of its day as a resource to construct and experience faith."[33]

For others, the spiritual is recognized in a deeply personal experience of art, literature, or music, whether Rembrandt or Francis Bacon, Dostoyevsky or Bob Geldof, Yo Yo Ma and Trevor Pinnock or Elton John. Or the transcendent may be found in an experience of community or in the contemplative moment, a time of meditation that goes beyond thought, word, and images and is characterized by a sense of wonderment as we resonate at the deepest level of our being with a reality beyond words.

For CD and countless others, the crucible of life-threatening illness presents yet another path. In presenting an experience of our frailty, it sweeps aside lesser preoccupations and opens a window on an experience of the soul.

THE MEDICAL MODEL AND SPIRITUAL DISTRESS

As a prelude to examining how we might recognize and respond to spiritual distress, let us consider current attitudes concerning the physician's mandate and the goals of health care in general. Two papers are enlightening in this regard: Anthony Reading's classic "Illness and Disease"[21] and H. Brownell Wheeler's landmark Shattuck Lecture, "Healing and Heroism."[34]

Reading has drawn attention to the importance of distinguishing between "illness" and "disease" if optimal health care is to be achieved. He points out that modern medical practice is based on a paradigm whose validity has generally passed unquestioned, that is, that "illness is the result of disease and is best dealt with by treating the underlying disease." Thus, "disease" (the various structural disorders of the individual's tissues and organs that give rise to the signs of ill health), the object of science and technology, has been accepted as the preeminent focus of medical care, and "illness" (the patient's experience of ill health) has been largely ignored or at most viewed as being of secondary importance, a simple by-product of disease. But disease is neither necessary nor sufficient to explain illness.[21] For the patient, it is his illness that he complains of and that causes him to seek medical attention. It is illness, not disease, that is his concrete reality. And how the illness, not the disease, is relived determines the patient's satisfaction and evaluation of physician competence.[35] *Illness both affects and is affected by all aspects of the sufferer's being,*[21,36] and therein lies the failure of the paradigm. In the absence of demonstrable disease, despite the persistence of illness, the doctor may conclude that, "there is nothing wrong," "there is nothing more I can do." The psychosocial and spiritual variables that at the very least color and may produce illness are not understood. The significance of the meaning of the illness for the sufferer is missed. The potential for healing in the face of progressive disease, a potential rooted in the special relationship formed between healer and sufferer,[37,38] so familiar to Osler,[34] the shamans of primitive cultures, and faith healers, remains an untapped resource. Cassell has eloquently expressed the reality underlying the flaw in modern medicine's paradigm, "same disease, different patient—different illness, pain, and suffering.[39]

Williams Osler, a professor at McGill at age 25 and subsequently professor of medicine at the University of Pennsylvania, Johns Hopkins, and, finally, Oxford University, was the dominant clinician of his era and is still regarded by many as the preeminent physician of modern times. He remains an illuminating reference point against which to judge our current, "more scientific" medical model—our propensity to focus on disease rather than on illness and the person. Osler had access to a relatively primitive diagnostic and therapeutic armamentarium. Indeed, Wheeler points out, Osler's place in history rests not on his diagnostic or therapeutic skills, but on his "profound embodiment of the role of the healer."[34] Osler was a great physician because he combined superb "scientific" competence with an adroit ability to communicate at a deeply personal level, to inspire hope, to establish a relationship with patients that arose out of a genuine deep interest in them as individuals, and thus to perceive the person as well as the disease.[35] But there was more than that. Osler was profoundly

aware of the spiritual dimension and its importance in health and illness. An obituary written at the time of his death stated in part, "His errand in life . . . not only concerned the bodies of men and women, but their spirits. He lived in constant contact with all manner of people, giving out incessantly the kindness and wisdom that were in him. . . . He was always directing human life, and wherever he touched it, it seemed to go lighter and more blithely."[40] Thomas Cullen, who knew Osler well at Johns Hopkins Hospital, rounded out these thoughts in commenting on Osler's life that "brotherly love became its dominant note." He added, "That, in my opinion, was William Osler's finest and most enduring contribution to American medicine."[41]

In assessing how Osler would view our contemporary medical model, Wheeler makes several observations relevant to these pages:

> Osler would be particularly concerned that medical care today does not place enough emphasis on treating patients first of all as human beings. He regarded life primarily as a journey of the spirit, and the body as its conveyance. He understood that when illness afflicts the body, the spirit is also afflicted, and that it is important to minister to both body and spirit. . . . He ministered effectively to the spirit of his patients simply through warm human contact, without the necessity of any shared theology. His was a one-to-one interaction, the concerned spirit of the physician reaching out to the troubled spirit of the patient. . . . Osler was regarded as a great physician because to some extent he represented the spiritual, as well as the physical basis for healing. To the power of medical knowledge, Osler added a soul.[34]

THE FEAR DYNAMIC AND THE ORIGINS OF SPIRITUAL PAIN

A simplified version of Carl Jung's map of the psyche[42] may be helpful in reflecting on the nature of spiritual pain. In this model, the psyche is seen as having two different and distinct levels, the *surface* and the *deep*. The surface level refers to the conscious aspects of the psyche, where the *ego*, that is, the aware and organizing aspect of the personality, and the language of rational, analytical, and linear thinking are dominant. The deep level, on the other hand, refers to the unconscious aspects of the psyche. This is the realm of intuition and imagination, and it is here that what Jung calls the *Self*, that is, the deep, inner center of personhood, which some would see as being continuous with the transcendent, is located.

The ego loves the surface level of psyche with an intensity equaled only by its terror of the deep. Why is this? Jung points toward an answer when he comments that the dread and resistance that human beings naturally experience when it comes to delving deeply into the unconscious is, at bottom, the fear of the journey to Hades.[42] In other words, from the perspective of the ego, the deep aspects of psyche are as unknown and terrifying as the underworld of death itself.

TERROR-MANAGEMENT THEORY

Solomon et al. have built on the work of Becker[43,44] to develop what they call terror-management theory,[45,46] a construct that is pertinent to an understanding of the genesis of spiritual pain.

Solomon et al. postulate that a defining characteristic of humanity is the capacity for mortality salience, that is, the ability to be aware of our own mortality. This awareness generates terror, which they describe not as an intense fear of death per se but rather as a profound and usually unconscious dread of death as absolute annihilation. We cope, they suggest, with such terror by developing what they term an "anxiety buffer." This is achieved by denying or repressing the terror at an individual unconscious level while simultaneously creating, maintaining, and participating in "culture" at a communal level. From this perspective, therefore, culture is seen as a symbolic construction that helps to minimize the anxiety associated with an awareness of death.[45] This it does by bestowing on the individual a sense of self-esteem. By having faith in the cultural world view and accepting the values inherent in that world view, the individual is rewarded by gaining a sense of meaning. Perceiving that one is meeting the adopted cultural standards and is therefore playing a significant role in the cultural conception of reality also brings with it a sense of personal value. Self-esteem, therefore, involves viewing oneself as a valued participant in a meaningful cultural drama. With the "anxiety buffer" intact, the individual has a sense of safety and of being part of something greater that will not die, that is, reassurance of immortality.[46]

It follows from this that one of the primary motivations of human behavior is to defend the death-anxiety buffer by maintaining self-esteem.

Solomon et al. have shown that threats to self-esteem heighten an individual's anxiety, which in turn activates defenses ("terror-management processes") that work to minimize the anxiety by restoring the status quo. In addition, in a fascinating series of studies,[45] they have shown that when healthy individuals become mortality salient, that is, when their denial is threatened by something that reminds them of their mortality, the same terror-management processes are also triggered. These defenses or terror-management processes have consistently been shown to maintain self-esteem and so to lessen anxiety in two principle ways: by reinforcing the dominant cultural world view and by distancing the individual from or denigrating alternative views. For example, subjects, including a group of municipal court judges, some of whom had been made mortality salient, were asked to recommend a dollar amount at which bail should be set for a woman accused of prostitution and, in a second study, to establish the reward for a woman who had risked her own safety by turning in a criminal. The first study found that if the mortality-salient subjects opposed prostitution, they were especially punitive to the accused woman, a person who threatened their cultural norms and, therefore, their self-esteem. In the second study, subjects with increased mortality salience were especially positive to the woman who had heroically attempted to uphold cultural values. Bail and reward were both significantly greater than the corresponding amounts set by control group subjects who did not have increased mortality salience.

What is the relevance of this to the genesis of spiritual pain in individuals close to death? In terms of the Western psyche, the dominant cultural values are those of the surface mind, that is, of rational, analytic, linear, and concrete thinking. The reaction of the ego, when it senses death's approach, bears striking resemblance to that of a mortality-salient judge in one of Solomon et al.'s studies. At an intrapsychic level, the mortality-salient ego clings to the values of the surface mind while simultaneously projecting onto the deep mind the face of a terrifying enemy, rejecting its values and distancing itself from what it sees as a threatening and potentially destructive aspect of psyche. In other words, in an attempt to lessen anxiety, the ego projects its fear of death onto the deep and unconscious aspects of mind, seeing in its unfamiliar and unpredictable depths a microcosm of death itself. In this reaction, aimed at ensuring its survival, the panicking ego flees from the deeper layers of the psyche, thereby alienating itself from the potential source of profound inner healing that contact with this aspect of the psyche can bring. This, in turn, generates feelings of isolation and terror, meaninglessness and hopelessness, that is, "spiritual pain."[10,11] The roots of spiritual distress can, therefore, be understood in this framework as a direct consequence of the ego's fear reaction (i.e., as a terror-management process), which, while perhaps having some short-term positive effects in lessening anxiety, may also lead to a damaging alienation from and conflict with the depths of ourselves.

RECOGNIZING SPIRITUAL PAIN

While spiritual pain can appear somatically, emotionally, religiously, or socially, at the root of such distress is a rupture, a disconnection, and a resulting alienation within individuals from that aspect of their deepest selves that gives meaning, hope, and purpose. The challenge is to make the diagnosis, to recognize spiritual pain for what it is. This recognition will, in turn, point toward appropriate ways of responding.

While it would be foolish to suppose that it is easy to recognize spiritual pain, it is, nonetheless, essential to attempt to do this if we are to help someone who is suffering in this way. As in any other aspect of medicine, there is an implicit value in accurately naming the source of symptoms. This tends to rob the symptoms of some of the tyrannical power that thrives on anonymity, helps both carers and patients to agree to realistic goals for treatment, and, perhaps most important, points the healing interventions in the right direction. Spiritual pain is a difficult diagnosis to make. There are, however, certain characteristic features that may allow recognition of this form of human suffering.

Spiritual pain can manifest as symptoms in any area of a patient's experience. These may be physical (intractable symptoms that continuously defy all usually successful forms of treatment or may actually be exacerbated by these interventions), psychological (especially fear, anxiety, panic, depression, despair, hopelessness, and meaninglessness), religious (such as a "crisis of faith" or the "fear of eternal damnation" that may accompany certain images of God), or social (as in a disintegration of previously close human relationships). It is usually not possible to recognize spiritual pain on the basis of these symptoms alone. It is the presence of such symptoms in combination with characteristic descriptions and behavior patterns that helps both carer and patient to accurately identify this form of human suffering.

When we are involved in caring for someone in spiritual pain, we instinctively begin to use words like "suffering," "anguished," and "tortured," rather than a more orthodox, scientific terminology. It is as if, even before we may be fully conscious of the fact, we seem to have an intuitive ability to sense when the source of a patient's suffering is more than the obvious bone pain, anxiety, or strife between the patient and family or carers. Its origins in depth from a "troubled" spirit is reflected in the language we use in our attempts to describe it to another.

The behavior patterns spiritual pain generates in patient and carers can be usefully understood as expressions of the "terror-management processes" discussed earlier. In this context, their behavior is aimed at bolstering what Solomon et al. call "self-esteem" by acting to preserve the status quo ("culture") while distancing patient and carer from the source of threat. Acting to "preserve the status quo" is seen in those patients who react to their symptoms by struggling desperately to find a way out of their awful situation, by an overreliance on the medical model, or by having impossibly high expectations of their carers; for the carers this may be evident in their "never giving up," in their continuing to try new treatments or administering escalating doses of analgesics and sedatives, despite the absence of any apparent success or even when such efforts are clearly counterproductive. Alternatively, or simultaneously, "distancing oneself from the source of threat" may appear in the patient who manifests psychological denial (which may include an absolute insistence that his or her problem is simply what it appears to be) or in the carers' attempts to get out of this painful situation as quickly as possible, usually through urgent referral to the social worker, counselor, or chaplain, who are "better suited than we are to deal with this type of problem."

SPIRITUAL PAIN AND CLINICAL DEPRESSION

Spiritual pain and clinical depression can, at times, have much in common. The characteristic fear and agitated struggle of a patient trying desperately to find a way out of spiritual pain, perhaps with associated feelings of alienation, have many overlapping features with acute agitated depression. Spiritual pain that has been present over a prolonged period of time, that causes individuals to feel utterly hopeless as they progressively withdraw from life and from living, can look like an apathetic depression. In the context of this chapter, however, our primary concern is not to debate whether spiritual pain is depression by another name, nor is it to debate whether spiritual pain is biologically or existentially generated; rather, it is to examine the language we use as clinicians to describe such an experience because this indicates and affects how we view that experience, which in turn influences how we act in response to it. The difficulty with labeling such suffering in an individual as "only an episode of depression" and then only prescribing antidepressant medication by way of response is that this constitutes at best a superficial response to the surface features of spiritual pain. Furthermore, it can prevent carers from seeing the full existential dimensions of the person's suffering and therefore ultimately have the effect of devaluing what such an individual is living.

The psychological and existential event that is spiritual pain may be associated with biological changes, and psychologically active medication, including antidepressants, may, in some cases, have a helpful role to play. However, such diagnosis and treatment is only one small, albeit on occasion a valuable, part of what needs to be a far more holistic response to the suffering at hand. What is needed is a way of responding that also addresses the deep, existential aspects of each individual's experience. Recognizing and naming such suffering as spiritual pain means acknowledging that something more than purely scientific medical skills and expertise are needed here.

RESPONDING TO SPIRITUAL PAIN

Given that terror-provoked disconnection from depth is what both has initially caused and sub-

sequently maintains the complex of symptoms and behavior that is spiritual pain, it is essential to plan a treatment strategy that will lessen fear and encourage and enable the individual to descend toward the healing depths of his or her psyche. To achieve this, the symptoms, be they physical, emotional, social, or religious, that are troubling the dying individual must be treated. That is, good palliative care and the skilled, multidisciplinary expertise that characterizes this approach must be used to achieve physical comfort, to open blocked channels of communication, to provide emotional and social support, and to address any specific religious issues that patient may have. For many patients, such an approach will also ease their spiritual distress. By lessening their fear and creating safety, good palliative care encourages these individuals to begin to lessen their resistance to the natural gravitational pull of their psyche toward a connectedness with the depths, the spirit domain, and its potential for centeredness and peace.

In the context of the map of the psyche we have presented, responses to spiritual pain can be discussed in terms of surface-work and depth-work. *Surface-work* refers to interventions aimed at easing distress at the surface, that is, the conscious and concrete level of an individual's experience. "Surface," used in this way, does not mean "superficial," nor does it convey a value judgment. Rather, the surface is the way to the deep, and surface-work is the essential first step in that direction. *Depth-work* describes any approach or intervention that brings an individual inward and downward toward the deeper layers of the psyche. While of value, it is also somewhat artificial to talk of surface-work and depth-work as if they were two completely distinct and separate entities. For many, as we have discussed, caring, effective surface-work is also depth-work and all that is needed to bring these individuals into depth. As Saunders reminds us, "the way care is given can reach the most hidden places."[10] Depth-work is also about helping the patient in spiritual distress to reconnect with those very simple and very ordinary aspects of life that have, in the past, brought them a sense of depth or significance, what Kreinheder calls "meaningful things done habitually."[47] This might involve encouraging patients to share memories, to spend time with people they love, to visit a place of special importance to them, to return home from the hospital or, if this is not possible, to bring something of home or something they especially value, for example, a photograph or a particular treasured object, to the hospital with them.

For a few, this skilled and compassionate approach is not enough. These are the patients who, despite all that good palliative care has to offer, remain stuck at the surface level of their psyche, trapped in a prison of spiritual pain. Such individuals need specific help and encouragement to let go to the deeper levels of their experience. Interventions that engage the imagination offer this potential, for imagery is the language of the deep mind and can bridge or link the surface and the deep aspects of the psyche. These interventions, which have been described as *depth skills*,[48] include imagework,[49] dream work,[50] art therapy,[51] music therapy,[52] reminiscence and biography therapy,[53] body work (including massage),[54] and certain forms of meditation.[55]

Two important assumptions underlie all such ways of working. The first is that the dynamic core of the suffering that is spiritual pain lies in the terrified ego's resistance to depth. Therefore, if the intervention allows that person to make the descent into depth, as a microcosm of death, in a way that feels safe and contained, it may enable the individual to re-emerge less frightened of depth and with less terror of death than before. Second, if these approaches enable that individual's movement toward depth and proximity to the Self, that is, the dynamic core at the depth of personhood, this will itself bring deep inner consolation. Such a person may experience healing of his or her spiritual pain. Carers may once again struggle to find words that describe the subtle but significant change that they now notice in such a patient. They may use phrases like "more real" or "more human," while the sufferer may describe feeling "more at peace," make comments concerning symptoms such as "my pain is still there, but it's different from before. . . . I can live with it now," and speak of the future in a way that makes it clear that fear is now a less formidable presence.

In terms of terror-management theory, the necessity for those in spiritual pain to move from the surface to the deep psyche echoes Solomon et al.'s observations of what may occur for individuals when their particular cultural world view becomes redundant: "One possibility for such people is to find an alternative shared cultural world view that is more compelling and better enables them to obtain self-esteem." Dramatic examples of this are individuals who experience religious conversions, join "cults" or emigrate to other cultures. Consistent with this analysis, Ullman found that religious conversions are often preceded by acute stress and feelings of low self-esteem, and Paloutzian found that after religious conversion, people report a greater purpose in life and a diminished fear of death.[56]

Sounding a cautionary note and countering any tendency towards unrealistic romanticism in this area, Solomon et al. add:

"However, for some individuals, such options are not readily available. Lacking an anxiety buffer, such individuals are completely overwhelmed with terror (i.e., become psychotic), or attempt to cope with terror in ways that the culture deems maladaptive and abnormal (e.g., neuroses, drug addictions). . . . From this perspective, mental illness can be viewed broadly as a failure in terror management that is ultimately shared by the individual and the culture.[15]

What a combination of good palliative care and appropriate depth skills can facilitate for the patient in spiritual pain is a safe and contained transition from one "culture" that is no longer relevant to another that more adequately meets the needs of that individual, thereby bringing inner consolation and healing and preventing the disorganized collapse from terror into chaos that might otherwise follow.

SPECIFIC ASPECTS OF THE RESPONSE TO SPIRITUAL PAIN

Accurate recognition and naming of an individual's suffering as spiritual pain and then reaching agreement, as a team, on this diagnosis is itself the beginnings of an effective response. Other aspects of the response include the following.

Value the Therapeutic Relationship

In responding to spiritual distress, it is essential to appreciate the healing potential of the relationship between carer and patient. For the dying patient, the inner descent to the deep psyche is as much a move into perilous territory as is a move toward the unknown future. The therapeutic relationship helps to create conditions that facilitate such moves toward unsafety. As Saunders puts it, "The real presence of another person is a place of security. We have to give all patients that feeling of security in which they can begin, when they are ready, to face unsafety."[57] The simple presence of one who is concerned, one who is willing to be a companion and to remain steadfast when there are no easy answers, is itself a form of powerful communication that goes beyond words. One of the most valuable ways of forming a connection with a stranger is to acknowledge and understand his or her reality in all its bleakness without conveying a sense of helplessness, despair, or defeat (Ormont LR, Ormont J, personal communication).

Who we are as carers, in terms of our relationship to our own inner depths, is also of relevance here.[58] The patient experiencing spiritual pain knows intuitively if the carer who sits by the bedside is someone familiar with depth. If so, such presence can bring reassurance to that person and encourage his or her own letting go, for, in the words of the Psalm, "Deep calls on deep, in the roar of waters."[59]

Establish Contact

Bridging the gap that exists between two strangers involves a process of active listening, discovering common ground, and exploring differences. The primary means of establishing contact with a person in spiritual pain is through active listening. This means deliberately and consciously "tuning in" to that patient's unique wavelength by attending to both the factual and the feeling content of what that person is communicating. The latter is crucially important. Feelings may connect to the depths of a person, and the experience of being heard at this profound level can result in a transformation of the terrifying isolation that is a hallmark of such spiritual distress into a sense of aloneness that is bearable and mysteriously permeated with hope. While the factual content of what a person is saying is relatively easily determined from the individual's verbal communication, the feeling content is less easily perceived. Feelings are "heard" through the nonverbal aspects of that person's communication—by how he says what he says, by his tone of voice, his posture, and how he is in the silences between his words. Active listening, therefore, includes noticing what we see and how we ourselves feel as we engage with

another in this way and is incomplete until we have checked with the person to determine whether our perceptions have been accurate.

Active listening to the patient and previously acquired information from other caregivers, family members, or medical records may suggest areas in which the caregiver and patient share common ground. Such areas may open the way for the growth of common bonds. Allen has provided a list of areas that are helpful in this regard: age, biorhythms (feelings during daily, monthly, and yearly cycles), socioeconomic class (childhood and present), position and relation within the family (childhood and present), grief experience, language(s) spoken and understood, marital status, nationality, personality structure (e.g., extroverted, introverted), regional experience (urban or rural), sex, state of health, and work or profession.[60]

Having discovered areas of common ground, the path is prepared to explore more openly differences of experience, personal philosophy, and context of values and meaning. At this point, the dialogue may naturally evolve from a one-sided presentation in which the caregiver is seen by both parties as the one more able to give into a more egalitarian exchange with two givers and two receivers. In this process, energies are exchanged and the potential is created for new insight and understanding and a deeper or altered sense of meaning.[60]

Respect the Patient's Otherness

This means adopting a stance that recognizes and honors the distinctiveness of the person being cared for. To acknowledge the uniqueness of the sufferer is to validate his or her personhood. This is accomplished through gestures, actions, questions, and assertions that demonstrate recognition that you are dealing with a unique human being whose essence is characterized by dignity. It is compromised by waiting lines, case numbers, institutional norms, lapses of privacy, unexplained delays in bedside care, investigations, or procedures, and a thousand other potentially invasive incidents that may pass unnoticed in a patient's day.

Control Symptoms Effectively

The control of pain and other symptoms is the foundation on which excellence in whole-person care is fashioned. Psychosocial interventions and the sorts of depth skills described earlier are much less likely to be effective if inadequate attention is given to the diagnosis and management of the patient's multiple symptoms. Should carers of whatever discipline—nurse, physician, cleaner, priest—identify unresolved distress such as pain, nausea, dyspnea, or constipation, this should be brought to the attention of colleagues on the team in order to ensure optimal management of the physical contributors to these symptoms while additional attention is paid to potential psychosocial and spiritual factors that may be involved. Attention should also be given to whatever meaning such symptoms hold for the patient. In parallel with this attention to physical symptoms, all other reversible aspects of the patient's suffering, whether in the area of communications, relationships, specifically religious issues, activities of daily living, or financial and other practical affairs, must be identified and treated using the broad and varied skills of the multidisciplinary team.

Obtain a "Clinical Biography"

There is a real therapeutic potential in broadening and deepening the case history of the patient in spiritual pain into a narrative tale that provides a "who" as well as a "what" and knowledge of a real person rather than simply a disease.[61] An understanding of the full "who" of the person being cared for depends on developing insight into the topography of the patient's individuality, remembering that all persons have personality and character, a past, a family, a cultural background, roles and relationships, a political identity, behaviors and actions, an inner world view, a body, a secret life, a perceived future and a transcendent dimension. Each of these domains shapes their identity and their experiences of illness, and each is affected by the illness.[25]

Determine the Meaning of the Illness for the Patient

This follows from the preceding step and involves gaining insight into the significance of the illness for the patient. This may not be immediately apparent. For an elderly, isolated immigrant, her illness was a catastrophic threat to her ability to care for and protect the secret existence of her 42-year-old mentally handicapped daughter. A young woman thought her breast cancer meant she would die with the uncontrolled pain she had observed when her grandmother had the same disease. A lonely widower experienced his cancer as a ticket to liberation from grief; an aging bachelor saw his as God's punishment for a life misspent. Only by gentle inquiry in an atmosphere of trust can the real meaning of illness for the patient be expressed, confronted, and dealt with.

Determine the Meaning of the Illness for the Family

This involves trying to understand the perceived implications of this life crisis for the patient's family and friends. For one young man, his friend's illness meant the inevitable public disclosure of their homosexual relationship. For four children, the loss of their alcoholic, often absent father meant anger, relief, and guilt; it also meant an unpaid mortgage, the need to sell their home, and a move that would leave all friends and familiar associations behind. The dimensions of the loss facing another grieving family could not be fully appreciated without knowing that the middle son of three, age 9, had died. The full scope of their distress was clarified only on seeing the family photographs. In each snapshot, the boy who had died was standing at the center of the family group. "Now I understand," the caregiver exclaimed. "You didn't lose the middle son of three; you lost the glue of the family, the center of gravity, the lynchpin." "Yes! Yes!" blurted out the father. "We lost the family's soul!" Further gentle inquiry led to a deepening understanding of this ruptured family system and more meaningful insight into the family's distress. When this was communicated to the family members, they recognized that they were with a carer who understood something of the enormity of their loss. This was a true connection over and above the emotional release the family experienced.

Explore Sources of Meaning in the Person's Life

At a time when life seems overwhelming and to have lost purpose, the patient has a fundamental need to once again experience a sense of meaning. Such a spark cannot be imposed or given by someone else. It must arise from within that individual. The caregiver can, however, be a catalyst in this process. This is achieved primarily by sitting down and taking the time to ask and to listen.

Frankl has suggested four areas where reflection may help the patient reconnect to a sense of meaning.[62] The four areas of questioning are: (1) What has been created or accomplished? ("You have driven a truck for 30 years. You must have transported a lot of goods in that time. Tell me about that."); (2) Who or what has been loved? (This includes the people, animals, the places, the sights, the ideas, the music, the books, and so forth that have been loved.); (3) What legacy is being left behind? (This may include family, life achievements, material things, organ donations, participation in experimental protocols, having a low-cost funeral, contributing to fellow patients or to caregivers.); and (4) What are the things believed in, and what ability to transcend suffering is unique to this patient? (Recalling that our transcendent dimension involves our need to identify with someone or something greater than ourselves, we might ask the question "Who is the transcendent figure the person is identifying with who can help him through this difficult time?")

Assist in Redefining Hope

The terminally ill may hope for an absence of pain and suffering, for caregivers whose continuing involvement can be relied on, for friends who will continue to visit, for a hospital bed without a parking meter on it if it is needed, and perhaps for longer life, although, as illness progresses, the hope for prolonged life usually gives way to hope for quality in the moment. Hope comes when a patient has the sense of having choice in some area of life, even if this has apparently little to do with the suffering the person is going through. Hope can thus be fostered by establishing concrete, realistic, short-term goals: "Why don't you decide when you would like your bath, this morning or this afternoon?" Hope and wishing are not the same thing. For the dying, there is an important difference. Hope bespeaks a perspective on reality, a point of view. It is a child of the human spirit. It arises out of an experience of personal meaning and thus reflects a degree of inner peace. Wishing, on the other hand, arises from a sense of need, dissatisfaction, and unrest. It reflects a sense of incompleteness. Hope is the product of adversity transcended, wishing of adversity denied. Hope is found in acceptance, the conscious attitude that accompanies integration. The one who accepts is freed to act, respond, and take control in new ways.

Examine Fears, Particularly Concerning the Unknown

In naming a fear, we rob it of much of its power. Uncertainty breeds anxiety, which, in turn, paralyzes coping mechanisms. Many fears are associated with the unknowns of illness. "Will I choke to death?" "Will I have a lot of pain?" "Will I die alone?" A discussion of symptom control options and the assurance of attentive continuity in care reassures and provides security, which, in turn, extinguishes anxiety.

A further unknown lies in the question of eternity. Is there an existence after death? This primordial issue arises for all who face death, whether or not it is expressed. Asking simply, "What do you think comes after death?" may enable a great release as the anxiety accompanying this most basic of human fears is shared in honesty with another person. It is important to remember that coping skills are enhanced not through hearing someone else's answers to such questions but through the asking of them and the subsequent working through of the patient's own answers with the help of one who cares enough to be involved.

Explore the Patient's Need for Reconciliation

The stress of terminal illness may accentuate inherent difficulties in family relationships. Old misunderstandings, resentments, jealousies, and prejudices are often inflamed. The caregiver is in a privileged position as an objective observer who may be able to point out opportunities for reconciliation at this time of changing reality in the family system. Like acceptance of forgiveness, reconciliation always starts with self, then involves others and, for many, God, however that ultimate reality may be perceived.

Celebrate the Transcendent

Transcendence is experienced when moments are illuminated by an awareness of the majesty and mystery of life through seeing, hearing, smelling, tasting, or touching the beauty that is always there. It may occur in prayer or meditation, as we have an experience of stillness, simplicity, and a power beyond ourselves yet within ourselves. Wholeness is the integration of the twin experience of transcendence and immanence. For those who have a particular faith and system of belief, transcendence may be fostered through the use of symbols, rituals, and other resources of that religion or philosophical perspective. For many this will be aided by involving a minister of religion capable of performing the sacramental rites of the religion involved. As Lunn reminds us, "The traditional rituals of religion have great power in the context of death and dying, separation and loss. This is true for the majority of people who are not regular participants in religious ritual at other times. . . . The profoundly spiritual and cultural need for ritual is most evident in the face of death."[11]

Actively Intervene if Patient Remains Stuck

The various aspects of response already discussed, in particular the control of physical suffering and the establishment of a relationship of trust between patient and carer, enable the majority of individuals in spiritual pain to descend to a place of inner consolation and peace. For others, however, this is not enough, and such individuals remain trapped in their surface prison of spiritual pain. It is in instances such as this that one of the depth skills mentioned earlier may be of particular relevance. It is essential that the individual who offers the patient the opportunity of working in this way be fully trained in that particular depth skill and adequately supervised and, ideally, already be part of the caring team and known to the patient. What is common to all such approaches is their ability to tackle the problem at the heart of spiritual pain, that is, the disconnection and subsequent alienation from depth, by safely bringing the patient from the surface mind to the deep mind and by encouraging the patient to open and experience there the healing power of depth. The appropriate use of religious ritual, as discussed, might also be seen as a depth skill from this perspective. The following is an example of the use of one such technique, imagework, in a patient with spiritual pain.

Case Example

Joyce was a 42-year-old woman who was known to have carcinomatosis peritonei from carcinoma of the caecum. Widowed 5 years previously when her husband died from malignant melanoma, she had two children and worked as a journalist. She had been brought up Roman Catholic but was no longer practicing. Her family doctor had referred her to the palliative home-care team for symptom control and emotional support.

When the doctor and nurse visited Joyce at home, they found a gaunt and frightened woman who complained of severe abdominal pain, nausea, and vomiting. These symptoms were thought to result from a combination of malignant subacute bowel obstruction and opioid-induced constipation. During the visit Joyce spoke openly of her advanced cancer and said that she knew death was not far off but that she "had no fears." As they drove from the home, the palliative-care nurse commented to the doctor that she felt Joyce's attitude seemed almost "too good to be true."

Over the following days Joyce's symptoms settled as she responded to the treatment regime suggested to her family doctor by the home-care team. Indeed, within a week of that initial assessment visit, she was so much improved that she was able to recommence part-time work.

Little was heard from Joyce for some weeks. Then her family doctor telephoned, requesting her admission to the palliative-care ward. On admission she was extremely weak but otherwise calm and comfortable. Physical examination showed that she had now developed massive hepatomegaly and ascites and that, in addition, she had a lot of palpable intra-abdominal tumor. Haematological investigation showed that she was not anemic. As no other possible causes were found, her profound weakness was felt to be the result of the systemic effects of her very advanced malignancy.

Three days after Joyce's admission she had an episode of massive fecal incontinence, spurious diarrhea from her subacute bowel obstruction. While her physical symptoms quickly responded to treatment, she suddenly became extremely emotionally distressed. "This is the last straw," she cried. "I feel utterly degraded. . . . Do you call this "dying with dignity?" . . . If this is a sign of what's to come, I want it over, now."

Over the next 24 hours, Joyce remained greatly distressed and seemed inconsolable, despite constant attention from her family and many of the ward staff (in particular, the nurses, the social worker/counselor, and the aromatherapist). By then, her demands for euthanasia had become persistent and increasingly desperate. She countered comments that such a measure was not legally permissible by asking to be transferred wherever necessary so that it could be performed. In addition, it was evident by then that she was physically a lot weaker and that her life expectancy was likely to be only a few days at most. Her only relief appeared to come with the sleep she got following intermittent sedative medication. However, each time she awoke she appeared even more distressed than before.

At this stage, a number of members of the ward team met to discuss what else could be done to help Joyce. Every one agreed that her emotional distress was a form of spiritual pain, and there was a shared sense of the inadequacy of our pharmacological and counseling efforts. The management options seemed limited at this point. Either her physician could prescribe regular sedative medication for her, or the team could try, once more, to reach the roots of her suffering. One of the team, a doctor, had experience working with imagework, a form of active imagination,[49,63] and he agreed to meet with Joyce. As he sat by her bedside in her darkened single room, she lay curled up on her side under her duvet. She looked skeletal, and her eyes were closed. When she spoke, her voice and face were filled with pain: "The only thing you could do is to help me to die, now. I want to die. I want to die *now*."

The doctor then told Joyce that time was very short for her and that she would probably die within the next day or so. It was evident from the tears and moaning that followed that this was of no consolation to her. The doctor then explained about imagework. He said that while he could not, and would not, do anything to physically accelerate her dying, if she was willing to try this particular way of working, it might well "help her in her dying." Joyce listened carefully to all of this. She had tried visualization in the early stages of her illness. "I am willing to try anything that might help," she replied. The doctor then asked her to close her eyes and led her through the following active imagination:

"Imagine yourself standing on a grassy hill. It's a summer evening and the sun is beginning to set in a clear sky. It's still warm. There is a very faint breeze, which you feel on your face and in your hair. As you look around, you can see, in the middle distance, a river. It's a large river, wide and obviously deep, as its surface is still and smooth and its black waters hardly appear to be moving. It's coming from hills to one side, and you can see it meandering its way to the sea on the far-distant western horizon. You look down the hill. You notice that between you and the river is a large green field. You begin to descend through the tall grass toward the river.

You know that waiting for you on the bank of the river is someone who knows you and cares deeply about you. You are now getting closer to the river. You can see the person standing there. It may be someone you know well, or it may be someone who is unfamiliar to you. You also know that this is someone wise, someone who knows the river and who will be your guide on the next stage of your journey. As you approach this person, he or she greets you and points toward a little wooden rowing boat tied at the riverbank nearby. This person is offering to take you in the boat. This is a choice you have to make—whether or not you will trust this person, whether or not you will get into the boat."

At this point Joyce began to weep quietly. The doctor asked her if she was all right. Without opening her eyes, she nodded. When he then asked her if it was her choice to get into the boat, she mumbled, faintly but clearly, "yes." The doctor then continued:

"Your guide gets into the boat before you. He or she is sitting in the middle seat and indicates to you to sit in the rear of the boat. You do, and your guide pulls the rope into the boat and, using an oar, pushes the little boat out toward the center of the enormous river. You know that you are with someone who cares deeply about you. You know that you are with someone who knows about the boat and who understands the river. You do not know where this will bring you, but you do know that you are with someone who knows the way there. You have done all you can. At this stage you can choose to trust yourself to this guide and to trust yourself to the river. Let your guide lead the way, the river carry you. Allow yourself to be carried, to be held by this deep and silent river that is flowing into the next stage of your journey. Be aware, notice, experience how this feels. Allow this experience. Allow yourself to be carried."

By then Joyce was lying utterly still, breathing slowly and evenly as if deeply asleep. "I met my husband by the riverside," she said, as she slowly began to open her eyes. Once again she began to weep, but the doctor felt her tears were now of sadness, in contrast to earlier tears of desperation. "I asked my husband to help me to die," she continued. "He said he was with me, and we would be together." She then smiled and looked very much more relaxed. She asked the doctor if she could sleep. As he left her room, he reassured her that everything possible would be done to keep her comfortable.

For several hours after this, despite receiving no further sedation, Joyce slept deeply. Her family sat by her bedside. During the night, when the nurses were turning her, she opened her eyes briefly and smiled. She died in the early hours of the following morning.

In Joyce's case, spiritual pain manifested preterminally as an acute and overwhelming emotional crisis. In terms of Solomon et al.'s terror-management framework, she was experiencing the consequences of a breakdown of her anxiety buffer as it became apparent to her that the cultural model that had served her so well until then had now become redundant. In this context, her request for euthanasia can be seen as a cry to others to help her move beyond the old cultural model. In terms of the surface/deep model of the psyche, Joyce's asking for euthanasia can also be seen metaphorically. Here was a woman who, despite all that skilled palliative care could offer, remained trapped at the surface level of the psyche. In this context, her plea to "help me to die" was also a request for help in moving beyond the surface and toward the deep psyche that she sensed would bring her the comfort she sought. The depth skill of imagework facilitated this process. By allowing her to move into depth, though the doorway of the imagination, this intervention enabled her to make the necessary culture change, helped her to cross into the unknown of the deep psyche as a microcosm of death, and appeared to heal her spiritual pain.

CONCLUSION

How do we know whether the observations we have made in the preceding pages are true or accurate? Our response to spiritual pain is not dependent on clinical trials or belief systems. How we see this arena depends on how such ideas and concepts relate to our individual experience of caring for others, as well as our own personal experience of living with and through spiritual pain, our own search for meaning and healing.

This is not an add-on luxury area of patient care. Rather, it is of central importance. Attending to a patient's spiritual distress has to do with the alleviation of suffering and healing in its deepest sense. These concepts are relevant in all areas of health care and call for a revision and a redefinition of the medical model.

To address these issues involves a cost, to both the patient and ourselves as caregivers. The widely accepted doctor-patient relationship is rooted in the biomedical model and focused on the biology of disease. With the adoption of terms of reference that include the spiritual domain, this status quo can never again be judged to be adequate. The new relationship involves more responsibility for the patient and more vulnerability for the doctor. In abandoning the narrow mandate that focuses on fighting disease in favor of a broader challenge, the alleviation of suffering, the physician is opting for the role of wounded healer rather than that of heroic combatant.[49]

We advocate "whole-person care." Recognition of the rich potential this embraces challenges us to reexamine medical education, to consider what whole-person education for doctors might look like. Our thesis is not that all doctors must become competent in the area of alleviating spiritual distress but that all doctors must be aware that existential issues are intrinsic to the experience of illness, that the issue of spiritual pain is an important consideration in establishing each differential diagnosis, and that such issues need to be recognized and attended to by each multidisciplinary team.

References

1. Yalom ID. *Existential Psychotherapy*. New York: Basic Books, 1980:25.
2. Mount BM. *Sightings*. Downer Grove: InterVarsity Press, 1983.
3. Cohen SR, Mount BM. Quality of life assessment in terminal illness: defining and measuring subjective well-being in the dying. *Journal of Palliative Care*, 1992; 8:40–45.
4. *Cancer Pain Relief and Palliative Care*. Technical Report Series 804. Geneva: World Health Organization, 1990.
5. *Oxford English Dictionary*. Oxford: Oxford University Press, 1988.
6. Onions CT, ed. *Oxford Dictionary of English Etymology*. Oxford: Oxford University Press, 1985.
7. Teihard de Chardin P. *The Heart of the Matter*. San Diego: Harcourt Brace and Co., 1980.
8. Hillman J. Re-Visioning Psychology. New York: Harper & Row, 1975:67–70.
9. Tournier P. *The Meaning of Persons*. London: SCM Press, 1957.

10. Saunders C. Spiritual Pain. *Journal of Palliative Care*, 1988; 4:29–32.

11. Lunn L. Spiritual concerns in palliation. In: Saunders C, ed, *The Management of Terminal Malignant Disease*. 3rd ed. London: Edward Arnold, 1993; 213–225.

12. Moore T. *Care of the Soul*. New York: HarperCollins, 1992:xi–xiii.

13. Buber M, RG Smith, trans. *I and Thou*. Edinburgh: T and T Clark, 1973.

14. Luke 17:21. *New Oxford Annotated Bible with the Apocrypha*, May HG, Metzger BM, eds, New York: Oxford University Press, 1977.

15. 1 Thessalonians 5:23. *New Oxford Annotated Bible with the Apocryphar*, May HG, Metzger BM, eds, New York: Oxford University Press, 1977.

16. Mascaro J. Introduction to *The Upanishads*. London: Penguin Books, 1965:13.

17. Mascaro J. Introduction to *The Dhammapada*. London: Penguin Books, 1973:15.

18. Lao-Tzu; Roberts RG. trans. intro., and commentary *Te-Tao Ching*. New York: Ballantine Books, 1989:xxiv.

19. Plato; Jowett B, trans. *Charmides: The Dialogue of Plato*. New York: Random House, 1937:6.

20. Cassell EJ. *The Nature of Suffering and the Goals of Medicine*. Oxford: Oxford University Press, 1991:33.

21. Reading A. Illness and disease. *Medical Clinics of North America*, 1977; 61(4):703–710.

22. Wasserstein AG. Toward a romantic science: the writings of Oliver Sacks. *Annals of Internal Medicine*, 1988; 1(September):440–444.

23. Bugental J. The third force in psychology. *Journal of Humanistic Psychology*. 1964; 4:19–26. Cited by Yalom ID. in *Existential Psychotherapy*. New York: Basic Books, 1980:18.

24. Saunders C. *The Management of Terminal Illness*. London: Edward Arnold, 1967.

25. Cassell EJ. *The Nature of Suffering and the Goals of Medicine*. Oxford: Oxford University Press, 1991: 37–43.

26. Yalom ID. *Existential Psychotherapy*. New York: Basic Books, 1980:3–26.

27. Chief Seattle *Letter to the Great Chief in Washington*, 1853. Cited in *Joseph Campbell: The Power of Myth*. BS. Flowers ed. New York: Doubleday, 1988:34.

28. Dillard A. *Teaching a Stone to Talk*. New York: Harper & Row, 1982.

29. *The Words of Gandhi* selected by R. Attenborough. New York: Newmarket press, 1982, 74.

30. 1 Kings 19:12 *The New Oxford Annotated Bible with the Apocrypha*, May HG, Metzger BM, eds, New York: Oxford University Press, 1977.

31. Psalm 139. *The New Oxford Annotated Bible with the Apocrypha*, May HG, Metzger BM, eds, New York: Oxford University Press, 1977.

32. Berry T. *The Dream of the Earth*. San Francisco: Sierra Club Books, 1988. Cited by McFague S. In *The Body of God*. Minneapolis: Fortress Press, 1993:70–71.

33. McFague S. *The Body of God*. Minneapolis: Fortress Press, 1993:66.

34. Wheeler HB. Shattuck Lecture—Healing and Heroism. *New England Journal of Medicine* 1990; 322:1540–1548.

35. Lazare A, Eisenthall S, Wasserman L. The customer approach to patienthood: attending to patient requests in a walk-in clinic. *Archives of General Psychiatry* 1975; 32:553–568.

36. Cassell EJ. *The Nature of Suffering and the Goals of Medicine*. Oxford University Press, 1991:30–47.

37. Frank JD. The faith that heals. *Johns Hopkins Medical Journal* 1975; 137:127.

38. Kiev A. *Magic, Faith and Healing*. New York: The Free Press, 1964.

39. Cassell EJ. *The Nature of Suffering and the Goals of Medicine*. Oxford University Press, 1991:48.

40. *Life Magazine*. The Best Doctor of All, 1920. Cited by Wheeler HB. Shattuck Lecture—Healing and Heroism. *New England Journal of Medicine* 1990; 322:1540–1548.

41. Cullen TS. The gay heart. *Archives of Internal Medicine* 1949; 84:41–45.

42. Jung C.G. (1953) Psychology and Alchemy, Voulme 12, The Collected Works, Pinceton, New Jersey, Princeton University Press, para 439, page 336.

43. Becker E. *The Birth and Death of Meaning*. 2nd ed. New York: Free Press, 1971.

44. Becker E. *The Denial of Death*. New York, 1973.

45. Solomon S, Greenberg J, Pyszczynski T. A terror management theory of social behaviour: The psychological functions of self-esteem and cultural worldviews. In: Zanna MP, ed, *Advances in Experimental Social Psychology*. San Diego: Academic Press, Inc., 1991:91–159.

46. Solomon S, Greenberg J, Pyszczynski T. Terror Management Theory of Self-Esteem. In Snyder CR, Forsyth D, eds, *Handbook of Social and Clinical Psychology: The Health Perspective*. New York: Pergamon, 1991:24–40.

47. Kreinheder A. (1991), Body and Soul—the other side of illness. In Studies in Jungian Psychology by Jungian Analysts. Toronto, Inner City Books, page 110.

48. Kearney M. *Mortally Wounded—Stories of Soul Pain, Death and Healing*. Dublin: Marino Books, 1996.

49. Kearney M. Imagework in a case of intractable pain. *Palliative Medicine*, 1992; 6:152–157.

50. Hillman J. *The Dream and the Underworld.* New York: Harper and Row, 1979.

51. Connell C. Art therapy as part of the palliative care programme. *Palliative Medicine*, 1992; 6:18–25.

52. Munro S, Mount B. Music therapy in palliative care. *Canadian Medical Association Journal*, 1978; 119:258–263.

53. Lichton L, Mooney J, Doyd M. Biography as therapy. *Palliative Medicine*, 1993; 7:133–137.

54. Wilkinson S. Aromatherapy and massage in palliative care. *International Journal of Palliative Nursing*, 1995; 1:21–30.

55. Levine S. *Who Dies?* Bath: Gateway Books, 1988.

56. Paloutzian R.F. Purpose in life and value changes following conversion. *Journal of Personality and Social Psychology*, 1981; 41:1153–1160, cited by Solomon S, Greenberg J, Pyszczynski T. A terror management theory of social behaviour: The psychological functions of self-esteem and cultural worldviews. In: Zanna MP, ed, Advances in Experimental Social Psychology. San Diego: Academic Press, Inc., 1991:91–159.

57. Saunders C. Appropriate treatment, appropriate death. In *The Management of Terminal Disease.* London: Edward Arnold, 1978:6.

58. Kearney M. Palliative medicine—just another specialty? *Palliative Medicine*, 1992; 6:39–46.

59. Psalm 42, vs. 7 in The Psalms, Grail Translation. Fontana, 1966.

60. Allen C. Bridging the gulf of meaning: a philosophical approach to palliative care. In: Ajemian I, Mount B, eds, RVH *Manual on Palliative Hospice Care.* Salem: New Hampshire, The Ayer Company, 1982:231–242.

61. Sacks O. *The Man Who Mistook His Wife for a Hat and Other Clinical Tales.* New York: Harper and Row, 1987.

62. Frankl V. *Man's Search for Meaning—an Introduction to Logotherapy.* London: Hodder and Stoughton, 1987.

63. Hannah B. *Encounters with the Soul: Active Imagination.* Boston: Sigo Press, 1981.

26

The Treatment of Suffering in Patients with Advanced Cancer

Nathan I. Cherny, MBBS, FRACP

For the patient with advanced incurable cancer, the goals of care are the alleviation of suffering, the optimization of quality of life until death ensues, and the provision of comfort in death.[1] The alleviation of suffering is universally acknowledged as a cardinal goal of medical care.[1-6] Persistent suffering that is inadequately relieved (or the anticipation of this situation) undermines the value of life for the sufferer.

The ability to formulate a clinical response to the problem of suffering in the cancer patient requires a clinically relevant understanding of the nature of the problem.[7-11] In an attempt to develop a clinically relevant definition, Cherny et al. have defined suffering as an aversive emotional experience characterized by the perception of personal distress that is generated by adverse factors that undermine quality of life.[11] According to this model, there are 3 defining characteristics of suffering: (1) perceptual capacity (sentience) must be present,[12,13] (b) the factors undermining quality of life must be appraised as distressing, and (c) the experience must be aversive. Suffering is not a diagnosis; rather, it is a phenomenon of conscious human existence.[12] The intensity of the experience is a variable that is determined by the number and severity of the factors diminishing quality of life, the processes of appraisal, and perception. Each of these factors is amenable to therapeutic interventions.

Advanced cancer is a potential cause of great distress to patients, their families, and the professional caregivers attending them. While at least two-thirds of patients with advanced cancer have significant pain,[14] numerous other physical symptoms can equally diminish the patient's quality of life.[15-22] Furthermore, many patients endure enormous psychological distress,[23-25] in some cases from an existential perspective that suggests that, even without pain or other physical symptoms, continued life is without meaning.[26] For the families and loved ones of patients there is, likewise, great distress in this process: anticipated loss, standing witness to the physical and emotional distress of the patient, and bearing the burdens of care.[27,28] Professional caregivers may potentially be stressed by the suffering they witness, which challenges their clinical and emotional resources.[29-32] According to this model, the suffering of each of these groups is inextricably interrelated, and the perceived distress of any one may amplify the distress of the others (Figure 26.1).

SUFFERING AND PERSONAL GROWTH

The potential for personal development and satisfaction in overcoming situations of adversity is a well-recognized phenomenon. The ability to rise

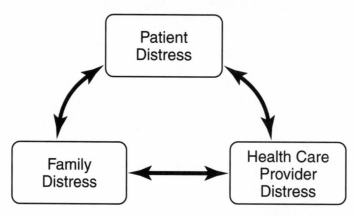

Figure 26.1 The Relationship Among the Distress of the Patient, Family and Health-care Providers

from adversity is predicated on a perception of self-efficacy and the ability to cope with prevailing problems. When, however, a person perceives the demands of a situation as exceeding the available coping resources, then stress, a sense of personal vulnerability, and associated emotional distress are triggered.[33] In the advanced cancer patient, this occurs when the factors diminishing the quality of life are excessively severe, or numerous or when the patient appraises the available resources for coping as inadequate to the task.

The phenomenon of coping generates the potential for growth and reward. Coping does not occur if the demands of the situation *are* overwhelming (as distinct from merely being appraised as overwhelming). The patient with inadequately relieved pain or dyspnea may be absolutely unable to address issues related to his or her offspring and spouse. The spouse and offspring who are overwhelmed by problems of daily care requirements may be absolutely unable to savor the remaining time with the patient. By understanding and addressing the factors that may potentially overwhelm the patient, family, and health-care providers, the necessary preconditions for coping and growth are established. Suffering in advanced cancer patients cannot be eliminated, but if adequate relief is achieved, then coping and growth can occur.

RELIEF OF SUFFERING AS A RIGHTS ISSUE

In patients with advanced cancer, a readiness to address pain and other intolerable symptoms is a medical and moral imperative.[1,34] The corollary of the right of the incurably ill to relief of pain and suffering is the responsibility of caregivers to ensure that adequate provisions are made for relief.[35] The formulation of a therapeutic response requires an understanding of the factors that contribute to it. Failure to appreciate or to effectively address the full diversity of contributing factors may confound effective therapeutic strategies.

From this perspective, the provision of adequate relief of symptoms is an overriding goal, which must be pursued even in the setting of a narrow therapeutic index for the necessary palliative treatments.[1,34,36–38] This concept has been endorsed by a presidential commission[6] and by consensus statements from major professional organizations in medicine and ethics.[4,39–45]

HIPPOCRATIC MEDICINE AND THE RELIEF OF SUFFERING

Hippocratic medicine has traditionally defined the purview of medical practice in normative situations. According to the Hippocratic paradigm, medicine is seen as a vocation of compassion in which the quality and quantity of human life are of critical concern. The imperative to alleviate suffering precludes the elimination of the sufferer, and the administration of "a deadly drug to any patient" falls beyond the normative practice of medicine.

The Hippocratic Charter may be summarized as follows:

1. To abhor suffering and preventable premature death

2. To strive to prevent or to cure illness that generates suffering and foreshortens survival
3. When cure is not possible, to find the optimal balance between relief of suffering and prolongation of survival
4. The relief of suffering should be achieved by means other than the termination of the life of the sufferer

The advocates of euthanasia and physician-assisted suicide challenge this construct. For some practitioners and ethicists, the data indicating that the treatment of pain and suffering are frequently ineffectual are sufficient to justify elective death by euthanasia or by assisted suicide as beneficent options when standard therapies have been inadequate to the task.[1,46–48]

Besides absolutist reservations about the deliberate termination of human life, standard objections to this approach include the so-called slippery-slope argument (of progressive precedent) and the argument of the potential for abuse.[49] Among palliative-medicine practitioners, three other approaches have taken increasing prominence.

1. *The "not-yet" argument.* Several clinicians have argued that the legalization of either of these options without first ensuring universal availability of expert care in symptom management or, at very least, the requirement of expert assessment of potential candidates may result in the maleficent foreshortening of the lives of some patients when other appropriate options were untested and unexplored.[2,50–59] They assert that the focus of public discussion on these life-curtailing options is inappropriate when so little has yet been done to ease suffering without having to kill patients or assist in their killing of themselves.
2. *The nature-of-rights objection.* Arguing from the nature of rights, some have challenged the contention that the ethical principle of autonomy can be extrapolated to claim a right to choose one's time and mode of death. Given that a valid right implies the existence of a duty to respond that cannot be *reasonably* refused[60,61] and that reasonable moral compunction about either killing patients or assisting in their suicide is acknowledged, it is argued that a right to die by euthanasia or physician-assisted suicide does not exist.[37]
3. *The argument from nonnecessity.* Proponents of this view argue that sedation for patients with refractory suffering provides adequate relief without intending the death of the patient.[62–64] In contrast to those practices, in which the death of the pa-

tient is intended and critical to the outcome, deep sedation obliterates the perception of distress. The death of the patient, when it occurs, is a foreseen contingency but not an intended or essential outcome. The use of sedating therapies recognizes the right of patients with advanced cancer to adequate relief of unendurable symptoms and the right of all patients to choose among therapeutic options within the purview of medical practice.[1,65,66] In the absence of such ethical equilibrium, the moral reservations of clinicians or family members may result in either the undertreatment of catastrophic symptoms or subsequent guilt and its morbid psychological sequelae.

Hippocratic purview of medicine, in summary, requires that suffering be acknowledged, its causes identified, and steps taken to provide adequate relief with haste and effect until adequate relief is achieved.

STUDIES ON THE RELIEF OF SUFFERING

It is widely held that the treatment of pain and suffering are frequently ineffectual and that, in some circumstances, this situation may render death the preferred option.[1,3] In one survey of public attitudes, 57% of respondents endorsed the statement that a painful death can be expected with cancer, and 69% endorsed the statement that cancer pain can be so bad that a person with cancer might consider suicide.[67] In a recent survey of 1308 outpatients treated by oncologists of the Eastern Cooperative Oncology Group, 67% of the patients reported that they had pain during the week preceding the study, and 36% had pain severe enough to impair their ability to function. Of those with pain, 42% were not given adequate analgesic therapy.[68] Among cancer patients, uncontrolled pain has been reported to be a significant determinant of suicidal ideation. A study at Memorial Sloan-Kettering Cancer Center that evaluated 185 cancer patients experiencing pain observed that suicidal ideation (thoughts of suicide with or without an immediate plan) occurred in 17%.[69] In a retrospective survey of the charts of 90 patients with advanced cancer, 20% of patients had expressed the view that suicide could be an option "somewhere in the future" if pain and other symptoms were uncontrolled or if the patients became an excessive burden on their families.[20] Indeed, one author has suggested that some of the non-physical causes of patient distress may be intrinsically refractory to comfort directed interventions and that these alone may be sufficient to suggest death as the preferred option.[70]

Inadequately relieved suffering can present as uncontrolled physical symptoms, depression or anxiety, severe existential distress, or family member and health-care provider fatigue, or it can manifest itself in the request for euthanasia or physician-assisted suicide.[51,71] Most often the contributing factors coexist in combinations; for example, the depressed patient with uncontrolled pain may be attended to by frustrated, distressed relatives and an exhausted, exasperated physician.

Uncontrolled suffering in a dying patient is a medical emergency.[1] When patients, their families, or other health-care providers request that the patient be killed or helped to kill himself, this

is usually in response to actual suffering that is inadequately relieved or to anticipated unrelieved suffering.[48,51,72-79] In the Hippocratic tradition, an appropriate response is to say, "I don't kill patients, but neither will I just stand by and watch inadequately treated suffering."

Assessment

Familiarity with the range of distressing factors that generate suffering can help to guide the clinician in the assessment process on which further interventions are predicated. On the basis of a review of the existing data on pain and symptoms in patients with advanced cancer and on psychosocial and existential distress among patients, their families, and professional caregivers, Cherny et al. proposed a taxonomy of the factors that contribute to suffering.[11] They assert that an appreciation of the full diversity of factors that may contribute to suffering underscores the need for a methodical approach to the assessment of each individual case (Table 26.1). Such an approach incorporates the identification of care

Table 26.1   Taxonomy of Factors Contributing to Distress

In Patients	In Family Members of Patients	Among Health-Care Providers
Physical symptoms	Empathic suffering from the distress	Empathic suffering from the
pain	of the patient	distress of the patient
lack of energy	(see Table 26.1a)	(see Table 26.1a)
feeling drowsy	Physical illness	Empathic suffering from the
dry mouth	symptoms	distress of the family
lack of appetite	disability	see Table 26.1b)
nausea	therapy	Physical illness
feeling bloated	Family dynamic	symptoms
change in the way food tastes	family stability	disability
numbness/tingling in hands/feet	intrafamily conflict	therapy
constipation	inability to work cohesively	Burdens of care
cough	Impending bereavement	emotional distress
swelling of arms or legs	loss	frequent life and death decisions
itching	the end of their life as they have	frequent exposure to death
weight loss	known it	frequent exposure to profound
weight gain	finding a way to living together in	emotional distress
diarrhea	anticipation of death	patient related
dizziness	role changes	high consumer expectations
problems with sexual interest or	Burdens of care	(patient and family)
activity	physical	severe patient dependency
shortness of breath	more than needs to be done	(physical, emotional)
vomiting	the things to be done involve	severe patient debilitation
problems with urination	heavy physical work	severe patient distress (physical
difficulty swallowing	sleep disturbance	emotional)
Psychological symptoms	psychological	aesthetic
anxiety	performance anxiety in provid-	severe patient disfigurement
depression	ing comfort	severe patient odor

Table 26.1 Taxonomy of Factors Contributing to Distress (*Continued*)

In Patients	In Family Members of Patients	Among Health-Care Providers
sleep disturbance	conflict	inadequate resources
irritability	performance anxiety in adminis-	inadequate training to manage
impaired concentration	tering medication	the prevailing patient and
nightmares	anxiety about emergencies such	family problems
delirium	as pain dyspnea or bleeding	inadequate assistance
Existential concerns	aesthetic	excessive workload
disrupted or distorted personal	toileting care	Conflict
integrity	wound care	with colleagues (substantive or
changes in body image	financial	style)
changes in body function	cost of care	with patient ± family (substantive
changes in intellectual function	lost income	or style)
changes in social and profes-	insurance concerns	with self decision making in
sional function	Conflicts	ambiguous circumstances
diminished attractiveness as a	adequate relief of distressing	duty to care for a patient vs. duty
person	symptoms vs preservation of	to care for oneself and one's
diminished attractiveness as a	alertness and avoiding the has-	other responsibilities
sexual partner	tening of death duty to care for	Psychological
increased dependency	a loved-one vs. duty to care for	anxiety
distress from retrospection	oneself and one's other respon-	depression
unfulfilled aspirations	sibilities	sleep disturbance
deprecation of the value of	Distress related to health-care	substance abuse
previous achievements	services	Existential Concerns
remorse from unresolved guilt	communication	distress from retrospection
distress from future concerns	availability	deprecation of the value of
separation	personal and cultural sensitivity	previous achievements
hopelessness	excessively candid	guilt about limitations of thera-
futility	inadequate information	peutic efficacy
meaninglessness	lack of availability	distress from future concerns
concern about death	lack of services	futility
religious concerns	invasive	meaninglessness
illness as a punishment	uncommitted services	concerns about death
fears of divine retribution	ineffectual services	
fears of a void	expense	
Empathic suffering from the	Psychological	
distress of the family	anxiety	
(see Table 26.1b)	depression	
Distress related to health-care	sleep disturbance	
services	irritability	
communication	impaired concentration	
availability	nightmares	
personal and cultural sensitivity	substance abuse	
excessively candid	Existential concerns	
inadequate information	distress from retrospection	
lack of availability	unfulfilled aspirations	
lack of services	remorse from unresolved guilt	
exhausted services	distress from future concerns	
uncommitted services	separation	
ineffectual services	hopelessness	
expense	futility	
	meaninglessness	
	concern about death	
	religious concerns	
	illness as a punishment	

Reproduced with permission from Cherny NI, Coyle N, Foley KM. Suffering in the advanced cancer patient: A definition and taxonomy. *Journal of Palliative Care* 1994;10(2):57–70.

needs, the formulation of multidisciplinary interventions to address those needs, and the provision of ongoing monitoring with readiness to reevaluate the care plan as problems arise or needs change.

Objectives

The objectives of the assessment are to identify current problems that are a source of distress to each of the parties, to assess the patient's care needs, and to evaluate the adequacy of the available resources. Evaluation should include medical variables in the patient, family, and available community medical system; psychological variables in the patient, family, and psychosocial community supports; and social and financial variables in the patient and family. Since both the patient and the family are part of the unit of care, assessment requires discussion with both. The clinician must maintain a clinical posture that affirms relief of suffering as the central goal of therapy and that encourages open and effective communication about perceived problems.

Patient Assessment

The prevalence of poorly controlled pain and other physical symptoms and the impact of these factors on the lives of all involved emphasize the importance of addressing these issues at the earliest opportunity. The early establishment of good symptom control conveys concern, builds the trust of patients and their families, and facilitates the ability to address other important issues. Patient variables that must be assessed include the disease status, expected disease progression, present functional level, symptoms, current therapies, and anticipated future problems. Of particular importance is the patient's level of function, reflecting his or her mobility (e.g., whether the patient is fully bedbound or fully mobile without aids), ability to communicate (impairment may be severe, as with brain tumors, or minimal), ability to perform the activities of daily living, bowel and bladder function (from incontinence to full self-care), level of alertness (from coma to full alertness), and emotional status. The use of validated pain and symptom assessment instruments can provide a format for communication between the patient and health-care professionals and facilitate outcome evaluation.[80–85]

Family Assessment

Family assessment should encompass medical variables, psychosocial concerns, and the adequacy and availability of supports. Evaluation of the willingness and ability of home carers to provide home care and the availability of supports is essential.[27,86–89] Concurrent medical problems in a family member, particularly a primary caregiver, need to be evaluated, since the viability of the home-care plan may depend on the family member's ability to participate in care. Since the ability of families to cope with home care is largely determined by the nature of the available home-care supports,[86,90–94] the family assessment must include an assessment of available health-care professional and community supports.

It is important to ascertain the family's understanding of the nature and extent of the patient's cancer and their expectations of treatment and outcome. Discrepancies between what is known and understood by the patient and the family should be identified, and the reasons for these discrepancies should be tactfully explored. Knowledge deficits may have been deliberately maintained; the family or patient may not want information overload, the patient may wish to protect the family from knowledge of a poor prognosis, or the family may wish to protect the patient from the impact of such information.[95–97] This part of the assessment requires a nonjudgmental posture and sensitivity to psychological and cultural factors that may influence the transmission of information.[95,96,98,99]

Evaluation of the Professional Caregiver Supports

Evaluation of the professional caregiver supports usually requires greater detail than that which can be provided by the patient and family alone. To effectively plan for ongoing care, the coordinating clinician must understand the limitations of the involved health-care professionals (knowledge, experience, and availability for home care), their difficulties in coping with the situation, and their perceived needs to improve the care outcome.

Family Meetings

Family meetings meetings can open communication, improve coordination in the formulation of a care plan, and facilitate better personal coping for each of the individuals involved. The coordination of a family meeting with relevant members of the professional health-care team provides a format for discussing the needs of all parties involved, clarifying care goals, sharing and exploring concerns, and developing a therapeutic plan that adequately addresses those needs.[38,100] The participants should be determined on an individual case basis. Since the family is an appropriate unit of care with its particular concerns and needs, and its members have a right to confidentiality, on occasion it may be appropriate to meet without the participation of the patient to address these issues.

Clarifying the Goals of Care

A common source of distress for patient, family, and professional carers occurs when there is a lack of coordination among the involved parties in the desired goals of patient care. The goals of care are often complex but can generally be grouped into three broad categories: prolonging survival, optimizing comfort, and optimizing function.[101] The relative priority of these goals provides an essential context for therapeutic decision making. The prioritization of these goals is a dynamic phenomenon that changes with the evolution of the disease; whereas the optimization of comfort, function, and survival may share equal priority during the phase of ambulatory palliation, the provision of comfort usually assumes overriding priority as death approaches.[101] When patients prioritize optimal comfort and function equally, the therapeutic intent is to achieve an adequate degree of relief without compromising cognitive and physical function. When comfort is the overriding goal of care, the overriding intent is to achieve relief. In the latter circumstance, there is a willingness to continue therapies that may impair function or even foreshorten life expectancy.

The assessment of patient and family will identify specific care needs to be addressed, as well as the strengths and weaknesses of available resources. This approach facilitates the development of a flexible care plan that addresses the spectrum of problems that have been identified, using the coordinated skills of a range of health-care providers[27,41,102] (Tables 26.2 and 26.3).

DIFFICULT PROBLEMS IN THE RELIEF OF SUFFERING

The problems that commonly underlie situations of uncontrolled suffering include severe anxiety or depression, profound existential distress, refractory symptoms, and profound family fatigue. Familiarity with clinical strategies in the management of these problems will enhance the physician's ability to respond to these problems.

Severe Anxiety or Depression

Depression represents a major source of patient morbidity. It is a factor in 50% of all suicides and is probably a factor in many requests for euthanasia or assisted suicide.[69,103,104] Undertreatment derives largely from problems of recognition and assessment and from the misconception that depression is a normal response to cancer.[104] Depressive symptoms may result from existential distress (discussed later), the empathic perception of family distress, psychiatric problems of adjustment disorder or major depression, or organic problems such as persistently unrelieved symptoms. The normal grief or sadness engendered by a diagnosis of cancer is usually associated with fluctuating feelings of mild or moderate depression, which gradually diminish in intensity as adaptive processes develop.[104]

Anxiety may be produced by a primary psychological disorder, by situational factors related to the disease, its treatment, and potential outcomes and to related existential concerns, or by organic processes related to the disease or its treatment.[23] Anxiety generally presents with either somatic or cognitive manifestations. Common themes in the anxieties of terminally ill patients include feelings of being overcome by threatening forces, preoccupation with the uncertainties of treatment outcomes and duration of survival, fears relating to the process of deteriorating health with loss of dignity and control, and fears about the mode of death (particularly with regard to pain and suffocation). In the face of uncertainty, it is normal to experience fluctuating feelings of mild or moderate anxiety, which gradually diminish in intensity as adaptive coping develops.

Depression or anxiety that is severe enough to interfere with the patient's ability to function, worsening rather than resolving, or that persists

Table 26.2 Dimensions of Patient Distress, Management Approaches, and Potential Therapeutic Resources

Dimension	Distress	Intervention(s)	Therapist(s)
Physical	Pain	Comprehensive pain management	MD, Nur, Anesth, PCS, Physiat, OT, PT.
	Other physical symptoms	Comprehensive therapy	
	Physical disability	Physiatric review and therapy	
Psychological	Anxiety	Careful assessment for reversible factors	Onc, Nur, SW, Psych, Neur, PCS
	Depression	Psychotherapy ± pharmacotherapy	
	Adjustment difficulties	Cognitive or behaviorial interventions	
	Cognitive impairment		
	Unresolved previous loss or separation		
	Control		
Social	Strained family relationships	Family assessment, supportive intervention	MD, Nur, SW, Psych, PCS
	Unsatisfactory communication regarding illness or treatment	Assessment and facilitation	
	Economic	Assessment and support	
	Family related	Address issues of family distress	See Table 3
	Feeling an excessive care burden		
	Feeling an excessive emotional burden		
	Feeling an excessive economic burden		
	Doctor related	Evaluate limits of available medical supports	PCS, Psych, SW, Nurs
	Lack of M.D. attention to current problems	Expert consultation	
	Lack of empathic support from M.D.		
	M.D. excessively hopeful or pessimistic		

Existential	Current personal integrity	Attention to reversible factors	MD, Nur, SW, Phys, Psych, Chap, PCS, Physiat, OT, PT, ST, Cosmet
	Changes in body image and function	Use of prosthetic, cosmetic, orthotic or functional supports	
	Changes in intellectual function		
	Changes in social and professional function	Cognitive, behavioral, and supportive	
	Changes in attractiveness as a sexual partner	Psychotherapies to enhance coping	
	Retrospective distress	Cognitive restructuring	SW, Psych, Chap, MD, Nurs, PCS, MT, RecT
	Disappointment	Life-review techniques	
	Remorse		
	Anticipation	Cognitive restructuring and goal reprioritization	Psych, SW, MD, Nur, Chap, PCS, ClinEth
	Hopelessness	Identification of short-term achievable goals	
	Futility	Abandonment of unachievable goals	
	Meaninglessness	Addressing fears associated with death	
	Death concerns		

Chap	Chaplain	PCS	Palliative Care Specialist
ClinEth	Clinical Ethicist	Physiat	Physiatrist
Cosmet	Cosmetician	Psych	Psychiatrist
MD	Doctor	PT	Physical Therapist
MT	Music therapist	RecT	Recreation Therapist
Nurs	Nurse	SW	Social worker
OT	Occupational Therapist		

Reproduced with permission from Cherny NI, Coyle N, Foley KM. Suffering in the advanced cancer patient: a definition and taxonomy. *Journal of Palliative Care* 1994;10(2):57–70.

Table 26.3   Dimensions of Family Member Distress, Management Approaches, and Potential Therapeutic Resources

Dimension	Distress	Intervention	Therapist(s)
Patient related	Patient in physical distress	Treat patient and support family	MD, Nurs, Psych,
	Patient in psychological distress	Treat patient and support family	Chap, ClinEth
	Patient in existential distress	Treat patient and support family	
Physical	Illness	Comprehensive therapy	MD, Nur,
	Physical disability	Physiatric review and therapy	
Psychological	Anxiety	Psychotherapy ± pharmacotherapy	MD, Nur, SW,
	Depression	Cognitive or behavioral interventions	Psych, Neur, PCS
	Adjustment difficulties		Chap
	Unresolved previous loss or separation		
	Uncertainty		
Social	Alteration in roles and lifestyles	Acknowledge difficulties	MD, Nur, SW,
	Unsatisfactory communication regarding illness or treatment	Explore specific problems of family and supports	Psych, PCS
		Assess information needs and address them	
	Lack of comfort and support from family members	Provide sensitive information and express readiness to provide appropriate supports	
	Lack of support and comfort from health care professionals	Express readiness to deal with whatever difficulties may arise	
	Nonconvergent needs among family members	Identify family members in need of psychological or psychiatric support	
	Economic/employment		
Personal resources	Excessive physical demands	Optimize home supports	SW, Nurs, MD
	Excessive complexity of care	Provide effective backup	
	Exhaustion	Consider alternative care arrangements	
		Consider respite care	

Chap	Chaplain	PCS	Palliative Care Specialist
ClinEth	Clinical Ethicist	Physiat	Physiatrist
Cosmet	Cosmetician	Psych	Psychiatrist
MD	Doctor	PT	Physical Therapist
MT	Music therapist	RecT	Recreation Therapist
Nurs	Nurse	SW	Social worker
OT	Occupational Therapist		

Reproduced with permission from Cherny NI, Coyle N, Foley KM. Suffering in the advanced cancer patient: a definition and taxonomy. *Journal of Palliative Care* 1994;10(2):57–70.

more than 7 days warrants skilled intervention.[105] As previously described, effective management is predicated on the development of a trusting relationship. Patient evaluation begins with an assessment of the patient's symptoms, mental status, and physical status; possible treatment effects; and all pertinent investigational studies. This process defines the pattern and the severity of the psychological symptoms, evaluates the presence of suicidal ideation, and identifies possible contributing factors that may be remediable.

The therapeutic plan is influenced by the specific psychological problem and by the severity of the symptomatology, disease, and situational factors. In all cases, the adequacy of symptom control and social supports must be addressed. Though mild depression or anxiety can be treated with short-term psychotherapy, more severe symptoms generally require a combined modality approach that also incorporates pharmacotherapy.[23,104] Anxiety is usually treated using anxiolytic pharmacotherapy selected from benzodiazepine, neuroleptic, or tricyclic antidepressant drugs, along with supportive psychotherapy, often using behavioral techniques of relaxation, guided imagery, and distraction.[23,105,106] Prolonged or severe depression requires an approach that combines antidepressive pharmacotherapy with psychotherapy; occasionally, electroconvulsive therapy may be indicated.[23,105] Cognitive strategies can be used to correct misconceptions, emphasize past strengths, improve coping strategies, and mobilize inner resources.[105,106]

Patients who express suicidality must be assessed urgently, since appropriate intervention may be critical.[23,103] Factors contributing to patient vulnerability to suicide include advanced illness with poor prognosis, depression and hopelessness, pain, delirium, loss of control with perceived helplessness, preexisting psychiatric disease, a personal or family history of suicide, and exhaustion.[23] It is important to ascertain the reasons underlying the suicidal thoughts and the seriousness of the intent. Evaluation of the patient's mental status and pain control is essential. If indicated, analgesics, antidepressants, or neuroleptics should be used for pain, severe depression, agitation, or psychosis.[23,103] Mobilization of as much of the patient's support system as possible is critical. In situations in which the support systems are inadequate or the suicidal risk is very high, the patient should be admitted for closely supervised care and the initiation of appropriate therapy.[23,103]

Existential Distress

Common existential issues for patients with advanced cancer include hopelessness, futility, meaninglessness, disappointment, remorse, death anxiety, and disruption of personal identity.[107–110] Existential distresses may also be related to past, present, or future concerns. Concerns regarding the past can trigger disappointment related to unfulfilled aspirations, a deprecation of the value of previous achievements, or remorse from unresolved guilt.[108,110,111] Present concerns may revolve around the sense of who one is as a person, which can be disrupted by changes in body image; in somatic, intellectual, social and professional function; and in perceived attractiveness as a person and as a sexual partner.[108,111,112] And, if future life is perceived to offer, at best, comfort in the setting of fading potency or, at worst, ongoing physical and emotional distress as days pass slowly until death, anticipation of the future may be associated with feelings of hopelessness, futility, or meaninglessness such that the patient sees no value in continuing to live.[110] Death anxiety is common among cancer patients; surveys have shown that 50% to 80% of terminally ill patients have concerns or troubling thoughts about death and that only a minority achieve an untroubled acceptance of death.[113–117] Although these existential issues are sometimes referred to as "spiritual,"[41,109,118–120] they appear to be universal and independent of religion and religious practice.[107,108,110,121,122] Therapeutic approaches have been developed to address concerns about current personal integrity, retrospective disappointment and remorse, death anxiety, and issues of hopelessness, futility, and meaninglessness.[109–111,119,123,124]

With attention to detail, steps can be undertaken to minimize the consequences of the somatic and social changes that have intruded on the patient's life.[109,111,119,123] Appropriately fitting clothes, cosmetic prostheses, and attention to patient grooming help maintain personal dignity. The provision of assistive or orthotic devices can help optimize the patient's level of social function. Issues of impeded intimacy and altered sexual function can be broached by a skilled sexual counselor.[28,125–129]

The use of cognitive techniques can facilitate changes in somatic and social functioning. Cognitive therapies can help patients and their families to modify their appraisal of their lives, to diminish distress, and to enhance a sense of positivity.[110,124,130] This is often referred to as cognitive restructuring.[123] For example, the distressing symbolism of the need for a wheelchair may be modified by altering the patient's focus to the contribution of enhanced mobility on participation in important relationships. Cognitive therapies need to be ego-syntonic with the patient's own coping mechanisms; the loss of employment may be seen as an opportunity to pursue more important activities by the patient who is ready to acknowledge imminent mortality, while for the patient with a need for hope of recovery, the loss of employment can be viewed as a temporary setback until satisfactory restoration of health and function. Maladaptive strategies, such as catastrophizing, need to be identified for specific targeted therapies.[131,132]

The maintenance or reestablishment of meaning is a central goal in the existential care of the incurably ill.[26,109,111,119,123] Exclusive focusing by the patient on unachievable long-term goals can enhance feelings of futility and distress. Cognitive restructuring can help the patient identify meaningful and achievable short-term goals, the fulfillment of which preserves a sense of self-efficacy.[26,124,133–135] As previously described, a harsh self-evaluation of the value of the patient's life may cause significant distress.[109,110,119,123] Life-review techniques can facilitate a constructive reappraisal of life events that focuses on positive feelings engendered by positive recollections, while also acknowledging, but not minimizing, negative recollections.[136–139] The reestablishment of purpose can be bolstered by the identification of unfulfilled aspirations, incomplete tasks, and unresolved issues that the patient can productively pursue.[137,139] Remorse can provide the motivation for achievable constructive pursuit; however, it is important to help the patient identify issues that are not remediable so as not to distract from more productive expenditure of time and energy.[26] Insight-directed therapy can help the patient to acknowledge that there are meaningful and fulfilling tasks to be done, joys to be shared, things to be said or completed, relationships to be savored, and animosities to be resolved.[26]

These methods may also be helpful for family members who are despairing of the value of the remaining time until the patient dies. So long as patient comfort is adequately preserved, the potential remains for meaningful communication and interaction. Situations when the patient is confused or unconscious due to advanced disease or when symptom control can be achieved only with therapies that induce sedation or cognitive impairment can be particularly difficult for families. In these situations, continued vigilance in attending to patient comfort and reassurance that comfort is being achieved are essential for the well-being of the bereaving family. This communication must be handled with sensitivity to individual differences in coping resources and styles; some family members may benefit from encouragement in continuing to communicate with both words and touch, while others need reassurance that their presence at the bedside is no longer essential for patient comfort (see the section on the profoundly fatigued family later in this chapter).

Many patients and their families turn to professional health-care providers to discuss issues relating to the nature of death and issues of after-life.[110,123] The anxiety engendered by these concerns requires careful assessment, provision for emotional faith support, and readiness for philosophical discussion. When the theological issues are complex or specific to a particular religion, the assistance of an appropriate religious chaplain or minister should be sought.[123,140]

Pain and Other Physical Symptoms

Effective strategies now exist for the routine management of pain and other physical symptoms in the majority of cases.[141–146] Patients with pain or other physical symptoms that are refractory to standard care must be reviewed by a specialist skilled in the symptomatic management of advanced cancer.[147] Among inpatients referred to the Pain Service at Memorial Sloan-Kettering Cancer Center, one survey demonstrated that careful evaluation by a pain expert revealed a previously undiagnosed lesion in 64% of patients; many of these tumors were amenable to a primary antitumor therapy.[148] Strategies for the management of patients who are unable to readily achieve an acceptable balance between analgesia and side effects have been reviewed elsewhere.[149]

Refractory Physical, Psychologic, or Existential Distress

For patients with advanced cancer, physical and psychological symptoms cannot be eliminated but are usually relieved enough to temper the suffering of the patient and family. The term "refractory" can be applied when a symptom cannot be adequately controlled despite aggressive efforts to identify a tolerable therapy that does not compromise consciousness.[62] In deciding that a symptom is refractory, the clinician must perceive that further invasive and noninvasive interventions are incapable of providing adequate relief, associated with excessive and intolerable acute or chronic morbidity, or unlikely to provide relief within a tolerable time frame.[62] For patients with advanced cancer, the designation of a symptom as refractory has profound implications, suggesting that suffering will not be relieved with routine measures.

Controlled sedation is routinely used to manage the severe pain and anxiety associated with noxious procedures that would otherwise be intolerable.[150] Obviously, the loss of interactional function associated with sedation precludes its application in the ongoing management of routine patient care to relieve chronic physical, psychological, or existential distress, since the therapeutic goal is to achieve adequate relief with preserved function. At the end of life, however, the goals of care may change such that the relief of suffering predominates over all other considerations. In this situation, the designation of a symptom as "refractory" justifies the use of induced sedation as an option of laser report to provide relief with certainty and speed.

Ethics

The use of sedating therapies recognizes the right of patients with advanced cancer to adequate relief of unendurable symptoms and the right of all patients to choose among appropriate therapeutic options.[1,65,66] The ethical validity of this approach derives from the "principle of double effect," which distinguishes between the compelling primary therapeutic intent (to relieve suffering) and unavoidable untoward consequences (the likely diminution of interactional function and the potential for accelerating death).[49] This principle is predicated on the axioms that intent is a critical ethical concern and that the distinction between foreseeing and intending an unavoidable maleficent outcome is ethically significant. The criticism, expressed by Quill,[151] that clinical intentions may sometimes be more complex and ambiguous than those presented in this argument does not diminish the observation that the invocation of this principle allows the patient, family, and treating clinician to maintain an ethical equilibrium in this difficult situation. In the absence of this ethical equilibrium, the moral reservations of clinicians or family members may result in either the undertreatment of catastrophic symptoms or subsequent guilt and its morbid psychological sequelae.

Patient Evaluation

Clinicians want neither to subject severely distressed patients to therapies that provide inadequate relief or excessive morbidity nor to sacrifice conscious function when viable alternatives remain unexplored. The refractory symptom must, therefore, be distinguished from "the difficult symptom" that might respond within a tolerable time frame to other approaches without excessive adverse effects. The difficulties inherent in distinguishing between "difficult symptoms" and "refractory symptoms" and the major clinical and ethical consequences of this distinction contribute to the onerous nature of clinical decision making in this setting. The challenge inherent in this decision making requires that patients with unrelieved symptoms undergo repeated evaluation prior to progressive application of routine therapies.

The evaluation of unrelieved and intolerable psychological, existential, or spiritual distress is more difficult because strategies for the management of some of these problems are less well established and the severity of distress may be highly fluid and idiosyncratic. Furthermore, standard treatments have low intrinsic morbidity, and the presence of these symptoms does not necessarily indicate a far advanced state of physiological deterioration. Nonetheless, the administration of routine approaches to the management of patients with severe anxiety,[23] depression,[23] or existential distress[109–111,119,123,124] may still eventuate in a small proportion of patients who continue to express a high level of distress. The designation of such symptoms as refractory can be done only after a period of repeated assessment by a knowledgeable clinician who has established a relationship with the patient and his or her family. As in the situation of refractory physical symptoms, this situation requires expert evaluation and a readiness to consider extraordinary therapeutic approaches including sedation.

Since individual clinician bias can influence decision making in these difficult deliberations, a case-conference approach is prudent when assessing a challenging case. This conference may involve the participation of oncologists, palliative-care physicians, anesthesiologists, neurosurgeons and psychiatrists, nurses, social workers, and others. The discussion attempts to clarify the remaining therapeutic options and the goals of care. When local expertise is limited, telephone consultation with expert physicians is encouraged.

If, after careful evaluation, the clinician concludes that there is no treatment capable of providing adequate relief of intolerable symptoms without compromising interactional function or that the patient would be unable to tolerate specific therapeutic interventions, refractoriness to standard approaches should be acknowledged.

The offer of sedation as an available thera-peutic option is often received as an empathic ac-knowledgment of the severity of the degree of pa-tient suffering. The enhanced patient trust in the commitment of the clinician to the relief of suf-fering may, in itself, influence decision-making, particularly if there are other tasks or life issues that need to be completed before a state of di-minished function develops. Patients sometimes decline sedation, acknowledging that symptoms will be unrelieved but secure in the knowledge that if the situation becomes intolerable this de-cision can be rescinded. Other patients reaffirm comfort as the predominating consideration and accept the initiation of sedation.

Consent to the use of sedation acknowledges the primacy of comfort as the dominant goal of care. Sedating pharmacotherapy for refractory symptoms at the end of life should not be initi-ated until a discussion about CPR has taken place with the patient or, if appropriate, with the pa-tient's proxy and until there is agreement that CPR will not be initiated. The initiation of car-diorespiratory recussitation (CPR) at the time of death is almost always futile in this situa-tion.[152,153] and, furthermore, is inconsistent with the agreed goals of care.[152]

Administration

When sedation is desired by the patient who is al-ready receiving an opioid for pain or dyspnea, an attempt is usually made to first escalate the opioid dose. Although some patients benefit from this in-tervention, inadequate sedation or the develop-ment of neuroexcitatory side effects, such as my-oclonus or agitated delirium, often necessitate the addition of a second agent.[154,155] The addition of a benzodiazepine is usually effective in this situa-tion. The short-half-life drugs, such as lorazepam,[23] midazolam,[156–161] and flunitrazepam,[162] are easy to titrate and are generally preferred. When rapid ef-fect is required, the selected drug should be administered by a parenteral route, preferably intravenous (IV) or subcutaneous (SC). Patients suffering from an agitated delirium who are inad-equately sedated by a neuroleptic agent such as haloperidol, metho-trimeprazine, or chlorpro-mazine can also benefit from addition of a ben-zodiazepine.[23]

Patients with refractory depression, anxiety, or existential distress at the end of life can usually be adequately sedated using a benzodiazepine alone. Similarly, a single-agent approach, using either a benzodiazepine[156–162] or one of the more sedating neuroleptic drugs, such as metho-trimeprazine[163] or chlorpromazine,[164] usually suf-fices for dying patients with terminal restlessness.

The severe anxiety associated with a massive terminal hemorrhage should be managed with an anesthetizing dose of a rapidly acting sedative that can, if necessary, be easily administered by a fam-ily member. Midazolam is recommended because of its rapid onset of action and versatility of ad-ministration (IV, SC, or IM) in an emergency.

Rarely, benzodiazepine drugs can cause a para-doxical agitation, and an alternative strategy is re-quired. Recently, experience in the management of refractory physical symptoms using barbiturates alone has been described. Greene and Davis[63] treated 17 imminently dying terminally ill patients with amobarbital (9 cases) or thiopental (8 cases) and reported adequate symptom relief in all cases. The median survival of these patients after initia-tion of the infusion was 23 hours (range 2 hr–4 days). Although most of the patients maintained interactional function for a time, all patients died in their sleep. This approach has recently been en-dorsed by Troug et al.,[64] who also described the potential utility of barbiturates for terminal agita-tion or terminal anguish.

Irrespective of the agent selected, administra-tion initially requires dose titration to achieve ad-equate relief, followed by provision of ongoing therapy to ensure maintenance of effect. On oc-casion, patients may need extraordinarily high doses; opioid doses equivalent to 35 000 mg of par-enteral morphine per day have been reported,[20] and the authors observed a terminally ill 44-year-old woman with severe chest wall pain who required midazolam 60 mg per hour to manage re-fractory dyspnea and anxiety. Regular, around-the-clock administration can be maintained by continuous infusion or intermittent bolus. The route of administration can be IV, SC, or rectal. In some situations, drugs can be administered via a stoma or gastrostomy. In all cases, provision for emergency bolus therapy to manage breakthrough symptoms is recommended.

The depth of sedation necessary to control symptoms varies greatly. For some patients, a state of "conscious sedation," in which they retain the ability to respond to verbal stimuli, may provide adequate relief without total loss of interactive function.[63,157] Some authors have suggested that doses can be titrated down to reestablish lucidity after an agreed interval or for preplanned family interactions.[63,64] This, of course, is a potentially unstable situation, and the possibility that lucidity may not be promptly restored or that death may ensue as doses are again escalated should be explained to both the patient and the family.

Once adequate relief is achieved, the parameters for patient monitoring and the role of further dose titration is determined by the goal of care. If the goal of care is to ensure comfort until death to an imminently dying patient, the only salient parameters for ongoing observation are those pertaining to comfort. Symptoms should be assessed until death; observations of pulse blood pressure and temperature do not contribute to the goals of care and can be discontinued. Since downward titration of drug doses places the patient at risk for recurrent distress and does not serve the goal of care, it is not recommended even as the patient approaches death.

The Profoundly Fatigued Family

The development of advanced cancer in a family member affects the entire family.[165–170] The challenges confronting the family—the need to acknowledge the end of life as they have known it and to define a new way of constructively living out their final days together as best possible—engender great stresses.[168] Among the factors contributing to the ensuing distress are empathic suffering with the patient, grief and bereavement, role changes, and the physical, financial, and psychological sequelae of the burdens of care.[165,168,171–174] The needs of the families of patients with advanced cancer have been surveyed by several researchers.[165,166,172,173,175] They are summarized in Table 26.3.

Severe family fatigue is commonly observed in four situations: (1) persistently inadequate relief of patient suffering,[27,28,176] (2) inadequate resources to cope effectively with home care without severely compromising the current or future welfare of the family members,[171,177,178] (3) family members' unrealistic expectations of themselves or of professional health-care supports, and (4) emotional distress that persists even in the face of adequate relief of patient suffering.[168,179]

The problem of family fatigue may indicate problems of undiagnosed patient distress, or a foundering home situation that is further intensifying the distress of the family and the patient. Assessment may identify specific problems of patient suffering, logistic problems related to home care that are amenable to simple intervention (i.e., a catheter for a newly incontinent patient), or exhausted family carers with inadequate assistance or respite. Planned multidisciplinary interventions can assist with the logistic problems of home care, improving the adequacy of supports, providing for family respite, providing contingency planning for anticipated emergent situations (such as bleeding, uncontrolled pain, or dyspnea), and planning for the time that death occurs.[27,55,102,180] Attentive follow-up to monitor the outcome of interventions facilitates the early detection of new problems and reinforces the perception of care and support. This, in turn, enhances patient and family security and facilitates a more positive appraisal of coping.

Inadequate Relief of Patient Suffering

When inadequate relief of patient suffering is the cause of family distress, the steps outlined in the previous sections should be considered. Difficulties may arise when the level of relief of a particular problem, such as pain, is adequate to the patient but deliberately incomplete so as to preserve the patient's interactional capacities. This situation can ultimately fatigue both the patient and the family, and alternative strategies to improve the therapeutic index should be considered. If none are available, patient well-being needs to be closely monitored, and the option of respite sedation therapy should be available if needed. It can be of value to reassure the patient's family that this situation reflects the patient's will to continue to participate in ongoing interaction despite adversity, that the therapy is being closely monitored, and that more effective comfort-directed measures are available if desired. In some cases, family members may need additional emotional, psychiatric, or respite support to bolster their coping.

Inadequate Resources and Unrealistic Expectations

The resources of family members and or professional services are both finite, and the care system thus far described seeks to find a balance among needs, expectations, and resources. After a careful needs assessment, care plans are instituted as a collaborative program using family and professional services to provide a level of support that facilitates optimization of quality of life for the patient and the family. Changing needs are met by changes in the therapeutic strategy and, when necessary and possible, with changes in allocation of care resources. Balance in this system is maintained by all parties having reasonable expectations of themselves, of what they can ask of others, and of what can be achieved. As previously described, the use of family meetings and the development of clearly defined goals contribute to this task.[38,100] These formal and informal meetings are also the appropriate forum to discuss the difficult issue of limit setting: How much can a family member really ask of himself or expect of the other family members? What are the limits of available nursing care? Is it going to be possible to achieve total pain relief and maintain perfect lucidity until death? This sort of discussion can relieve the guilt of family members who are exhausted from pursuing excessively high goals for themselves in the care role, diminish tensions among the parties involved in care, and facilitate the reevaluation of the goals of care if they are not reasonably achievable.

Emotional Distress that Persists
Even in the Face of Adequate
Relief of Patient Suffering

Even in situations when patient suffering is well controlled, the persistent unresolved grief of impending death can cause enormous fatigue. This is especially true when the process of death is protracted.[28] Factors contributing to exhaustion in this situation include continuing concern for patient comfort, perceived need to be with the patient at the time of death, and emotional discomfort with the ambiguity of the situation of a loved one who is neither interactionally alive or resolutely dead. In some situations, the family members of dying patients may be concerned that rapid, labored, or noisy respiration or restlessness indicate patient distress. Even when the patient is comatose and therefore insentient, the apparent suffering can invoke great distress for family members, other patients, and the health-care providers. In the absence of any means to verify

patient comfort, pharmacotherapeutic intervention to achieve the appearance of comfort remains an imperative. Professional carers can ease the distress of this situation with empathic support that acknowledges the sadness of the impending death, continued vigilance in patient care, reassurance that patient suffering is well controlled, unambiguous, culturally sensitive, goal-oriented therapy, and cognitive restructuring techniques that focus on the blessing of comfort in death.

CONCLUSION

An appreciation of the diversity of factors that may contribute to suffering underscores the need for methodical assessment and familiarity with a range of therapeutic strategies. Application of this approach enables health-care providers to formulate a treatment approach that encompasses the needs of patients, their families, and health-care providers and that preserves the moral values of all involved parties. The current community focus on the issue of inadequately relieved suffering should be harnessed to work toward the provision of care that diminishes the impression that elective death is necessary to ensure adequate relief from suffering.

References

1. Wanzer SH, Federman DD, Adelstein SJ, et al. The physician's responsibility toward hopelessly ill patients—a second look. *New England Journal of Medicine*, 1989; 120:844–849.
2. Roy DJ. Relief of suffering: the doctor's mandate. *Journal of Palliative Care*, 1991; 7(4):3–4. Editorial.
3. Angell M. The quality of mercy. *New England Journal of Medicine*, 1982; 306:98–99.
4. American Medical Association Council on Ethical and Judicial Affairs. Decisions near the end of life. *Journal of the American Medical Association*, 1992; 267:2229–2233.
5. American Nursing Association. *Position Statement on Promotion of Comfort and Relief of Pain in Dying Patients*. Kansas City: American Nursing Association, 1991.
6. President's Commission for the Study of Ethical Problems in Medical and Biomedical and Behavioral Research. *Deciding to Forgo Life-Sustaining Treatment: Ethical and Legal Issues in Treatment De-

cisions. Washington, DC: US Government Printing Office, 1983.

7. Burge F. The epidemiology of palliative care in cancer. *Journal of Palliative Care*, 1992; 8(1):18–23.

8. Van Eys J. The ethics of palliative care. *Journal of Palliative Care*, 1991; 7(3):27–32.

9. Churchill LR. Why we need a theory of suffering and lots of other theories as well. *Journal of Clinical Ethics*, 1991; 2(2):95–97.

10. Copp LA. Pain and suffering. The spectrum of suffering. *American Journal of Nursing*, 1974; 74(3):491–495.

11. Cherny NI, Coyle N, Foley KM. Suffering in the advanced cancer patient: a definition and taxonomy. *Journal of Palliative Care*, 1994; 10(2):57–70.

12. Loewy EH. The role of suffering and community in clinical ethics. *Journal of Clinical Ethics*, 1991; 2(2):83–89.

13. Chapman CR, Gavrin J. Suffering and its relationship to pain. *Journal of Palliative Care*, 1993; 9(2):5–13.

14. Foley KM. The treatment of cancer pain. *New England Journal of Medicine*, 1985; 313:84–95.

15. Johanson GA. Symptom character and prevalence during cancer patients' last days of life. *American Journal of Hospital Palliative Care*, 1991; 8(2):6–8.

16. Ventafridda V, Ripamonti C, De Conno F, Tamburini M, Cassileth BR. Symptom prevalence and control during cancer patients' last days of life. *Journal of Palliative Care* 1990; 6(3):7–11.

17. Brescia FJ, Adler D, Gray G, Ryan MA, Cimino J, Mamtani R. Hospitalized advanced cancer patients: a profile. *Journal of Pain and Symptom Management* 1990; 5(4):221–227.

18. Dunlop GM. The study of the relative frequency and importance of gastrointestinal symptoms and weakness in patients with far advanced cancer: student paper. *Palliative Medicine* 1989; 4:37–43.

19. Curtis EB, Krech R, Walsh TD. Common symptoms in patients with advanced cancer. *Journal of Palliative Care* 1991; 7(2):25–29.

20. Coyle N, Adelhardt J, Foley KM, Portenoy RK. Character of terminal illness in the advanced cancer patient: pain and other symptoms during last four weeks of life. *Journal of Pain and Symptom Management* 1990; 5:83–89.

21. Reuben DB, Mor V, Hiris J. Clinical symptoms and length of survival in patients with terminal cancer. *Archives of Internal Medicine* 1988; 148(7):1586–1591.

22. Fainsinger R, Miller MJ, Bruera E, Hanson J, Maceachern T. Symptom control during the last week of life on a palliative care unit. *Journal of Palliative Care* 1991; 7(1):5–11.

23. Breitbart W, Passik SD. Psychiatric aspects of palliative care. In: Doyle D, Hanks GW, MacDonald N, ed. *Oxford Textbook of Palliative Medicine*. Oxford: Oxford University Press, 1993:609–626.

24. Bukberg J, Penman D, Holland JC. Depression in hospitalized cancer patients. *Psychosomatic Medicine* 1984; 46:199–212.

25. Massie MJ, Holland JC, Glass E. Delirium in terminally ill cancer patients. *American Journal of Psychiatry* 1983; 140:1048–1050.

26. Yalom ID. Meaninglessness and psychotherapy. In: *Existential Psychotherapy*. New York: Basic Books, 1980:461–486.

27. Coyle N, Loscalzo M, Bailey L. Supportive care for the advanced cancer patient and family. In: Holland JC, Rowland JH, ed. *Handbook of Psychooncology*. New York: Oxford University Press, 1989:598–611.

28. Vachon MLS. Emotional problems in palliative medicine: patient, family and professional. In: Doyle D, Hanks GW, MacDonald N, ed. *Oxford Textbook of Palliative Medicine*. Oxford: Oxford University Press, 1993:577–605.

29. Saunders C. *The Management of Terminal Malignant Disease* (2nd ed.) Baltimore: Arnold Publishers, 1984.

30. Herman JF. Psychosocial support: interventions for the physician. *Seminars in Oncology* 1985; 12(4):466–471.

31. Mount BM. Dealing with our losses. *Journal of Clinical Oncology* 1986; 4:1127–1134.

32. Billings JA. On being a reluctant physician-strains and rewards in caring for the dying at home. In: Billings JA, ed. *Outpatient Management of Advanced Cancer*. Philadelphia: Lippincott, 1985:309–318.

33. Lazarus RS, Folkman C. *Stress, Appraisal and Coping*. New York: Springer, 1984.

34. Smith RS. Ethical issues in cancer pain. In: Chapman CR, Foley KM, eds. *Current and Emerging Issues in Cancer Pain: Research and Practice*. New York: Raven Press, 1993:385–392.

35. Roy DJ. Need they sleep before they die? *Journal of Palliative Care* 1991; 6(3):3–4.

36. Latimer E. Ethical challenge in cancer care. *Journal of Palliative Care* 1992; 8(1):65–70.

37. Pollard BJ. Dying: rights and responsibilities. *Medical Journal of Australia*, 1988; 149(3):147–149.

38. Scanlon C, Fleming C. Ethical issues in caring for the patient with advanced cancer. *Nursing Clinics of North America* 1989; 24(4):977–986.

39. American College of Physicians Health and Public Policy Committee. Drug therapy for severe chronic pain in terminal illness. *Annals of Internal Medicine* 1983; 99:870–880.

40. American Pain Society. *Principles of Analgesic Use in the Treatment Acute Pain and Chronic Cancer Pain. A Concise Guide to Medical Practice.* (3rd ed.) Skokie, Illinois: American Pain Society, 1992.

41. World Health Organization. *Cancer Pain Relief and Palliative Care.* Geneva: World Health Organization, 1990.

42. American Pain Society Committee of Quality Assurance Standards. American Pain Society quality assurance standards for the relief of acute pain and cancer pain. In: Bond MR, Charlton JE, Woolf CJ, eds. *Proceedings of the VIth World Congress on Pain.* Amsterdam: Elsevier, 1991:185–190. *Pain Research and Clinical Management* vol 4.

43. Spross JA, McGuire DB, Schmitt RM. Oncology Nursing Society Position Paper on Cancer Pain. Part I. *Oncology Nursing Forum* 1990; 17(4):595–614.

44. Spross JA, McGuire DB, Schmitt RM. Oncology Nursing Society Position Paper on Cancer Pain. Part II. *Oncology Nursing Forum* 1990; 17(5):751–760.

45. American College of Physicians Ethics Committee. *American College of Physicians Ethics Manual,* 3rd ed. *Annals of Internal Medicine* 1992; 117:947–960.

46. Quill TE, Cassell CK, Meier DE. Care of the hopelessly ill: proposed criteria for physician assisted suicide. *New England Journal of Medicine* 1992; 327(19):1380–1383.

47. Smith G. Recognizing personhood and the right to die with dignity. *Journal of Palliative Care* 1990; 6(2):24–32.

48. Brody H. Assisted death—compassionate response to medical failure. *New England Journal of Medicine* 1992; 327(19):1384–1388.

49. Latimer EJ. Ethical decision-making in the care of the dying and its applications to clinical practice. *Journal of Pain and Symptom Management* 1991; 6:329–336.

50. Brescia FJ. Killing the known dying: notes of a death watcher [editorial]. *Journal of Pain and Symptom Management* 1991; 6(5):336–339.

51. Foley KM. The relationship of pain and symptom management to patient requests for physician-assisted suicide. *Journal of Pain and Symptom Management* 1991; 6(5):289–297.

52. Latimer EJ. Euthanasia: a physician's reflections. *Journal of Pain and Symptom Management* 1991; 6(8):487–91.

53. Cundiff D. Euthanasia is Not The Answer: A Hospice Physician's View of the "Death With Dignity" Debate. Totowa, NJ: Humana Press, 1992.

54. Twycross RG. Assisted death: a reply. *The Lancet* 1990; 336:796–798.

55. Saunders C, ed. *Hospice and Palliative Care: An Interdisciplinary Approach.* London: Edward Arnold, 1990:120.

56. Foley KM. Pain, physician-assisted suicide and euthanasia. *Proceedings, American Pain Society.* p. 1–8, 1994.

57. Pollard B, Winton R. Why doctors and nurses must not kill patients. *Medical Journal of Australia* 1993; 158(6):426–429.

58. Conolly ME. Alternative to euthanasia: pain management. *Issues in Law and Medicine* 1989; 4(4):497–507.

59. Wilkinson J. The ethics of euthanasia. *Palliative Medicine* 1990; 4:81–86.

60. Feinberg J. Rights: I. Systematic analysis. In: Reich WT, ed. *Encyclopedia of Bioethics.* New York: Macmillan, 1978:1507–1511.

61. Macklin R. Rights: II. Rights in bioethics. In: Reich WT, ed. *Encyclopedia of Bioethics.* New York: Macmillan, 1978:1511–1516.

62. Cherny NI, Portenoy RK. Sedation in the treatment of refractory symptoms: guidelines for evaluation and treatment. *Journal of Palliative Care* 1994; 10(2):31–38.

63. Greene WR, Davis WH. Titrated intravenous barbiturates in the control of symptoms in patients with terminal cancer. *Southern Medical Journal* 1991; 84(3):332–337.

64. Truog RD, Berde CB, Mitchell C, Greir HE. Barbiturates in the care of the terminally ill. *New England Journal of Medicine* 1992; 327(23):1678–1682.

65. Edwards RB. Pain management and the values of health care providers. In: Hill CS, Fields WS, ed. *Drug Treatment of Cancer Pain in a Drug Oriented Society.* New York: Raven Press, 1989:101–112. *Advances in Pain Research and Therapy,* vol 11.

66. Martin RS. Mortal values: healing, pain and suffering. In: Hill CS, Fields WS, ed. *Drug Treatment of Cancer Pain in a Drug Oriented Society.* New York: Raven Press, 1989:19–26. *Advances in Pain Research and Therapy,* vol 11.

67. Levin DN, Cleeland CS, Dan R. Public attitudes towards cancer pain. *Cancer* 1985; 56:2337–2339.

68. Cleeland CS, Gonin R, Hatfield A, et al. Pain and its treatment in outpatients with metastatic cancer. *New England Journal of Medicine* 1994; 330(9):592–596.

69. Breitbart W. Cancer pain and suicide. In: Foley KM, Bonica JJ, Ventafridda V, ed. *Second International Congress on Cancer Pain.* New York: Raven Press, 1990:399–412. *Advances in Pain Research and Therapy,* vol 16.

70. Quill T. *Death and Dignity: Making Choices and Taking Charge.* Norton: New York, 1992.

71. Cassem NH. Treatment decisions in irreversible illness. In: Cassem NH, ed. *Massachusetts General Hospital Handbook of General Hospital Psychiatry.* St. Louis: Mosby-Year Book, 1991:618–639.

72. Brahams D. Euthanasia in The Netherlands. *The Lancet* 1990; 335(8689):591–592.

73. Dickey NW. Euthanasia: a concept whose time has come? *Issues in Law and Medicine* 1993; 8(4): 521–532.

74. Doerflinger R. Mercy, murder, & morality: perspectives on euthanasia. Assisted suicide: prochoice or anti-life? *Hastings Center Report* 1989; 19(1):16–19.

75. Engelhardt HJ. Mercy, murder, & morality: perspectives on euthanasia. Fashioning an ethic for life and death on a post-modern society. *Hastings Center Report* 1989; 19(1):7–9.

76. Kurtz P. The case for euthanasia: a humanistic perspective. *Issues in Law and Medicine* 1992; 8(3):309–316.

77. Miller FG. Is active killing of patients always wrong? *Journal of Clinical Ethics* 1991; 2(2):130–132.

78. Quill TE. Death and dignity. *New England Journal of Medicine* 1991; 324:691–694.

79. Somerville MA. Pain, suffering and ethics. In: 7th World Congress on Pain: *Congress Abstracts.* Seattle: I.A.S.P. Publications, 1993.

80. Melzack R. The McGill pain questionnaire: Major properties and scoring methods. *Pain* 1975; 1:277–299.

81. Daut RL, Cleeland CS. The prevalence and severity of pain in cancer. *Cancer* 1982; 50: 1913–1918.

82. Fishman B, Pasternak S, Wallenstein SL, Houde RW, Holland JC, Foley KM. The Memorial Pain Assessment Card: A valid instrument for the evaluation of cancer pain. *Cancer* 1987; 60: 1151–1158.

83. Portenoy R, Thaler HT, Kornblith AB, et al. The Memorial Symptom Assessment Scale: an instrument for the evaluation of symptom prevalence, characteristics and distress. *European Journal of Cancer and Clinical Oncology* 1994; 30: 1326–1336.

84. Foley KM. Pain assessment and cancer pain syndromes. In: Doyle D, Hanks GW, MacDonald N, ed. *Oxford Textbook of Palliative Medicine.* Oxford: Oxford University Press, 1993:148–165.

85. Bruera E, Kuehn N, Miller MJ, Selmser P, Macmillan K. The Edmonton Symptom Assessment System (ESAS): a simple method for the assessment of palliative care patients. *Journal of Palliative Care* 1991; 7(2):6–9.

86. Brown P, Davies B, Martens N. Families in supportive care—Part II: Palliative care at home: a viable care setting. *Journal of Palliative Care* 1990; 6(3):21–27.

87. Coyle N. A model of continuity of care for cancer patients with chronic pain. *Medical Clinics of North America* 1987; 71:259–270.

88. Coyle N, Monzillo E, Loscalzo M, Farkas C, Massie MJ, Foley KM. A model for continuity of care for cancer patients with pain and neurological complications. *Cancer Nursing* 1985; 8: 111–119.

89. Hull M. Family needs and supportive nursing behaviors during terminal cancer: a review. *Oncology Nursing Forum* 1989; 16:787–792.

90. Grobe M, Ahmann D, Ilstrup D. Needs assessment for advanced cancer patients and their families. *Oncology Nursing Forum* 1982; 9(4):26–30.

91. Stetz K. Caregiving demands during advanced cancer. *Cancer Nursing* 1987; 10(5):260–268.

92. Nugent LS. The social support requirements of family caregivers of terminal cancer patients. *Canadian Journal of Nursing Research* 1988; 20(3): 29–37.

93. Welch D. Planning nursing interventions for family members of adult cancer patients. *Cancer Nursing* 1981; 5:365–370.

94. Kristjanson L. Needs assessment for advanced cancer patients and their families. *Oncology Nursing Forum* 1986; 9(4):26–30.

95. Freedman B. Offering truth. One ethical approach to the uninformed cancer patient. *Archives of Internal Medicine* 1993; 153(5):572–576.

96. Della-Vorgia P, Katsouyanni K, Garanis TN, et al. Attitudes of a Mediterranean population to the truth-telling issue. *Journal of Medical Ethics* 1992; 18:67–74.

97. Buckman R. Communication in palliative care: a practical guide. In: Doyble D, Hanks GW, MacDonald N, ed. *Oxford Textbook of Palliative Medicine.* Oxford: Oxford University Press, 1993: 47–61.

98. Manos N, Chistakis K. Attitudes of cancer specialists towards their patients in Greece. *International Journal of Psychiatry in Medicine* 1981; 10:305–313.

99. Manos N, Chistakis J. Coping with cancer: Psy-

chological dimensions. *Acta Psychiatrica Scandinavica* 1985; 72:1–5.

100. Krech MR, Walsh TD. The role of a palliative care service family conference in the management of the patient with advanced cancer. *Palliative Medicine* 1990; 5:34–39.

101. Cherny NI, Portenoy RK. Practical issues in the management of cancer pain. In: Wall PD, Melzack R, ed. *Textbook of Pain.* 3rd ed. Edinburgh: Churchill Livingstone, 1994:1437–1467.

102. Ajemian I. The interdisciplinary team. In: Doyle D, Hanks GW, MacDonald N, ed. *Oxford Textbook of Palliative Medicine.* Oxford: Oxford University Press, 1993:17–28.

103. Breitbart W. Suicide in the cancer patient. *Oncology* 1987; 1:49–54.

104. Valente SM, Saunders JM, Cohen MZ. Evaluating depression among patients with cancer. *Cancer Practice* 1994; 2(1):65–71.

105. Massie MJ. Depression. In: Holland JC, Rowland JH, ed. *Handbook of Psychooncology.* New York: Oxford University Press, 1990:283–290.

106. Kissane DW. Reducing fear in cancer survivors. *Australian Family Physician* 1994; 23(5):888–892.

107. Rowland JH. Developmental stage and adaption: adult model. In: Holland JC, Rowland JH, ed. *Handbook of Psychooncology.* New York: Oxford University Press, 1990:25–43.

108. Cassell EJ. The nature of suffering and the goals of medicine. *New England Journal of Medicine* 1982; 306(11):639–645.

109. Mobert DO, Brusek PM. Spiritual well-being: a neglected subject in quality of life research. *Social Indicators Research* 1978; 5:303–323.

110. Yalom ID. *Existential Psychotherapy.* Basic Books, 1980.

111. Doyle D. Have we looked beyond the physical and psychosocial? *Journal of Pain and Symptom Management* 1992; 7(5):302–311.

112. Hopwood P, Maguire GP. Body image problems in cancer patients. *British Journal of Psychiatry* (Suppl) 1988; July(2):47–50.

113. Hinton J. Comparison of places and policies for terminal cases. *The Lancet* 1979; (Jan 6):29–32.

114. Vachon MLS, Conway B, Lancee WJ, Adair WK. *Final Report on the Needs of Persons Living with Cancer in Quebec.* Toronto: Canadian Cancer Society, 1991.

115. Vachon MLS, Conway B, Lancee WJ, Adair WK. *Final Report on the Needs of Persons Living with Cancer in Manitoba.* Toronto: Canadian Cancer Society, 1990.

116. Vachon MLS, Conway B, Lancee WJ, Adair WK. *Report on the Needs of Persons Living with Cancer*

in Prince Edward Island. Toronto: Canadian Cancer Society, 1989.

117. Byrne CM. Needs assessment and hospice planning in a rural setting. *Evaluation and Health Professionals* 1984; 7:205–219.

118. Highfield MF, Cason C. Spiritual needs of patients: are they recognized? *Cancer Nursing* 1983; 6:187–192.

119. International Work Group for Death and Dying. Assumptions and principles of spiritual care. *Death Studies* 1990; 14:75–81.

120. Vastyan EA. Spiritual aspects of the care of cancer patients. *CA: A Cancer Journal of Clinicians* 1986; 36(2):110–114.

121. Copp LA, Copp JD. Illness and the human spirit. *Quality of Life—A Nursing Challenge* 1993; 2(3): 50–55.

122. Cohen MZ. Spirituality, quality of life, and nursing care. *Quality of Life—A Nursing Challenge* 1993; 2(3):47–49.

123. Speck PW. Spiritual issues in palliative care. In: Doyle D, Hanks GW, MacDonald N, ed. *Oxford Textbook of Palliative Medicine.* Oxford: Oxford University Press, 1993:517–525.

124. Scanlon C. Creating a vision of hope: the challenge of palliative care. *Oncology Nursing Forum* 1989; 16(4):491–496.

125. Schover LR, Montague DK, Schain WS. Sexual problems. In: DeVita VT, Hellman S, Rosenberg SA, eds. *Cancer Principles and Practice of Oncology.* 4th ed. Philadelphia: Lippincott, 1993:2464–2479.

126. Ganz PA. Current issues in cancer rehabilitation. *Cancer* 1990; 3(1):742–51.

127. Aso R, Yasutomi M. Urinary and sexual disturbances following radical surgery for rectal cancer, and pudendal nerve block as a countermeasure for urinary disturbance. Am J Proctol 1974; 25(3):60–9.

128. Ofman US. Psychosocial and sexual implications of genitourinary cancers. *Seminars in Oncology Nursing* 1993; 9(4):286–92.

129. Filiberti A, Audisio RA, Gangeri L, et al. Prevalence of sexual dysfunction in male cancer patients treated with rectal excision and coloanal anastomosis. *European Journal of Surgical Oncology* 1994; 20(1):43–46.

130. Fishman B. The treatment of suffering in patients with cancer pain: cognitive behavioral approaches. In: Foley KM, Bonica JJ, Ventafridda V, eds. *Second International Congress on Cancer Pain.* New York: Raven Press, 1990:301–316. *Advances in Pain Research and Therapy,* vol 16.

131. Wilkie DJ, Keefe FJ. Coping strategies of patients

with lung cancer–related pain. *Clinical Journal of Pain* 1991; 7(4):292–299.

132. Meyerowitz BE, Heinrich RL, Schag CA. Helping patients cope with cancer. *Oncology (Huntingt)* 1989; 3(11):120–129.

133. Greer S, Moorey S, Baruch JD, et al. Adjuvant psychological therapy for patients with cancer: a prospective randomised trial. *British Medical Journal* 1992; 304:675–80.

134. Greer S, Moorey S, Baruch J. Evaluation of adjuvant psychological therapy for clinically referred cancer patients. British *Journal of Cancer* 1991; 63(2):257–260.

135. Jones SA. Personal unity in dying: alternative conceptions of the meaning of health. *Journal of Advances in Nursing* 1993; 18(1):89–94.

136. Viederman M, Perry S3. Use of a psychodynamic life narrative in the treatment of depression in the physically ill. *General Hospital Psychiatry* 1980; 2(3):177–185.

137. Bennett SL, Maas F. The effect of music based life review on the life satisfaction and ego integrity of elderly people. *British Journal of Occupational Therapy* 1988; 51(12):433–436.

138. Lichter I, Mooney J, Boyd M. Biography as therapy. *Palliative Medicine* 1993; 7(2):133–137.

139. O'Callaghan C. Communicating with brain-impaired palliative care patients through music therapy. *Journal of Palliative Care* 1993; 9(4):53–55.

140. Dorff EN. Religion at a time of crisis. *Quality of Life—A Nursing Challenge* 1993; 2(3):56–59.

141. Billings JA, ed. *Outpatient Management of Advanced Cancer.* Philadelphia: Lippincott, 1985.

142. Doyle D, Hanks GW, MacDonald N, eds. *Oxford Textbook of Palliative Medicine.* Oxford: Oxford University Press, 1993:845.

143. Twycross RG, Lack SA. *Therapeutics in Terminal Cancer* 2nd ed. Edinburgh: Churchill Livingstone, 1990.

144. Walsh TD, ed. *Symptom Control.* London: Blackwell, 1989.

145. Woodruff R. *Palliative Medicine.* Melbourne: Asperula, 1993.

146. Saunders C, Baines M, ed. *Living with Dying: The Management of Terminal Illness,* 2nd ed. Oxford: Oxford University Press, 1989.

147. Cherny NI, Portenoy RK. Cancer pain management: current strategy. *Cancer* (Suppl) 1993; 72(11):3393–3415.

148. Gonzales GR, Elliot KJ, Portenoy RK, Foley KM. The impact of a comprehensive evaluation in the management of cancer pain. *Pain* 1991; 47:141–144.

149. Cherny NI, Portenoy RK. The management of cancer pain. *CA—A Cancer Journal for Clinicians* 1994; 44(5):263–303.

150. Agency for Health Care Policy and Research: Acute Pain Management Panel. *Acute Pain Management: Operative or Medical Procedures and Trauma.* Washington, D.C.: U.S. Dept. of Health and Human Services., 1992: Clinical Practice Guideline.

151. Quill TE. The ambiguity of clinical intentions. *New England Journal of Medicine* 1993; 329(14):1039–1040.

152. Haines IE, Zalcberg J, Buchanan JD. Not-for-resuscitation orders in cancer patients: principles of decision making. *Medical Journal of Australia* 1990; 153(7):225–229.

153. Rosner F, Kark PR, Bennett AJ, et al. Medical futility. Committee on Bioethical Issues of the Medical Society of the State of New York. *New York State Journal of Medicine* 1992; 92(11):485–488.

154. Portenoy RK, Moulin DE, Rogers A, Inturrisi CE, Foley KM. IV infusion of opioids for cancer pain: clinical review and guidelines for use. *Cancer Treatment Reports* 1986; 70(5):575–581.

155. Dunlop RJ. Excitatory phenomena associated with high dose opioids. *Current Therapy in Endocrinology and Metabolism* 1989; 30(6):121–123.

156. Amesbury BDW. Use of SC midazolam in the home care setting. *Palliative Medicine* 1989; 3:299–301.

157. Burke AL, Diamond PL, Hulbert J, Yeatman J, Farr EA. Terminal restlessness—its management and the role of midazolam. *Medical Journal of Australia* 1991; 155(7):485–487.

158. Johanson GA. Midazolam in terminal care. *American Journal of Hospice and Palliative Care* 1993; 10(1):13–14.

159. Enck RE. The last few days. *American Journal of Hospice and Palliative Care* 1992; 9(4):11–13.

160. McNamara P, Minton P, Twycross RG. The use of midazolam in palliative care. *Palliative Medicine* 1991; 5:244–249.

161. Bottomly DM, Hanks G. Subcutaneous midazolam infusion in palliative care. *Pain and Symptom Management* 1990; 5(4):259–261.

162. Smales OR, Smales EA, Sanders HG. Flunitrazepam in terminal care. *Journal of Pediatric and Child Health* 1993; 29(1):68–69.

163. Oliver OJ. The use of methotrimeprazine in terminal care. *British Journal of Clinical Practice* 1985; 39:339–340.

164. McIver B, Walsh D, Nelson K. The use of chlorpromazine for symptom control in dying cancer

patients. *Journal of Pain and Symptom Management* 1994; 5:341–345.

165. Kristjanson L. Quality of terminal care: salient factors identified by families. *Journal of Palliative Care* 1989; 5(1):21–30.

166. Hampe SO. Needs of the grieving spouse in a hospital setting. *Nursing Research* 1975; 24:113–119.

167. Skorupka P, Bohnet N. Primary caregivers' perceptions of nursing behaviors that best meet the needs in a home care hospice setting. *Cancer Nursing* 1982; 5(5):371–374.

168. Davies B, Reimer JC, Martens N. Families in supportive care—Part 1. The transition of fading away: the nature of the transition. *Journal of Palliative Care* 1990; 6(3):12–20.

169. Smith N. The impact of terminal illness on the family. *Palliative Medicine* 1990; 4:127–135.

170. Beck-Friis B, Strang P. The family in hospital-based home care with special reference to terminally ill cancer patients. *Journal of Palliative Care* 1993; 9(1):5–13.

171. Schachter S. Quality of life for families in the management of home care patients with advanced cancer. *Journal of Palliative Care* 1992; 8(3):61–66.

172. Ferrell BR, Rhiner M, Cohen MZ, Grant M. Pain as a metaphor for illness. Part I: Impact of cancer pain on family caregivers. *Oncology Nursing Forum* 1991; 18(8):1303–1309.

173. Ferrell BR, Cohen MZ, Rhiner M, Rozek A. Pain as a metaphor for illness. Part II: Family caregivers' management on pain. *Oncology Nursing Forum* 1991; 18(8):1315–1321.

174. Dar R, Beach CM, Barden PL, Cleeland CS. Cancer pain in the marital system: a study of patients and their spouses. *Journal of Pain and Symptom Management* 1992; 7(2):87–93.

175. Sykes NP, Pearson SE, Chell S. Quality of care of the terminally ill: the carer's perspective. *Palliative Medicine* 1992; 6:227–236.

176. Stam HJ, Bultz BD, Pittman CA. Psychosocial problems and interventions in a referred sample of cancer patients. *Psychosomatic Medicine* 1986; 48:539–548.

177. West SR, Harris BJ, Warren A, Wood H, Montgomery B, Belsham V. A retrospective study of persons with cancer in their terminal year. *New Zealand Medical Journal* 1986; 99:197–200.

178. Lewis FM. The impact of cancer on the family: a critical analysis of the research literature. *Patient Education and Counseling* 1986; 269–289.

179. Chochinov H, Holland JC. Bereavement: a special issue in oncology. In: Holland JC, Rowland JH, ed. *Handbook of Psychooncology*. New York: Oxford University Press, 1989: 609–626.

180. Ahles TA, Martin JB. Cancer pain: a multidimensional perspective. *Hospice Journal* 1992; 8(1–2):25–48.

PART VII
Research Issues

27

Quality Assurance and Audit in Palliative Care

Irene J. Higginson, B.Med.Sci., B.M.B.S., M.F.P.H.M., Ph.D.

Throughout the world, interest in quality assurance and clinical audit is growing, driven by a need to ensure the quality of health care and value for money. Higher public expectations and the move toward quality service in many public and private companies have contributed to this change.[1] In response, clinicians, managers, and governments have sought to standardize clinical practice to that which is the best possible practice or that which is proven to be the most effective and efficient.[1]

However, the idea of ensuring quality of health care has existed for centuries. Probably the first reference to quality assurance is from 1700 B.C., when King Hannurabi of Egypt proposed drastic penalties and in some instances death for surgical incompetence. In the sixteenth century in Spain, Juan Cuidad Duarte, appalled by existing conditions, proposed improved standards of care for mental illness. In 1518 the Charter of the Royal College of Physicians included doctors' pledge "to uphold the standards of medicine both for their own honour and public benefit."[2] Writing in 1911, George Bernard Shaw advised people to "treat persons who profess to cure diseases as you treat fortune tellers," and said that "nothing is more dangerous than a poor doctor, not even a poor employer or a poor landlord."

In the twentieth century, ward rounds, postgraduate lectures, and clinical presentations have contributed to the review of medical, nursing, and social work performance. However, the new emphasis on audit and quality assurance has led to four new standards of practice:

1. Explicit criteria for good practice should be applied by all clinicians, rather than only by those in exemplary centers.
2. All patients in care should be included in quality monitoring, rather than a few "interesting" cases.
3. Patients and their families should be able to seek empowerment.
4. Funding or accreditation may be withheld from those units that do not comply with quality standards or that are found to be ineffective or inefficient.[2]

References in the medical and nursing literature to quality assurance and medical and nursing audit began to appear in the late 1970s. The number of such references continues to rise. Quality assurance has been by far the most commonly used term since the 1980s (see Table 27.1).

DEFINITIONS

Although definitions of quality assurance vary, one that is commonly used defines it as the setting of standards, the measurement of their achievement, and the development of mechanisms to improve performance.[2] Quality assurance is a cycle whereby

Table 27.1   Number of Medline Citations for the Terms "Quality Assurance," "Medical Audit," and "Nursing Audit," 1966–1995.

Year	Quality Assurance	Medical Audit	Nursing Audit
1966	0	0	0
1970	0	24	18
1975	2	76	34
1980	154	74	26
1985	387	85	34
1990	790	203	37
1995	945	340	64

standards are set, practice is measured against those standards, and quality is improved (see Figure 27.1). However, quality assurance also implies that the organization has a planned program for improving the quality of care, which can include several different individual audits or other quality assurance activities. Other common definitions and terms are shown in Table 27.2.[2–5]

Clinical audit is a cycle of setting standards, measuring whether these standards are achieved, and then, as necessary, changing practice that lies within a quality assurance program. It has been more simply defined as "doing the right things well." The cycle can be entered at any point, for example it is possible to begin by observing practice and acting on the results and then to proceed to setting standards.[1–3,6]

QUALITY ASSURANCE AND AUDIT OF PSYCHOSOCIAL AND PSYCHIATRIC ASPECTS OF PALLIATIVE CARE

Quality assurance and clinical audit are fairly well established in both palliative care and psychiatric care. Many methods of clinical audit and quality assurance are described for palliative care.[7,8] Early programs were described in the early 1980s, along with the first hospice services. Since then, standardized methods have evolved, regional or national groups have banded together to undertake audit, and several well-validated systems have come into existence.[7,8] For example, registrations of the use of the Support Team Assessment Schedule, an outcome measure that is frequently used to audit care, comprise registrants in more than 15 different countries, in inpatient, home, and day-care settings (see Table 27.3). Similarly, quality assurance in psychiatric care is well established, including suicide audits, quality inspection of inpatient units, audits of discharge procedures, and establishment of treatment policies.

However, the audit of the psychiatric and psychosocial aspects of palliative care is not well developed. Between 1966 and 1996 there were 17,441 references on Medline that included audit or quality assurance; of these, 517 (3%) included psychological aspects, mental health, depression, or anxiety. However, of these, only 7 were for palliative care, and 4 were audit studies that included psychological or psychiatric aspects as part of a larger audit, 2 were review articles suggesting a need for psychosocial audit, and 1 was a study that concluded that audit was needed. Quality assurance in palliative care has often concentrated on symptom relief rather than on psychological relief, which may be more difficult to measure than care of other symptoms, such as pain, or measurement of clinical indicators, such as hemoglobin.

Nevertheless, audit of psychological and psychiatric aspects of palliative care is needed. From the outset, psychological and psychiatric aspects of care have been an important component of palliative care. Psychological and psychiatric

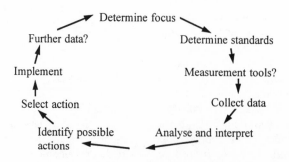

Figure 27.1. Quality Assurance Cycle

Table 27.2   Common Definitions: Audit and Quality Assurance

Term	Definition
Medical audit	The systematic critical analysis of the quality of medical care, including the procedures used for diagnosis and treatment, the use of resources, and the resulting outcome and quality of life of the patient
Clinical audit	The systematic critical analysis of the quality of clinical care, including the procedures used for diagnosis and treatment, the use of resources, and the resulting outcome and quality of life of the patient, like medical audit except for involvement of all professionals and volunteers, rather than only doctors
Nursing audit	Audit of methods used by nurses to compare their actual practice against pre-agreed guidelines and identify areas for improving their care
Prospective audit	Audit of standards and measures recorded on patients and their families during their care
Retrospective audit	Review of care given to patients who have been discharged or have died; standards are applied to the information available from case notes or by asking families about the care after the patient has died
Quality assurance	The definition of standards, the measurement of their achievement, and the mechanisms to improve performance. The quality-assurance cycle is as for medical audit or clinical audit. However, quality assurance implies a planned program involving the whole unit or health services. Clinical or medical audit is usually described as one part of a quality-assurance program.

needs are common among both patients and their families or carers. Palliative practice varies from one place to another, even in simple aspects such as staffing levels and composition (e.g., whether staff includes practitioners with psychiatric or psychological training) and mix within the hospice or home-care team, the catchment populations, the operational policies, and the follow-up care.[9-11] We need to know which psychological and psychiatric models of care work best and for which types of problems.

Hospices and palliative services bring new therapies, such as new treatments for psychological and psychiatric symptoms, support and counseling services, or complimentary therapies. However, new therapies and approaches must be evaluated and audited to determine when and in whom they are useful. Otherwise, hospices' resources and patients' time will be wasted. There is a great danger on concentrating on only current concerns without reviewing previous failings and using those findings to plan improved care in the future.

Table 27.3   Registered Users of the Support Team Assessment Schedule by Country

Country	Number of Users
United Kingdom	89
Italy	7 (one registrations covers study of 61 users)
Canada	5
Belgium	3
Ireland	2 (one registration covers study of 6 users)
Spain	2 (one registration covers users in Catalan)
Sweden	2
Poland	2
Also: Australia, Germany, France, Singapore, Hong Kong, South Africa, United States	

Settings where STAS is used are: 51 home care, 34 hospital team, 30 community unit, 29 hospice, 10 day care, 5 oncology unit, 5 GP, 12 other.

ASPECTS OF PSYCHIATRIC CARE THAT MIGHT BE AUDITED

Components of audit can be based on the structure (resource) or process (use of resources) of care or on clinical indicators or outcome (e.g., results, change in health or psychological status), as in clinical audit. Examples are shown in Table 27.4.

APPROACHES TO QUALITY ASSURANCE AND AUDIT

Common methods used in quality assurance and audit are outlined in this section. Two of these,

Table 27.4   Potential Measures of Structure, Process, or Outcome for Assessing Psychiatric Aspects of Palliative Care

Type of Measure	Examples
Structure	Values or aims of the service
	Financial resources—% on psychiatric care, psychological care
	Home care/hospital/hospice services—psychiatric input
	Day hospice places—psychiatric input
	Number of psychiatrists or psychologists per cancer patient in the population
	Staffing mix, grades
	Drugs and equipment available—e.g., antidepressants
	Physical environment—e.g., safety, pleasantness of surroundings
Process	Number of attendances at counseling sessions
	Number of admissions
	Procedures followed—e.g., assessment of psychiatric problems
	Documentation—e.g., of psychiatric and psychological problems
	Policies and procedures for staff training and working
	Mechanism for handling complaints and the documentation of this
	Adherence to ethical and legal codes
	Staff support given
Output	Rate of discharge
	Completed consultant episodes
	Follow-up care
	Completed courses of treatment—e.g., drugs given; appropriate prescribing of antidepressants; course completed; completed counseling sessions
	Well-coordinated care—e.g., telephone communication
	Supply of medicines after discharge
	Completed patient management plans
	Early arrival of discharge information to GP
	Satisfaction of professionals referring to the service
Outcome	Reduction in depression/anxiety
	Improved mental health of patient and carer
	Patient and carer satisfaction
	Satisfaction with place of care
	Open and honest communication as the patient wishes
	Resolved communication, fears, grief, anger
	Resolved need to plan future events—e.g., funeral or meetings
	Good use of remaining time
	Reduced carer strain
	Improved carer health
	Resolved grief after death (if appropriate)

key indicators and topic review, are commonly used in palliative care, and confidential inquiry into adverse events is often used to audit suicide in mental-health care.

Retrospective Case Review

In this method either an individual case is reviewed or case notes are selected at random and critically reviewed by a group that includes staff not involved in the patient's care. If individual records are chosen, the patient may be chosen be-cause he or she has a particular problem that the group wants to investigate. However, self-selection of certain individual cases may not fulfil the requirement that the audit be widely relevant, rather than concentrate on special cases, as in the medical grand round. Random selection of cases can fulfil this criterion better but may lose direction if the aims and criteria for quality are not clear. One way to focus the audit is to develop ahead of time a checklist for use in the critical review. The method can be linked with key indicators or topic review; a random sample of notes are examined for the key indicators or for the particular topic.

Key Indicators

Routinely collected data, such as follow-up care, number of psychiatric visits, or re-admission rates, can be used in some areas of health care, but in palliative care these may not be appropriate criteria, and the clinical record may have to be amended to include relevant items. Indicators are chosen and recorded prospectively and examined after a period of care or assessed by peers. Examples audit tools that use key indicators in palliative care include the organizational audit of the Cancer Relief Macmillan Fund or, in clinical audit, the Support Team Assessment Schedule, the Edmonton Symptom Assessment System, and the Palliative Care Core Standards.[7,8] All of these key indicators have some psychological or psychiatric components, although these are often rudimentary. Quality-of-life measures or measures of depression and anxiety such as the EORTC QLQ C30, the Rotterdam Symptom Checklist, or the Hospital Anxiety and Depression Scale could also be administered and monitored routinely, like other key indicators.[7]

When using key indicators, it is important to include a representative sample of all patients in care or in a particular group. The measures can be collected for everyone, for a random sample of admissions, or for a group meeting specific criteria, such as patients admitted with some depression (as determined by a standardized measure). Use of key indicators has several advantages:

- Key indicators give a larger picture and include the main components of care considered important in palliative care.
- Important aspects of care are less likely to be overlooked.
- The list of indicators can serve as a checklist to assist in monitoring day-to-day clinical care.
- Several components of care can be considered at once.

Disadvantages of using key indicators for quality assurance are these:

- The large number of components included can make data collection cumbersome and time consuming.
- There is a temptation to try to include everything that is important; this is impossible.

- Analysis of the data can be time consuming, and data are complex and therefore difficult to interpret.

Topic Review

In this type of audit a topic is chosen and reviewed prospectively or retrospectively. Although retrospective review often reveals inadequacies in the clinical records, it is frequently valuable in providing a baseline for later comparison. Examples of data that can be used to evaluate psychological and psychiatric aspects of care are medical records and letters (do these include psychiatric information?), referral or admission procedures (are psychiatric aspects assessed?), detection of particular symptoms (e.g., depression, delirium), control of particular symptoms, prescribing practice, or diagnostic procedures used. This technique has also been used successfully in palliative care.[8] Its main advantages are that it allows auditors to examine one aspect of care in depth, it is fairly easy to start, and, at least initially, it can be contained and limited. Problems can arise if not all team members are happy with the area selected for study, and some prefer to look at different aspects. In addition, it may be difficult to see the topic in the context of other problems and symptoms that are affecting the patient and family. Topics can snowball, so that they end up being studied in greater and greater depth, leaving other important factors overlooked.

Patient or Family Satisfaction

The simplest method of evaluating care is to analyze patient and family complaints. However, in palliative care patients may die before they are able to complain. Surveys of patients' or families' views may be included in the overall quality improvement plan of a hospice or hospital. A national survey of families' views after the death has also examined care,[12] although detailed surveys tend to be beyond the resources of single units.

Adverse Patient Events

This audit method systematically identifies events during a patient's treatment that indicate some lapse in the quality of care. Patients' clinical records are reviewed retrospectively by a health professional or a ward clerk for examples of agreed adverse events. One of the most common forms of investigation into adverse events is the confidential inquiry. When an agreed adverse event occurs, it is investigated retrospectively by two or more peers, who assess the clinical records and reports about the case. Their report is confidential and therefore cannot be used for litigation. Three main forms of confidential inquiry exist in the United Kingdom. The first involves maternal deaths, all of which are subject to confidential inquiry. These events are rare, and therefore a fairly major investigation occurs for each maternal death; the hospitals and other services are expected to take action if any deficiencies are identified. The second type of inquiry involves perioperative deaths. This type of investigation was first undertaken as part of a national study, in which all deaths occurring during the first 28 days after an operation were investigated by peers using information in the clinical record. This investigation showed that a small proportion of deaths were due to surgeon failure, particularly in cases where junior, inexperienced doctors operated at night, although the case would have been better managed by deferring medical treatment until the following morning, when the operation could have been performed by a more senior surgeon.

The third type of confidential inquiry is the suicide audit. This is the most recent development. The Department of Health in England and Wales proposed that all suicides in which the individual was known to health or social services be subject to a confidential inquiry, in which peers examine the documentation regarding the case and determine whether the services could have taken steps to prevent the suicide. Although suicide is rare in palliative care, given the evidence that depression is underdetected and the association between the presence of depression and requests for euthanasia, such an audit may be helpful.

Other adverse events, such as severe delirium, could also be monitored. But it may be difficult to identify some of the less striking events in palliative care, unless these can be systematically recorded in patients' clinical records. This may require standardized, enhanced records.

Inspection and Accreditation

This form of quality assurance has as a main focus the survey or inspection of a service by an ex-ternal team. For many years health services provided to elderly people in the United Kingdom were subject to inspection by the hospital advisory services (HAS). After inspection, usually lasting several days, the multiprofessional team produced a written report and recommendations for change. The team often met with local representatives after their visit to discuss their findings. There was a rolling program of visits, and most districts were visited every 5 years or so. Physical and mental health services were included in the investigations, along with the links with social services. The program was discontinued in 1992 shortly after the introduction of National Health Service (NHS) reforms in the United Kingdom. Purchasers of health services were expected to undertake quality visits locally and match quality standards with services.

Several countries have also developed organizational standards, which are part of an accreditation or inspection program, undertaken by organizations either voluntarily or to ensure entitlement to funding. In the United States, the National Hospice Organization has developed standards of care to which units are to adhere. Canada has developed similar standards, which are under discussion.

In the United Kingdom, two main countrywide organization audit programs exist: the King's Fund Organisational Audit and the Bristol Hospital Accreditation Programme (HAP).[7] Both are voluntary programs. The King's Fund worked voluntarily with NHS and private hospitals to come to consensus on lengthy document of standards. In its first 3 years, to the end of 1992, the program measured more than 130 acute general hospitals against published standards. It is now piloting standards for primary care.[1] The Hospital Accreditation Programme (HAP), established at the Clinical Audit Unit in South Western Region in Bristol, was designed to assess smaller hospitals or community based services. In its first 3 years as a pilot scheme limited to general-practitioner hospitals in one region, the HAP completed 61 surveys on 70% of eligible hospitals and accredited 75% against standards based on action research. This program became available nationally in April 1993 for community hospitals, which are generally smaller than those eligible for the King's Fund hospital program.[1]

The Cancer Relief Macmillan Fund developed an organizational audit for specialist-care services with and following the King's Fund organizational audit program. A working group consisting of six regional coordinators for palliative care, five of whom were nurses, and a representative from Cancer Relief Macmillan Fund, developed an initial draft of standards. The 11 standards cover service values; organization and management; organizational and operational policy; physical environment for care; self-determination and climate for care; direct patient and family care; multidisciplinary working and team work; staffing and skill mix; education, training, and staff development; staff support; and ethics and law. Each of these standards has a rationale and specific criteria, which are used by a team of external surveyors to determine the extent that each standard is achieved. When this protocol is used for assessing a criterion, guidance is provided for auditors on what questions to ask, but the validity, reliability, practicality, and sensitivity of the questions are unreported. The audit is in its relatively early stages; an independent evaluation or one similar to that undertaken for the HAP would help to assess the audit's utility and problems.

EXAMPLES OF QUALITY ASSURANCE AND AUDITS UNDERTAKEN FOR PSYCHIATRIC AND PSYCHOSOCIAL ASPECTS

Although quality assurance in this area of palliative care is relatively rare, some examples that are consistent with the quality assurance approach can be found. However, many of these began as research projects, not as audits. These examples may be helpful if planning quality assurance in this field.

Detection of Depression and Psychological Problems

Depression and anxiety are more prevalent among cancer patients than in the general population; however, these problems are frequently underdetected by clinicians. Recommended guidelines for the management of psychological and psychiatric problems in other chapters of this book could be used to set standards and to audit care.

Family Anxiety and Needs

In multicenter audits of palliative care teams in the United Kingdom and in Ireland, family anxiety was found to be the most severe problem among patients and families in the last week of a patient's life. As part of an audit of key indicators, using STAS, units collected data on the severity of family anxiety weekly on all patients in care, from referral until the last week of care. Although family anxiety appears to be initially alleviated by care from a palliative care team, it increased during the last weeks of life. About 30% of families had severe or overwhelming anxiety during this period (see Figure 27.2). Using data collected on the demographic and clinical characteristics of patients and families at referral, it is possible to develop a clinical algorithm, which

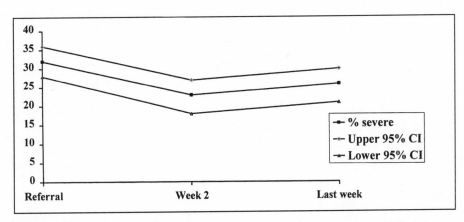

Figure 27.2. Percentage Rated with Severe Family Anxiety. Severe anxiety (rated 3 or 4) Wilcoxon: referral v. week 2 z-3.6, $p < .005$; referral v. last week, z-4, $p < .005$

correctly identifies 75% of those cases in which family anxiety will occur.[13] However, the validity of this model is lower, and a fairly large number of cases identified do not go on to have severe anxiety. It may be useful in oncology or acute settings, where there is insufficient time to gather full details about family characteristics. Using additional information about family needs, the predictive model could be developed further.[13]

CONCLUSIONS

Although quality assurance and audit are well developed in both palliative care and psychiatric care, audit of the psychiatric aspects of palliative care is underdeveloped. Available methods sometimes include psychosocial assessments, but better approaches are needed. Clinical audit may be helpful in developing clinical protocols to help to identify and treat problems or algorithms to predict patient problems and the need for specialized care. Audit is here to stay and is now widely accepted. But it requires resources, so it must be sure to benefit patients and families, be kept as simple and efficient as possible, and have a strong educational component.

References

1. Shaw CD. Quality assurance in the United Kingdom. *Quality Assurance Health Care*, 1993;5(2): 107–118.
2. Shaw CD. Medical Audit. In: *A hospital handbook*. London: King's Fund Centre, 1989.
3. Rosser RM. A history of the development of health indices. In: Smith GT, ed, *Measuring the social benefits of medicine*. London: Office of Health Economics, 1985.
4. Shaw CD. Aspect of audit. 1. The background. *British Medical Journal*, 1980; 280:1256–1258.
5. Higginson I, Edmonds P. Services, costs and appropriate outcomes in end of life care. *Annals of Oncology*, 1999; 10:135–136.
6. Butters E, Higginson I, George R, Smits A, McCarthy M. Assessing the symptoms, anxiety and practical needs of HIV/AIDS patients receiving palliative care. *Quality of Life Research*, 1992; 1(1):47–51.
7. Higginson I. Are we doing the right thing well?: clinical and organisational audit in palliative care. In: Doyle D, Hanks GWC, MacDonald N, eds, *Oxford Textbook of Palliative Medicine*, 2nd ed. Oxford: Oxford University Press, 1998; 26:67–82.
8. Higginson I, ed. *Clinical Audit in Palliative Care*. Oxford: Radcliffe Medical Press, 1993.
9. Johnson I, Rogers C, Biswas B, Ahmedzai S. What do hospices do? A survey of hospices in the United Kingdom and Republic of Ireland. *British Medical Journal*, 1990; 300:791–793.
10. Kirkham S, Davis M. Bed occupancy, patient throughput and size of independent hospice units in the UK. *Palliative Med*, 1992; 6:47–53.
11. Eve A, Smith AM. Palliative care services in Britain and Ireland—update 1991. *Palliative Medicine*, 1994; 8(1):19–27.
12. Addington Hall J, McCarthy M. Regional study of care of the dying: methods and sample characteristics. *Palliative Medicine*, 1995; 9:27–35.
13. Higginson I, Priest P. Predictors of family anxiety in the weeks before bereavement. *Social Science and Medicine*. 1997; 46:43, 1621–1625.

28

New Directives for Psychosocial Research in Palliative Medicine

Eduardo Bruera, M.D.

The development of palliative-care medicine[1] and psychooncology[2] has greatly increased the body of knowledge on the assessment and management of psychosocial complications in cancer patients. This increased focus has also demonstrated the unique characteristics of terminally ill patients and their families and the unique nature of their problems. These characteristics make psychosocial assessment and treatment techniques used in other populations only partially applicable. The purpose of this chapter is to address some of the areas on which future research efforts should focus.

PATIENT ASSESSMENT

Regular assessment of patients' conditions and charting of physical and laboratory variables are common practice in almost all inpatient and outpatient settings. Adequate charting allows the team of physicians, nurses, and other professionals to adequately plan the different diagnostic and treatment interventions for a given patient. In many cases, such as checks of vital signs or diabetic and neurological assessments, a graphic display allows for an immediate visualization of the course of the problem over time. However, in the areas of symptom control and psychosocial support, the development of similar assessment forms has been quite slow.

There are probably two reasons for this: (1) Physicians and nurses are much more used to measuring objective end-points such as blood pressure, pulse, or glucose in blood or urine than to monitoring the subjective end-points of palliative care; and (2) they are not comfortable with multidimensional interpretation of the intensity expressed by patients. In the case of blood pressure and glucose in blood, we are measuring simple dimensions that require a simple response. In the case of pain or nausea, the equivalent would be measuring nociception at the level of the tumor or nausea at the level of the stomach; we do not have the ability to measure the generation of the symptom, and this generation is quite variable between individuals. We are also unable to measure the second step in the symptom production, the brain perception, which can also be modulated by factors such as descending inhibiting pathways or endorphins in the case of pain. Finally, what we are measuring is the expression of the patient; individual perceptions can vary greatly depending on the individual's beliefs (e.g., whether pain is due to cancer or is simply a headache), intrapsychic factors (somatization), and cultural ethnic factors. For these reasons, the intensity of a given symptom should be interpreted as a multidimensional construct; while in a given patient 90% or 100% of the pain expression may be nociception, in another patient somatization or addiction may be the main component. All assessment tools should assist us in characterizing the components of the symptom expression in a given patient, and their reactive contribution to the total intensity.[3,4]

Table 28.1 summarizes some of the assessments that should take place in all terminally ill patients. This comprehensive assessment likely will be achieved not by a single tool but by a combination of tools. In addition, the tools may differ significantly according to the setting (e.g., whether staff is available to administer the different tools) and the patient populations; while the great majority of patients admitted to a tertiary palliative-care unit develop cognitive failure,[5] only a small proportion of patients present these abnormalities in outpatient palliative-care clinics.[6] The different instruments to be developed will need to have the following characteristics:

1. *They should be simple.* Ideally, they should be self-report forms or forms that can be administered by relatives or volunteers.
2. *They should be quick to complete.* Asthenia, psychological distress, and lethargy are highly prevalent in these patients.[7-9] Extensive interviews can exhaust patients and families and will not be useful for follow-up. Excellent tools previously used for psychiatric screening or diagnosis are not appropriate for routine use in this population.[10] Financial constraints also impede the implementation of extensive questionnaires.
3. *They should be valid and reliable.* Ideally, they should have been validated on the population on which they will be used clinically.
4. *They should be sensitive.* Many quality-of-life

questionnaires that emphasize function[11] and performance-status tools[12,13] result in clustering of terminally ill patients at one end of the scale and therefore have limited usefulness.
5. *They should be clinically relevant.* The information obtained during the assessment should be of value to teams in their management of the patient and families.
6. They should be graphic. The graphic display of information like that which has proved to be successful in the recoding of vital signs, body weight, and some laboratory values would help in the interpretation and monitoring of changes over time and as a result of different interventions.

Physicians and nurses could complete part of these tests after their own assessment. For routine follow-up or for more time-consuming assessments, a technician could perform evaluations on a regular basis.

Assessing Specific Problems

- *Delirium.* Partial aspects of this syndrome such as distorted cognitive function can be easily assessed with reproducible tools.[14,15] Tools that contemplate most diagnostic criteria for this syndrome need to be completed by psychiatrists or specially trained physicians.[16,17] It is important to develop simple, comprehensive tools for screening and follow-up of this highly prevalent syndrome.
- *Affective disorders.* The presence of physical symptoms complicates the assessment of follow-up depression in advanced cancer patients.[18,19] Good tools exist but are lengthy to administer. Simpler tools are needed.
- *Somatization.* This is one of the recognized dimensions in the expression of pain and other symptoms.[20,21] It is also part of affective disorders.[22] Because of its role as an independent poor

Table 28.1   Multidimensional Assessment of Palliative-Care Patients

1. Physical Symptoms	2. Psychological Symptoms	3. Other Issues
• Pain • Anorexia • Nausea • Dyspnea • Asthenia • Constipation • Physical function • Other (e.g., pruritus, hiccups)	• Coping resources • Anxiety • Depression • Cognition • Somatization • Alcohol/addiction • Comfort • Quality of life	• Expected length of life • Financial issues • Spiritual concerns • Family structure and function • Preferred setting for care

prognostic factor for pain control, somatization should be part of the routine multidimensional assessment. Simple and reliable tools must be developed for this purpose.

- *Alcohol and drug addiction.* Screening for alcohol is useful,[23] since most physician assessments miss alcoholic patients.[24] However, a history of alcoholism or drug addiction does not necessarily mean that the patient is coping chemically at a given time. More comprehensive assessments are required for these symptoms.
- *High-risk populations.* Because of the magnitude of the problem in this era of decreasing financial resources, it is impossible to expect that every patient will be referred to a psychooncologist. For this reason, it is particularly important to develop effective tools to detect high-risk patients that will allow for a rapid assessment and management of the most difficult cases.[25] Such tools, by defining prognostic factors, will allow for characterization of patients in research studies, comparison of results from different groups, and care planning and quality control.

MANAGEMENT OF PALLIATIVE CARE

In recent years, major improvements have taken place in the pharmacological and nonpharmacological management of the psychosocial complications of advanced cancer. Numerous meetings, journals, and even major textbooks[2] have had a major role in disseminating these improvements. However, there are several areas in which the level of evidence for therapeutic interventions is poor. Some of these areas are the following.

The Impact of Multidimensional Assessment on Management

While it would be logical to expect that better management will result from comprehensive assessment and regular charting, this needs to be demonstrated in prospective studies. These studies may provide the evidence required to generate the changes in medical and nursing behaviours.

Treating Delirium

The role of benzodiazepines, major tranquilizers, and psychostimulants needs to be better clarified. While some evidence suggests that benzodi-

azepines are not indicated for treatment of this syndrome,[26] these drugs continue to be among the most frequently used. Randomized, controlled trials are need in order to better define the most effective type, dose, and modality of administration for different major tranquilizers. The role of adjuvant interventions such as opioid rotation[27] and hydration[28] also needs to be better defined. Methodologically, it is important to develop consensus on appropriate characterization of patients and on sensitive monitoring of responses to treatment. For example, it is likely that a sedative phenothiazine will be more effective in patients with hyperactive symptoms, while a psychostimulant might be more effective in lethargic patients.[28] However, this can be tested only if we have tools that are able to characterize and monitor the different components of delirium.

The role of newer antipsychotics in cancer delirium should also be evaluated in randomized, controlled trials. The mechanisms for patient accrual and consent should be addressed. Because of the complex nature of these studies and the great relevance of the subject, multicenter protocols should be developed. The impact of delirium on conflict between members of the staff and between staff and families[29] should be addressed in both epidemiological and prospective clinical trials of conflict prevention and management. Delirium is one of the most distressing syndromes for families.[29] Future studies should assess the family's perception of the patient's symptoms, especially their interpretation of physical or emotional suffering. More effective counseling would result from this research.

Treating Depression

Depressed terminally ill patients with cancer and other diseases present unique management challenges. Malnutrition,[28] cognitive failure,[5] autonomic failure,[30] and treatment with numerous drugs, including opioids, all increase the likelihood that antidepressants will have serious side effects. A long latency period before improvement is also not practical, given the short-life duration. Finally, the complex interaction with other physical symptoms results in different treatment goals. For these reasons, it is very difficult to extrapolate from studies conducted among psychiatric patients. Randomized, controlled trials that focus on terminally ill patients should be designed. The best type and dose of antidepressant should be established. The role of psychostimulants[31] and corticosteroids,[32] used instead of traditional antidepressants or in addition to them, should be addressed in randomized, controlled trials. The pharmacological management of depression in patients with borderline cognition is a major issue in the care of the terminally ill and should be addressed in prospective studies.

Finally, the effect of treatment for depression on patients' expressions of physical symptoms such as pain, nausea, or dyspnea should be addressed in clinical trials, with careful monitoring of symptom intensity and somatization.

COMMUNICATION/COUNSELING INTERFACE

We anticipate a 50% increase in the number of terminal cancer patients in the next decade,[33] with no major change in the approximate 50% mortality rate. With currently existing resources, it is impossible to expect that all or even a significant number of patients will be able to receive counseling by psychiatrists or psychologists. Even if it were possible to provide counseling, there would still be the problem of care delivery before the specialized referral. In addition, there are concerns and symptoms that occur in terminally ill patients and their families that do not constitute psychiatric diagnoses.[34,35] The area of medical communication is starting to emerge in response to some of these issues. It is crucial that effective techniques for counseling and communication be developed that can then be applied by nonspecialists. These techniques need to be developed and tried first by psychooncologists, much in the way that pain assessment and treatment techniques were initially developed by pain specialists for later use by all nonspecialists. Educational programs for counseling training and the results of the clinical application of counseling techniques by nonspecialists should be assessed in prospective trials.

CONCLUSIONS

The increasing interest in the care of palliative-care patients and their families has increased awareness of the lack of research to back up many commonly employed diagnostic and therapeutic approaches. The grant support and scholarship programs of initiatives such as "Death in America"[36] have provided, for the first time, a faculty and resources to begin to address some of these issues. This chapter has suggested some areas in which research is badly needed.

References

1. Doyle D, Hanks GWC, MacDonald RN, eds. *Oxford Textbook of Palliative Medicine*. Second Edition. Oxford: Oxford University Press, 1998.
2. Holland J, ed. *Psycho-oncology*. New York: Oxford University Press, 1998.
3. Bruera E, MacDonald S. Audit methods: the Edmonton Symptom Assessment System. In: Higginson I, ed, *Clinical Audit in Palliative Care*. Oxford: Radcliffe Medical Press, 1993:61–77.
4. Higginson, I. Audit methods: a community schedule. In: Higginson I, ed, *Clinical Audit in Palliative Care*. Oxford: Radcliffe Memorial Press, 1993.
5. Bruera E, Miller L, McCallion J, Macmillan K, Krefting L, Hanson J. Cognitive failure in patients with terminal cancer: a prospective study. *Journal of Pain and Symptom Management*, 1992; 7(4):192–195.
6. Bruera E. Unpublished results.
7. Neuenschwander H, Bruera E, Asthenia. In: Doyle D, Hanks GWG, MacDonald LN, eds. *Oxford Textbook of Palliative Medicine*. 2nd ed. London: Oxford Medical Publications, 1998:573–582.
8. Bruera E, Fainsinger RL. Clinical management of cachexia and anorexia. In: Doyle D, Hanks GWC, MacDonald RN, eds, *Oxford Textbook of Palliative Medicine*. London: Oxford Medical Publications, 1993:4.3.6:330–37.
9. Higginson I, Winget C. Psychological impact of cancer cachexia on the patient and family. In: Higginson I, Bruera E, eds, *Cachexia-Anorexia Syndrome in Advanced Cancer*, in press.
10. Rowland JH. Intrapersonal resources: coping. In: Holland J, Rowland JH, eds, *Handbook of Psychooncology. Psychological Care of the Patient with Cancer*. New York: Oxford University Press, 1990; 4:44–57.
11. Mount BM, Cohen SR. Quality of life in the face of life-threatening illness: what should we be measuring? *Current Oncology*, 1995; 2(3):121–125.
12. Mor V, Laliberte L, Morris JN, et al. The Karnofsky Performance Status Scale, an examination of its reliability and validity in a research setting. *Cancer*, 1984; 53:2002–2007.

13. Tulman L, Fawcett J, McEvoy MD. Development of the inventory of functional status—cancer. *Cancer Nursing*, 1991; 14(5):254–260.

14. Folstein MF, Folstein S, McHugh PR. "Mini-mental state": a practical method for grading the cognitive state of patients for the clinician. *Journal of Psychiatric Research*, 1975; 12:189–198.

15. Pereira J, Hanson J, Bruera E. The frequency and clinical course of cognitive impairment in terminal cancer patients. *Cancer*, 1997; 79:835–841.

16. Trzepacz PT, Baker RW, Greenhouse J. A symptom rating scale for delirium. *Psychiatry Research* 1988; 23:89–97.

17. Inouye SK, van Dyke CH, Alessi CA, et al. Clarifying confusion: the confusion assessment method. A new method for detection of delirium. *Annals of Internal Medicine*, 1990; 113:941–948.

18. Billings JA, Block S. Depression. *Journal of Palliative Care*, 1995; 11(1):48–54.

19. Chochinov HM, Wilson KG, Enns M, et al. The prevalence of depression in the terminally ill: effects of diagnostic criteria and symptom threshold judgements. *American Journal of Psychiatry* 1994; 151:537–540.

20. Bruera E, Schoeller T, Wenk R, MacEachern T, Marcelino S, Suarez-Almazor M, Hanson J. A prospective multi-center assessment of the Edmonton Staging System for cancer pain. *Journal of Pain and Symptom Management* 1995; 10(5):348–355.

21. Turk DC, Fernandez E. Pain: a cognitive-behavioural perspective. In: M Watson, ed. *Cancer Patient Care: Psychosocial Textbook Methods.* Cambridge: Cambridge University Press, 1991.

22. Lynch ME. The assessment and prevalence of affective disorders in advanced cancer. *Journal of Palliative Care*, 1995; 11(1):10–18.

23. Bruera E, Moyano J, Seifert L, Fainsinger RL, Hanson J, Suarez-Almazor M. The frequency of alcoholism among patients with pain due to terminal cancer. *Journal of Pain and Symptom Management,* 1995; 10(8):599–603.

24. Moore R, Bone L, Geller G, et al. Prevalence, detection and treatment of alcoholism in hospitalized patients. *JAMA* 1989; 261:403–407.

25. Loscalzo M. Psychological approaches to the management of pain in patients with advanced cancer. In: Cherny NI, Foley KM, eds. *Hematology/Oncol-*
ogy *Clinical of North America.* Philadelphia: W.B. Saunders Company 1996; 139–154.

26. Breitbart W, Passik SD. Psychiatric aspects of palliative care. In: Doyle D, Hanks GWC, MacDonald N, eds. *Oxford Textbook of Palliative Medicine,* Oxford: Oxford University Press, 1993:607–626.

27. de Stoutz ND, Bruera E, Suarez-Almazor M. Opioid rotation (OR) for toxicity reduction in terminal cancer patients. *Journal of Pain and Symptom Management,* 1995; 10(5):378–384.

28. Watanabe S, Bruera E. Anorexia and cachexia, asthenia, and lethargy. In: Cherny NI, Foley KM, eds. *Hematology/Oncology Clinics of North America.* 1996:189–206.

29. Bruera E, Fainsinger R, Miller MJ, Kuehn N. The assessment of pain intensity in patients with cognitive failure: a preliminary report. *Journal of Pain and Symptom Management,* 1992; 7(5):267–270.

30. Roca E, Bruera E, Politi P, Barugel M, Cedaro L, Carraro S, Chacon R. Vinca alkaloids-induced cardiovascular autonomic neuropathy. *Cancer Treatment Report,* 1985; 69(2):149–151.

31. Breitbart W, Bruera E, Chochinov H, Lynch M. A National Cancer Institute of Canada Workshop on symptom control and supportive care in patients with advanced cancer: methodological and administrative issues. Neuropsychiatric syndromes and psychological symptoms in patients with advanced cancer. *Journal of Pain and Symptom Management* 1995; 10(2):131–141.

32. Bruera E, Brenneis C, Chadwick S, Hanson J, MacDonald RN. Methylphenidate associated with narcotics for the treatment of cancer pain. *Cancer Treatment Report,* 1987; 71(1):67–70.

33. Cancer pain relief and palliative care. Report of a WHO Expert Committee, Geneva, Switzerland: World Health Organization, 1990.

34. Maguire P, Faulkner A. Communicate with cancer patients: 1 Handling bad news and difficult questions. *British Medical Journal,* 1988; 297:907–909.

35. Butow PN, Dunn SM, Tattersall MHN. Communication with cancer patients: does it matter? *Journal of Palliative Care,* 1995; 11(4):34–38.

36. Building Open Societies. Open Society Institute, Soros Foundations 1994. New York: Open Society Institute, 1995.

Index

effect on patient's family, 282–283
endorphin role in, 407
fatigue with, 117, 177
fear effects on, 225–226
gate control model of, 224
inadequate control of, 134
intensity measurements of, 101, 102, 133, 135, 224,
   225, 261
management of, 103–115, 248, 340–341, 351–352
NSAID use for, 103, 104, 105, 106–107
opioid use for, 103, 104–105, 108–113
patient control of, 226
in pediatric patients, 259, 261–262
primary treatments for, 103
procedural, 261, 262
psychological factors in, 135–136
psychosocial management of, 261, 407
psychotropic analgesics for, 143–144
as reason for requests for suicide, 56, 57–58
resistant syndromes of, 13
in schizophrenia patients, 92
severe vs. moderate, 110
supportive therapy of, 248
"total pain" concept of, 132–133
Palliation, definition of, 338
Palliative care. *See* Hospice/palliative care
Palliative Care Core Standards, 403
Palliative medicine, research needs in, 407–411
Pamidronate, use for bone pain, 114
Pancreatic cancer
   anorexia/cachexia in, 162, 164
   depression with, 36, 166
Pancreatic pain, in AIDS patients, 132
Panic disorder
   diagnosis of, 29
   in dying patients, 17, 178
   in end-stage lung disorder, 178
   fatigue in, 176
   symptoms and causes of, 66–67
   treatment of, 71, 182
Paraminophenol, use for pain control, 106
Paraneoplastic syndrome
   autonomic neuropathy in, 119
   delirium in, 75, 82
Paranoid disorders
   appetite loss in, 165
   DSM-IV criteria for, 17–18
   in mental patients, 95
Parathyroid tumors, anxiety induced by, 65
Parental death, children's views of, 284–285
Parenteral catheters, for patient feeding, 170, 171
Parkinson's disease, antidepressant use in, 40
Paroxetine
   as antidepressant, 71, 144
   side effects of, 40
   use in pain control, 113, 144, 145
   use in terminal illness, 38, 40
Passive-aggressive disorder, DSM-IV criteria for, 17–18
Passive-avoidant strategies, of cancer patients, 26

Passive relaxation, in management of anxiety, 69
Patient-controlled administration, of analgesics, 111, 142,
   226
Patient focus, in hospice facility, 8
Pediatric patients
   anorexia in, 161, 179, 258
   anticipatory grief in, 268–270
   anxiety in, 258–259
   behavioral changes in, 261
   caregivers of, 255, 258, 312
   death concerns of, 256–257, 261, 266, 268
   depression in, 259, 260
   diagnosis and therapy of, 258–262
   family needs of, 257–258, 263
   fatigue in, 260
   food aversions in, 167
   insomnia in, 261
   medical expenses of, 257
   pain in, 259, 261–262
   palliative care of, 253–272
   parent role in care of, 255, 258, 266, 270–271
   preexisting psychopathology in, 262
   psychotherapy of, 189, 265–272
   siblings of, 255, 257, 258, 269
   social support systems for, 260
   suicide ideation in, 259–260
   treatment-induced illness in, 263
Pemoline
   use for opioid side effects, 143
   use in fatigue therapy, 118
   use in pain control, 145, 146
   use in terminal illness, 38, 41
Pentazocine, use for pain control, 105, 141
Pentoxifylline, use for cachexia, 169
Perceptual disturbances, in delirium, 78
Periactin. *See* Cyproheptadine
Peripheral neuropathy
   after chemotherapy, 132
   in AIDS patients, 132, 136
Perls, Fritz, existential psychotherapy of, 205
Personality disorders
   DSM-IV criteria for, 17–18
   in dying patients, 13
Pethidine, side effects of, 39
Phantom pain, 132
   analgesics for, 114
Phases of dying, of Kübler-Ross, 4
Phencyclidine (PCP), delirium from, 77
Phenelzine, use in terminal illness, 38
Phenomenology
   influence on existentialism, 200
   influence on existential psychotherapy, 202
Phenophthalein, for constipation management, 121
Phenothiazines
   discovery of, 4
   nausea control by, 123
   as sedatives, 409
   side effects of, 39, 40, 84
Phenylbutazone, use for pain control, 107